Thrombosis: Assessment and Management

Thrombosis: Assessment and Management

Edited by Morgan Bell

hayle
medical

New York

Hayle Medical,
750 Third Avenue, 9th Floor,
New York, NY 10017, USA

Visit us on the World Wide Web at:
www.haylemedical.com

ISBN: 978-1-63241-631-5

Cataloging-in-Publication Data

Thrombosis : assessment and management / edited by Morgan Bell.
p. cm.
Includes bibliographical references and index.
ISBN 978-1-63241-631-5
1. Thrombosis. 2. Blood--Coagulation. 3. Thrombosis--Diagnosis.
4. Thrombosis--Treatment. 5. Blood vessels--Diseases. I. Bell, Morgan.
RC694.3 .T47 2019
616.135--dc23

Table of Contents

Preface

Over the recent decade, advancements and applications have progressed exponentially. This has led to the increased interest in this field and projects are being conducted to enhance knowledge. The main objective of this book is to present some of the critical challenges and provide insights into possible solutions. This book will answer the varied questions that arise in the field and also provide an increased scope for furthering studies.

The condition in which a blood clot is formed within a blood vessel is known as thrombosis. It obstructs the blood flow through the circulatory system. The two primary types of thrombosis are venous thrombosis and arterial thrombosis. Venous thrombosis occurs in the veins and results in the congestion of the affected body part. Arterial thrombosis impacts the supply of the blood and could also lead to tissue damage. Anticoagulation, antiplatelet drugs, thrombolysis and surgery are some common methods for treating thrombosis. The various advances in the treatment of thrombosis are glanced at in this book and their applications and ramifications are looked at in detail. Most of the topics introduced herein cover new techniques of assessment of this condition. Students, researchers, doctors and hematologists will benefit alike from this book.

I hope that this book, with its visionary approach, will be a valuable addition and will promote interest among readers. Each of the authors has provided their extraordinary competence in their specific fields by providing different perspectives as they come from diverse nations and regions. I thank them for their contributions.

Editor

External validation of prognostic rules for early post-pulmonary embolism mortality: assessment of a claims-based and three clinical-based approaches

Erin R. Weeda[1,2], Christine G. Kohn[3,2], Gregory J. Fermann[4], W. Frank Peacock[5], Christopher Tanner[3], Daniel McGrath[3], Concetta Crivera[6], Jeff R. Schein[6] and Craig I. Coleman[1,2]*

Abstract

Background: Studies show the In-hospital Mortality for Pulmonary embolism using Claims daTa (IMPACT) rule can accurately identify pulmonary embolism (PE) patients at low-risk of early mortality in a retrospective setting using only claims for the index admission. We sought to externally validate IMPACT, Pulmonary Embolism Severity Index (PESI), simplified PESI (sPESI) and Hestia for predicting early mortality.

Methods: We identified consecutive adults admitted for objectively-confirmed PE between 10/21/2010 and 5/12/2015. Patients undergoing thrombolysis/embolectomy within 48 h were excluded. All-cause in-hospital and 30 day mortality (using available Social Security Death Index data through January 2014) were assessed and prognostic accuracies of IMPACT, PESI, sPESI and Hestia were determined.

Results: Twenty-one (2.6 %) of the 807 PE patients died before discharge. All rules classified 26.1–38.3 % of patients as low-risk for early mortality. Fatality among low-risk patients was 0 % (sPESI and Hestia), 0.4 % (IMPACT) and 0.6 % (PESI). IMPACT's sensitivity was 95.2 % (95 % confidence interval [CI] = 74.1–99.8 %), and the sensitivies of clinical rules ranged from 91 (PESI)-100 % (sPESI and Hestia). Specificities of all rules ranged between 26.8 and 39.1 %. Of 573 consecutive patients in the 30 day mortality analysis, 33 (5.8 %) died. All rules classified 27.9–38.0 % of patients as low-risk, and fatality occurred in 0 (Hestia)-1.4 % (PESI) of low-risk patients. IMPACT's sensitivity was 97.0 % (95%CI = 82.5–99.8 %), while sensitivies for clinical rules ranged from 91 (PESI)-100 % (Hestia). Specificities of rules ranged between 29.6 and 39.8 %.

Conclusion: In this analysis, IMPACT identified low-risk PE patients with similar accuracy as clinical rules. While not intended for prospective clinical decision-making, IMPACT appears useful for identification of low-risk PE patient in retrospective claims-based studies.

Keywords: Mortality, Pulmonary embolism, Prognosis, Risk assessment, Severity of illness index

* Correspondence: Craig.Coleman@hhchealth.org
[1]School of Pharmacy, University of Connecticut, 69 North Eagleville Road, Storrs, CT 06269, USA
[2]University of Connecticut/Hartford Hospital Evidence-Based Practice Center, Hartford, CT, USA
Full list of author information is available at the end of the article

Background

Guidelines suggest that patients with pulmonary embolism (PE) who are identified to have a low-risk of early post-PE all-cause mortality may be candidates for abbreviated hospital admission or outpatient treatment if appropriate follow-up can be arranged [1, 2]. Data from randomized trials and observational studies suggest that early discharge or outpatient treatment of low-risk PE patients is feasible and safe [3, 4].

A prior meta-analysis suggested at least one-third of acute PE patients could be classified as low-risk for early mortality according to clinical prediction rules [5]. This same meta-analysis identified the Pulmonary Embolism Severity Index (PESI), simplified PESI (sPESI) and Hestia clinical prediction rules as having high sensitivities and negative predictive values (NPVs) for identifying low-risk PE patients. In order to use PESI [6], sPESI [7] and Hestia [8] in the risk stratification of a patient with PE, access to vital signs, laboratory values, comorbid conditions and a cognitive evaluation at presentation is necessary. While PESI, sPESI and Hestia can be helpful in clinical practice, the extensive clinical data required to score these rules are not commonly found in claims databases or easily accessible to individual hospitals/health-systems. As a result, the utility of PESI, sPESI or Hestia for retrospective identification of low-risk patients with PE is limited.

While not originally derived to aid in prognostication in a prospective clinical setting, the In-hospital Mortality for Pulmonary embolism using Claims daTa (IMPACT) multivariable prediction rule utilizes data accessible within claims databases and/or claims from individual hospitals to retrospectively risk stratify patients with PE for early mortality [9]. Prior validation studies suggest IMPACT can accurately identify pulmonary embolism (PE) patients at low-risk of early mortality [10, 11]. The ability of IMPACT to correctly identify patients at low- and higher-risk of early mortality has not previously been compared to analogous clinical prediction rules. Therefore, using data from a single center, this study sought to externally validate IMPACT, PESI, sPESI and Hestia for predicting in-hospital and 30 day post-PE mortality.

Methods

Preparation of this study report was in accordance with the Transparent reporting of a multivariable prediction model for individual prognosis or diagnosis (TRIPOD) statement [12]. For this retrospective cohort study, we identified consecutive patients diagnosed with acute PE between October 21, 2010 and May 12, 2015 using computerized claims records for admissions to Hartford Hospital (Hartford, Connecticut, USA). The hospital's computerized claims system contains information on source of admission, International Classification of Diseases, Ninth Revision, Clinical Modification (ICD-9-CM) diagnosis and procedure codes, admission and discharge dates and discharge status. To be eligible for inclusion into this study, patients ≥18 years of age presenting to our institution had to have a primary diagnosis of PE (ICD-9-CM code = 415.1x). Consistent with prior studies, we excluded patients lacking objective confirmation of acute PE according to clinical guidelines. The following were considered confirmatory studies for the diagnosis of acute PE: high probability perfusion-ventilation lung scan (V/Q scan), computed tomography pulmonary angiography (CTPA) or pulmonary angiography diagnostic for PE, or a non-diagnostic V/Q scan or CTPA in combination with an abnormal compression ultrasonography of the lower extremities. Consistent with many prior studies of PE clinical prediction rules [5], subjects that received thrombolysis and/or pulmonary embolectomy within the 48 h of presentation were excluded as clinical guidelines do not consider such patients low-risk [1, 2]. All patients included in this study were managed according to usual clinical practice for our institution.

Risk stratification of patients with acute PE using IMPACT, PESI, sPESI and Hestia was performed according to published methods (Additional file 1) [6–9]. Patients with an IMPACT predicted mortality risk ≤1.5 % [9], PESI score ≤85 [6] or a sPESI or Hestia scores =0 [7, 8] were classified as low-risk for early mortality. Estimated mortality risk according to the claims-based IMPACT prediction rule [estimated % absolute risk = $1/(1 + \exp(-x)$; where $x = -5.833 + (0.026 \ast age) + (0.402 \ast myocardial\ infarction) + (0.368 \ast chronic\ lung\ disease) + (0.464 \ast stroke) + (0.638 \ast prior\ major\ bleeding) + (0.298 \ast atrial\ fibrillation) + (1.061 \ast cognitive\ impairment) + (0.554 \ast heart\ failure) + (0.364 \ast renal\ failure) + (0.484 \ast liver\ disease) + (0.523 \ast coagulopathy) + (1.068 \ast cancer)]$ was determined using all available hospital claims data (i.e., ICD-9-CM diagnosis and procedural codes) for each patient's index PE encounter along with their age at time of presentation. ICD-9-CM coding for relevant IMPACT co-morbidities were performed according to the original IMPACT derivation paper [9]. Data necessary to classify patients as low- or high-risk of early mortality according to the PESI, sPESI and Hestia clinical prediction rules [6–8] were obtained by linking all included patients identified through hospital claims to the hospital's electronic health record (EHR). We used vital signs (heart rate, blood pressure, respiratory rate, oxygen [O2] saturation, body temperature), laboratory values (serum creatinine, platelet count, total bilirubin) and mental status assessments obtained as close to the time of presentation for the index PE encounter as possible to score each of the clinical prediction rules [6]. For all patients admitted through the emergency department, the first vital sign, laboratory value and/or mental status assessment upon presentation (but within 24 h) was utilized. For patients directly admitted to the hospital we used the first values recorded on the day of hospital admission. Consistent with previous studies of this type, missing vital, laboratory and mental status assessment data were assumed to be normal [6]. For PESI, sPESI and Hestia, the presence of cancer, heart failure, chronic lung disease, severe liver disease (defined as a total bilirubin ≥2.5 mg/dL), heparin-induced thrombocytopenia and recent clinical events (gastrointestinal bleeding within 14 days, stroke with 4 weeks, surgery with 2 weeks) were assessed at time of hospital admission for the index PE encounter. All required data was abstracted from the electronic health record (including vital signs, laboratory values and emergency department, admission and consult notes) by trained study personnel blinded to study outcome.

All-cause in-hospital and 30 day post-PE mortality served as *a priori* endpoints for this study. In-hospital mortality was determined using the discharge status field for the index admission within the hospital billing system and electronic health record. Thirty-day mortality was based upon searches of the Social Security Death Index (SSDI) [11] performed >6 months after the last day of eligible inclusion in this analysis. Computerized health-system encounter data from our hospital's billing records were queried for subsequent emergency visit claims, clinic visits and/or hospital readmissions outside of 30 days. These were used as confirmatory markers of vital status at 30 days. Beginning in March 2014, rules regarding access to data within the SSDI changed; restricting the release of three most recent years of data [13, 14]. For this reason, our 30 day mortality endpoint was assessed only in the subset of consecutive patients presenting to the hospital prior to January 31, 2014.

Baseline characteristics are described with means ± SDs for continuous data and counts and proportions for categorical data. Sensitivity, specificity and negative and positive predictive values for predicting early mortality were calculated for IMPACT, PESI, sPESI and Hestia along with 95 % confidence intervals (CIs). C-statistics were computed to evaluate each rule's overall discriminative power. All database management and statistical analyses were performed using IBM SPSS Statistics version 22.0 (IBM Corp., Armonk, NY, USA). The study was approved by the Hartford Hospital institutional review board.

Results

A total of 861 patients with a primary ICD-9-CM code for acute PE and objective confirmation of diagnosis were identified (Fig. 1). Of these, 54 received thrombolytic therapy/embolectomy within 48 h of presentation,

leaving 807 for analysis. Baseline characteristics of the cohort, stratified by low- and high-risk for each rule are shown in Table 1. Two-hundred and thirty-four patients presented with PE after January 2014 and were excluded from the 30 day mortality endpoint analysis, as SSDI data are not available for patients past this time point. The baseline characteristics of the 30 day mortality analysis patient subset were similar to the overall population (Additional file 1: Table S1).

The IMPACT, PESI, sPESI and Hestia scores (mean ± SD) for the complete cohort of 807 PE patients were 3.9 ± 4.3, 96.4 ± 33.3, 1.1 ± 0.9 and 1.3 ± 1.1, respectively. While mean age for patients was 64.1 ± 16.57; when dichotomized into risk groups, high-risk patients were considerably older, regardless of prediction rule used. At time of presentation, mean vital sign values were within normal ranges in the overall analysis population; but more than half of the subjects required O2 supplementation to maintain saturations >90 %. The use of thrombolysis and/or embolectomy after 48 h was infrequent, occurring in only 4 (0.5 %) of patients.

The overall incidence of all-cause in-hospital mortality was 2.6 % (21/807). IMPACT, PESI, sPESI and Hestia classified 26 % (Hestia)-38 % (PESI) of the cohort as low-risk for early post-PE mortality. Fatality among low-risk patients was low (0–0.6 %), corresponding to NPVs of 99.4 (PESI)-100 % (sPESI and Hestia) (Table 2). IMPACT's sensitivity was 95.2 % (95 % CI = 74.1–99.8 %), and the sensitivities of clinical rules ranged from 91 (PESI)-100 % (sPESI and Hestia). Specificities of all rules ranged between 26.8 (Hestia)-39.1 % (PESI) and C-statistics from 0.76 (sPESI)-0.86 (Hestia). Additional file 1: Table S2 describes the characteristics of patients who died in-hospital and had discordant risk categorization across any of the four prediction rules.

Among the subset of 573 patients accessible within the SSDI, 33 (5.8 %) died of any cause within 30 days of presentation for PE. All rules classified 27.9 (Hestia)-38.0 % (PESI) of PE patients as low-risk, and fatality occurred in 0.0 % (Hestia)-1.4 % (PESI) of low-risk patients (NPVs = 98.6–100 %) (Table 3). IMPACT's sensitivity for predicting 30 day mortality was 97.0 % (95%CI = 82.5–99.8 %), while sensitivities for clinical rules ranged from 91 (PESI)-100 % (Hestia). Specificities of rules ranged between 29.6 % (Hestia)-39.8 % (PESI) and their C statistics ranged from 0.73 (sPESI)-0.81 (PESI). Additional file 1: Table S3 describes the characteristics of patients who died within 30 days of presentation and had discordant risk categorization across any of the 4 prediction rules.

Discussion

In this analysis, the claims-based IMPACT prediction rule displayed prognostic accuracy similar to that of commonly used clinical risk stratification rules, including PESI and

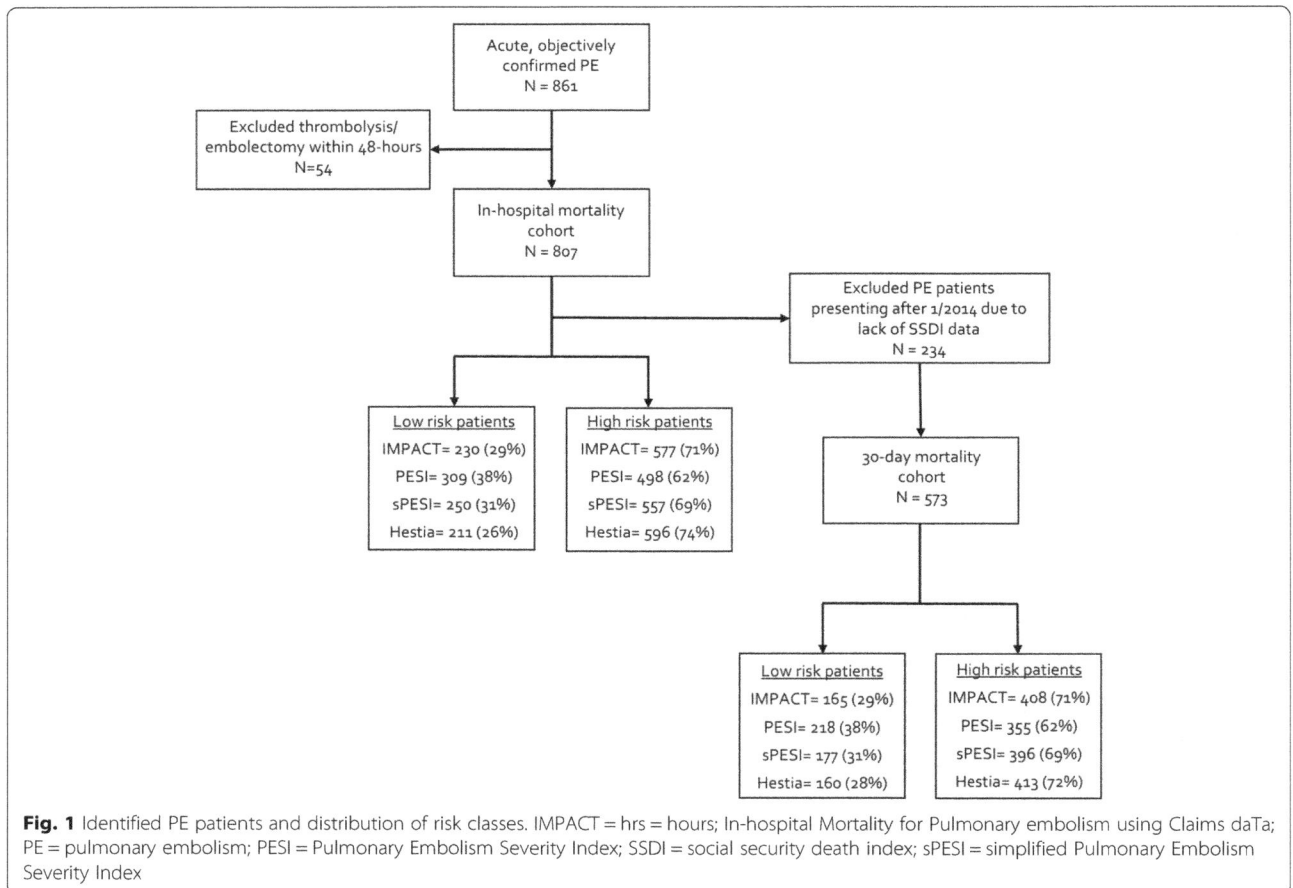

Fig. 1 Identified PE patients and distribution of risk classes. IMPACT = hrs = hours; In-hospital Mortality for Pulmonary embolism using Claims daTa; PE = pulmonary embolism; PESI = Pulmonary Embolism Severity Index; SSDI = social security death index; sPESI = simplified Pulmonary Embolism Severity Index

sPESI (which have been prospectively validated for identification of low-risk PE patients) and the Hestia criteria (which was prospectively designed to identify patients whom could be treated as outpatients). The 4 rules evaluated in this study classified between 1/4th and 2/5ths of patients as low-risk. Each exhibited sensitivities >90 %, NPVs >98.6 % and specificities <40 % for predicting in-hospital or 30 day all-cause mortality, and these findings are consistent with prior derivation and validation studies. To our knowledge, this is the first external validation study of Hestia [5, 9–11]. Taken together, our results suggests each of the four rules can identify a cohort of low-risk PE patients whom are unlikely to die within the first 30 days of presentation. However, because a minority of patients with PE (<6 % in our study) die within 30 days, these prognostic rules classify a substantial number of patients who ultimately survive into higher-risk groups (hence their lower specificities). Prognostic tests seldom have both high sensitivity and specificity. Therefore, when using a prognostic test to decide upon implementing a less conservative treatment strategy (e.g., discharging a patient with acute PE directly from the emergency department) higher sensitivity and NPV values are preferable.

The American College of Chest Physicians and the European Society of Cardiology guidelines support early discharge and/or home treatment of PE patients at low-risk for early mortality as long as they have adequate home circumstances [1, 2]. These guidelines suggest that clinicians use validated clinical prediction rules to assist in identification and selection of low-risk patients. Although in this analysis IMPACT displayed a similar ability to identify low-risk PE patients as PESI, sPESI and Hestia; IMPACT was not originally derived or validated to assist in prospective clinical decision-making (and is relatively more computationally complex compared to clinical prediction rules), and it should not be used for individual patient decision-making [9]. However, IMPACT appears valid for retrospective identification of low-risk PE patients and therefore could be used to aid in the performance of real-world outcomes studies and to enable payer/institution benchmarking of rates of low-risk PE patients treated at home or following an abbreviated admission. Using claim s data as described by IMPACT may have advantages over obtaining highly granular clinical information from the EHR (including reduced time and effort requirements).

Table 1 Characteristics of pulmonary embolism patients

Characteristic	Total Cohort[a]	IMPACT Low-Risk	IMPACT Higher-Risk	PESI Low-Risk	PESI Higher-Risk	sPESI Low-Risk	sPESI Higher-Risk	Hestia Low-Risk	Hestia Higher-Risk
	N (%)	N (%)	N (%)	N (%)	N (%)	N (%)	N (%)	N (%)	N (%)
	N = 807	N = 230	N = 577	N = 309	N = 498	N = 250	N = 557	N = 211	N = 596
Age (years, mean ± SD)	64.1 ± 16.47	46.4 ± 11.36	71.2 ± 12.38	51.9 ± 14.39	71.6 ± 12.76	56.3 ± 14.49	67.6 ± 16.12	59.9 ± 17.10	65.6 ± 16.00
> 80 years	145 (18.0)	0 (0)	145 (25.1)	9 (2.9)	136 (27.3)	0 (0)	145 (26.0)	27 (12.8)	118 (19.7)
Male gender	372 (46.1)	114 (49.6)	258 (44.7)	135 (43.7)	237 (47.6)	140 (56.0)	232 (41.7)	99 (46.9)	273 (45.8)
Cancer	254 (31.5)	18 (7.8)	236 (40.9)	15 (4.9)	239 (48.0)	0 (0)	254 (45.5)	51 (24.2)	203 (34.1)
Cancer (ICD-9-CM)	154 (19.1)	0 (0)	154 (26.7)	10 (3.2)	144 (28.9)	3 (1.2)	151 (27.1)	25 (11.8)	129 (21.6)
Chronic cardiopulmonary disease	230 (28.5)	29 (12.6)	201 (34.3)	42 (13.6)	188 (37.8)	0 (0)	230 (41.3)	37 (17.5)	193 (32.4)
Chronic lung disease	198 (24.5)	27 (11.7)	171 (29.6)	40 (12.9)	158 (31.7)	0 (0)	198 (35.5)	34 (16.1)	164 (27.5)
Chronic lung disease (ICD-9-CM)	224 (27.8)	22 (9.6)	202 (35.0)	47 (15.2)	177 (35.5)	7 (2.8)	217 (39.0)	36 (17.1)	188 (31.5)
Heart failure	62 (7.7)	2 (0.9)	60 (10.3)	3 (1.0)	59 (11.8)	0 (0)	62 (11.1)	4 (1.9)	58 (9.7)
Heart failure (ICD-9-CM)	75 (9.3)	1 (0.4)	74 (12.8)	9 (2.9)	66 (13.3)	5 (2.0)	70 (12.6)	8 (3.8)	67 (11.2)
Altered mental status at presentation	42 (5.2)	3 (1.3)	39 (6.8)	0 (0)	42 (8.4)	6 (2.4)	36 (6.5)	4 (1.9)	38 (6.4)
Cognitive impairment (ICD-9-CM)	60 (7.4)	0 (0)	60 (10.4)	7 (2.3)	53 (10.6)	6 (2.4)	54 (9.7)	7 (3.3)	53 (8.9)
Pulse (beats/min, mean ± SD)	93.2 ± 18.92	94.0 ± 18.51	92.9 ± 19.10	91.6 ± 17.35	94.1 ± 19.78	85.6 ± 13.38	96.6 ± 20.04	87.6 ± 17.73	95.2 ± 18.96
Pulse ≥ 110 beats/min	169 (20.9)	56 (24.3)	113 (19.6)	47 (15.2)	122 (24.5)	0 (0)	169 (30.3)	29 (13.7)	140 (23.5)
Systolic blood pressure (mmHg, mean ± SD)	133.6 ± 22.90	134.4 ± 21.75	133.3 ± 23.35	136.4 ± 21.32	131.9 ± 23.69	136.8 ± 21.60	132.2 ± 23.33	139.8 ± 22.30	131.4 ± 22.70
Systolic blood pressure <100 mmHg	36 (4.5)	7 (3.0)	29 (5.0)	3 (1.0)	33 (6.6)	0 (0)	36 (6.5)	3 (1.4)	33 (5.5)
O2 saturation (%, mean ± SD)	96.3 ± 3.50	96.8 ± 3.83	96.1 ± 3.34	96.3 ± 2.42	95.9 ± 3.97	97.0 ± 2.35	96.0 ± 3.87	97.1 ± 2.12	96.0 ± 3.83
O2 saturation <90 %	32 (4.0)	6 (2.6)	26 (4.5)	1 (0.3)	31 (6.2)	0 (0)	32 (5.7)	0 (0)	32 (5.4)
Oxygen needed to maintain O2 saturation >90 % for >24 h	412 (51.1)	79 (34.3)	333 (57.7)	112 (36.2)	300 (60.2)	90 (36.0)	322 (57.8)	0 (0)	412 (69.1)
Respiratory rate (breaths/min, mean ± SD)	19.1 ± 3.56	18.7 ± 3.31	19.3 ± 3.64	18.5 ± 2.20	19.5 ± 4.14	18.5 ± 2.51	19.4 ± 3.90	18.2 ± 2.37	19.5 ± 3.84
Respiratory rate ≥30 breaths/min	19 (2.4)	2 (0.8)	17 (2.9)	0 (0)	19 (3.8)	2 (0.8)	17 (3.1)	2 (0.9)	17 (2.9)
Temperature (degrees Celsius, mean ± SD)	97.6 ± 1.38	97.8 ± 1.29	97.6 ± 1.41	97.9 ± 1.38	97.4 ± 1.47	97.6 ± 1.28	97.6 ± 1.40	97.4 ± 1.24	97.7 ± 1.42
Temperature <36° Celsius	206 (25.5)	47 (20.4)	159 (27.6)	40 (12.9)	166 (33.3)	68 (27.2)	138 (24.8)	60 (28.4)	146 (24.5)
Thrombolysis or embolectomy > 48 h	4 (0.5)	2 (0.9)	2 (0.3)	3 (1.0)	1 (0.2)	3 (1.2)	1 (0.2)	0 (0)	4 (0.7)
High risk of bleeding[b]	101 (12.5)	37 (16.1)	64 (11.1)	48 (15.5)	53 (10.6)	37 (14.8)	64 (11.5)	0 (0)	101 (16.9)
PE on anticoagulation	62 (7.7)	17 (7.4)	45 (7.8)	21 (6.7)	41 (8.2)	11 (4.4)	51 (9.2)	0 (0)	62 (10.4)
History of heparin-induced thrombocytopenia	5 (0.6)	1 (0.4)	4 (0.7)	2 (0.6)	3 (0.6)	2 (0.8)	3 (0.5)	0 (0)	5 (0.8)
Medical or social reason for admission[c]	237 (29.3)	43 (18.7)	194 (33.6)	64 (20.7)	173 (34.7)	42 (16.9)	195 (34.9)	0 (0)	237 (39.8)
Need for intravenous pain medication for > 24 h	87 (10.8)	43 (18.7)	44 (7.6)	48 (15.5)	39 (7.8)	32 (12.8)	55 (9.9)	0 (0)	87 (14.6)
Severe liver impairment[d]	10 (1.2)	3 (1.3)	7 (1.2)	3 (1.0)	7 (1.4)	3 (1.2)	7 (1.3)	0 (0)	10 (1.7)

Table 1 Characteristics of pulmonary embolism patients (*Continued*)

Liver disease (ICD-9-CM)	6 (0.7)	0 (0)	6 (1.0)	3 (1.0)	3 (0.6)	2 (0.8)	4 (0.7)	0 (0)	6 (1.0)
Creatinine clearance <30 mL/min	31 (3.8)	2 (0.9)	29 (5.0)	11 (3.6)	20 (4.0)	7 (2.8)	24 (4.3)	0 (0)	31 (5.2)
Renal failure (ICD-9-CM)	60 (7.4)	2 (0.9)	58 (10.1)	18 (5.8)	42 (8.4)	16 (6.4)	44 (7.9)	8 (3.8)	52 (8.7)
Hemodynamically unstable[e]	94 (11.6)	24 (10.4)	70 (12.1)	30 (9.7)	64 (12.9)	17 (6.8)	77 (13.8)	0 (0)	94 (15.8)
Myocardial infarction (ICD-9-CM)	40 (5.0)	4 (1.7)	36 (6.2)	15 (4.9)	25 (5.0)	16 (6.4)	24 (4.3)	2 (0.9)	38 (6.4)
Cerebrovascular disease (ICD-9-CM)	11 (1.4)	0 (0)	11 (1.9)	5 (1.6)	6 (1.2)	4 (1.6)	7 (1.3)	2 (0.9)	9 (1.5)
Prior major bleeding (ICD-9-CM)	28 (3.5)	1 (0.4)	27 (4.7)	8 (2.6)	20 (4.0)	5 (2.0)	23 (4.1)	3 (1.4)	25 (4.2)
Atrial fibrillation (ICD-9-CM)	87 (10.8)	2 (0.9)	85 (14.7)	15 (4.9)	72 (14.5)	11 (4.4)	76 (13.6)	18 (8.5)	69 (11.6)
Coagulopathy (ICD-9-CM)	41 (5.1)	3 (1.3)	38 (6.6)	11 (3.6)	30 (6.0)	12 (4.8)	29 (5.2)	6 (2.8)	35 (5.9)

[a]Of the 807 patients, 3 (0.4 %) patients had unknown values for respiratory rate; 2 (0.2 %) for pulse, systolic blood pressure, O2 saturation, and temperature; 516 (63.9 %) for bilirubin (component of liver disease); 1 (0.1 %) for platelets (component of bleed risk); and 1 (0.1 %) for glomerular filtration rate (creatinine clearance estimate)

Hrs hours, *ICD-9-CM* International Classification of Diseases-Ninth Revision-Clinical Modification, *min* minutes, *SD* standard deviation, *O2* oxygen

[b]Gastrointestinal bleeding in the preceding 14 days, stroke in the preceding 4 weeks, procedure in the preceding 2 weeks, bleeding disorder or thrombocytopenia (platelet count <75 × 109/L), or uncontrolled hypertension (systolic blood pressure > 180 mmHg or diastolic blood pressure > 110 mmHg)

[c]Medical or social reason for hospital treatment was determined by trained study personnel using all data available in the electronic health record including vital signs, laboratory values, and emergency department, admission and consult notes

[d]Cirrhosis or bilirubin > 2.5 mg/dL

[e]Pulse ≥ 100 beats/minute and systolic blood pressure ≤ 100 mmHg or condition requiring admission to an intensive care unit

Table 2 Prognostic test characteristics for in-hospital mortality

	IMPACT	PESI	sPESI	Hestia
Low-Risk Mortality	1/230	2/309	0/250	0/211
n/N (%)	(0.4 %)	(0.6 %)	(0 %)	(0 %)
High-Risk Mortality	20/577	19/498	21/557	21/596
n/N (%)	(3.5 %)	(3.8 %)	(3.8 %)	(3.5 %)
Sensitivity	95.2 %	90.5 %	100 %	100 %
(95 % CI)	(74.1–99.8 %)	(68.2–98.3 %)	(80.8–100 %)	(80.8–100 %)
Specificity	29.1 %	39.1 %	31.8 %	26.8 %
(95 % CI)	(26.0–32.5 %)	(35.6–42.6 %)	(28.6–35.2 %)	(23.8–30.1 %)
PPV	3.5 %	3.8 %	3.8 %	3.5 %
(95 % CI)	(2.2–5.4 %)	(2.4–6.0 %)	(2.4–5.8 %)	(2.2–5.4 %)
NPV	99.6 %	99.4 %	100 %	100 %
(95 % CI)	(97.2–100 %)	(97.4–99.9 %)	(98.1–100 %)	(97.8–100 %)
C-statistic	0.766	0.792	0.762	0.857
(95 % CI)	(0.685–0.848)	(0.696–0.889)	(0.682–0.842)	(0.796–0.918)

CI confidence interval, IMPACT In-hospital Mortality for Pulmonary embolism using Claims data, NPV negative predictive value, PESI Pulmonary Embolism Severity Index, PPV positive predictive value, sPESI simplified Pulmonary Embolism Severity Index

Our study has limitations that require consideration. First, this validation study was performed retrospectively and therefore may be subject to biases, particularly due to missing data. Nonetheless, our study had similar rates of missing data than reported in prior prospective derivation/external validation papers of clinical prediction rules [5–7]. Second, this was a single-center study limiting its generalizability and sample size. However, baseline characteristics and mortality rates were consistent with national estimates [10, 15] and our sample size (573–807 patients) was large relative to many previously published external validation studies of PE clinical prediction rules [5]. Third, we could not assess 30 day mortality in our entire study cohort due to restrictions on the availability of SSDI data [14]. Despite this, the sample size of patients with objectively confirmed PE available for final analysis was robust. Moreover, we are unaware of any programmatic changes in evaluation and treatment of patients with PE at our institution since February 2014. Consequently, the likelihood of selection bias resulting from the unavoidable exclusion of patients after this date is low. Next, the more subjective nature of certain criteria in Hestia (i.e., medical or social reason for hospital admission and the need for intravenous pain

Table 3 Prognostic test characteristics for 30 day mortality

	IMPACT	PESI	sPESI	Hestia
Low-Risk Mortality	1/165	3/218	1/177	0/160
n/N (%)	(0.6 %)	(1.4 %)	(0.6 %)	(0 %)
High-Risk Mortality	32/408	30/355	32/396	33/413
n/N (%)	(7.8 %)	(8.5 %)	(8.1 %)	(8.0 %)
Sensitivity	97.0 %	90.9 %	97.0 %	100 %
(95 % CI)	(82.5–99.8 %)	(74.5–97.6 %)	(82.5–99.8 %)	(87.0–100 %)
Specificity	30.4 %	39.8 %	32.6 %	29.6 %
(95%CI)	(26.6–34.5 %)	(35.7–44.1 %)	(28.7–36.8 %)	(25.8–33.7 %)
PPV	7.8 %	8.5 %	8.1 %	8.0 %
(95 % CI)	(5.5–11.0 %)	(5.9–12.0 %)	(5.7–11.3 %)	(5.6–11.1 %)
NPV	99.4 %	98.6 %	99.4 %	100 %
(95 % CI)	(96.2–100 %)	(95.7–99.6 %)	(96.4–100 %)	(97.1–100 %)
C-statistic	0.804	0.805	0.731	0.791
(95 % CI)	(0.749–0.859)	(0.731–0.879)	(0.653–0.810)	(0.721–0.860)

CI confidence interval, IMPACT In-hospital Mortality for Pulmonary embolism using Claims data, NPV negative predictive value, PESI Pulmonary Embolism Severity Index, PPV positive predictive value, sPESI simplified Pulmonary Embolism Severity Index

medication for >24 h), make retrospective scoring challenging. This being said, the proportion of patients in our study classified as higher-risk because of these "subjective" criteria was not inconsistent with the Hestia derivation study [8]. Lastly, the 48 h cut-off used to exclude patients undergoing thrombolysis and/or embolectomy is somewhat arbitrary. We excluded patients receiving thrombolysis and/or embolectomy in less than 48 h because such patients likely had hemodynamic instability at presentation and would not be considered low-risk per guidelines [1, 2]. Of note, numerous studies evaluating the prognostic accuracy of clinical prediction rules have similarly excluded patients undergoing early thrombolysis and/or embolectomy [5]. However, when these procedures are performed later in a hospital stay (day 3 onwards), they are more likely an indicator of a therapeutic failure resulting in a poor clinical course (i.e., respiratory failure or cardiac arrest). In addition, the need for and timing of thrombolysis and/or embolectomy can easily be detected in a claims database and a clinical setting, allowing it to be implemented in our evaluation of IMPACT and clinical prediction rules. The 48 h cut-off was chosen *a priori* to approximate the likely timing used for assessing the similar Hestia criterion (i.e., the Hestia study required discharge within 24 h of PE diagnosis, likely resulting in the assessment of the 11 Hestia criteria within 48 h of initial PE presentation) [8].

Conclusion

IMPACT identified low-risk PE patients with similar accuracy as PESI, sPESI and Hestia. While not designed for prospective clinical decision-making, IMPACT appears useful for identification of low-risk PE patient in retrospective claims-based studies.

Abbreviation

CI: Confidence intervals; CTPA: Computed tomography pulmonary angiography; EHR: Electronic health record; ICD-9-CM: International classification of diseases, ninth revision, clinical modification; IMPACT: In-hospital mortality for pulmonary embolism using claims daTa; NPV: Negative predictive value; O2: Oxygen; PE: Pulmonary embolism; PESI: Pulmonary embolism severity index; PPV: Positive predictive value; sPESI: Simplified pulmonary embolism severity index; SSDI: Social security death index; TRIPOD: Transparent reporting of a multivariable prediction model for individual prognosis or diagnosis; USA: United States of America; V/Q: Ventilation/perfusion.

Competing interest

The authors declare that they have no competing interests.

Authors' contributions

Study concept and design: ERW, CGK, GJF, WFP, CC, JRS, CIC. Acquisition of data: ERW, CGK, CT, DM, CIC. Analysis and interpretation of data: ERW, CGK, GJF, WFP, CT, DM, CC, JRS, CIC. Drafting the manuscript: ERW, CGK, CT, DM,

CIC. Critical Revision of the manuscript for important intellectual content: ERW, CGK, GJF, WFP, CT, DM, CC, JRS, CIC. Administrative, technical or material support: ERW, CGK, CIC. Study supervision: CIC. CIC had full access to all the study data and take full responsibility for the integrity of the data and the accuracy of the data analysis. All authors read and approved the final manuscript. The authors meet criteria for authorship as recommended by the International Committee of Medical Journal Editors (ICJME) and were fully responsible for all content and editorial decisions, and were involved in all stages of manuscript development. All authors read and approved the final manuscript.

Acknowledgements
None.

Funding

This study was funded by Janssen Scientific Affairs, LLC, Raritan, NJ, USA CIC has received grant funding and consultancy fees from Janssen Scientific Affairs, LLC; Bayer Pharma AG; and Boehringer-Ingelheim Pharmaceuticals, Inc. CC, JRS are employees of Janssen Scientific Affairs LLC. GJF has received grant funding for Novartis, Cardiorentis, Cardioxyl, Cempra Pharmaceuticals, Trevena, Intersection Medical, Siemens, The Mayday Foundation, Pfizer; and is on the advisory board and speakers bureau for Janssen Scientific Affairs. FWP has received grant funding and consultancy fees from Abbott, Alere, Banyan, Cardiorentis, Janssen Pharmaceuticals, Portola, Roche, The Medicine's Company, Prevencio and Singulex.

Author details

School of Pharmacy, University of Connecticut, 69 North Eagleville Road, Storrs, CT 06269, USA. ²University of Connecticut/Hartford Hospital Evidence-Based Practice Center, Hartford, CT, USA. ³University of Saint Joseph School of Pharmacy, Hartford, CT, USA. ⁴Department of Emergency Medicine, University of Cincinnati, Cincinnati, OH, USA. ⁵Department of Emergency Medicine, Baylor College of Medicine, Houston, TX, USA. ⁶Janssen Scientific Affairs LLC, Raritan, NJ, USA.

References

1. Kearon C, Akl EA, Ornelas J, Blaivas A, Jimenez D, Bounameaux H, Huisman M, King CS, Morris T, Sood N, Stevens SM, Vintch JRE, Wells P, Woller SC, Moores CL, Antithrombotic Therapy for VTE Disease: CHEST Guideline, CHEST (2016), doi: 10.1016/j.chest.2015.11.026.
2. Konstantinides SV, Torbicki A, Agnelli G, Danchin N, Fitzmaurice D, Galiè N, et al. 2014 ESC guidelines on the diagnosis and management of acute pulmonary embolism. Eur Heart J. 2014;35:3033–69.
3. Zondag W, Kooiman J, Klok FA, Dekkers OM, Huisman MV. Outpatient versus inpatient treatment in patients with pulmonary embolism: a meta-analysis. Eur Respir J. 2013;42:134–44.
4. Aujesky D, Roy PM, Verschuren F, Righini M, Osterwalder J, Egloff M, et al. Outpatient versus inpatient treatment for patients with acute pulmonary embolism: an international, open-label, randomised, non-inferiority trial. Lancet. 2011;378:41–8.
5. Kohn CG, Mearns ES, Parker MW, Hernandez AV, Coleman CI. Prognostic accuracy of clinical prediction rules for early post-pulmonary embolism all-cause mortality: A bivariate meta-analysis. Chest. 2015;147:1043–62.
6. Aujesky D, Obrosky DS, Stone RA, Auble TE, Perrier A, Cornuz J, et al. Derivation and validation of a prognostic model for pulmonary embolism. Am J Respir Crit Care Med. 2005;172:1041–6.
7. Jiménez D, Aujesky D, Moores L, Gómez V, Lobo JL, Uresandi F, et al. Simplification of the pulmonary embolism severity index for prognostication in patients with acute symptomatic pulmonary embolism. Arch Intern Med. 2010;170:1383–9.
8. Zondag W, den Exter PL, Crobach MJ, Dolsma A, Donker ML, Eijsvogel M, et al. Comparison of two methods for selection of out of hospital treatment in patients with acute pulmonary embolism. Thromb Haemost. 2013;109:47–52.
9. Coleman CI, Kohn CG, Bunz TJ. Derivation and validation of the In-hospital mortality for pulmonary embolism using claims daTa (IMPACT) prediction rule. Curr Med Res Opin. 2015;31:1461–8.

10. Coleman CI, Kohn CG, Crivera C, Schein JR, Peacock WF. Validation of the multivariable in-hospital mortality for pulmonary embolism using claims daTa (IMPACT) prediction rule within an all-payer inpatient administrative claims database. BMJ Open. 2015;5:e009251.

11. Kohn CG, Peacock WF, Fermann GJ, Bunz TJ, Crivera C, Schein JR, et al. External validation of the in-hospital mortality for pulmonary embolism using claims data (IMPACT) multivariable prediction rule. Int J Clin Pract. 2016;70:82–8.

12. Moons KG, Altman DG, Reitsma JB, Ioannidis JP, Macaskill P, Steyerberg EW, et al. Transparent reporting of a multivariable prediction model for individual prognosis or diagnosis (TRIPOD): explanation and elaboration. Ann Intern Med. 2015;162:W1–73.

13. Social Security Administration. Social Security Death Index, Master File. Social Security Administration. Available at: http://www.ntis.gov/products/ssa-dmf.aspx (Last accessed on August 2, 2015).

14. Bipartisan Budget Act of 2013. Public Law 113–67. Sec. 203. Restriction on access to the death master file. Available at: https://www.congress.gov/113/plaws/publ67/PLAW-113publ67.pdf (Last accessed on August 2, 2015).

15. Wiener RS, Schwartz LM, Woloshin S. Time trends in pulmonary embolism in the United States: evidence of overdiagnosis. Arch Intern Med. 2011;171:831–7.

2

Pro-coagulant activity during exercise testing in patients with coronary artery disease

Joanna Cwikiel[1,3,4]* (iD), Ingebjorg Seljeflot[1,2,3], Eivind Berge[2], Harald Arnesen[1,3], Kristian Wachtell[5], Hilde Ulsaker[6] and Arnljot Flaa[2,4]

Abstract

Background: Strenuous exercise may trigger myocardial infarction through increased pro-coagulant activity. We aimed to investigate whether patients referred for exercise testing, who were found to have angiographically verified coronary artery disease (CAD), have a more hypercoagulable profile during exercise testing than those without CAD.

Methods: Patients with symptoms of stable CAD were examined with exercise electrocardiography on bicycle ergometer. Venous blood samples were taken at rest and within 5 min after end of exercise. The following haemostatic variables were analyzed: tissue factor pathway inhibitor (TFPI) activity and antigen, prothrombin fragment 1 + 2 (F1 + 2), D-dimer and endogenous thrombin potential (ETP). All participants underwent conventional coronary angiography. CAD was defined as having any degree of atherosclerosis.

Results: Out of the 106 patients enrolled, 70 were found to have CAD. Mean exercise duration was $10:06 \pm 4:11$ min, with no significant differences between the groups. A significant increase from baseline to after exercise testing was observed in all measured markers in the total population ($p \leq 0.002$ for all). In patients with angiographically verified CAD, total TFPI was significantly lower at baseline compared to patients without CAD (median value 67.4 and 76.6 ng/ml respectively, $p = 0.027$). However, no significant differences in changes of any of the measured markers during exercise were observed between the two groups.

Conclusion: Pro-coagulant activity increased during short-term strenuous exercise testing in patients with symptoms suggestive of CAD. However the hypercoagulable state observed, was not more pronounced in patients with angiographically verified CAD compared to patients without CAD. NCT01495091.

Keywords: Coagulation, Atherosclerosis, Angina, Exercise testing, Coronary angiography

Background

Atherosclerotic coronary artery disease (CAD) is a chronic inflammatory process caused by accumulation of low-density lipoproteins (LDL) and plaque formation, activation of intimal inflammation and immune response initiated by endothelial injury and dysfunction, and activation of the haemostatic system [1]. These vascular alterations with subsequent plaque instability may lead to an acute coronary event with fatal consequences. While coronary artery plaques are known to develop over several years, the haemostatic activation is thought to be more prominent in the acute phase of a myocardial infarction [2].

With endothelial injury at plaque site, the haemostatic process is initiated with platelet activation by collagen and von Willebrand factor in the vessel wall, and simultaneously, tissue factor (TF) from the necrotic core of the plaque binds to factor VII, inducing the coagulation cascade [3, 4]. Tissue factor pathway inhibitor (TFPI) synthesized by vascular endothelial, smooth muscle cells and possibly by platelets [5], is the main inhibitor of TF-mediated coagulation, thus mainly reflecting anticoagulant activity. Prothrombin fragment 1 + 2 (F1 + 2) which is generated through the conversion of prothrombin to

* Correspondence: jcwikiel@gmail.com
[1]Department of Cardiology, Center for Clinical Heart Research, Oslo University Hospital Ullevaal, PB 4956 Nydalen, 0424 Oslo, Norway
[3]Faculty of Medicine, University of Oslo, Oslo, Norway
Full list of author information is available at the end of the article

thrombin reflects the amount of in vivo thrombin formed, while on-going coagulation and fibrinolysis can be assessed by D-dimer, a fibrin degradation product. Ex vivo thrombin generation potential, which lately has been given attention as a measure of the degree of hypercoagulability, can be estimated through endogenous thrombin potential (ETP). The ETP is provided through a thrombogram measuring a set of parameters reflecting speed and amount of thrombin generated after standardized activation [6].

It is well recognized that strenuous physical exercise may provoke symptoms of angina or an acute coronary syndrome. During acute heavy physical load simultaneous activation of the coagulation and fibrinolytic processes is believed to occur. An exercise induced transient hypercoagulable state is known to take place in all individuals [7, 8], especially in those who are untrained [9]. Previous studies have suggested an imbalance between coagulation and fibrinolysis in favor of coagulation, in patients with CAD during strenuous exercise [10]. Changes in various haemostatic markers during heavy physical load have previously been investigated, mainly focusing on F1 + 2 and D-dimer [9, 11–13], although mapping of these is far from complete. Previous studies with observations of increased amounts of free and total TFPI in CAD have mainly focused on patients with acute coronary syndrome while sparse studies include patients with stable angina [14–16].

To provide more insight into mechanisms of haemostatic activity among patients with CAD, the aim of our study was to investigate whether patients with angiographically verified CAD, undergoing strenuous exercise, have an increase in markers of pro-coagulant activity different from those without verified CAD.

Methods
Study population
Patients referred for exercise testing due to symptoms suspected of stable CAD enrolled in the on-going CADENCE study (clinicaltrials.gov NCT01495091) at the outpatient clinic at the Department of Cardiology, Oslo University Hospital Ullevaal, Oslo Norway. Eligible patients were those ≥ 18 years of age, with symptoms suspected of CAD and intermediate or high risk (Morise risk score [17] ≥ 9 points). Exclusion criteria were the following: acute coronary syndrome, clinical heart failure, on-going arrhythmia or implanted pacemaker, moderate to severe valvular heart disease, renal insufficiency (S-creatinine >150 μmol/L), inability to perform exercise testing or coronary angiography. For the purpose of the present investigation, patients on oral anticoagulant therapy were excluded. All participants have given written informed consent to participate. The study has been conducted in accordance with the Declaration of Helsinki, and the Regional

Ethics Committee in South Eastern Health Region in Norway approved the protocol.

A thorough medical history was recorded before inclusion. Prior to exercise testing a physical examination including blood pressure, weight and waist circumference was performed. Hypertension and hyperlipidemia were defined according to known diagnosis or use of specific medication.

Exercise stress test
Exercise testing was performed using an electrical bicycle ergometer, monitored by physician and nursing staff. Registration of a resting 12-lead ECG was taken before exercise, while continuous 12-lead ECG monitoring using a computerized electrocardiogram was used during the test. According to protocol the initial workload was 30 watts (W) for women and 50 W for men, with a gradual increase of 10 W per min and participant maintaining a pedaling rate (cadence) of about 65 rpm. Every third min patients were asked about their perceived exhaustion using Borg scale [18]. Auscultatory blood pressure measurements were performed every third min of the test. One physician assessed the test results. Patients were exercised to exhaustion, if there were no clinical signs of ischemia developed prior to reaching high intensity level. The test was stopped after a recovery time of 5 min. A positive test result was defined as having horizontal or down-sloping ST-segment > 1.0 mm (0.1 mV) at 60 milliseconds after the J point and/or chest pain or discomfort. Reasons for terminating the test were development of suspected pathological ECG changes such as ST-segment elevation, ST-segment depression in leads without Q waves, arrhythmias increasing through exercise, chest pain, desire of patient to stop the test and insufficient chronotropic response to exercise, insufficient or exaggerative hypertensive response (systolic blood pressure ≥ 250 mmHg or diastolic blood pressure ≥ 115 mmHg) [19].

Blood sampling and laboratory methods
Blood samples were collected prior to exercise at rest and within 5 min of terminating workload, while patients were still seated on the bicycle ergometer. Citrated blood (0.129 M trisodium citrate in dilution 1:10) was separated within 30 min by centrifugation at 2500 x g at 4 °C and kept frozen at ÷80 °C until analyzed. The following commercially available enzyme immunoassays were used to determine levels of TFPI, F1 + 2 and D-dimer: Asserachrom free and total TFPI antigen, recognizing full-length and truncated TFPI molecules associated to lipoproteins, respectively (Stago Diagnostica, Asniere, France), Enzygnost® F1 + 2 (monoclonal) (Siemens, Marburg, Germany) and Asserachrom D-dimer (Stago Diagnostica). The inter assay coefficients of variation (CV) in our laboratory

were 5.6, 5.7, 4.9 and 6.7%, respectively. ETP was determined by the Calibrated Automated Thrombogram (CAT) assay according to the manufacturer's instructions (Thrombinoscope BV, Maastricht, The Netherlands) and thrombin generation was analyzed on the Fluoroscan Ascent fluorometer (Thermo Fisher Scientific OY, Vantaa, Finland). A reagent mixture of rTF and phospholipids in addition to a thrombin-specific fluorogenic substrate in Hepes buffer containing $CaCl_2$ was added to the plasma to obtain a final concentration of 5 pM, 4 µM and 2.5 mM, respectively. To calculate the final results, plasma was measured together with a thrombin calibrator. The software (version 3.0.0.29; Thrombinoscope BV) enabled the calculation of the lag time (LT), peak thrombin generation (pTG), ETP (area under the curve) and time to peak (TTP). Further, Velo (Velocity Index) = TP/(TTP-LT), indicating the average net rate of pro-thrombin activation during the propagation phase. All experiments were run in duplicates. The inter assay CVs for the different CAT variables were 14.2, 4.6, 5.0 and 8.0%, respectively.

Coronary angiography

All study participants were referred to coronary angiography, performed using the standard Seldinger technique, mostly by using radial artery access. Quantitative coronary angiography (QCA) was analyzed in all angiograms by a single investigator. According to protocol, if a luminal artery stenosis was ≥30%, fractional flow reserve (FFR) was to be performed. Significant coronary stenosis was considered when minimal luminal diameter was >50% according to QCA measures or FFR ≤0.80.

For the purpose of this study CAD was defined as any degree of angiographically verified atherosclerosis, i.e. coronary angiographies described by the operator as having either minimal atherosclerotic changes to significant stenosis.

Statistical analysis

Data was analyzed using IBM SPSS Statistics version 22.0. Laboratory values were mainly not normally distributed and are therefore presented with median value, 25th and 75th percentiles. Continuous data are otherwise presented as mean and standard deviation, and categorical data are presented as numbers (%). Depending on distribution of the continuous data either Student T-test or Mann–Whitney U test were used for comparisons between groups, while Wilcoxon signed rank test was used for pairwise comparisons of continuous data within the groups. For assessment of categorical variables Chi-square test was used. P-values ≤ 0.05 were considered statistically significant.

Results

Demographic and angiography data

Demographic, clinical and medical characteristics are described in Table 1, in the total cohort and according to having CAD or not. In total 120 of the patients enrolled in the CADENCE study were considered for this study of whom 3 patients were excluded due to anticoagulant therapy, 6 patients resigned before completing the study protocol, 5 patients were found to have ≥ 1 exclusion criteria not seen prior to inclusion. Remaining patients (n = 106) constituted the effective study sample. Out of the total population, 70 (66%) patients were found to have angiographically verified CAD and 28 (26.4%) patients were revascularized with either percutaneous coronary intervention or coronary artery bypass graft. The majority of the patients had one or more cardiovascular risk factors such as smoking (58%), hypertension (63%) and hyperlipidemia (79%), which were not significantly differently distributed between the two groups. A significantly lower number of men were found in the group without CAD compared to those with CAD ($p = 0.012$). Previous history of CAD was observed significantly more common in patients also diagnosed with CAD in this study. This is also illustrated by a significantly larger number of patients with CAD being treated with aspirin, statins or beta blockers ($p ≤ 0.03$ for all) compared to those without CAD (Table 1).

Exercise performance

Mean exercise duration was 10:06 ± 4:11 min, exercise capacity 134 ± 48 W and mean metabolic equivalent (MET) 6.7 ± 1.8, with non-significant differences between the two groups. Positive exercise test results were found in 31 (44.3%) patients with CAD and in 7 (19.4%) patients without CAD. Comparable results were found between the revascularized (n = 28) versus non-revascularized (n = 78) groups performing an exercise test, with a sensitivity of 39.3% and specificity of 73.1% for CAD. Maximal heart rate was significantly lower in patients with CAD (137 ± 21 beats per minute (bpm)), Compared to those without CAD (150 ± 19 bpm) ($p = 0.003$).

Markers of pro-coagulant activity

Baseline levels of the haemostatic markers in the total population and according to having CAD or not are shown in Table 2. We observed a significant increase during exercise testing in most of the measured markers in the total population ($p ≤ 0.002$ for all) (Figure 1). When adjusting for change in hematocrit, the increase remained significant in all markers presented in Figure 1, except for D-dimer ($p = 0.071$). Median value of change in hematocrit during exercise was 0.03 (0.02, 0.04) units. As for the CAT assay parameters, only ETP was found to increase significantly (Fig. 1). LT, ttPeak and PeakH changed during exercise

Table 1 Baseline characteristics of the total population and stratified into groups according to angiographically verified CAD or not

	Overall (*n* = 106) (%)	CAD (*n* = 70)	No CAD (*n* = 36)	*P*-value
Age (years)	62 ± 10	63 ± 10	60 ± 10	0.132
Sex (male)	62 (58.5)	47 (67.1)	15 (41.7)	*0.012*
Smoking (current/past)(%)	61 (57.5)	40 (57.1)	21 (58.3)	0.907
Diabetes (%)	19 (17.9)	15 (21.4)	5 (11.1)	0.190
Hypertension (%)	67 (63.2)	44 (62.9)	23 (63.9)	0.917
Hyperlipidemia (%)	84 (79.2)	59 (84.3)	25 (69.4)	0.074
BMI (kg/m^2)	27.8 ± 4	27.9 ± 3.9	27.6 ± 3.8	0.726
Previous CAD (%)				
1.Previous angina	31 (29.2)	27 (38.6)	4 (11.1)	*0.003*
2.Previous MI	14 (13.2)	12 (17.1)	2 (5.6)	0.132
3.Previous interv.	27 (25.5)	25 (35.7)	2 (5.6)	*0.001*
Resting SBP (mmHg)	133 ± 22	133 ± 22	133 ± 21	0.928
Resting DBP (mmHg)	84 ± 10	84 ± 11	85 ± 9	0.621
Resting heart rate (bpm)	70 ± 13	68 ± 12	73 ± 13	0.050
ACE-inhib./ARB	43 (40.6)	30 (42.9)	13 (36.1)	0.503
Betablocker	45 (42.5)	35 (50)	10 (27.8)	*0.028*
Nitrate	9 (8.5)	9 (12.9)	0	*0.025*
Statin	68 (64.2)	50 (71.4)	18 (50)	*0.029*
Aspirin	71 (67)	55 (78.6)	16 (44.4)	*<0.001*

however, results were not significant after adjustment for hematocrit (data not shown). Velocity index did not change.

In patients with verified CAD compared to patients without CAD, significantly lower baseline levels of total TFPI (median value 67.4 versus 76.6 ng/ml respectively, *p* = 0.027) and platelet counts (median value 222 x 10^{e9} and 251 x 10^{e9} respectively, *p* = 0.003) were found (Table 2). Platelet counts were also significantly less increased during exercise in patients with CAD during exercise (*p* = 0.023), also when adjusted for hematocrit (*p* ≤ 0.001) (Figure 2). There were, however, no other

Table 2 Baseline haemostatic markers in the total population and stratified into groups according to angiographically verified CAD or not

	Overall (*n* = 106)	CAD (*n* = 70)	No CAD (*n* = 36)	*P*-value
Hb (g/dL)	14.6 (13.6, 15.1)	14.7 (13.6, 15.2)	14.3 (13.4, 15.1)	0.481
Hematocrit (units)	0.43 (0.40, 0.44)	0.43 (0.40, 0.44)	0.42 (0.40, 0.44)	0.711
Leucocytes (x 10^{e9})	6.60 (5.80, 7.90)	6.4 (5.8, 7.8)	6.8 (5.7, 8.3)	0.502
Platelets (x 10^{e9})	234 (201, 273)	222 (192, 261)	251 (232, 294)	*0.003*
Lactate (mmol/L)	1.40 (1.20, 2.00)	1.4 (1.2, 2.0)	1.4 (1.0, 2.0)	0.759
LT (min)	3.09 (2.68, 3.67)	3.0 (2.7, 3.3)	3.2 (2.9, 3.7)	0.301
ETP (nM*min)	1406 (1283, 1554)	1397 (1281, 1546)	1420 (1279, 1581)	0.667
PeakH (nM)	271.2 (243.3, 307.8)	265 (246, 308)	280 (233, 321)	0.662
ttPeak (min)	5.68 (5.17, 6.36)	289 (247, 329)	286 (253, 324)	0.346
Velo (nM/min^{-1})	103 (87, 132)	103 (88, 131)	110 (82, 135)	0.949
F1 + 2 (pmol/L)	280 (216, 341)	282 (216, 338)	275 (214, 359)	0.679
D-dimer (ng/ml)	348 (210, 581)	381 (221, 583)	296 (196, 578)	0.412
Free TFPI (ng/ml)	16 (13, 20)	15 (13, 19)	16 (12, 20)	0.741
Total TFPI (ng/ml)	71 (60, 81)	67 (58, 79)	77 (64, 84)	*0.027*

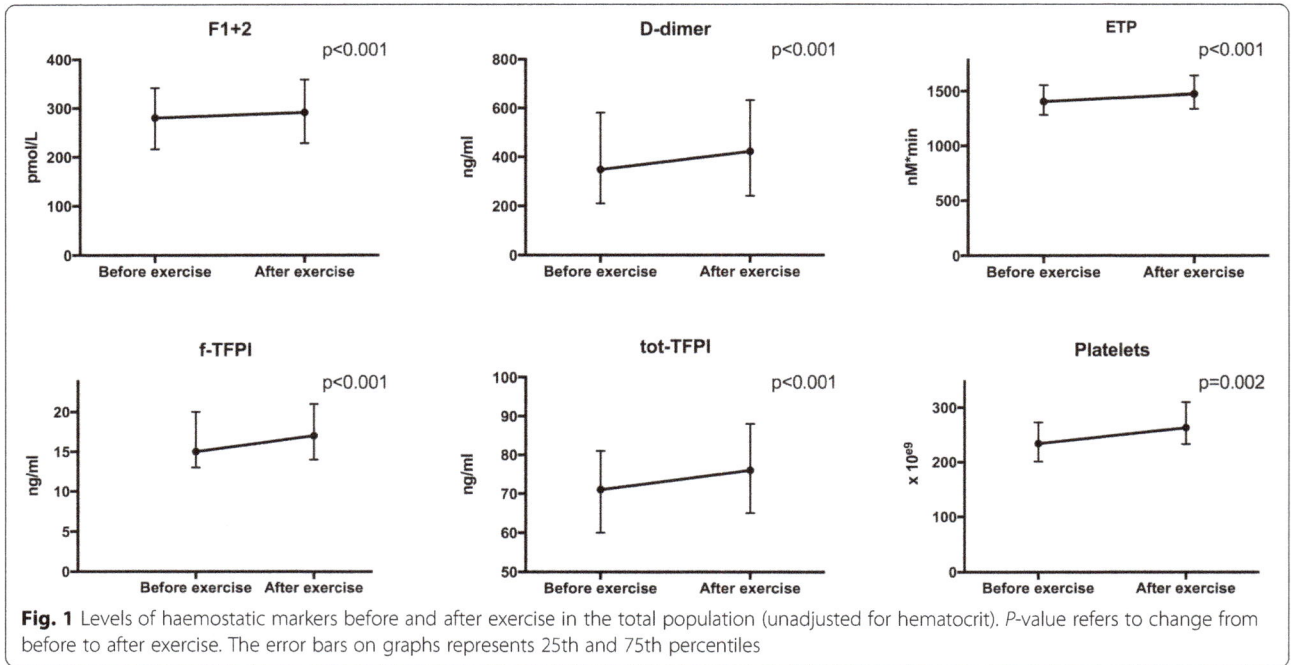

Fig. 1 Levels of haemostatic markers before and after exercise in the total population (unadjusted for hematocrit). *P*-value refers to change from before to after exercise. The error bars on graphs represents 25th and 75th percentiles

significant differences in changes of the measured markers during exercise, between the two groups (Fig. 2). Neither was there any significant difference in changes of these markers comparing patients that were revascularized versus not (data not shown).

In patients with the longest time of exercise duration (≥12:46 min), according to the highest quartile, there was a significant increase in free TFPI during exercise. In this group, patients with CAD had significantly lesser increase in levels of free TFPI compared to patients without CAD

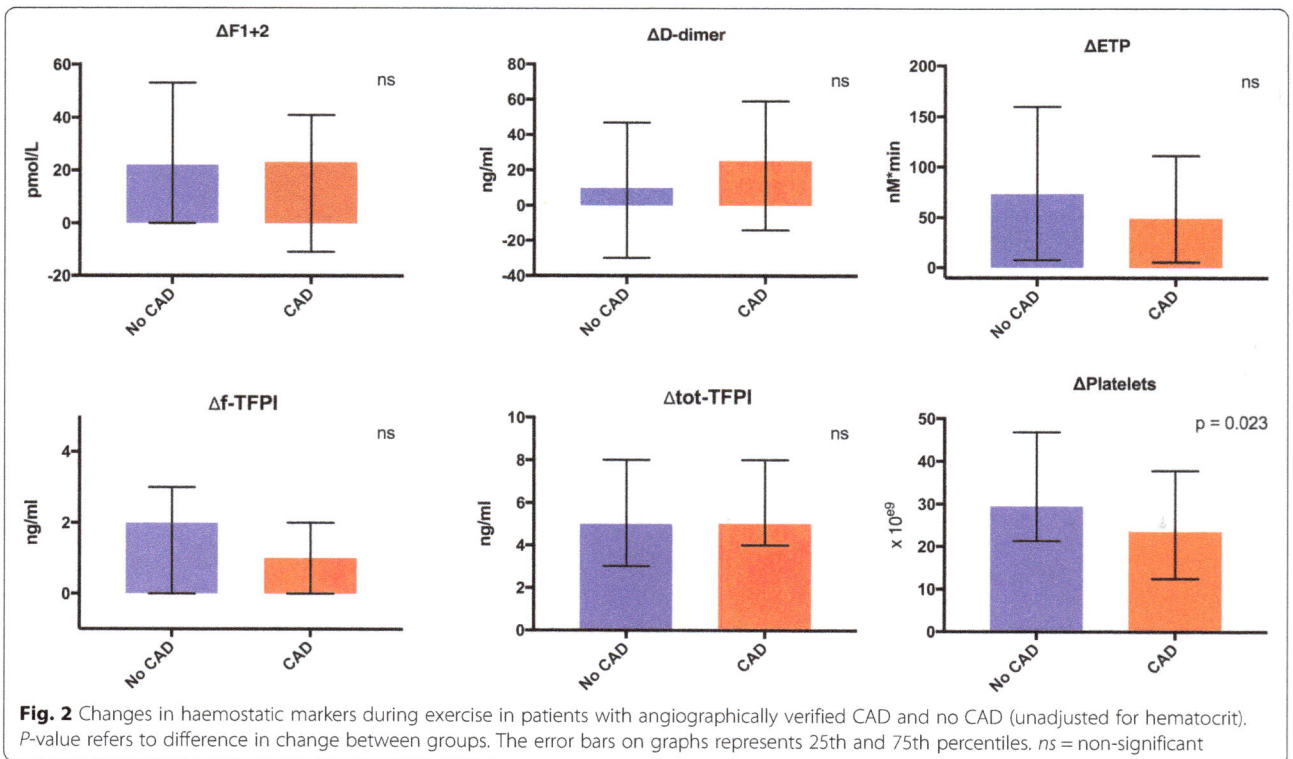

Fig. 2 Changes in haemostatic markers during exercise in patients with angiographically verified CAD and no CAD (unadjusted for hematocrit). *P*-value refers to difference in change between groups. The error bars on graphs represents 25th and 75th percentiles. *ns* = non-significant

(median value 0.4 and 1.6 ng/ml respectively, $p = 0.047$). However these results did not remain significant after adjustment for hematocrit ($p = 0.09$).

Otherwise, no other variables were related to exercise duration.

Discussion

Our study demonstrates that among patients with symptoms of CAD there was a significantly increased pro-coagulant activity during short-term strenuous exercise. Our results show that free and total TFPI, ETP and $F1 + 2$ increased considerably during exercise and these results remain significant despite acknowledged hemoconcerntration during physical exercise. This considered hypercoagulable state was, however, not more pronounced in patients who were angiographically diagnosed with CAD or in need of revascularization compared to those without verified CAD.

It might be suggested that TFPI, being the main inhibitor of TF, would be consumed during a hypercoagulable state, such as in acute coronary syndrome (ACS) or strenuous exercise, or even to an increased extent when the two coincide. To our knowledge the present study is the first to report on the effect of exercise on TFPI in patients with CAD, and we have demonstrated a significant increase in both free and total TFPI. As TFPI is released from endothelial cells, under different stimuli, it has been claimed to be released upon endothelial activation [20]. Our results could therefore be discussed to be related to exercise induced endothelial activation.

However, some studies have shown lower levels of TFPI in patients with CAD, as also was found in our study [21–23]. Arguments of possibly wide inter-individual variation of TFPI levels as well as the known association of TFPI to cardiovascular risk factors or influence of use of medication may be responsible for the diverging data [15, 24]. Two previous studies have concluded that subjects with lower levels of TFPI have an increased risk of developing ACS over a 5-year period [25, 26]. This supports our findings of lower baseline TFPI levels in patients with CAD, considering that patients who developed ACS most likely have atherosclerotic arterial changes long before their first cardiovascular event. Other studies including patients with stable angina pectoris have shown that TFPI levels mostly do not differ from controls [15, 16, 27]. These varying data necessitate further research in this field.

Exercise intensity rather than exercise duration has been supported to affect the haemostatic profile [7, 9]. Our results on increased pro-thrombotic markers, $F1 + 2$ as well as increased ex vivo thrombin generation shown by ETP, are partly in line with previous studies. The borderline significant increased levels of D-dimer might also be discussed as part of the acute phase response. Several previous studies have established that healthy, well-trained individuals have lower ETP levels and higher $F1 + 2$ levels than untrained subjects [28–30]. This has partly been explained by a decrease of ex vivo thrombin generation in the presence of decreasing amounts of prothrombin by its conversion to thrombin in vivo, potentially an exhaustion phenomenon [31]. This did not correspond to findings in our CAD population as our results showed an increase in both markers, which might be discussed along with the exercise performance of relatively short duration. No data on exercise habits of our population was gathered; hence this might have influenced our results. Similar exercise performance was seen in both groups (CAD vs. no CAD), however this does probably not reflect upon exercise capacity of the individuals as they had different reasons for terminating the exercise test. Our finding of lower maximal heart rate in patients with CAD may be explained by worse chronotropic response due to CAD, premature limitation of exercise test due to ECG changes and symptoms or, most likely, by the significantly increased use of beta blockers in this group. Beta blocker use may also explain the overall significantly lower platelet counts in patients with CAD. Catecholamine activation leading to splanchnic activation and subsequent platelet release might be suppressed due to higher incidence of chronic use of beta blockers in the CAD patients [32, 33].

Conclusion

Selected markers of pro- and anticoagulant activity investigated in our study on patients with symptoms of CAD, confirm a haemostatic activation with hypercoagulable response during strenuous exercise, however, this was not more pronounced in patients who presented with angiografically verified CAD.

Acknowledgements
The study group would like to thank medical laboratory technologists Vibeke Kjaer, Vibeke Bratseth and Sissel Akra as well as study nurse Charlotte H Hansen, for their much appreciated help performing this study. A special thank you to my colleague Ida U. Njerve for all wonderful help and support.

Funding
Funding of this study is made by the Stein Erik Hagen foundation for Clinical Heart Research.

Authors' contributions
JC was involved in interpretation of clinical and laboratory data, drafting and finalizing the manuscript. HU recruited study participants and was involved in planning of the study. AF was involved in designing and planning the study. AF, IS and EB interpreted data and intellectually contributed to drafting and discussion of the manuscript. HA and KW were involved in discussion of the manuscript. All authors read and approved the final manuscript.

Competing interests
The authors declare that they have no competing interests.

Author details

[1]Department of Cardiology, Center for Clinical Heart Research, Oslo University Hospital Ullevaal, PB 4956 Nydalen, 0424 Oslo, Norway. [2]Department of Cardiology, Oslo University Hospital Ullevaal, Oslo, Norway. [3]Faculty of Medicine, University of Oslo, Oslo, Norway. [4]Section of Cardiovascular and Renal research, Oslo University Hospital Ulleval, Oslo, Norway. [5]Department of Cardiology, Division of Cardiovascular and Pulmonary diseases, Oslo University Hospital, Oslo, Norway. [6]Modum Bad, Vikersund, Norway.

References

1. Ross R. Atherosclerosis - inflammatory disease. NEJM. 1999;340
2. Lusis AJ. Atherosclerosis. Nature. 2000;407:233–41.
3. Okafor ON, Gorog DA. Endogenous Fibrinolysis: An Important Mediator of Thrombus Formation and Cardiovascular Risk. J Am Coll Cardiol. 2015;65:1683–99.
4. Ardissino D, Merlini PA, Ariëns R, Coppola R, Bramucci E, Mannucci PM. Tissue-factor antigen and activity in human coronary atherosclerotic plaques. Lancet. 1997;349:769–71.
5. Rendu F, Brohard-Bohn B. The platelet release reaction: granules' constituents, secretion and functions. Platelets. 2001;12:261–73.
6. Hemker HC, Al Dieri R, De Smedt E, Béguin S. Thrombin generation, a function test of the haemostatic-thrombotic system. Thromb Haemost. 2006;96:553–61.
7. Posthuma JJ, van der Meijden PE, Ten Cate H, Spronk HM. Short- and Long-term exercise induced alterations in haemostasis: a review of the literature. Blood Rev. 2015;29:171–8.
8. Womack CJ, Nagelkirk PR, Coughlin AM. Exercise-induced changes in coagulation and fibrinolysis in healthy populations and patients with cardiovascular disease. Sports Med. 2003;33:795–807.
9. Acil T, Atalar E, Sahiner L, Kaya B, Haznedaroglu IC, Tokgozoglu L, Ovunc K, Aytemir K, Ozer N, Oto A, Ozmen F, Nazli N, Kes S, Aksoyek S. Effects of acute exercise on fibrinolysis and coagulation in patients with coronary artery disease. Int Heart J. 2007;48:277–85.
10. Smith JE. Effects of strenuous exercise on haemostasis. Br J Sports Med. 2003;37:433–5.
11. Weiss C, Velich T, Niebauer J, Hauer K, Kälberer B, Kübler W, Bärtsch P. Activation of coagulation and fibrinolysis after rehabilitative exercise in patients with coronary artery disease. Am J Cardiol. 1998;81:672–7.
12. Gorog DA. Prognostic value of plasma fibrinolysis activation markers in cardiovascular disease. J Am Coll Cardiol. 2010;55:2701–9.
13. Sedaghat-Hamedani F, Kayvanpour E, Frankenstein L, Mereles D, Amr A, Buss S, Keller A, Giannitsis E, Jensen K, Katus HA, Meder B. Biomarker changes after strenuous exercise can mimic pulmonary embolism and cardiac injury–a metaanalysis of 45 studies. Clin Chem. 2015;61:1246–55.
14. Morange PE, Blankenberg S, Alessi MC, Bickel C, Rupprecht HJ, Schnabel R, Lubos E, Münzel T, Peetz D, Nicaud V, Juhan-Vague I, Tiret L, Atherogene I. Prognostic value of plasma tissue factor and tissue factor pathway inhibitor for cardiovascular death in patients with coronary artery disease: the AtheroGene study. J Thromb Haemost. 2007;5:475–82.
15. Golino P, Ravera A, Ragni M, Cirillo P, Piro O, Chiariello M. Involvement of tissue factor pathway inhibitor in the coronary circulation of patients with acute coronary syndromes. Circulation. 2003;108:2864–9.
16. Falciani M, Gori AM, Fedi S, Chiarugi L, Simonetti I, Dabizzi RP, Prisco D, Pepe G, Abbate R, Gensini GF, Neri Serneri GG. Elevated tissue factor and tissue factor pathway inhibitor circulating levels in ischaemic heart disease patients. Thromb Haemost. 1998;79:495–9.
17. Morise AP, Haddad WJ, Beckner D. Development and validation of a clinical score to estimate the probability of coronary artery disease in men and women presenting with suspected coronary disease. Am J Med. 1997;102:350–6.
18. Borg GA. Psychophysical bases of perceived exertion. Med Sci Sports Exerc. 1982;14:377–81.
19. Fletcher GF, Ades PA, Kligfield P, Arena R, Balady GJ, Bittner VA, Coke LA, Fleg JL, Forman DE, Gerber TC, Gulati M, Madan K, Rhodes J, Thompson PD, Williams MA, American Heart Association Exercise CR, and Prevention Committee of the Council on Clinical Cardiology, Council on Nutrition, Physical Activity and Metabolism, Council on Cardiovascular and Stroke Nursing, and Council on Epidemiology and Prevention. Exercise standards for testing and training: a scientific statement from the American Heart Association. Circulation. 2013;128:873–934.
20. Lupu C, Lupu F, Dennehy U, Kakkar VV, Scully MF. Thrombin induces the redistribution and acute release of tissue factor pathway inhibitor from specific granules within human endothelial cells in culture. Arterioscler Thromb Vasc Biol. 1995;15:2055–62.
21. Kawaguchi A, Miyao Y, Noguchi T, Nonogi H, Yamagishi M, Miyatake K, Kamikubo Y, Kumeda K, Tsushima M, Yamamoto A, Kato H. Intravascular free tissue factor pathway inhibitor is inversely correlated with HDL cholesterol and postheparin lipoprotein lipase but proportional to apolipoprotein A-II. Arterioscler Thromb Vasc Biol. 2000;20:251–8.
22. Saigo M, Abe S, Ogawa M, Yamashita T, Biro S, Minagoe S, Maruyama I, Tei C. Imbalance of plasminogen activator inhibitor-I/tissue plasminogen activator and tissue factor/tissue factor pathway inhibitor in young Japanese men with myocardial infarction. Thromb Haemost. 2001;86:1197–203.
23. Blann AD, Amiral J, McCollum CN, Lip GY. Differences in free and total tissue factor pathway inhibitor, and tissue factor in peripheral artery disease compared to healthy controls. Atherosclerosis. 2000;152:29–34.
24. Mitchell CT, Kamineni A, Palmas W, Cushman M. Tissue factor pathway inhibitor, vascular risk factors and subclinical atherosclerosis: the Multi-Ethnic Study of Atherosclerosis. Atherosclerosis. 2009;207:277–83.
25. Morange PE, Simon C, Alessi MC, Luc G, Arveiler D, Ferrieres J, Amouyel P, Evans A, Ducimetiere P, Juhan-Vague I, PRIME SG. Endothelial cell markers and the risk of coronary heart disease: the Prospective Epidemiological Study of Myocardial Infarction (PRIME) study. Circulation. 2004;109:1343–8.
26. Empana JP, Canoui-Poitrine F, Luc G, Juhan-Vague I, Morange P, Arveiler D, Ferrieres J, Amouyel P, Bingham A, Montaye M, Ruidavets JB, Haas B, Evans A, Ducimetiere P, PRIME SG. Contribution of novel biomarkers to incident stable angina and acute coronary syndrome: the PRIME Study. Eur Heart J. 2008;29:1966–74.
27. Soejima H, Ogawa H, Yasue H, Kaikita K, Nishiyama K, Misumi K, Takazoe K, Miyao Y, Yoshimura M, Kugiyama K, Nakamura S, Tsuji I, Kumeda K. Heightened tissue factor associated with tissue factor pathway inhibitor and prognosis in patients with unstable angina. Circulation. 1999;99:2908–13.
28. Cimenti C, Schlagenhauf A, Leschnik B, Schretter M, Tschakert G, Gröschl W, Seibert FJ, Hofmann P, Muntean WE. Low endogenous thrombin potential in trained subjects. Thromb Res. 2013;131:e281–5.
29. Hilberg T, Prasa D, Stürzebecher J, Gläser D, Gabriel HH. Thrombin potential and thrombin generation after exhaustive exercise. Int J Sports Med. 2002;23:500–4.
30. Huskens D, Roest M, Remijn JA, Konings J, Kremers RM, Bloemen S, Schurgers E, Selmeczi A, Kelchtermans H, van Meel R, Meex SJ, Kleinegris MC, De Groot PG, Urbanus RT, Ninivaggi M, de Laat B. Strenuous exercise induces a hyperreactive rebalanced haemostatic state that is more pronounced in men. Thromb Haemost. 2016;115:1109–19.
31. Lamprecht M, Moussalli H, Ledinski G, Leschnik B, Schlagenhauf A, Koestenberger M, Polt G, Cvirn G. J Appl Physiol. 2013;115:57–63. 1985.
32. Bakovic D, Pivac N, Eterovic D, Palada I, Valic Z, Paukovic-Sekulic B, Dujic Z. Changes in platelet size and spleen volume in response to selective and non-selective beta-adrenoceptor blockade in hypertensive patients. Clin Exp Pharmacol Physiol. 2009;36:441–6.
33. Winther K, Willich SN. Beta 1-blockade and acute coronary ischemia. Possible role of platelets. Circulation. 1991;84:VI68–71.

3

The adaptor protein Disabled-2: new insights into platelet biology and integrin signaling

Hui-Ju Tsai[1,2] and Ching-Ping Tseng[1,2,3,4]*

From The 9th Congress of the Asian-Pacific Society on Thrombosis and Hemostasis
Taipei, Taiwan.

Abstract

Multiple functions of platelets in various physiological and pathological conditions have prompted considerable attention on understanding how platelets are generated and activated. Of the adaptor proteins that are expressed in megakaryocytes and platelets, Disabled-2 (Dab2) has been demonstrated in the past decades as a key regulator of platelet signaling. Dab2 has two alternative splicing isoforms p82 and p59. However, the mode of Dab2's action remains to be clearly defined. In this review, we highlight the current understanding of Dab2 expression and function in megakaryocytic differentiation, platelet activation and integrin signaling. Accordingly, Dab2 is upregulated when the human K562 cells, human CD34[+] hematopoietic stem cells, and murine embryonic stem cells were undergone megakaryocytic differentiation. Appropriate level of Dab2 expression is essential for fate determination of mesodermal and megakaryocytic differentiation. Dab2 is also shown to regulate cell-cell and cell-fibrinogen adhesion, integrin αIIbβ3 activation, fibrinogen uptake, and intracellular signaling of the megakaryocytic cells. In human platelets, p82 is the sole Dab2 isoform present in the cytoplasm and α-granules. Dab2 is released from the α-granules and forms two pools of Dab2 on the outer surface of the platelet plasma membrane, one at the sulfatide-bound and the other at integrin αIIbβ3-bound forms. The balance between these two pools of Dab2 controls the extent of clotting reaction, platelet-fibrinogen interactions and outside-in signaling. In murine platelets, p59 is the only Dab2 isoform and is required for platelet aggregation, fibrinogen uptake, RhoA-ROCK activation, adenosine diphosphate release and integrin αIIbβ3 activation stimulated by low concentration of thrombin. As a result, the bleeding time is prolonged and thrombus formation is impaired for the megakaryocyte lineage-restricted Dab2 deficient mouse. Although discrepancies of Dab2 function and isoform expression are noted between human and murine platelets, the studies up-to-date define Dab2 playing a pivotal role in integrin signaling and platelet activation. With the new tools such as CRISPR and TALEN in the generation of genetically modified animals, the progress in gaining new insights into the functions of Dab2 in megakaryocyte and platelet biology is expected to accelerate.

Keywords: Disabled-2, Integrin αIIbβ3, Megakaryocyte, Platelet

(Continued on next page)

* Correspondence: ctseng@mail.cgu.edu.tw
[1]Department of Medical Biotechnology and Laboratory Science, Collage of Medicine, Chang Gung University, Kweishan, Taoyuan 333, Taiwan, Republic of China
[2]Molecular Medicine Research Center, Chang Gung University, Kweishan, Taoyuan 333, Taiwan, Republic of China
Full list of author information is available at the end of the article

(Continued from previous page)

Abbreviations: ADP, Adenosine diphosphate; CSF-1, Colony-stimulating factor-1; Dab2, Disabled-2; ESCs, Embryonic stem cells; ITAM, Immunoreceptor tyrosine-based activation motif; PARs, Protease-activated receptors; PKC, Protein kinase C; PRD, Proline rich domain; PTB, Phosphotyrosine binding domain; TPA, 12-O-tetradecanoylphorbol-13-acetate; TXA_2, Thromboxane A_2

Background

Platelets are the second most abundant blood cells and are derived from the cytoplasm of megakaryocytes [1]. The crucial role of platelet in haemostasis and thrombosis has prompted extensive attentions on unveiling the underlying mechanisms of platelet activation induced by soluble agonists [2–4]. Platelet activation is mainly mediated by binding of ligands to the membrane receptors such as the immunoglobulin family of glycoproteins for collagen and the G-protein coupled receptors for thrombin, thromboxane A2 (TXA_2) and adenosine diphosphate (ADP) [5]. Collagen interacts with glycoprotein VI which contains an immunoreceptor tyrosine-based activation motif (ITAM). The ITAM is phosphoryated by two Src kinases (Lyn and Fyn) and recruits the protein tyrosine kinase Syk to the plasma membrane for phosphorylation of downstream substrates at the tyrosine residue that are essential for platelet activation [5]. Other soluble agonists such as thrombin, TXA_2 and ADP bind to the respective G protein-coupled receptors and cause an increase in intracellular calcium and protein kinase C (PKC) activity, Rho activation, inhibition of adenylyl cyclase and activation of phosphoinositide 3-kinase-Akt through the $G\alpha_q$-, $G\alpha_{12/13}$-, $G\alpha_i$-, and $G\beta\gamma$-dependent pathway, respectively [5, 6]. The inside-out signaling induced by different platelet agonists activates integrin $\alpha IIb\beta 3$ followed by the binding of fibrinogen to integrin $\alpha IIb\beta 3$ and activation of outside-in signaling. These intracellular events ultimately lead to platelet activation, secretion and aggregation [7]. Despite extensive studies, the underlying mechanisms of platelet signaling networks still wait to be fully elucidated.

Adaptor protein is a type of proteins mediating protein-protein and protein-lipid interactions. It has been clearly demonstrated that adaptor proteins are essential for coupling membrane receptors to intracellular signaling pathways and the assembly of signaling scaffolds within the cells. Many adaptor proteins expressed in the platelets are involved in inside-out and outside-in signaling of integrin during platelet activation [8]. Disabled-2 (Dab2) is a newly identified adaptor protein that is known to express in megakaryocytes and platelets from a variety of species [9, 10]. The current knowledge about the roles of Dab2 in megakaryocytic differentiation and platelet signaling is still in the beginning. This review will focus on the expression and functional aspects of Dab2 in megakaryocytic differentiation, platelet activation and integrin signaling.

Review

Discovery and the protein properties of Dab2

Human *dab2* gene is located at the chromosome 5p13 and was first identified by Mok et al. as the tumor suppressor gene of the ovary cancer in 1994 [11]. The mouse Dab2 protein was then revealed in 1995 during the analysis of phosphoproteins induced by colony-stimulating factor-1 (CSF-1) in macrophage [12]. In 1998, Tseng et al. further defined rat *dab2* as the differentially expressed gene that was up-regulated in the castrated rat prostate [13]. At least two Dab2 isoforms with the molecular weight of 82 and 59 kDa, referred to p82-Dab2 and p59-Dab2, respectively, are generated through alternative splicing (Fig. 1) [14]. Because of the undefined post-translational protein modification, the protein bands of p82-Dab2 and p59-Dab2 are up-shifted to the positions at 96 and 67 kDa on sodium dodecyl sulfate-polyacrylamide gel electrophoresis. Hence, p82-Dab2 and p59-Dab2 sometimes are referred to p96-Dab2 and p67-Dab2, respectively. The ninth coding exon corresponding to the amino acids 230–447 of p82-Dab2 is not present in the protein of p59-Dab2. As a result, several binding sites for endocytic proteins are absent in p59-Dab2. Particular motifs mediating protein-protein and protein-lipid interactions are present in Dab2, allowing them to communicate with other signaling molecules. The phosphotyrosine binding (PTB) domain is located at the N-terminus of Dab2, playing a role in the interaction of Dab2 with DIP1/2, Smad2/3, Dishevelled-3, phosphatidylinositol 4,5-bisphosphate (PI(4,5)P_2), and a subset of receptors such as integrin, low density lipoprotein receptor, megalin and related receptors that contain the non-tyrosine-phosphorylated NPXY motif [14–21]. The aspartic acid-proline-phenylalanine (DPF) motif of Dab2 interacts with the α-adaptin subunit of the clathrin adaptor protein 2 (AP-2) [21]. The C-terminal proline-rich domain (PRD) interacts with Grb2, c-Src, Akt and c-Cbl-interacting protein of 85 kDa [22–26]. By interacting with other cellular factors through these motifs, Dab2 elicits its functions in endocytosis, differentiation, and immune response and is involved in the cell signaling pathways of Ras-mitogen activated protein kinase (MAPK), Wnt, TGF-β, c-Src and RhoA-ROCK [24, 27–36]. Dab2 is also known to regulate cytoskeleton reorganization by binding to non-muscle myosin heavy chain IIA, myosin VI, actin, and dynein [12, 37–39].

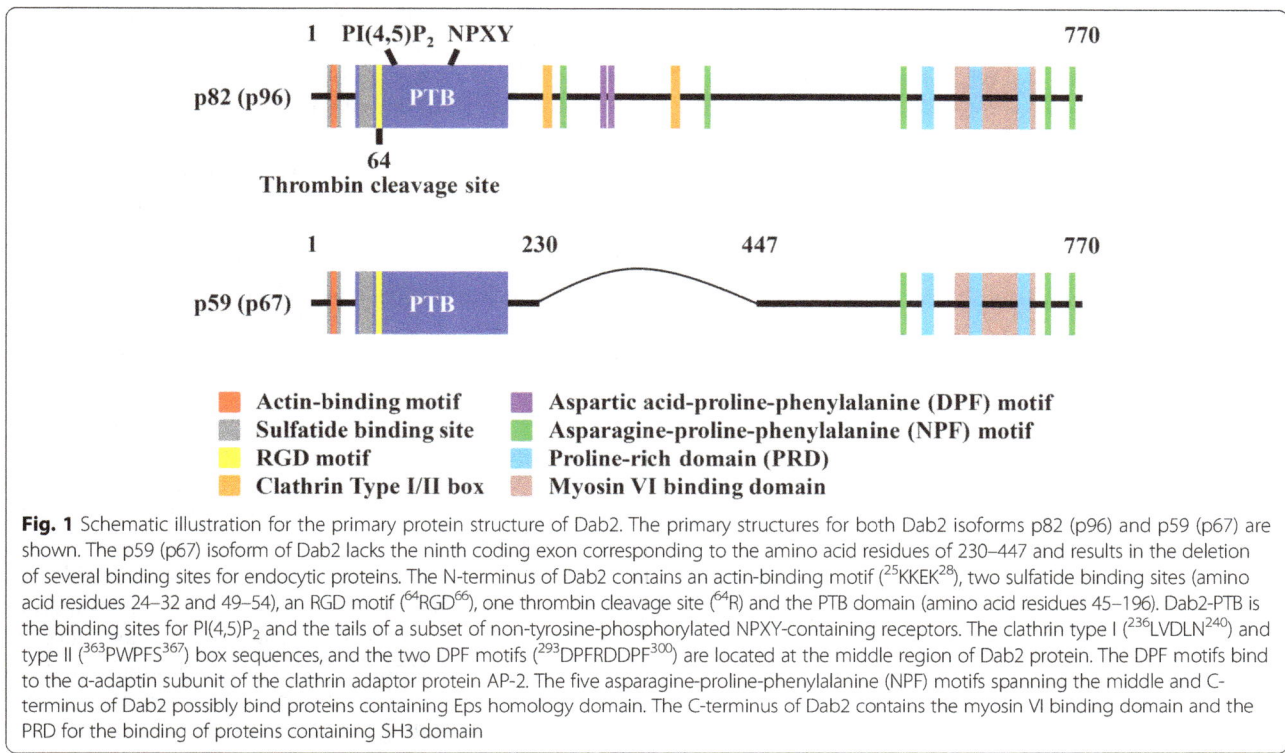

Fig. 1 Schematic illustration for the primary protein structure of Dab2. The primary structures for both Dab2 isoforms p82 (p96) and p59 (p67) are shown. The p59 (p67) isoform of Dab2 lacks the ninth coding exon corresponding to the amino acid residues of 230–447 and results in the deletion of several binding sites for endocytic proteins. The N-terminus of Dab2 contains an actin-binding motif (^{25}KKEK^{28}), two sulfatide binding sites (amino acid residues 24–32 and 49–54), an RGD motif (^{64}RGD^{66}), one thrombin cleavage site (^{64}R) and the PTB domain (amino acid residues 45–196). Dab2-PTB is the binding sites for PI(4,5)P_2 and the tails of a subset of non-tyrosine-phosphorylated NPXY-containing receptors. The clathrin type I (^{236}LVDLN^{240}) and type II (^{363}PWPFS^{367}) box sequences, and the two DPF motifs (^{293}DPFRDDPF^{300}) are located at the middle region of Dab2 protein. The DPF motifs bind to the α-adaptin subunit of the clathrin adaptor protein AP-2. The five asparagine-proline-phenylalanine (NPF) motifs spanning the middle and C-terminus of Dab2 possibly bind proteins containing Eps homology domain. The C-terminus of Dab2 contains the myosin VI binding domain and the PRD for the binding of proteins containing SH3 domain

Dab2 is a phosphoprotein with several phosphorylation sites having been identified. Dab2 is phosphorylated at serine residues in murine macrophage cell line in response to mitogenic stimulation by CSF-1 [12]. Dab2-Ser24 is phosphorylated by PKCβII, γ and δ but not by casein kinase II, playing a critical role in the inhibition of 12-O-tetradecanoylphorbol-13-acetate (TPA)-induced AP-1 activity and integrin activation [33, 40]. Dab2 is hyperphosphorylated by the cyclin-dependent serine/threonine kinase Cdc2 during the mitosis phase of the cell cycle in HeLa S3 cells [41]. The phosphorylated Dab2 interacts with the peptidylprolyl isomerase Pin1 that facilitates Dab2 dephosphorylation immediately after the end of mitosis phase [42]. Similarly, Akt interacts with PRD domain of Dab2 and phosphorylates Ser448/Ser449 to regulate albumin endocytosis and mediate albumin uptake in proximal tubule [25, 43]. These distinct protein properties facilitate the involvement of Dab2 in diverse signaling network in response to extracellular responses.

Expression pattern of Dab2 in megakaryocytes and platelets

The first study addressing Dab2 expression and function in megakaryocytes and platelets was published in 2001 [31]. Dab2 is upregulated when the human leukemic K562 cells, human CD34$^+$ hematopoietic pluripotent stem cells, and murine embryonic stem cells (ESCs) are undergone megakaryocytic differentiation (Table 1) [31–33, 35]. Among the platelets from the species of murine, rat, and human, murine platelets have the least amount of Dab2 [9]. This is in accord with the genome-wide RNA-seq analysis of platelet transcriptomes that revealed several thousands-fold differences for the expression of Dab2 transcripts between human and mouse platelets [44]. Moreover, Dab2 isoforms are differentially expressed in human, rat and murine platelets. Both p82-Dab2 and p59-Dab2 are detectable in the rat platelets, while p82-Dab2 and p59-Dab2 is mainly expressed in the platelets from human and murine, respectively [9].

The evolutionary roles for an increase in Dab2 expression from mouse to rat and human platelets and the species-specific expression of Dab2 isoforms are not yet understood. Distinctive functions of p82-Dab2 and p59-Dab2 have been unveiled in several studies. p82-Dab2 is known to regulate receptor-mediated endocytosis, while p59-Dab2 is a transcriptional regulator when the F9 cells are undergone differentiation [18, 20, 45, 46]. Knock-in expression of p59-Dab2 only partially compromises the absence of Dab2 in the Dab2-knockout mice [14]. The increased expression of p82-Dab2 protein in human platelets may fine tune platelet response to soluble agonists and provide a superior way to prevent excessive blood loss in the large mammals. Future study using an in vivo animal model expressing human platelet p82-Dab2 should provide new insight for the aforementioned hypothesis.

Table 1 Dab2 expression and function in megakaryocytes and platelets

Experimental systems	Reported Dab2 expression/function	References
Human K562 cells	Increased Dab2 expression during TPA-induced megakaryocytic differentiation	[19, 31–34]
	Positive regulation of fibrinogen uptake	
	Dab2 interacts with integrin β3 and inhibits integrin αIIbβ3 activation	
Human CD34+ stem cells	Increased Dab2 expression during TPO-induced megakaryocytic differentiation	[10]
Mouse embryonic stem cells/OP9 co-culture	Increased Dab2 expression during mesodermal and megakaryocytic differentiation	[35]
	Dab2 is required for mesodermal differentiation	
Human platelets	High expression of p82-Dab2 in the cytoplasm and α-granule	[10, 33, 47–49]
	Dab2 interacts with the cytoplamic tail of platelet integrin	
	Secreted Dab2 interacts with integrin αIIb and sulfatide; is a substrate of thrombin	
	Dab2 regulates fibrinogen binding and homotypic and heterotypic platelet interactions	
Mouse platelets	Low expression of p59-Dab2	[9]
	Dab2-deficient mice display a prolonged bleeding time and impaired thrombus formation	
	Dab2 is required for platelet aggregation, fibrinogen uptake, RhoA-ROCK activation, ADP release and integrin αIIbβ3 activation stimulated by low concentration of thrombin	

Dab2 functions in megakaryocytic differentiation and platelet signaling

Dab2 has been shown to elicit multiple functions in mega-karyocytic differentiation and platelet signaling (Table 1 and Fig. 2). The human K562 leukemic cells induced by TPA to form megakaryocyte-like cells have been used to define the role of Dab2 in integrin activation, cell adhesion, fibrinogen uptake, and megakaryocytic differentiation [31–34]. Dab2 is crucial in cell-cell adhesion of K562 cells and negatively regulates integrin αIIbβ3 activation and cell adhesion to fibrinogen. A mutual regulation between Dab2 and MAPK was also unveiled when the K562 cells are undergone megakaryocytic differentiation [31, 32]. Dab2 colocalizes with clathrin and mediates fibrinogen uptake in the primary megakaryocytes and megakaryocytic differentiating K562 cells [34]. Dab2-

associated regulatory circuit controls mesoderm and megakaryocytic differentiation by regulating β-catenin and plakoglobin cellular distribution through the interaction between the PTB domain of Dab2 and the Asn-Pro-Asp-Tyr motif of plakoglobin [35]. Accordingly, down-regulation of Dab2 in murine ESCs disrupts cell-cell adhesion and affects embryoid body and colony formation leading to impaired mesodermal and megakaryocytic differentiation. Multiple roles of Dab2 in intracellular signaling, integrin activation and fibrinogen uptake of the megakaryocytic cells, and the fate determination of mesodermal and megakaryocytic differentiation were defined by these studies.

Dab2 is present in the cytoplasm and α-granules of human platelets and is released from the platelets in response to platelet activation [10]. Dab2 is shown in a number of studies playing a pivotal role in the activation of human platelets. Dab2 interacts with the cytoplasmic tail of the platelet integrin and regulates inside-out signaling [33]. On the other hand, Dab2 released from the α-granules is able to bind the extracellular region of αIIbβ3 integrin through the Dab2 cell-adhesion Arg-Gly-Asp (RGD) motif (amino acid residues 64–66) and the fibrinogen binding region of integrin αIIb. Such interactions compete for the integrin αIIb-fibrinogen interactions and inhibit platelet aggregation induced by soluble agonists except thrombin. Thrombin renders Dab2 inactive by cleavage of Dab2 at the amino acid residue 64 [10]. Notably, the action of thrombin on Dab2 cleavage is suppressed when Dab2 binds to the phospholipid sulfatide through four positively charged residues (Lys25, Lys49, Lys51, and Lys53) located at the PTB domain [47]. Hence, two pools of Dab2 is present at the outer surface of the platelet plasma membrane, one at the sulfatide-bound and the other at the integrin αIIbβ3-bound states. The balance between these two Dab2 states is involved in the regulation of clotting reaction, platelet aggregation and the interactions of platelet and fibrinogen in response to stimulation by platelet agonists [10, 47–49].

Megakaryocyte/platelet lineage-restricted Dab2 knock-out (Dab2$^{-/-}$) mice have been generated by using the Cre-loxP transgenic system driven by the platelet factor 4 promoter to elucidate Dab2 functions in vivo [9]. Dab2$^{-/-}$ platelets, when stimulated by low concentrations of thrombin, are defective in platelet aggregation, clot retraction, and spreading on fibrinogen. The functional imperfection of Dab2$^{-/-}$ platelets is related to the defective responses to thrombin-induced RhoA-ROCKII and Akt-mTOR activation, ADP release and integrin αIIbβ3 activation [9]. Although Dab2 elicits a restrictive function to the murine platelets stimulated by low concentrations of thrombin, defective Dab2 expression has profound effects on hemostasis and thrombosis in vivo.

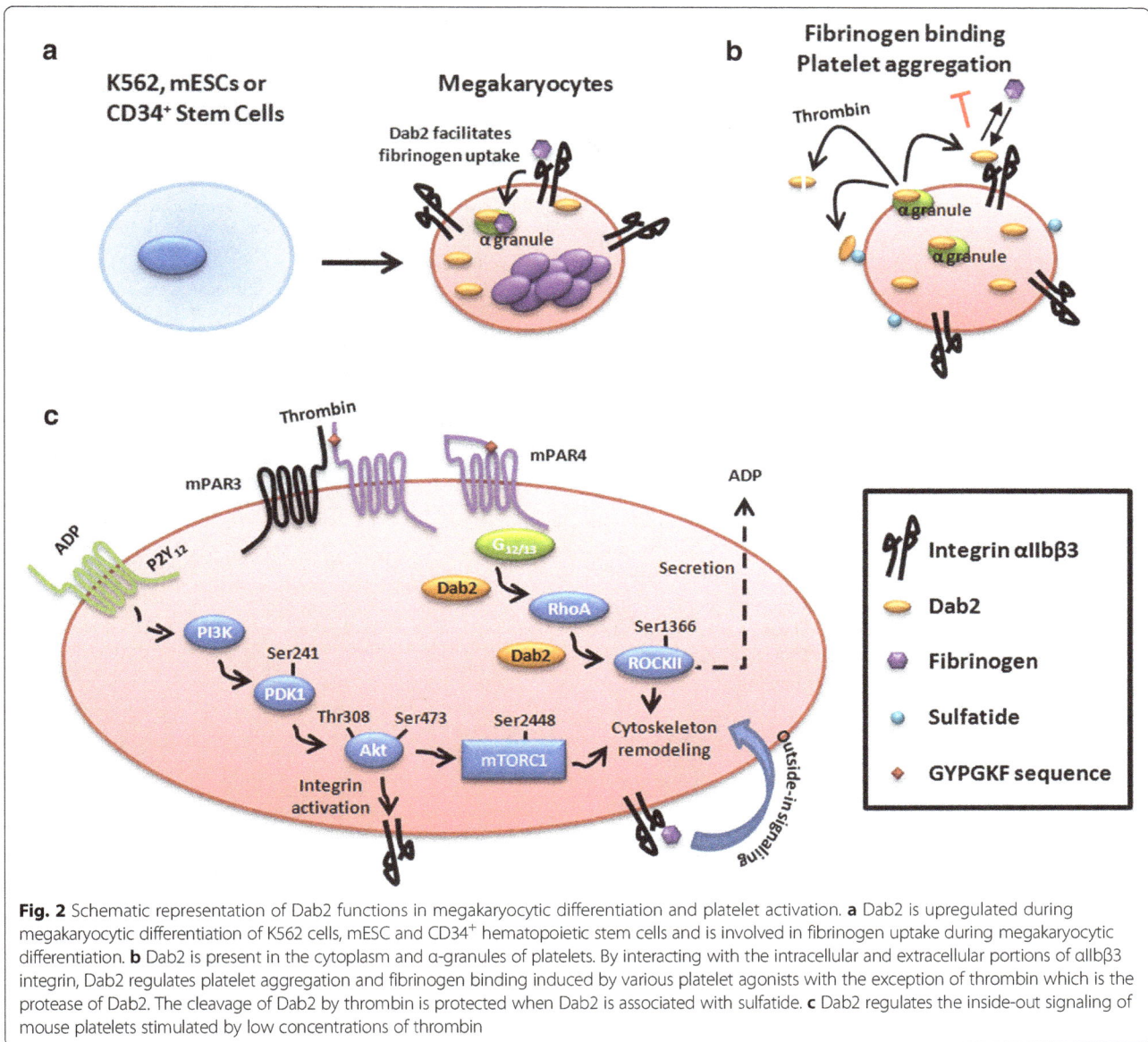

Fig. 2 Schematic representation of Dab2 functions in megakaryocytic differentiation and platelet activation. **a** Dab2 is upregulated during megakaryocytic differentiation of K562 cells, mESC and CD34+ hematopoietic stem cells and is involved in fibrinogen uptake during megakaryocytic differentiation. **b** Dab2 is present in the cytoplasm and α-granules of platelets. By interacting with the intracellular and extracellular portions of αIIbβ3 integrin, Dab2 regulates platelet aggregation and fibrinogen binding induced by various platelet agonists with the exception of thrombin which is the protease of Dab2. The cleavage of Dab2 by thrombin is protected when Dab2 is associated with sulfatide. **c** Dab2 regulates the inside-out signaling of mouse platelets stimulated by low concentrations of thrombin

This is evidenced by the observations that bleeding time is prolonged and thrombus formation is impaired in the Dab2$^{-/-}$ mice. These findings are consistent with the perception that protease-activated receptors (PAR) 3- and PAR4-deficient mice, despite eliciting a partial decrease in thrombin-induced platelet aggregation, are impaired in hemostasis and are protected against thrombosis [50, 51]. These studies support the notion that Dab2 is a key regulator in hemostasis and thrombosis.

The consensuses, controversies and future prospects

The study linking Dab2 functions with megakaryocytic differentiation, platelet signaling and integrin activation was first reported 15 years ago [31]. The studies up-to-date support extensively that Dab2 is a regulator of megakaryocytic differentiation and platelet function. Nevertheless, distinctive functions of Dab2 in human and mouse megakaryocytes and platelets are noted. Knockdown of Dab2 results in an increase in αIIbβ3 activation and cell adhesion to fibrinogen in the K562 cells [33]. Dab2 is, however, required for murine platelet aggregation and integrin αIIbβ3 activation when the platelets are stimulated by low concentrations of thrombin [9]. Dab2 negatively regulates human platelet-fibrinogen interaction and platelet aggregation induced by soluble agonists except thrombin [10, 47–49]. The complexity in the abundance and species-specific expression of Dab2 isoforms and the diverse thrombin signaling in human and murine platelets [6, 9] likely contribute to the reported heterogeneity of Dab2 function. Alternatively, the discrepancy in these findings could be due to the different assay systems being used in these studies. In the studies of human platelets, recombinant Dab2 protein was the main tool for analyzing the effects of Dab2 function on platelet response by in vitro experiments [10, 47–49]. There are no Dab2 mutants or Dab2-deficient human platelets available for in vivo study. On the other hand, Dab2-deficient murine platelets have been generated for analysis of Dab2 function in vivo [9]. An animal model expressing human platelet Dab2 should help us to understand the distinctive Dab2 functions in human and murine platelets.

Dab2 is known as a phosphoprotein in a variety of cellular processes [12, 25, 33, 40–43]. Due to the lack of appropriate tools, the physiological functions of Dab2 phosphorylation in platelet signaling have not yet been elucidated. We have addressed these issues in our recent work and revealed that Dab2 is phosphorylated during agonist-stimulated human platelet activation (unpublished data). With the new tools such as CRISPR and TALEN [52–55] in the generation of genetically modified animals, the progress in gaining new insights into the signaling network involving Dab2 expression and phosphorylation in megakaryocyte, platelet biology and integrin signaling is expected to accelerate.

Conclusions

Multiple functions of platelets in hemostasis, thrombosis, immunology, cancer progression, microorganism infections call for considerable attention on understanding how the activated platelets transmit intracellular signal to elicit their roles in different biological responses. Extensive evidence from the studies in the past decades demonstrates that Dab2 is a key regulator of platelet signaling, in particular, the endocytosis and the activation of thrombin-stimulated inside-out signaling of platelet integrin. With the complicated nature of the signaling network within megakaryocytes and platelets, the definitive roles of Dab2 in megakaryocytic differentiation, platelet activation and integrin signaling remain to be explored further.

Declaration
Publication fees for this article have been funded by APSTH 2016.
This article has been published as part of Thrombosis Journal Volume 14 Supplement 1, 2016. The full contents of the supplement are available at https://thrombosisjournal.biomedcentral.com/articles/supplements/volume-14-supplement-1

Funding
The work performed in the authors' laboratory was supported in part by the Ministry of Science and Technology grants MOST102-2628-B-182-009-MY3, MOST102-2628-B-182-010-MY3, MOST105-2320-B-182-029-MY3, MOST105-2320-B-182-030, the Chang Gung Memorial Hospital grants (CMRPD1C0551-3, CMRPD1B0391-3, CMRPD1E0181-3, and BMRP466), and the Chang Gung Molecular Medicine Research Center grant (EMRPD1E1491) to C.-P. Tseng; the Ministry of Science and Technology post-doctoral fellowship grants 104-2811-B-182-004 and 104-2811-B-182-006 to H.-J. Tsai.

Authors' contributions
HJT and CPT contributed in the conception and the design of the article and have given final approval of the version to be submitted.

Competing interests
The authors declare that they have no competing interests.

Author details
[1]Department of Medical Biotechnology and Laboratory Science, Collage of Medicine, Chang Gung University, Kweishan, Taoyuan 333, Taiwan, Republic of China. [2]Molecular Medicine Research Center, Chang Gung University, Kweishan, Taoyuan 333, Taiwan, Republic of China. [3]Graduate Institute of Biomedical Science, Collage of Medicine, Chang Gung University, Kweishan, Taoyuan 333, Taiwan, Republic of China. [4]Department of Laboratory Medicine, Chang Gung Memorial Hospital, Kweishan, Taoyuan 333, Taiwan, Republic of China.

References
1. George JN. Platelets. Lancet. 2000;355:1531–9.
2. Chong AJ, Pohlman TH, Hampton CR, Shimamoto A, Mackman N, Verrier ED. Tissue factor and thrombin mediate myocardial ischemia-reperfusion injury. Ann Thorac Surg. 2003;75:S649–55.
3. Schonberger T, Ziegler M, Borst O, Konrad I, Nieswandt B, Massberg S, Ochmann C, Jurgens T, Seizer P, Langer H, et al. The dimeric platelet collagen receptor GPVI-Fc reduces platelet adhesion to activated endothelium and preserves myocardial function after transient ischemia in mice. Am J Physiol Cell Physiol. 2012;303:C757–66.
4. White HD. Oral antiplatelet therapy for atherothrombotic disease: current evidence and new directions. Am Heart J. 2011;161:450–61.
5. Li Z, Delaney MK, O'Brien KA, Du X. Signaling during platelet adhesion and activation. Arterioscler Thromb Vasc Biol. 2010;30:2341–9.
6. Coughlin SR. Thrombin signalling and protease-activated receptors. Nature. 2000;407:258–64.
7. Shen B, Delaney MK, Du X. Inside-out, outside-in, and inside-outside-in: G protein signaling in integrin-mediated cell adhesion, spreading, and retraction. Curr Opin Cell Biol. 2012;24:600–6.
8. Leo A, Schraven B. Networks in signal transduction: the role of adaptor proteins in platelet activation. Platelets. 2000;11:429–45.
9. Tsai HJ, Huang CL, Chang YW, Huang DY, Lin CC, Cooper JA, Cheng JC, Tseng CP. Disabled-2 is required for efficient hemostasis and platelet activation by thrombin in mice. Arterioscler Thromb Vasc Biol. 2014;34:2404–12.
10. Huang CL, Cheng JC, Stern A, Hsieh JT, Liao CH, Tseng CP. Disabled-2 is a novel alphaIIb-integrin-binding protein that negatively regulates platelet-fibrinogen interactions and platelet aggregation. J Cell Sci. 2006;119:4420–30.
11. Mok SC, Wong KK, Chan RK, Lau CC, Tsao SW, Knapp RC, Berkowitz RS. Molecular cloning of differentially expressed genes in human epithelial ovarian cancer. Gynecol Oncol. 1994;52:247–52.
12. Xu XX, Yang W, Jackowski S, Rock CO. Cloning of a novel phosphoprotein regulated by colony-stimulating factor 1 shares a domain with the Drosophila disabled gene product. J Biol Chem. 1995;270:14184–91.
13. Tseng CP, Ely BD, Li Y, Pong RC, Hsieh JT. Regulation of rat DOC-2 gene during castration-induced rat ventral prostate degeneration and its growth inhibitory function in human prostatic carcinoma cells. Endocrinology. 1998;139:3542–53.
14. Maurer ME, Cooper JA. Endocytosis of megalin by visceral endoderm cells requires the Dab2 adaptor protein. J Cell Sci. 2005;118:5345–55.
15. Wang Z, Tseng CP, Pong RC, Chen H, McConnell JD, Navone N, Hsieh JT. The mechanism of growth-inhibitory effect of DOC-2/DAB2 in prostate cancer. Characterization of a novel GTPase-activating protein associated with N-terminal domain of DOC-2/DAB2. J Biol Chem. 2002;277:12622–31.
16. Hocevar BA, Smine A, Xu XX, Howe PH. The adaptor molecule Disabled-2 links the transforming growth factor beta receptors to the Smad pathway. EMBO J. 2001;20:2789–801.
17. Hocevar BA, Mou F, Rennolds JL, Morris SM, Cooper JA, Howe PH. Regulation of the Wnt signaling pathway by disabled-2 (Dab2). EMBO J. 2003;22:3084–94.
18. Mishra SK, Keyel PA, Hawryluk MJ, Agostinelli NR, Watkins SC, Traub LM. Disabled-2 exhibits the properties of a cargo-selective endocytic clathrin adaptor. EMBO J. 2002;21:4915–26.

19. Calderwood DA, Fujioka Y, de Pereda JM, Garcia-Alvarez B, Nakamoto T, Margolis B, McGlade CJ, Liddington RC, Ginsberg MH. Integrin beta cytoplasmic domain interactions with phosphotyrosine-binding domains: a structural prototype for diversity in integrin signaling. Proc Natl Acad Sci U S A. 2003;100:2272–7.

20. Keyel PA, Mishra SK, Roth R, Heuser JE, Watkins SC, Traub LM. A single common portal for clathrin-mediated endocytosis of distinct cargo governed by cargo-selective adaptors. Mol Biol Cell. 2006;17:4300–17.

21. Morris SM, Cooper JA. Disabled-2 colocalizes with the LDLR in clathrin-coated pits and interacts with AP-2. Traffic. 2001;2:111–23.

22. Zhou J, Hsieh JT. The inhibitory role of DOC-2/DAB2 in growth factor receptor-mediated signal cascade. DOC-2/DAB2-mediated inhibition of ERK phosphorylation via binding to Grb2. J Biol Chem. 2001;276:27793–8.

23. Xu XX, Yi T, Tang B, Lambeth JD. Disabled-2 (Dab2) is an SH3 domain-binding partner of Grb2. Oncogene. 1998;16:1561–9.

24. Zhou J, Scholes J, Hsieh JT. Characterization of a novel negative regulator (DOC-2/DAB2) of c-Src in normal prostatic epithelium and cancer. J Biol Chem. 2003;278:6936–41.

25. Koral K, Erkan E. PKB/Akt partners with Dab2 in albumin endocytosis. Am J Physiol Renal Physiol. 2012;302:F1013–24.

26. Kowanetz K, Terzic J, Dikic I. Dab2 links CIN85 with clathrin-mediated receptor internalization. FEBS Lett. 2003;554:81–7.

27. Huang CH, Cheng JC, Chen JC, Tseng CP. Evaluation of the role of Disabled-2 in nerve growth factor-mediated neurite outgrowth and cellular signalling. Cell Signal. 2007;19:1339–47.

28. Jiang Y, He X, Howe PH. Disabled-2 (Dab2) inhibits Wnt/beta-catenin signalling by binding LRP6 and promoting its internalization through clathrin. EMBO J. 2012;31:2336–49.

29. Jain N, Nguyen H, Friedline RH, Malhotra N, Brehm M, Koyanagi M, Bix M, Cooper JA, Chambers CA, Kang J. Cutting edge: Dab2 is a FOXP3 target gene required for regulatory T cell function. J Immunol. 2009;183:4192–6.

30. Penheiter SG, Singh RD, Repellin CE, Wilkes MC, Edens M, Howe PH, Pagano RE, Leof EB. Type II transforming growth factor-beta receptor recycling is dependent upon the clathrin adaptor protein Dab2. Mol Biol Cell. 2010;21:4009–19.

31. Tseng CP, Huang CH, Tseng CC, Lin MH, Hsieh JT, Tseng CH. Induction of disabled-2 gene during megakaryocyte differentiation of k562 cells. Biochem Biophys Res Commun. 2001;285:129–35.

32. Tseng CP, Huang CL, Huang CH, Cheng JC, Stern A, Tseng CH, Chiu DT. Disabled-2 small interfering RNA modulates cellular adhesive function and MAPK activity during megakaryocytic differentiation of K562 cells. FEBS Lett. 2003;541:21–7.

33. Huang CL, Cheng JC, Liao CH, Stern A, Hsieh JT, Wang CH, Hsu HL, Tseng CP. Disabled-2 is a negative regulator of integrin alpha(IIb)beta(3)-mediated fibrinogen adhesion and cell signaling. J Biol Chem. 2004;279:42279–89.

34. Hung WS, Huang CL, Fan JT, Huang DY, Yeh CF, Cheng JC, Tseng CP. The endocytic adaptor protein Disabled-2 is required for cellular uptake of fibrinogen. Biochim Biophys Acta. 1823;2012:1778–88.

35. Huang CL, Cheng JC, Kitajima K, Nakano T, Yeh CF, Chong KY, Tseng CP. Disabled-2 is required for mesoderm differentiation of murine embryonic stem cells. J Cell Physiol. 2010;225:92–105.

36. Tseng CP, Chang P, Huang CL, Cheng JC, Chang SS. Autocrine signaling of platelet-derived growth factor regulates disabled-2 expression during megakaryocytic differentiation of K562 cells. FEBS Lett. 2005;579:4395–401.

37. Morris SM, Arden SD, Roberts RC, Kendrick-Jones J, Cooper JA, Luzio JP, Buss F. Myosin VI binds to and localises with Dab2, potentially linking receptor-mediated endocytosis and the actin cytoskeleton. Traffic. 2002;3:331–41.

38. Inoue A, Sato O, Homma K, Ikebe M. DOC-2/DAB2 is the binding partner of myosin VI. Biochem Biophys Res Commun. 2002;292:300–7.

39. Hosaka K, Takeda T, Iino N, Hosojima M, Sato H, Kaseda R, Yamamoto K, Kobayashi A, Gejyo F, Saito A. Megalin and nonmuscle myosin heavy chain IIA interact with the adaptor protein Disabled-2 in proximal tubule cells. Kidney Int. 2009;75:1308–15.

40. Tseng CP, Ely BD, Pong RC, Wang Z, Zhou J, Hsieh JT. The role of DOC-2/DAB2 protein phosphorylation in the inhibition of AP-1 activity. An underlying mechanism of its tumor-suppressive function in prostate cancer. J Biol Chem. 1999;274:31981–6.

41. Olsen JV, Vermeulen M, Santamaria A, Kumar C, Miller ML, Jensen LJ, Gnad F, Cox J, Jensen TS, Nigg EA, et al. Quantitative phosphoproteomics reveals widespread full phosphorylation site occupancy during mitosis. Sci Signal. 2010;3:ra3.

42. He J, Xu J, Xu XX, Hall RA. Cell cycle-dependent phosphorylation of Disabled-2 by cdc2. Oncogene. 2003;22:4524–30.

43. Koral K, Li H, Ganesh N, Birnbaum MJ, Hallows KR, Erkan E. Akt recruits Dab2 to albumin endocytosis in the proximal tubule. Am J Physiol Renal Physiol. 2014;307:F1380–9.

44. Rowley JW, Oler AJ, Tolley ND, Hunter BN, Low EN, Nix DA, Yost CC, Zimmerman GA, Weyrich AS. Genome-wide RNA-seq analysis of human and mouse platelet transcriptomes. Blood. 2011;18:e101–11.

45. Teckchandani A, Toida N, Goodchild J, Henderson C, Watts J, Wollscheid B, Cooper JA. Quantitative proteomics identifies a Dab2/integrin module regulating cell migration. J Cell Biol. 2009;186:99–111.

46. Cho SY, Jeon JW, Lee SH, Park SS. p67 isoform of mouse disabled 2 protein acts as a transcriptional activator during the differentiation of F9 cells. Biochem J. 2000;352(Pt 3):645–50.

47. Drahos KE, Welsh JD, Finkielstein CV, Capelluto DG. Sulfatides partition disabled-2 in response to platelet activation. PLoS One. 2009;4:e8007.

48. Welsh JD, Charonko JJ, Salmanzadeh A, Drahos KE, Shafiee H, Stremler MA, Davalos RV, Capelluto DG, Vlachos PP, Finkielstein CV. Disabled-2 modulates homotypic and heterotypic platelet interactions by binding to sulfatides. Br J Haematol. 2011;154:122–33.

49. Xiao S, Charonko JJ, Fu X, Salmanzadeh A, Davalos RV, Vlachos PP, Finkielstein CV, Capelluto DG. Structure, sulfatide binding properties, and inhibition of platelet aggregation by a disabled-2 protein-derived peptide. J Biol Chem. 2012;287:37691–702.

50. Weiss EJ, Hamilton JR, Lease KE, Coughlin SR. Protection against thrombosis in mice lacking PAR3. Blood. 2002;100:3240–4.

51. Sambrano GR, Weiss EJ, Zheng YW, Huang W, Coughlin SR. Role of thrombin signalling in platelets in haemostasis and thrombosis. Nature. 2001;413:74–8.

52. Barrangou R, Birmingham A, Wiemann S, Beijersbergen RL, Hornung V, Smith A. Advances in CRISPR-Cas9 genome engineering: lessons learned from RNA interference. Nucleic Acids Res. 2015;43:3407–19.

53. Gaj T, Gersbach CA, Barbas 3rd CF. ZFN, TALEN, and CRISPR/Cas-based methods for genome engineering. Trends Biotechnol. 2013;31:397–405.

54. Flintoft L. Animal models: mastering RNAi in mice. Nat Rev Genet. 2011;12:380.

55. Singer O, Verma IM. Applications of lentiviral vectors for shRNA delivery and transgenesis. Curr Gene Ther. 2008;8:483–8.

4

DOACs – advances and limitations in real world

Lai Heng Lee

From The 9th Congress of the Asian-Pacific Society on Thrombosis and Hemostasis
Taipei, Taiwan.

Abstract

The group of new oral anticoagulants or NOACs, now termed direct oral anticoagulants or DOACs, with their favourable results from large scale phase III clinical trials, represent a major advancement and expanded armamentarium in antithrombotic therapy. Dabigatran, rivaroxaban, apixaban and edoxaban are now in clinical routine use for prevention and treatment of arterial and venous thrombotic diseases as addressed in their clinical trials. Usage of the DOACs is expected to increase as clinicians gain more experience and reassurance with data from the real world studies which are generally consistent with that from clinical trials. Development of specific antidotes in management of bleeding complications and development of coagulation assays for their plasma levels will further boost the confidence in the DOACs. Nonetheless, there are still limitations associated with the DOACs. Many patients in need of anticoagulant therapy for indications not studied in the clinical trials will not be eligible for treatment with a DOAC. Conditions where more data is required include DOACs use in the paediatric age group, patients with atrial fibrillation and valvular heart disease, thrombosis associated with the anti-phospholipid syndrome and cancer associated thrombosis. The affordability and access to these drugs may pose an issue for many patients under healthcare systems not providing for these medications. With four new anticoagulants coming onboard very quickly, the focus has shifted to the practical approach and management in real life as many clinicians are not yet familiar with the DOACs. Clinicians need to be educated on how to manage this new class for drugs, from choosing the appropriate drug to prevention and managing bleeding complications as a lack of knowledge and understanding in these drugs will lead to inappropriate use and compromise on patient safety.

Keywords: Oral anticoagulation, Atrial fibrillation, Stroke, Venous thromboembolism, Bleeding

Abbreviations: AF, Atrial fibrillation; DOACS, Direct oral anticoagulants; GT, Gastrointestinal; ICH, Intracranial haemorrhage.; NOACs, New oral anticoagulants; VTE, Venous thromboembolism

Background

Oral anticoagulation is essential for treatment of arterial and venous thromboembolic diseases. Vitamin K antagonists such as warfarin and Coumadin were the only oral anticoagulant available for decades until the introduction of a group of new and novel oral anticoagulants, initially coined as NOACs. Their favourable pharmacological properties and convenient administration overcome many of the problems associated with the vitamin K antagonists such as frequent coagulation blood tests, dose adjustments

Correspondence: Lee.lai.heng@singhealth.com.sg
Department of Haematology, Singapore General Hospital, 20, College Road, Academia Level 3, Singapore 169856, Singapore

and perceived dietary restrictions. In addition, the NOACs, as a class have been shown to have significantly less intracranial haemorrhage (ICH) than warfarin, thus mitigating the most feared complication of anticoagulation treatment. Subsequently, the term DOACs or 'direct oral anticoagulants" was preferred to refer this class of oral anticoagulants with similar pharmacological properties that directly inhibit a single target [1]. Currently, four DOACs, namely Dabigatran, Rivaroxaban, Apixaban and Edoxaban are registered for use in prevention of stroke and systemic embolism in atrial fibrillation (AF), venous thromboembolism (VTE) prophylaxis in major orthopaedic surgery, treatment of acute VTE and prevention of recurrent VTE. In addition, Rivroxaban is also registered for use in prevention of cardiovascular deaths after acute coronary syndrome. With the DOACs becoming commercially available and more widely used, the focus has shifted to their practical use in real life. The purpose of this article is to highlight available phase IV or post marketing real world data and their consistency with their prior clinical trials and to highlight the limitations and challenges in using these agents in real world.

Review
Stroke prevention in non-valvular atrial fibrillation
Anticoagulation therapy is necessary to prevent stroke, systemic embolization and all-cause mortality in patients with AF. THE CHADS2 score (Cardiac Failure, Hypertension, Age, Diabetes, and Stroke [double]) was widely used in risk stratification to identify patients who will benefit from anticoagulation [2]. However, even within the score "0", the risks of stroke ranged from 0.84 to 3.4 per year, hence missing out on those with increased risks who would have benefitted from anticoagulation. This gap was addressed with the CHA2DS2-VASc score (congestive heart failure, hypertension, age ≥ 75 years [doubled], diabetes mellitus, stroke [doubled], vascular disease, age 65–74 years, sex category [female]) which can better identify truly low risk AF patients, who are unlikely to benefit from antithrombotic therapy [3]. CHASDS2-VASc score is currently the preferred tool for risk stratification for stroke risk in AF patients.

Currently 4 DOACs available are dabigatran, rivaroxaban, apixaban and edoxaban have each shown similar efficacy and safety when compared to warfarin [4–7]. A meta-analysis of the phase III trials of these four DOACs showed a consistent favourable risk-benefit profile across a wide range of patients with significant reductions in stroke or systemic embolism, intracranial haemorrhage, and mortality but increased gastrointestinal bleeds when compared with warfarin [8]. Coupled with their convenient usage as fixed dose oral medications without the need for frequent laboratory tests and dose adjustments, DOACs have emerged as the preferred treatment option in some guidelines [9]. Large scale real world data of these drugs is has become available with increasing use of DOACs in routine care.

Dabigatran, in a review of 9 publications, involving more than 200,000 AF patients over 5 years [10], showed that data for dabigatran in 'real world' clinical practice were largely replicative of the main findings in the RE-LY phase III trial [4]. In particular, both dabigatran doses at 150 mg and 110 mg twice daily were associated with lower major extra-cranial bleeding rates than warfarin in patients less than75 years old and similar event rates in those above 75 years old. The 110 mg dose was associated with lower and similar gastrointestinal (GI)

bleeding rates, and the 150 mg dose yielded similar and higher GI bleeding rates in patients less than 75 years and more than 75 years old, respectively. A more recent systematic review and meta-analysis studied 348 750 patients (56.65 % warfarin, 40.2 % dabigatran-150 mg and 3.2 % dabigatran-110 mg) in routine care and this is 20 times the size of RE-LY patient population [11]. It included heterogeneous study cohorts regarding history of stroke, hypertension, or diabetes mellitus and did not exclude patients with severe renal impairment (creatinine clearance ≤30 mL/min), active liver disease, or conditions associated with an increased risk of bleeding. Patients receiving dabigatran-110 mg in routine clinical practice, tended to be older than patients in the RE-LY trial on this dose. In pooled analyses, dabigatran-150 mg was similar to warfarin in preventing stroke (hazard ratio, 0.92; 95 % confidence interval, 0.84–1.01; $P = 0.066$) and a significantly lower risks of intracranial bleeding (0.44; 0.34–0.59; $P < 0.001$). However risks of GI bleeding was significantly higher than warfarin (1.23; 1.01–1.50; $P = 0.041$), particularly in studies of older versus younger populations (median/mean age, ≥75 versus <75 years; $\beta = 1.53$; 95 % confidence interval, 1.10–2.14; $P = 0.020$). Again the findings were consistent with the RE-LY trial. Another observational study provided some insights on the use of Dabigatran 75 mg dose which was not studied in the RE-LY trial but approved in the USA for use in the renal impaired patients with CrCl 15-30 ml/min [12]. The use of dabigatran 75 mg was associated with significantly reduced risk of intracranial haemorrhage and similar rates of stroke, bleeding and mortality compared to warfarin. Interestingly, majority of patients on dabigatran 75 mg twice daily appeared not to have severe renal impairment as only 33 % had a diagnosis of chronic kidney disease, and 20 % of these with severe renal impairment, thus suggesting a possible off-label use of the 75 mg dose in many patients in the real world. While not advocating off label dose reduction, the observational data are nonetheless reassuring. Other findings noted from such real world observations include the observations that new starters of warfarin has a higher bleeding risk when compared to new starters of dabigatran, warfarin experienced switchers or patients remaining on warfarin [13], higher bleeding rates in the first 90 days of treatment in elderly new starters of dabigatran or warfarin [12, 14] and the higher bleeding risk with renal impairment regardless of which oral anticoagulant [15–17].

Rivaroxaban, in the Xantus prospective observational study for 6784 AF patients across 311 centres in Europe reported a lower thrombotic and bleeding rates for Rivaroxaban compared to its Rocket phase III clinical trial [18]. While the phase III ROCKET AF trial did not include patients with CHADs score of 0-1, Xantus had 12.7 % of patients had a CHA2DS2-VASc score of either 0 or 1. Generally, patients in Xantus had lower stroke risks, with a mean CHADS2 score of 2.0 and 19.0 % experiencing prior stroke/TIA or SE, compared with 3.5 and 55 % respectively in the Rocket AF trial. The overall bleeding incidence of 2.1 per 100 patient-years in Xantus was notably lower than 3.6 per 100 patient-years reported in Rocket AF. Similarly fewer major GI bleeds and ICH were observed in Xantus when compared to Rocket-AF. Recent analysis from the Dresden Registry [19] showed the overall rates of stroke and systemic embolism at 2.03/100 patient-years in the intention-to-treat analysis and 1.7/100 patient-years in the on-treatment analysis which were considerably lower than those in the ROCKET AF trial [5]. In addition, event rates for patients receiving 20 mg OD (1.25/100 patient-years), was considerably lower than patients on 15 mg OD (2.7/100 patient-years). Bleeding complications associated with rivaroxaban was addressed in a meta-analysis of 9 studies involving 51,533 patients in real world [20]. It showed the mean pooled rates of any major bleeding, major GI bleeding or ICH with rivaroxaban were 3.32, (95 % CI¼2.28–4.25); 2.41, (95 % CI¼1.25–3.56) and 0.40, (95 % CI¼0.17–0.74) events/100 patient-years. The pooled real-world rates of these bleeding rates largely mirrored those reported for rivaroxaban in the phase 3 ROCKET AF trial [5]. However, there were significant variability and heterogeneity variability in major bleeding rates across the studies. Five studies were retrospective claims analyses and identified bleeding using International Classification of Diseases–9/10 codes, while four were prospective registry studies and identified bleeding clinically using the International Society on Thrombosis and Haemostasis (ISTH) definition. Major bleeding rates and major GI bleeding rates as per 100 patient-years in studies that relied on claims were (2.86 to 12.79) and (2.53 to 9.5) respectively and these are substantially higher than (0.96 to 3) and (0.19 to 0.9) as reported in prospective studies using clinical identification. Such differences underscore the substantial heterogeneity across the studies and the inherent weaknesses associated with retrospective and observational studies. Nonetheless, the pooled rates of major bleeding with rivaroxaban estimated were generally low and consistent with those reported in ROCKET AF. This finding of a lower major bleed rate than Rocket AF was also seen in a large US study of electronic medical records of 27 467 patients (2.9 events per 100 patient-years) [18] as well as an earlier report from Dresden NOAC Registry involving 1200 AF patients treated with rivaroxaban(3.1 events per 100 patient-years) [21, 22].

Besides these published large scale real world comparisons of a single DOAC versus warfarin, evidence relating to the overall effectiveness and safety of all oral anticoagulant drugs used in clinical practice is emerging. An observational nationwide cohort study in Denmark had involved 61, 678 patients with non-valvular AF who were naïve to oral anticoagulants and had no previous indication for valvular AF or VTE [23]. The study population was distributed according to treatment type with 57 % warfarin, 21 % dabigatran 150 mg, 20 % on rivaroxaban 20 mg, and 10 % apixaban 5 mg. The baseline characteristics of patients in apixaban and rivaroxaban has more previous strokes, systemic embolism vascular disease and bleeding while dabigatran patients were younger and less renal impaired, warfarin has more patients with vascular disease hypertension, renal impairment, COPD and cancer. During 1 year follow-up, when compared to warfarin, annual rates of ischaemia strokes and systemic embolism were significantly lower for rivaroxaban (hazard ratio 0.83 (95 % confidence interval 0.69 to 0.99), while not significantly different for dabigatran and apixaban.(hazard ratios of 2.8 % and 4.9 % respectively) The mortality risk was significantly lower with apixaban (5.2 %) and dabigatran (2.75 %) when compared with warfarin (8.5 %), but not with rivaroxaban (7.7 %). No significant difference was found between DOACs and warfarin for ischaemic stroke. The bleeding endpoints for rivaroxaban 5.3 % was comparable to warfarin 5 %, while apixaban 2.3 % and dabigatran 2.4 % were both lower than warfarin. The risks of death, any bleeding, or major bleeding were significantly lower for apixaban and dabigatran compared with warfarin. This real world study concluded that all three DOACs seem to be safe and effective alternatives to warfarin in a routine care setting.

Real-life studies have their inherent weaknesses such as non-controlled and heterogeneous patient groups, uncontrolled influence of non-compliance, other concomitant medications and co-morbidities. However, they provide a wealth of data and insight into how DOACs are used in the real world. Despite the reassuring real world data on use of DOACs in routine care, the benefits of DOACs are not applicable to all patients. As shown in a smaller scale study involving 468 patient with AF from the UZ Brussel Stroke Registry, it was found that less than half of real life patients are eligible for therapy with one of the DOACs [24]. Reasons for non-eligibility include concomitant use of antiplatelet agents with apixaban, impaired renal function in dabigatran, concomitant use of rifampicin and anti-fungal drugs and presence of valvular heart diseases. More data are also required for AF patients on DOACs undergoing cardioversion or ablation. There are ongoing trials addressing some of these issues and their results together with more real world data can add more clarity to these limitations.

DOACs in Asia for AF patients

AF with its risks for ischaemic stroke is expected to pose a huge health burden in Asia. Although the DOACs are emerging as the preferred class of anticoagulant for stroke prevention in AF, there are concerns if the results of their global clinical trials are applicable to Asians. Subgroups analysis of more than 8000 Asian patients was performed in a meta-analysis of 5 pivotal phase III trials for the four available DOACs, namely RE-LY, ROCKET AF, J-ROCKET AF, ARISTOTLE, and ENGAGE AF-TIMI 48 [25]. The results showed greater benefits of DOACs in Asians with a greater reduction in stroke and systemic emboli when compared to non-Asians. As for bleeding complications, Asians also fared better with fewer bleeds than non-Asians. This is despite Asian patients on the warfarin comparator arm having less optimal time in therapeutic range, with more having international normalized ratio <2.0 and fewer had international normalized ratio >3.0. In particular, bleeding from the gastrointestinal track was similar between Asians on DOACs and vitamin K antagonists, but increased in non-Asians who were on DOACs. In studying the differences between Asians and non-Asians individually in each of the four DOACs [26], the relative risk reduction in stroke and systemic embolization, hemorrhagic stroke as well as all-cause mortality showed a greater numerical reduction in Asians compared to non-Asians for Dabigatran at 150 mg, 110 mg, Rivaroxaban 20 mg, Apixaban 5 mg and Edoxaban 60 mg. There was no evidence of increased risk of GI bleeding associated with DOACs in Asians. Hence it is expected that DOACs will become the preferred class of anticoagulant in the stroke prevention for AF in Asians.

In the real world, data the Taiwan National Health Insurance Research Database with close to 10,000 AF patients on each arm of treatment with either warfarin or dabigatran, has shown that Dabigatran significantly reduced risk of ischemic stroke, ICH, all hospitalized major bleeding and all-cause mortality compared with warfarin [27]. Rates of major GI bleeding and myocardial infarction were not increased in dabigatran when compared with warfarin. A multicenter retrospective cohort study of 241 stroke centers in Japan, patients with AF treated with a DOAC when compared with those on warfarin, had a lower rates of intracranial haemorrhage (17 % vs 26 %) and mortality (16 % vs 35 %) [28]. Such real world reports further bolster the confidence in the safety and efficacy of DOACs treatment for AF patients in Asia.

Thrombo-prophylaxis in major orthopaedic surgeries

In the phase III clinical trials for thromboprophylaxis in major orthopaedic surgeries, rivaroxaban, dabigatran and apixaban were found to be effective and safe without a significant increase in bleeding complications when compared to enoxaparin 40 mg once daily [25] and edoxaban was found to be more effective when compared with enoxaparin 20 mg once daily [29–31]. With early discharge after surgery, the DOACs make a very attractive option for continued prophylaxis after hospital discharge.

In an observational study in routine practice using dabigatran for thrombo-prophylaxis in 5292 hip and knee replacement surgeries [32], for patients with pre-specified age, renal function and body mass index (BMI), the composite incidence of symptomatic VTE events and all-cause mortality was 1.04 % (95 % CI 0.78, 1.35) and the post hoc analysis incidence of major bleeding events to be consistent with the findings in clinical trials, thus providing reassurance with regards to efficacy and safety of its use in routine practice. A three-fold increase in symptomatic VTE and all-cause mortality was seen in patients with moderate renal impairment of creatinine clearance of 30–49/ml who received dabigatran and a 2 fold increase in major bleeding was seen in the severely obese patients with BMI above 35 kg/m2. High level of satisfaction with dabigatran use was also reported despite the difficult and time consuming process of implementing dabigatran into routine practice [33].

Rivaroxaban in routine care for thromboprophylaxis post major orthopaedic surgery was similarly evaluated. XAMOS, a phase IV, non-interventional study in 17,701 patients across 37 countries showed that the incidence of symptomatic thromboembolic events was significantly lower in patients who received rivaroxaban compared with standard of care (0.9 % vs 1.4 %) [34] Treatment related major bleeding events as defined in the RECORD programme were similar between the rivaroxaban and standard of care groups at 0.4 % and 0.3 %, respectively. However, non-major bleeding and any bleeding rates were higher in the rivaroxaban group compared with the standard of care group (2.9 % vs 1.7 %, and 4.7 % vs 3.2 %, respectively). Nonetheless the overall data from XAMOS confirmed the favourable benefit–risk profile of rivaroxaban when used in routine clinical care. From the ORTHO-TEP registry of about 5000 patients in a single centre, rivaroxaban vs fondaparinus or low molecular weight heparin was retrospectively evaluated for the prevention of VTE [35, 36]. The rivaroxaban group demonstrated a significant reduction in symptomatic VTE and a numerical reduction in pulmonary embolism. Significant reduction in major bleeding rates, number of surgical revisions due to bleeding complications, blood transfusion rates and length of hospital stay were also seen in the rivaroxaban group. Notwithstanding the inherent bias and inadequacies in retrospective study designs, ORTHO-TEP confirmed that the efficacy of rivaroxaban was at least not offset by any increase in surgical complications.

Treatment of acute VTE

Similar to stroke prevention in patients with non-valvular AF, the DOACs have demonstrated excellent efficacy and safety in large scale phase III trials in the treatment of VTE

[37–41]. Evidence from real life studies are pending from ongoing studies such as : (i) Dresden Noac Registry (clinicaltrials.gov identifier: NCT01588119), (ii) XALIA study which is a non-interventional observational cohort study investigating rivaroxaban in VTE treatment in routine clinical practice (clinicaltrials. gov identifier: NCT01619007), (iii) PREFER in VTE, a multicentre, prospective observational disease registry for quality of life and treatment satisfaction for 4000 patients with VTE across Europe [42] and (iv) The GARFIELD-VTE registry, an observational study for about 10,000 patients to look at the acute and long term management of VTE, its complications and healthcare resource utilization.

The use of DOACs in the treatment of VTE associated with Antiphospholipid requires more clarity as this condition is associated with much increased risks for recurrences. A prospective phase II/III clinical trial using Rivaroxaban in antiphospholipid syndrome is currently in progress to address these efficacy and safety issues [43]. Cancer associated VTE represents a good proportion of VTE patients for which low molecular weight treatment is regarded as the gold standard. While these patients are at higher risks of recurrence and bleeding, they may also be on medications which may interact with DOACs via the CYP3A4 and P-gp metabolic pathways. The main limitation in using DOACs is the lack of efficacy and safety data from clinical trials specific for use of DOACs in the treatment of cancer associated VTE. Although subgroup analysis of cancer patients from meta-analysis of the major clinical trials for DOACs in the treatment of VTE showed similar efficacy and safety when compared to warfarin, it is not clear if these cancer patients had active cancer, what were the risks of bleeding and recurrence specific to their cancer types and whether they are on cancer treatment with potential drug interaction with DOACs [44].

Real life management issues

While it is reassuring that the body of emerging "real world data" from the routine use of NOACs largely mirrors that in clinical trials, there remains many concerns on the limitations of this new armamentarium for better management of thrombotic diseases.

Appropriate choice of anticoagulant and patient care when using DOACs

Choosing a particular DOAC for a patient can be difficult as not all DOACs are the same [45]. There is no evidence to recommend one agent over another because the DOACs have never been compared in head-to-head trials. Hence the guiding principle has been to match the right drug to the right patient based on the dosing properties of each drug, the efficacy and safety and side effect profile as demonstrated in phase III trials and real world

data, as well as the compliance, affordability and accessibility of the DOACs. Therefore understanding the properties of the drugs is fundamental to ensure safe and appropriate prescribing practice (Table 1). All DOACs depend variably on renal excretion; they are contraindicated in renal failure and should be used with caution with dose reductions in the renal impaired patients. The relative lack of drug interactions in DOACs is an advantage but clinicians must be mindful of the few important drug interactions with some anti-fungal, anti-microbial and anti-viral medications involving the CYP3A4 and P-gp metabolic pathways. The dosing regimen and dose adjustments for renal impairment are DOAC specific and different from each other and thus predispose to dosing and prescription errors if clinicians are not familiar with these anticoagulants. There are also clinical situations where DOACs are not suitable because of insufficient data on its efficacy and safety such as thromboembolism associated with anti-phospholipid syndrome and the unstable cancer patient, or where there are safety concerns as during pregnancy and for patient with mechanical heart valves. The notion of a simplified coagulation treatment approach is actually more complicated than anticipated and guidelines such as the NICE guidelines (https://www.nice.org.uk/guidance/cg180/resources/nic-consensus-statement-on-the-use-of-noacs-243733501) and the EHRA practical guide [46] are useful resources for clinicians prescribing DOACs. In situations when transiting between DOACs and other anticoagulants and during the peri-operative periods, due caution should be exercised taking into consideration the patient's renal function and the half-life of the DOAC for appropriate drug dosing and time of administration. To minimise the bleeding risks, these agents should be used in the appropriate patients and managed well when transiting between DOAC and other anticoagulants and during the peri-operative periods [46].

Laboratory coagulation tests

Patients on DOACs do not need routine coagulation monitoring. However, there are certain clinical scenarios in which coagulation testing and measurement of drug levels are necessary, such as episodes of bleeding, peri-operative management, suspected over dosage either from drug interactions or intentional overdose, renal impairment or a measure of suspected non-compliance. The effects of DOACs on routinely available clot-based tests such as APTT, PT and TT are variable and the degree of prolongation is highly dependent on the reagent used for the assay [47]. These widely available tests may be used to detect peak or supra-therapeutic drug levels, but should not be used for quantitation. Such routine coagulation tests may also appear normal during trough drug levels. In situations where drug levels are required and these are

Table 1 Pharmacological properties of the DOACs

	Dabigatran [9, 38]	Rivaroxaban [9, 40, 41]	Apixaban [9, 37]	Edoxaban [9, 39]
Target	Factor IIa	Factor Xa	Factor Xa	Factor Xa
Half-life (hour)	12-17	5-9	12	6-10
Time to peak effect (hour)	1-3	2-4	1-3	1-2
Renal clearance as unchanged drug (%)	80	33	27	50
Drug Interactions Pathways	P-gp	3A4/P-gp	3A4/P-gp	3A4/P-gp
Dosing in non-valvular AF	150 mg BID	20 mg OD	5 mg BID	60 mg OD
Dosing in VTE treatment	150 mg BID after 5-10 days of parenteral anticoagulation	15 mg BID for 21 days followed by 20 mg OD	10 mg BID for 7 days followed by 5 mg BID	60 mg OD after 5 days of parenteral anticoagulation

OD-once daily, BID-twice daily, P-gp – P-glycoprotein, 3A4 – cytochrome P450 3A4 isoenzyme

measured with specialized tests [48]. Dabigatran can be measured by the dilute thrombin time, ecarin assay and chromogenic anti-IIa assay. The anti-Xa DOACs can be measured by STA Neoplastin test and the anti-Xa assays. Unfortunately, such specialised laboratory facilities are not widely available, except in major hospitals, and very often not available when required.

In addition to influencing the results of clotting times, DOACs may also cause potential errors in some specialized coagulation tests, particularly, the clot based assays [49]. DOACs can falsely prolong the dilute Russels Vipers Venom Time (dRVVT) in lupus anticoagulant tests, falsely reduced levels of plasma clotting factors in one staged assays and falsely elevate the functional protein S levels. Generally, clinicians may not appreciate the impact of DOACs on coagulation tests, hence guidance from the local laboratory is important for appropriate requests, timing and interpretation of these tests for patients on DOAC treatment [50].

Management of DOAC associated bleeding

All anticoagulants, including the DOACs are associated with bleeding. Unlike warfarin and heparins where established reversal protocols with known antidotes are readily available for managing bleeds, clinicians may not be equipped with the bleeding management and reversal strategies in DOACs [51]. It is imperative that clinicians be equipped to manage bleeds by means of a local management plan stratified according to the severity of bleeds and availability of treatment agents [52] Exact identification of which DOAC, location and severity of bleeds, renal function and the time of last ingestion of DOAC are important factors to note in the management of bleeding associated with DOACs.

For mild bleeding events such as bruises or menorrhagia, the DOAC could be suspended and the drug restarted later at a lower dose and resuming full dose when bleed risks had resolved. For moderate to severe bleeds, symptomatic treatment such as mechanical compression of bleeding site, appropriate surgical or radiological intervention and blood transfusion may be necessary. Plasma and cryoprecipitate do not reverse the anticoagulant effect of novel agents, but may be required for correction of volume loss or coagulopathy associated with other co-morbidities. Adsorption of remnant DOACs by oral activated charcoal may be helpful if the last ingested dose of is within 2 h at presentation to the hospital [53]. Haemodialysis, with its logistic challenges, can be considered for removal of residual dabigatran [54] but not for the anti-Xa inhibitors like rivaroxaban or apixaban.

In the events of life threatening bleeds, off label use of pharmacological haemostatic agents such as prothrombin concentration complex and recombinant factor VIIa can be considered. However, such measures are controversial and without good supportive evidence [55]. Clinical development for specific antidotes to the DOACs took place only after DOACs reached routine use. The humanized monoclonal Fab BI 655075 or Idarucizumab specific for reversal of the anticoagulant effects of dabigatran has completed its phase III trial [56]. It has now been registered for use in many countries. Andexanet alfa [57], a FXa inhibitor antidote, is in advanced stages of clinical trial development. It is a recombinant modified human factor Xa decoy protein that is catalytically inactive but binds factor Xa inhibitors in the active site with high affinity, hence restoring the activity of endogenous factor Xa and reducing levels of anticoagulant activity. The availability of specific antidotes for the DOACs will certainly provide a better sense of security into their routine use. However, it is prudent to highlight the appropriate use of such antidotes [58]. Reasonable indications include life threatening and critical organ bleeds, bleeding that did not respond to conventional supportive and hemostatic measures, and for urgent surgical and invasive interventions with high risks of bleed that cannot be delayed. In the decision to reverse anticoagulation completely, one must take into consideration the pro-thrombotic risks that the patient has which required anticoagulation in the first place, hence such reversal should be taken lightly for trivial reasons just because reversal agents are available.

Cost effectiveness of DOACs

Affordability and accessibility for DOACs remains an issue in Asia. While some studies have advocated the positive cost savings and cost-effectiveness of DOACs in routine clinical practices [59–61], these may not be applicable to many countries with different healthcare systems. Also, the cost effectiveness as calculated from healthcare providers' perspective may not be portable to the full paying individual without subsidized healthcare benefits [62].

Conclusion

DOACs represent an important advancement in antithrombotic management. Real world data consistent with their clinical trial data is reassuring. However, a significant number of patients may not be eligible for treatment with a DOAC from a lack of data in conditions not addressed in their clinical trials. In addition, costs of these medications may limit their accessibility to a good number of patients. In routine clinical care, much has to be done to familiarize the clinicians on the use of these drugs. It is the careful patient selection, appropriate management and the ability to prevent and manage the bleeding complications that will permit optimization on the use of DOACs.

Acknowledgements
Not applicable.

Authors' contributions
Sole authorship.

Competing interests
Had received educational grants and lecture honorariums from Bayer, Boehringer Ingelheim, Bristol-Myers Squibb and Pfizer during the past 5 years.

References

1. Barnes GD, Ageno W, Ansell J, Kaatz S. Recommendation on the nomenclature for oral anticoagulants: communication from the SSC of the ISTH. J Thromb Haemost. 2015;13:1154–6.
2. Keogh C, Wallace E, Dillon C, Dimitrov BD, Fahey T. Validation of the CHADS2 clinical prediction rule to predict ischaemic stroke. A systematic review and meta-analysis. Thromb Haemost. 2011;106:528–38.
3. Olesen JB, Torp-Pedersen C, Hansen ML, Lip GY. The value of the CHA2DS2-VASc score for refining stroke risk stratification in patients with atrial fibrillation with a CHADS2 score 0-1: a nationwide cohort study. Thromb Haemost. 2012;107:1172–9.
4. Connolly SJ, Ezekowitz MD, Yusuf S, Eikelboom J, Oldgren J, Parekh A, et al. Dabigatran versus warfarin in patients with atrial fibrillation. N Engl J Med. 2009;361:1139–51.
5. Patel MR, Mahaffey KW, Garg J, Pan G, Singer DE, Hacke W, et al. Rivaroxaban versus warfarin in nonvalvular atrial fibrillation. N Engl J Med. 2011;365:883–91.
6. Granger CB, Alexander JH, McMurray JJ, Lopes RD, Hylek EM, Hanna M, et al. Apixaban versus warfarin in patients with atrial fibrillation. N Engl J Med. 2011;365:981–92.
7. Giugliano RP, Ruff CT, Braunwald E, Murphy SA, Wiviott SD, Halperin JL, et al. Edoxaban versus warfarin in patients with atrial fibrillation. N Engl J Med. 2013;369:2093–104.
8. Ruff CT, Giugliano RP, Braunwald E, Hoffman EB, Deenadayalu N, Ezekowitz MD, et al. Comparison of the efficacy and safety of new oral anticoagulants with warfarin in patients with atrial fibrillation: a meta-analysis of randomised trials. Lancet. 2014;383:955–62.
9. Camm AJ, Lip GY, De Caterina R, Savelieva I, Atar D, Hohnloser SH, et al. 2012 focused update of the ESC Guidelines for the management of atrial fibrillation: an update of the 2010 ESC Guidelines for the management of atrial fibrillation–developed with the special contribution of the European Heart Rhythm Association. Europace. 2012;14:1385–413.
10. Potpara TS. Dabigatran in 'real-world' clinical practice for stroke prevention in patients with non-valvular atrial fibrillation. Thromb Haemost. 2015;114:1093–8.
11. Romanelli RJ, Nolting L, Dolginsky M, Kym E, Orrico KB. Dabigatran versus warfarin for atrial fibrillation in real-world clinical practice: A systematic review and meta-analysis. Circ Cardiovasc Qual Outcomes. 2016;9:126–34.
12. Graham DJ, Reichman ME, Wernecke M, Zhang R, Southworth MR, Levenson M, et al. Cardiovascular, bleeding, and mortality risks in elderly Medicare patients treated with dabigatran or warfarin for nonvalvular atrial fibrillation. Circulation. 2015;131:157–64.
13. Larsen TB, Gorst-Rasmussen A, Rasmussen LH, Skjoth F, Rosenzweig M, Lip GY. Bleeding events among new starters and switchers to dabigatran compared with warfarin in atrial fibrillation. Am J Med. 2014;127:650–6. e655.
14. Avgil-Tsadok M, Jackevicius CA, Essebag V, Eisenberg MJ, Rahme E, Behlouli H, et al. Dabigatran use in elderly patients with atrial fibrillation. Thromb Haemost. 2016;115:152–60.
15. Hernandez I, Baik SH, Pinera A, Zhang Y. Risk of bleeding with dabigatran in atrial fibrillation. JAMA Intern Med. 2015;175:18–24.
16. Lauffenburger JC, Farley JF, Gehi AK, Rhoney DH, Brookhart MA, Fang G. Effectiveness and safety of dabigatran and warfarin in real-world US patients with non-valvular atrial fibrillation: a retrospective cohort study. J Am Heart Assoc. 2015;4:e001798.
17. Seeger JD, Bykov K, Bartels DB, Huybrechts K, Zint K, Schneeweiss S. Safety and effectiveness of dabigatran and warfarin in routine care of patients with atrial fibrillation. Thromb Haemost. 2015;114:1277–89.
18. Camm AJ, Amarenco P, Haas S, Hess S, Kirchhof P, Kuhls S, et al. XANTUS: a real-world, prospective, observational study of patients treated with rivaroxaban for stroke prevention in atrial fibrillation. Eur Heart J. 2016;37:1145–53.
19. Hecker J, Marten S, Keller L, Helmert S, Michalski F, Werth S, et al. Effectiveness and safety of rivaroxaban therapy in daily-care patients with atrial fibrillation. Results from the Dresden NOAC Registry. Thromb Haemost. 2016;115:939–49.
20. Weeda ER, White CM, Peacock WF, Coleman CI. Rates of major bleeding with rivaroxaban in real-world studies of nonvalvular atrial fibrillation patients: a meta-analysis. Curr Med Res Opin. 2016;32:1117–20.
21. Tamayo S, Frank Peacock W, Patel M, Sicignano N, Hopf KP, Fields LE, et al. Characterizing major bleeding in patients with nonvalvular atrial fibrillation: a pharmacovigilance study of 27 467 patients taking rivaroxaban. Clin Cardiol. 2015;38:63–8.
22. Beyer-Westendorf J, Forster K, Pannach S, Ebertz F, Gelbricht V, Thieme C, et al. Rates, management, and outcome of rivaroxaban bleeding in daily care: results from the Dresden NOAC registry. Blood. 2014;124:955–62.
23. Larsen TB, Skjoth F, Nielsen PB, Kjaeldgaard JN, Lip GY. Comparative effectiveness and safety of non-vitamin K antagonist oral anticoagulants and warfarin in patients with atrial fibrillation: propensity weighted nationwide cohort study. BMJ. 2016;353:i3189.
24. Desmaele S, Steurbaut S, Cornu P, Brouns R, Dupont AG. Clinical trials with direct oral anticoagulants for stroke prevention in atrial fibrillation: how

representative are they for real life patients? Eur J Clin Pharmacol. 2016; 72(9):1125–134.

25. Wang KL, Lip GY, Lin SJ, Chiang CE. Non-vitamin K antagonist oral anticoagulants for stroke prevention in Asian patients with nonvalvular atrial fibrillation: meta-analysis. Stroke. 2015;46:2555–61.

26. Chiang CE, Wang KL, Lin SJ. Asian strategy for stroke prevention in atrial fibrillation. Europace. 2015;17 Suppl 2:ii31–9.

27. Chan YH, Yen KC, See LC, Chang SH, Wu LS, Lee HF, et al. Cardiovascular, bleeding, and mortality risks of dabigatran in Asians with nonvalvular atrial fibrillation. Stroke. 2016;47:441–9.

28. Saji N, Kimura K, Aoki J, Uemura J, Sakamoto Y. Intracranial hemorrhage caused by non-vitamin K antagonist oral anticoagulants (NOACs)-multicenter retrospective cohort study in Japan. Circ J. 2015;79:1018–23.

29. Adam SS, McDuffie JR, Lachiewicz PF, Ortel TL, Williams Jr JW. Comparative effectiveness of new oral anticoagulants and standard thromboprophylaxis in patients having total hip or knee replacement: a systematic review. Ann Intern Med. 2013;159:275–84.

30. Fuji T, Wang CJ, Fujita S, Kawai Y, Kimura T, Tachibana S. Safety and efficacy of edoxaban, an oral factor xa inhibitor, for thromboprophylaxis after total hip arthroplasty in Japan and Taiwan. J Arthroplasty. 2014;29:2439–46.

31. Fuji T, Wang CJ, Fujita S, Kawai Y, Nakamura M, Kimura T, et al. Safety and efficacy of edoxaban, an oral factor Xa inhibitor, versus enoxaparin for thromboprophylaxis after total knee arthroplasty: the STARS E-3 trial. Thromb Res. 2014;134:1198–204.

32. Rosencher N, Samama CM, Feuring M, Brueckmann M, Kleine E, Clemens A, et al. Dabigatran etexilate for thromboprophylaxis in over 5000 hip or knee replacement patients in a real-world clinical setting. Thromb J. 2016;14:8.

33. Kendoff D, Perka C, Fritsche HM, Gehrke T, Hube R. Oral thromboprophylaxis following total hip or knee replacement: review and multicentre experience with dabigatran etexilate. Open Orthop J. 2011;5:395–9.

34. Turpie AG, Haas S, Kreutz R, Mantovani LG, Pattanayak CW, Holberg G, Jamal W, et al. A non-interventional comparison of rivaroxaban with standard of care for thromboprophylaxis after major orthopaedic surgery in 17,701 patients with propensity score adjustment. Thromb Haemost. 2014;111:94–102.

35. Beyer-Westendorf J, Lutzner J, Donath L, Radke OC, Kuhlisch E, Hartmann A, et al. Efficacy and safety of rivaroxaban or fondaparinux thromboprophylaxis in major orthopedic surgery: findings from the ORTHO-TEP registry. J Thromb Haemost. 2012;10:2045–52.

36. Beyer-Westendorf J, Lutzner J, Donath L, Tittl L, Knoth H, Radke OC, et al. Efficacy and safety of thromboprophylaxis with low-molecular-weight heparin or rivaroxaban in hip and knee replacement surgery: findings from the ORTHO-TEP registry. Thromb Haemost. 2013;109:154–63.

37. Agnelli G, Buller HR, Cohen A, Curto M, Gallus AS, Johnson M, et al. Oral apixaban for the treatment of acute venous thromboembolism. N Engl J Med. 2013;369:799–808.

38. Schulman S, Kakkar AK, Goldhaber SZ, Schellong S, Eriksson H, Mismetti P, et al. Treatment of acute venous thromboembolism with dabigatran or warfarin and pooled analysis. Circulation. 2014;129:764–72.

39. Buller HR, Decousus H, Grosso MA, Mercuri M, Middeldorp S, Prins MH, et al. Edoxaban versus warfarin for the treatment of symptomatic venous thromboembolism. N Engl J Med. 2013;369:1406–15.

40. Bauersachs R, Berkowitz SD, Brenner B, Buller HR, Decousus H, Gallus AS, et al. Oral rivaroxaban for symptomatic venous thromboembolism. N Engl J Med. 2010;36326:2499–510.

41. Buller HR, Prins MH, Lensin AW, Decousus H, Jacobson BF, Minar E, et al. Oral rivaroxaban for the treatment of symptomatic pulmonary embolism. N Engl J Med. 2012;366:1287–97.

42. Agnelli G, Gitt AK, Bauersachs R, Fronk EM, Laeis P, Mismetti P, et al. The management of acute venous thromboembolism in clinical practice - study rationale and protocol of the European PREFER in VTE Registry. Thromb J. 2015;13:41.

43. Cohen H, Dore CJ, Clawson S, Hunt BJ, Isenberg D, Khamashta M, et al. Rivaroxaban in antiphospholipid syndrome (RAPS) protocol: a prospective, randomized controlled phase II/III clinical trial of rivaroxaban versus warfarin in patients with thrombotic antiphospholipid syndrome, with or without SLE. Lupus. 2015;24:1087–94.

44. van der Hulle T, den Exter PL, Kooiman J, van der Hoeven JJ, Huisman MV, Klok FA. Meta-analysis of the efficacy and safety of new oral anticoagulants in patients with cancer-associated acute venous thromboembolism. J Thromb Haemost. 2014;12:1116–20.

45. Schaefer JK, McBane RD, Wysokinski WE. How to choose appropriate direct oral anticoagulant for patient with nonvalvular atrial fibrillation. Ann Hematol. 2016;95:437–49.

46. Heidbuchel H, Verhamme P, Alings M, Antz M, Diener HC, Hacke W, et al. Updated European Heart Rhythm Association Practical Guide on the use of non-vitamin K antagonist anticoagulants in patients with non-valvular atrial fibrillation. Europace. 2015;17:1467–507.

47. Tripodi A. The laboratory and the direct oral anticoagulants. Blood. 2013;121:4032–5.

48. Dale BJ, Chan NC, Eikelboom JW. Laboratory measurement of the direct oral anticoagulants. Br J Haematol. 2016;172:315–36.

49. Tsakiris DA. Direct oral anticoagulants–interference with laboratory tests and mechanism of action. Semin Hematol. 2014;51:98–101.

50. Wong WH, Yip CY, Sum CL, Tan CW, Lee LH, Yap ES, et al. A practical guide to ordering and interpreting coagulation tests for patients on direct oral anticoagulants in Singapore. Ann Acad Med Singapore. 2016;45:98–105.

51. Siegal DM, Garcia DA, Crowther MA. How I treat target-specific oral anticoagulant-associated bleeding. Blood. 2014;123:1152–8.

52. Ng HJ, Chee YL, Ponnudurai K, Lim LC, Tan D, Tay JC, et al. Consensus recommendations for preventing and managing bleeding complications associated with novel oral anticoagulants in singapore. Ann Acad Med Singapore. 2013;42:593–602.

53. Wang X, Mondal S, Wang J, Tirucherai G, Zhang D, Boyd RA, et al. Effect of activated charcoal on apixaban pharmacokinetics in healthy subjects. Am J Cardiovasc Drugs. 2014;14:147–54.

54. Khadzhynov D, Wagner F, Formella S, Wiegert E, Moschetti V, Slowinski T, et al. Effective elimination of dabigatran by haemodialysis. A phase I single-centre study in patients with end-stage renal disease. Thromb Haemost. 2013;109:596–605.

55. Cuker A, Siegal D. Monitoring and reversal of direct oral anticoagulants. Hematology Am Soc Hematol Educ Program. 2015;2015:117–24.

56. Pollack Jr CV, Reilly PA, Eikelboom J, Glund S, Verhamme P, Bernstein RA, et al. Idarucizumab for Dabigatran Reversal. N Engl J Med. 2015;373:511–20.

57. Siegal DM, Curnutte JT, Connolly SJ, Lu G, Conley PB, Wiens BL, et al. Andexanet Alfa for the reversal of Factor Xa inhibitor activity. N Engl J Med. 2015;373:2413–24.

58. Levy JH, Ageno W, Chan NC, Crowther M, Verhamme P, Weitz JI. When and how to use antidotes for the reversal of direct oral anticoagulants: guidance from the SSC of the ISTH. J Thromb Haemost. 2016;14:623–7.

59. Amin A, Bruno A, Trocio J, Lin J, Lingohr-Smith M. Real-world medical cost avoidance when new oral anticoagulants are used versus warfarin for venous thromboembolism in the United States. Clin Appl Thromb Hemost. 2016;22:5–11.

60. Jugrin AV, Ustyugova A, Urbich M, Lamotte M, Sunderland T. The cost-utility of dabigatran etexilate compared with warfarin in treatment and extended anticoagulation of acute VTE in the UK. Thromb Haemost. 2015;114:778–92.

61. Amin A, Stokes M, Makenbaeva D, Wiederkehr D, Wu N, Lawrence JH. Estimated medical cost reductions associated with use of novel oral anticoagulants vs warfarin in a real-world non-valvular atrial fibrillation patient population. J Med Econ. 2014;17:771–81.

62. Wang Y, Xie F, Kong MC, Lee LH, Ng HJ, Ko Y. Cost-effectiveness of dabigatran and rivaroxaban compared with warfarin for stroke prevention in patients with atrial fibrillation. Cardiovasc Drugs Ther. 2014;28:575–85.

5

Proposal for new diagnostic criteria for DIC from the Japanese Society on Thrombosis and Hemostasis

Hidesaku Asakura[1][*] [iD], Hoyu Takahashi[2], Toshimasa Uchiyama[3], Yutaka Eguchi[4], Kohji Okamoto[5], Kazuo Kawasugi[6], Seiji Madoiwa[7], Hideo Wada[8] and DIC subcommittee of the Japanese Society on Thrombosis and Hemostasis

Abstract

Disseminated intravascular coagulation (DIC) is a serious disease that, in the presence of underlying disease, causes persistent, generalized, marked coagulation activation. Early treatment based on an appropriate diagnosis is very important for improving patients' prognosis, to which end diagnostic criteria play a key role. Several criteria have been proposed, but each has its strengths and weaknesses, and improved criteria are needed. Widespread use of coagulofibrinolytic markers has elucidated that the pathology of DIC differs greatly as a function of the underlying disease. Thus, discriminating use of DIC diagnostic criteria that take underlying diseases into account is important. DIC diagnostic criteria that are well known in Japan include the Japanese Ministry of Health and Welfare's old DIC diagnostic criteria (JMHW criteria), the International Society on Thrombosis and Haemostasis's DIC diagnostic criteria (ISTH criteria), and the Japanese Association for Acute Medicine's acute-stage DIC diagnostic criteria (JAAM criteria). Those criteria have their respective drawbacks: the sensitivity of the ISTH criteria is poor, the JAAM criteria cannot be applied to all underlying diseases, and the JMHW criteria have poor sensitivity in the case of infections, do not use molecular markers, and result in misdiagnosis. The Japanese Society on Thrombosis and Hemostasis's newly proposed provisional draft DIC diagnostic criteria (new criteria) use diagnostic criteria classifications of "hematopoietic disorder type", "infectious type", and "basic type" based on the underlying pathology. For the hematopoietic disorder type the platelet count is omitted from the score, while for the infectious type, fibrinogen is omitted from the score. Also, points are added if the platelet count decreases with time. In the new criteria, molecular markers and antithrombin activity have been newly included, and as a countermeasure for misdiagnosis, 3 points are deducted if there is liver failure. In this paper, we discuss various problems encountered with DIC diagnosis, and we describe the new criteria together with the events that led to their creation.

These new diagnostic criteria take into account the underlying diseases of wide area, and we expect that they will serve clinicians well due to the above adaptations and improvements.

Keywords: Disseminated intravascular coagulation, DIC, Diagnostic criteria, Suppressed-fibrinolytic-type DIC, Enhanced-fibrinolytic-type DIC

* Correspondence: hasakura@staff.kanazawa-u.ac.jp
[1]Department of Internal Medicine (III), Kanazawa University School of Medicine, 13-1, Takaramachi, Kanazawa 920-8641, Japan
Full list of author information is available at the end of the article

Background

Disseminated intravascular coagulation (DIC) is a serious disease that, in the presence of underlying disease, causes persistent, generalized, marked coagulation activation and frequent formation of microthrombi in microvessels. Both coagulation activation and fibrinolytic activation are seen, but the severity of the fibrinolytic activation differs considerably as a function of the underlying disease(s). Progression of DIC causes decreases in hemostatic factors such as platelets and clotting factors and leads to consumption coagulopathy [1–5]. The two major symptoms of DIC are bleeding symptoms and organ symptoms, and the prognosis becomes very poor if the clinical symptoms become apparent. For that reason, it is ideal to initiate treatment of DIC before clinical symptoms manifest.

The Scientific Standardization Committee (SSC) of the International Society on Thrombosis and Haemostasis (ISTH) defined DIC as follows: "DIC is an acquired syndrome characterized by the intravascular activation of coagulation with loss of localization arising from different causes. It can originate from and cause damage to the microvasculature, which if sufficiently severe, can produce organ dysfunction" [6]. The view of the ISTH can be considered to represent the world's general perception regarding DIC. In fact, the pathology of DIC complicated by sepsis or some other severe infection is accurately presented. However, serious bleeding symptoms may occur due to marked fibrinolytic activation, as in the case of DIC secondary to acute leukemia (especially acute promyelocytic leukemia), aortic aneurysm, giant hemangioma, placental abruption, and metastatic prostate cancer. Although organ symptoms are usually not seen, there is a problem in that consideration has not been given to DIC with severe bleeding symptoms [7, 8].

DIC is a serious condition, and early treatment based on an appropriate diagnosis is very important for improving patients' prognosis, in which effective diagnostic criteria play a key role. In this paper, we discuss the diversity in DIC, as well as various problems encountered with DIC diagnosis, and describe the provisional draft DIC diagnostic criteria that have been proposed by the Japanese Society on Thrombosis and Hemostasis (JSTH) (the new criteria).

Review

DIC disease type classification

There are various DIC disease types, depending on the underlying disease. The concept of DIC disease type classification is important to understanding that diversity [9]. Marked coagulation activation is the primary pathology of DIC and seen in all cases, but in regard to other aspects, the pathology (especially the degree of fibrinolytic activation) differs considerably as a function of the underlying disease. The degree of fibrinolytic activation is controlled by plasminogen activator inhibitor-1 (PAI-1), which is one of the important factors characterizing DIC.

In suppressed-fibrinolytic-type DIC, coagulation activation is high, whereas fibrinolytic activation remains mild. This type of DIC is seen in cases complicated by sepsis. Lipopolysaccharide (LPS) and inflammatory cytokines act on the vascular endothelium, thereby enhancing production of fibrinolysis inhibitory factor PAI-1 and creating a potent state of inhibition of fibrinolysis. Dissolution of multiple microthrombi becomes difficult, increasing the risk of organ failure due to failure of the microcirculation, but bleeding symptoms are relatively mild. Laboratory findings include elevated levels of thrombin-antithrombin complex (TAT), soluble fibrin (SF), and prothrombin fragment $1 + 2$ (F_{1+2}), which are coagulation activation markers, but plasmin-α_2-plasmin inhibitor complex (PIC), a fibrinolytic activation marker, is only slightly elevated [10, 11]. Other characteristic findings are relatively mild increases in fibrin/fibrinogen degradation products (FDP) and D-dimer, which reflect lysis of microthrombi. Intrinsically, α_2-plasmin inhibitor (α_2PI) is consumptively decreased in DIC. However, in suppressed-fibrinolytic-type DIC, α_2PI is generally slightly below or almost normal because plasmin production is low, and α_2PI is a protein that increases in inflammation. FDP and D-dimer are recognized as the most important markers for DIC diagnosis. However, in suppressed-fibrinolytic-type DIC, it is not unusual for their elevation to be mild, leading to concern that diagnosis of DIC might be delayed if too much emphasis is placed only on these markers. Conversely, early diagnosis is possible if attention is paid to elevation of TAT and SF as blood markers, together with a decrease in the platelet count with time. Because of the inflammatory reaction, fibrinogen often does not decrease.

Enhanced-fibrinolytic-type DIC is characterized by marked fibrinolytic activation that is out of balance with coagulation activation. Characteristic patients have underlying diseases such as acute promyelocytic leukemia (APL), aortic aneurysm, and prostate cancer. PAI-1 is hardly elevated, while the strong fibrinolytic activation and hemostatic plugs (thrombi for hemostasis) are readily dissolved. As a result, bleeding symptoms are likely to be severe, but organ failure is almost never seen. In APL and some cancers, annexin II is involved in strong fibrinolytic activation [12, 13]. Laboratory findings include marked increases in the coagulation activation markers, TAT (SF, F_{1+2}), and the fibrinolytic activation marker, PIC, while FDP and D-dimer (especially FDP) are also increased [10, 11]. It is also characteristic for fibrinogen and α_2PI to be markedly decreased. Even if the platelet count is only slightly decreased, caution is needed in regard to potential massive bleeding. Furthermore, when treating enhanced- fibrinolytic-type DIC, it is not unusual for administration of only a heparin to promote bleeding, and in such cases it is effective to concomitantly administer nafamostat mesylate (a potent anti-thrombin agent that also has anti-plasmin activity) or tranexamic acid with a heparin [14–17].

Balanced-fibrinolytic-type DIC is characterized by balance between the coagulation and fibrinolytic activations and is thus an intermediate pathology between the two types of DIC described above. With the exception of advanced cases, bleeding symptoms and organ symptoms are relatively rare. Although this type is seen in many DIC cases with solid cancers, in the case of some cancers such as prostate cancer and blood vessel-associated malignant tumors, the disease type is enhanced-fibrinolytic-type DIC.

Gando et al. reported that DIC seen at the time of trauma is DIC with the fibrinolytic phenotype in which the initial fibrinolytic activation is high, but at 24–48 h post-trauma, the pathology changes to a thrombotic phenotype due to the activity of PAI-1 [18, 19]. For DIC caused by trauma, the fact that tranexamic acid is used only at the time of enhanced-fibrinolytic-type DIC can be considered to be the point. The concept is that DIC with the fibrinolytic phenotype is close to enhanced-fibrinolytic-type DIC, while DIC with the thrombotic phenotype is close to suppressed-fibrinolytic-type DIC.

The commonly used conventional animal models of DIC are induced with LPS or tissue factor (TF) (especially LPS), but the actual situation is that little conscious distinction has been made between them as the same DIC model. However, our group recently showed that the pathology differs greatly depending on the DIC inducer used [9]. The LPS-induced DIC model is characterized by a state of suppression of fibrinolysis due to markedly elevated PAI-1 activity and only mild elevation of D-dimer. It is easy to pathologically demonstrate multiple microthrombi. Whereas organ disorders such as hepatorenal disorder are advanced, bleeding symptoms are hardly seen, even though the platelet count and fibrinogen are markedly reduced [20]. Meanwhile, the TF-induced DIC model is characterized by only a mild increase in PAI-1 activity, while D-dimer is sharply increased, reflecting the fact that there is adequate fibrinolytic activation. It is difficult to pathologically demonstrate microthrombi due to enhanced thrombolysis. Interestingly, whereas there is almost no hepatorenal failure, severe hematuria is seen as a bleeding symptom. Moreover, the high degree of fibrinolytic activation results in progression of not only fibrin degradation, but also fibrinogen degradation [21]. In this way, it can be thought that the LPS-induced DIC model is similar in pathology to clinical suppressed-fibrinolytic-type DIC, while the TF-induced DIC model is pathologically similar to enhanced-fibrinolytic-type - balanced-fibrinolytic-type DIC.

Representative DIC diagnostic criteria

Three DIC diagnostic criteria are well known in Japan: the Japanese Ministry of Health and Welfare's DIC diagnostic criteria (JMHW criteria), the ISTH's DIC diagnostic criteria (ISTH criteria), and the Japanese Association for Acute Medicine's DIC diagnostic criteria (JAAM criteria) [6, 22, 23] (Table 1).

Those criteria have their respective drawbacks, such as the poor sensitivity of the ISTH criteria and that the JAAM criteria cannot be applied to all underlying diseases (e.g., DIC complicated by a hematopoietic malignancy

Table 1 Comparison of existing DIC diagnostic criteria

	JMHW	ISTH	JAAM
Underlying disease Clinical symptoms	1 p bleeding: 1 p organ failure: 1 p	0 p(essential) 0 p 0 p	0 p(essential) SIRS score ≥3: 1 p
Platelet count (X10^4/μL)	8 < − ≤12 : 1 p 5 < − ≤8 : 2 p ≤5 : 3 p	5–10 : 1 p <5 : 2 p	8 - ≤12 or >30 % reduction/24 h: 1 p <8 or >50 % reduction/24 h: 3 p
Fibrin-related marker	FDP (μg/ml) 10 ≤ − <20: 1 p 20 ≤ − <40: 2 p ≥40 : 3 p	FDP, D-dimer, SF moderate increase: 2 p strong increase: 3 p	FDP (μg/ml) 10 ≤ − <25: 1 p ≥25 : 3 p
Fibrinogen (mg/dl)	100 < − ≤150: 1 p ≤100: 2 p	<100: 1 p	None
PT	PT ratio 1.25 ≤ − <1.67: 1 p ≥1.67: 2 p	Prolonged PT(sec) 3–6: 1 p >6: 2 p	PT ratio ≥1.2: 1 p
Diagnosis of DIC	≥7 p	≥5 p	≥4 p

p: points
JMHW: JMHW criteria; ISTH: JMHW criteria; JAAM: JMHW criteria; PT: prothrombin time
JMHW criteria: When there is leukemia/related diseases, aplastic anemia, or marked bone marrow megakaryocyte reduction, such as after administration of an anti-tumor agent, and a high degree of thrombocytopenia, the bleeding symptom and platelet count items should be calculated as 0 points, and DIC is diagnosed if the score is ≥4 points

cannot be diagnosed). To date, the JMHW criteria have the longest history and a solid reputation.

However, the JMHW criteria have also been noted to have various problems because they have poor sensitivity in the case of infections, do not use molecular markers that reflect coagulation activation (which is at the heart of DIC), and result in misdiagnosis of liver failure. With the aim of developing better DIC diagnostic criteria, the SSC/DIC subcommittee of the Japanese Society on Thrombosis and Hemostasis (JSTH) held numerous discussions over the years, but a consensus was not reached. For that reason, in July 2012, the JSTH established a committee charged with creating DIC diagnostic criteria.

That committee also carried out numerous in-depth discussions, both in meetings and via e-mail exchanges. The committee had 13 members, consisting of 6 from the SSC/DIC subcommittee and 7 others. The members represented various medical fields: internal medicine, surgery, obstetrics and gynecology, pediatrics, clinical laboratory medicine, and emergency medicine. In addition, the SSC/DIC subcommittee members put in a collective effort and carried out a thorough literature search.

This culminated, in October 2014, with publication of the JSTH's provisional draft DIC diagnostic criteria (hereinafter, new criteria) [24]. The criteria are considered to be provisional, because they are likely to be modified on the basis of the results of future studies. Since that paper was published in a Japanese journal, the new criteria remain largely unknown internationally. We hope to remedy that situation through publication of the present English manuscript.

Basic concept of these DIC diagnostic criteria

Three main methods exist for creating diagnostic criteria. The first method is creation of criteria based on the definition of DIC. The ISTH's overt DIC criteria are equivalent to this. Since DIC is a domain that is evidence-poor, the approach is to try to create criteria by defining the portions for which there is no evidence [6]. The second method aims to create criteria that reflect the prognosis. In fact, most existing diagnostic criteria reflect the prognosis. No DIC diagnostic criteria have been drawn up based on prognosis as the endpoint, but there are a number of papers of DIC diagnostic criteria that secondarily reflect the prognosis [25–28]. The third method is to compile cases of DIC diagnosed by experts and then create diagnostic criteria. The JMHW criteria used this approach [29, 30].

Because there are no specific markers for DIC, it makes sense to diagnose DIC using a scoring method that combines multiple markers that show characteristic changes in DIC. The DIC clinical practice guidelines of the United Kingdom, Japan, and Italy that have been published as academic papers in English all recommend

using a scoring method to diagnose DIC [5, 31–33]. The JMHW criteria, ISTH criteria, and JAAM criteria all carry out diagnosis using a scoring method [6, 22, 23] (Table 1). Japan has a long history of DIC clinical trials of various drugs that have been performed using the JMHW criteria. For that reason, it can be thought that, even when the objective is to create new, improved diagnostic criteria, it would be inappropriate to create totally new criteria, and that the JMHW criteria should be kept as the core. Thus, even the new criteria must inevitably use a scoring method.

The background of creation of the JAAM criteria was that diagnosis by the JMHW criteria was often too late in the fields of emergency medicine and surgery [29]. However, it was often pointed out that, while the sensitivity of the JAAM criteria is high, their specificity is low [27], and they also do not incorporate the molecular markers associated with coagulation activation that reflect the nature of DIC. Verification of the JAAM criteria was performed by collecting cases in the emergency medicine field, and it was named the acute phase DIC diagnostic criteria, but originally the criteria were positioned only for the emergency medicine field (not all acute phase). The ISTH criteria were developed by modeling the Japanese JMHW criteria, but they were even less sensitive than the JMHW criteria [23].

Today, we know from analyses using molecular markers that the pathology of DIC differs greatly depending on the underlying disease [7, 9–11]. This means that there are limitations on the ability of any one set of criteria to diagnose all presentations of DIC. It can be thought that the DIC criteria should be selected and used in the light of a patient's underlying disease(s). However, because the numerous classifications of underlying diseases might complicate DIC diagnostic criteria, diagnosis should be performed using a set of criteria for the basic type and then adding different diagnostic items that are appropriate for the hematopoietic disorder type and infectious type of DIC. In particular, since the JMHW criteria are excellent for blood diseases but have weak diagnostic capacity for infectious diseases, there is a need for modification to address this point.

With the JMHW criteria, it is not uncommon for a coagulation abnormality that is accompanied by liver disease to be misdiagnosed as DIC, and that has to be considered.

The two major clinical symptoms of DIC are bleeding symptoms and organ symptoms. However, the clinical symptoms are non-specific, and it can be difficult to determine if they are symptoms due to an underlying disease or a complication other than DIC or are symptoms caused by DIC. Also, if no symptoms manifest and DIC is thus not diagnosed, that is an obstacle to early diagnosis of the disease. It can thus be thought that the clinical symptoms used in the JMHW criteria should be removed from the diagnostic criteria.

Significance of various markers for DIC diagnosis
FDP, D-dimer

FDP and D-dimer have great significance in the diagnosis of DIC, and they are, in fact, included as important test items in almost all DIC diagnostic criteria [6, 22, 29]. However, it must be kept in mind that, while FDP and D-dimer are high in sensitivity, they are low in specificity. For example, these markers are often elevated even in such diseases as deep vein thrombosis, pulmonary thromboembolism, massive hydrothorax/ascites, and large subcutaneous hematomas [34–36].

Since FDP and D-dimer do not necessarily coincide with the molecular species of interest, there is medical significance in measuring both. For example, not only fibrin but also fibrinogen is broken down in DIC [37], and fibrinogen degradation is increased when the fibrinolytic system is highly activated. FDP increases markedly, but D-dimer rises only moderately. This results in a dissociation phenomenon between FDP and D-dimer (i.e., the D-dimer/FDP ratio decreases) [13, 37–39]. However, we should refrain from aimlessly measuring both FDP and D-dime.

In the case that fibrin/fibrinogen degradation is advanced due to strong fibrinolytic activation, the reaction with the D-dimer fraction may be reduced depending on the D-dimer reagent that is used [39]. Accordingly, for the DIC diagnostic criteria, it can be thought that emphasis should be placed on FDP rather than D-dimer.

Platelet count

As noted earlier, the platelet count cannot be used in the diagnostic criteria for diagnosis of the hematopoietic disorder type, and sufficient caution is necessary in this regard.

Except for the hematopoietic disorder type, the platelet count, like FDP and D-dimer, is an important test item for DIC diagnosis. However, there are also many patients with a decreased platelet count that is not due to DIC, and it is necessary to raise awareness regarding diseases that need to be differentiated from DIC. A decreased platelet count has high sensitivity for diagnosis of DIC, but it can be said that its specificity is low [23, 27, 31, 40].

Changes in the platelet count with time are also important. For example, even if the platelet count is above $12 \times 10^4/\mu L$, DIC may be present if the count decreases with time. For this reason, there is significance in assigning a score to the thrombocytopenia rate, separate from the platelet count [41, 42].

Fibrinogen

For diagnosis of DIC, fibrinogen is a marker with high specificity, but low sensitivity [29, 30, 43–45]. Especially in inflammatory diseases, fibrinogen does not decrease even in patients thought to have DIC, and in some cases it actually increases [46]. The JAAM criteria were initially created using fibrinogen for DIC diagnosis at ≥5 points, but in actual application, fibrinogen could not be shown to have diagnostic significance. The criteria were thus modified by eliminating fibrinogen for DIC diagnosis at ≥4 points [29]. This is probably because the validation of JAAM criteria was performed in many cases with concurrent infection. There are underlying diseases for which fibrinogen is valuable as a marker. For example, fibrinogen readily decreases in patients with hematopoietic malignancies, obstetric complications, head trauma, aortic aneurysm, and solid cancers, and is an important finding [47–51].

Against this background, one approach would be to change the test items in the diagnostic criteria to fit each underlying disease. That is, in the case that the infectious type is the underlying disease, it is desirable to exclude fibrinogen, which fluctuates as an acute-phase reactive protein, from the score.

Prothrombin time (PT)

PT can reflect organ failure, and the prognosis is poor in patients with an infection and a prolonged PT [29, 30, 52–55]. On the other hand, since PT is also prolonged in liver disease and vitamin K deficiency, it is not a characteristic marker for DIC.

Most studies that investigated the sensitivity and specificity of PT in the diagnosis of DIC examined cases of infection, and almost none examined other underlying diseases [29, 30, 43, 44, 46]. Ordinarily, verification of significance of PT in diagnostic criteria should be performed in various underlying diseases such as infectious disease, hematopoietic malignancy, and solid cancer. Because PT has been used for many years and has a proven track record, it was decided to include it in the new criteria.

There is a problem as to the notation that should be used for PT in the new criteria, i.e., PT ratio or INR. INR values using different PT reagents converge in patients on warfarin but not in patients with liver disease or DIC. INR (liver) has been proposed [56, 57], and these values converges in liver disease but not in DIC. In the case of using PT for DIC diagnosis, the PT ratio must be used at present. However, given the current situation that the INR notation is widely used, if the ISI of the PT reagent is close to 1, it can be thought that INR can be substituted for the PT ratio.

Molecular markers of coagulation activation

TAT, SF, and F_{1+2} are molecular markers that reflect coagulation activation, which can be said to be at the heart of DIC. Incorporation of these molecular markers in DIC diagnostic criteria can be expected to improve both the sensitivity and specificity of the criteria [58–63]. Furthermore, TAT and SF are significant in that, if both are completely normal, then they can be used for exclusion of the diagnosis, that is, to determine that DIC is not present. At present, many institutions still do not measure these markers in-hospital, but that can be expected to change if they are included in the DIC diagnostic criteria. Even institutions that do not perform in-hospital assays will be able to confirm the test results at a later date, and it can be thought that this will help reduce misdiagnoses.

On the other hand, we can anticipate that contrary opinions will also be expressed, such as that there are many institutions that would not get the results for these molecular markers on the same day, and especially in pediatric departments, which have many patients for whom blood sampling is difficult, it is easy for many false high values to be generated [64].

These molecular markers of coagulation activation were also subjected to extensive discussions in the JSTH's committee for creating DIC diagnostic criteria, and in the end it was decided to include markers in the criteria because they had the support of many of the committee members. However, which molecular markers are the best to be included has not yet been settled and will require further discussion. For that reason, it was decided to include all three of these molecular markers of coagulation activation in the new criteria. However, the cutoff values for the molecular markers have yet to be set, and scores were given based on the degree of elevation above the upper limit of the standard range. Using the markers for exclusion diagnosis also seems to make sense. However, if a minus score were assigned when a molecular marker remains within its standard range, there is concern that the diagnosis might be reversed when test results are returned at a later date. Accordingly, this approach was not adopted.

Antithrombin (AT) activity

The JSTH's committee for creating DIC diagnostic criteria discussed many pros and cons regarding incorporation of AT activity into the criteria.

Multiple committee members expressed opinions explaining their being in favor of inclusion of AT activity in the criteria: measurement of AT activity is directly linked to treatment selection (use of AT concentrate for DIC finds AT activity in ≤70 % of cases in Japan); in cases of infection, the sensitivity of DIC diagnosis would be improved by adopting AT activity; the prognosis could be evaluated [46, 65–75].

Negative opinions were also expressed by multiple committee members: it is rare for AT activity to decrease due to DIC mechanisms, and AT activity is not a specific indicator for DIC (the diagnostic specificity would be reduced) [42, 43, 58, 76]; AT activity generally reflects a protein synthesis disorder in the liver or extravasation during inflammation; AT activity correlates with serum albumin [77–80]; the degree of decrease in AT activity differs with the underlying disease; incorporation would complicate the diagnostic criteria.

The committee's conclusion was as follows: AT activity would be incorporated in the new criteria, but the decision would be re-visited in the future at a time when the results of validation of the new criteria are in hand.

Considerations for the fields of obstetrics and pediatrics

In Japan, the obstetric DIC score is frequently used in obstetrics. Obstetric DIC takes a very rapid course and requires prompt diagnosis and treatment of the underlying disease(s) and clinical symptoms. The obstetric DIC score enables early initiation of treatment and is thus extremely useful. It is widely used in Japan (The Japan Society of Obstetrical, Gynecological & Neonatal Hematology; http://www.jsognh.jp/dic/). Moreover, since such DIC-associated markers as FDP, D-dimer, TAT, SF, and F_{1+2} increase even in normal pregnancy [81], DIC cannot be said to be present merely because these markers are elevated. An opinion of committee was expressed that, if the new criteria become diagnostic criteria consisting mainly of blood coagulation and fibrinolysis tests, they will not be able to be applied to obstetric DIC.

Also, an opinion was expressed that, if the new criteria are based on the JMHW criteria, it is highly likely that they will not be able to be applied to diagnosis of DIC in newborn infants. The reason is that some items for coagulation activation and fibrinolytic activation differ greatly between newborns and adults. In addition, since only a limited amount of blood can be drawn from children, especially newborns, it is desirable to keep the number of test items as small as possible. Coagulation activation-related markers such as TAT and SF, are prone to show false high values (leading to misdiagnosis) by ex vivo coagulation for patients for whom blood collection is difficult (such as children) [64]. The consensus reached on the basis of these opinions was that the new criteria would not be applied to newborns.

Countermeasures for misdiagnoses

With the JMHW criteria, misdiagnosis readily occurred for patients showing PT prolongation, decreased fibrinogen, and decreased platelet count due to liver failure, as well as patients with elevated FDP and D-dimer when they had liver failure and also massive ascites [36]. It is necessary to make adjustments to avoid misdiagnosis in liver failure cases.

Other molecular markers

Once DIC has been diagnosed, other markers are known to be useful for the subsequent steps of disease type

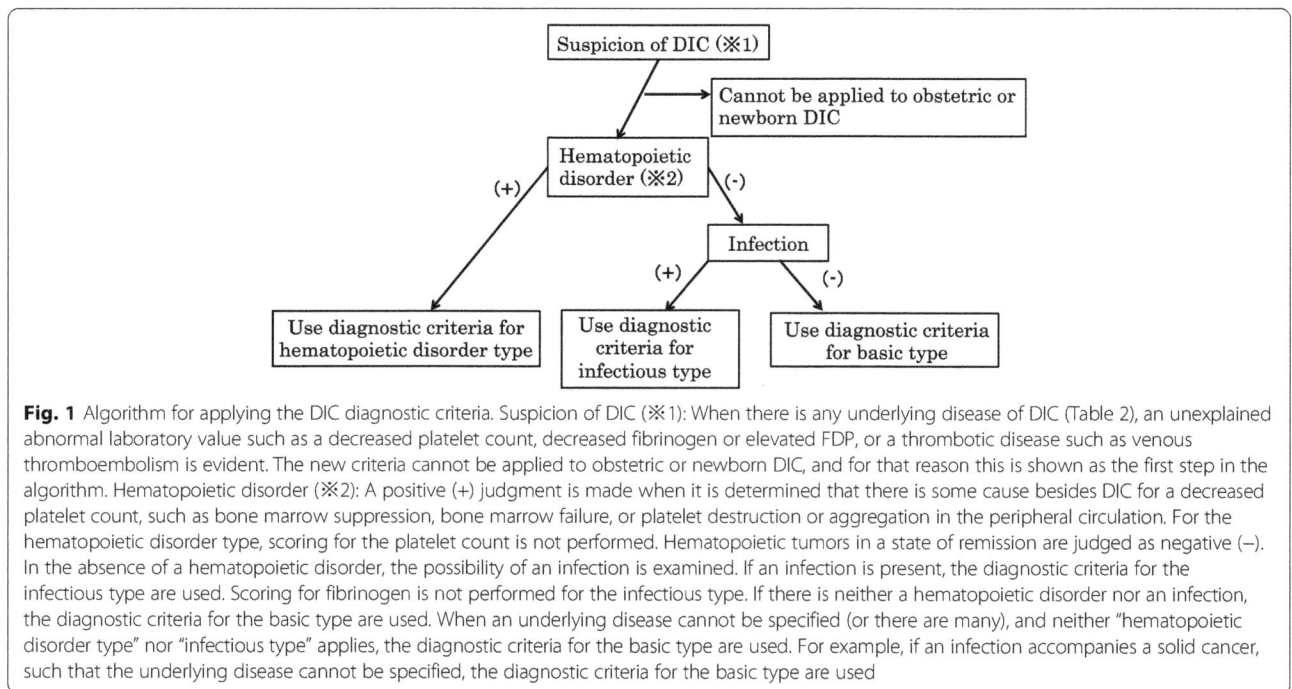

Fig. 1 Algorithm for applying the DIC diagnostic criteria. Suspicion of DIC (※1): When there is any underlying disease of DIC (Table 2), an unexplained abnormal laboratory value such as a decreased platelet count, decreased fibrinogen or elevated FDP, or a thrombotic disease such as venous thromboembolism is evident. The new criteria cannot be applied to obstetric or newborn DIC, and for that reason this is shown as the first step in the algorithm. Hematopoietic disorder (※2): A positive (+) judgment is made when it is determined that there is some cause besides DIC for a decreased platelet count, such as bone marrow suppression, bone marrow failure, or platelet destruction or aggregation in the peripheral circulation. For the hematopoietic disorder type, scoring for the platelet count is not performed. Hematopoietic tumors in a state of remission are judged as negative (−). In the absence of a hematopoietic disorder, the possibility of an infection is examined. If an infection is present, the diagnostic criteria for the infectious type are used. Scoring for fibrinogen is not performed for the infectious type. If there is neither a hematopoietic disorder nor an infection, the diagnostic criteria for the basic type are used. When an underlying disease cannot be specified (or there are many), and neither "hematopoietic disorder type" nor "infectious type" applies, the diagnostic criteria for the basic type are used. For example, if an infection accompanies a solid cancer, such that the underlying disease cannot be specified, the diagnostic criteria for the basic type are used

classification and pathological evaluation. It was thus decided to also include statements regarding "testing and significance related to DIC diagnosis".

Various excellent markers are known: PIC and α_2PI are essential markers for evaluating fibrinolytic activation [7, 9–11]; protein C is an anticoagulant factor for evaluating the prognosis [74, 82–84]; PAI-1 is a fibrinolytic inhibitory factor [73, 85–89]; HMGB-1 is a nuclear molecule [90, 91]; and e-XDP is a fibrin degradation product of granulocyte elastase [92–97].

The new DIC diagnostic criteria (JSTH's provisional draft DIC diagnostic criteria)
Algorithm of application of the DIC diagnostic criteria (Fig. 1)

This algorithm should be followed from the time that DIC is suspected.

Underlying diseases of DIC
Many underlying diseases of DIC are known. Table 2 shows representative underlying diseases. Obstetric complications and even diseases of the newborn are known to be characteristic underlying diseases of DIC. Specific examples of obstetric complications include placental abruption, amniotic fluid embolism, DIC-type afterbirth bleeding, and eclampsia, while diseases of newborns include neonatal asphyxia, infection, placental abruption, in utero death of one fetus in a multiple pregnancy, respiratory distress syndrome, and intraventricular hemorrhage.

Table 2 Underlying diseases of DIC

1. Infections
   - Sepsis
   - Other severe infections (of the respiratory organs, urinary tract, biliary system, etc.)

2. Hematopoietic malignancies
   - Acute promyelocytic leukemia (APL)
   - Other acute leukemia
   - Malignant lymphoma
   - Other hematopoietic malignancies

3. Solid cancers (usually advanced cancer with metastasis)

4. Tissue damage: trauma, burns, heat stroke, rhabdomyolysis

5. Post-surgery

6. Vascular-related diseases
   - Thoracic and abdominal aortic aneurysms
   - Giant hemangioma
   - Blood vessel-associated tumors
   - Collagen disease (cases of vasculitis complications)
   - Other vascular-related diseases

7. Liver injury: acute liver failure, acute hepatitis, liver cirrhosis

8. Acute pancreatitis

9. Shock

10. Hemolysis, incompatible blood-type transfusion

11. Snake bite

12. Hypothermia

13. Other

Note: There are characteristic underlying diseases of DIC in the fields of obstetrics and newborns, but they are not shown in this table because these diagnostic criteria are not applicable to either of those fields

Table 3 Representative underlying diseases and pathologies that must be differentiated

Decreased platelet count

1. Enhancement of platelet destruction and aggregation

   - Thrombotic microangiopathy (TMA): thrombotic thrombocytopenic purpura (TTP), hemolytic uremic syndrome (HUS), HELLP syndrome, TMA after hematopoietic stem cell transplantation

   - Heparin-induced thrombocytopenia (HIT)

   - Idiopathic thrombocytopenic purpura (ITP), systemic lupus erythematosus (SLE), antiphospholipid antibody syndrome (APS)

   - Extracorporeal circulation

2. Pathologies that lead to bone marrow suppression/bone marrow failure

   - Hematopoietic malignancies (acute leukemia, blastic crisis of chronic myelogenous leukemia, myelodysplastic syndrome, multiple myeloma, bone marrow infiltration of malignant lymphoma)

   - Hemophagocytic syndrome

   - Solid cancers (with bone marrow infiltration)

   - Chemotherapy or radiation therapy with bone marrow suppression

   - Bone marrow suppression due to drugs

   - Some viral infections

   - Some blood diseases besides hematopoietic malignances (aplastic anemia, paroxysmal nocturnal hemoglobinuria, megaloblastic anemia)

3. Liver failure, cirrhosis, hypersplenism

4. Sepsis

5. Bernard-Soulier syndrome, MYH9 disorder (e.g., May-Hegglin disorder), Wiskott-Aldrich syndrome

6. Dilution

   - Massive bleeding

   - Massive transfusion, massive infusion

   - Pregnancy thrombocytopenia

7. Pseudo-thrombocytopenia

Elevated FDP

1. Thrombosis: deep vein thrombosis, pulmonary thromboembolism

2. Massive hydrothorax/ascites

3. Large hematoma

4. Fibrinolytic therapy

Decreased fibrinogen

1. Congenital afibrinogenemia, congenital hypofibrinogenemia, dysfibrinogenemia

2. Liver failure, malnutrition

3. Drug-induced: L-asparaginase, corticosteroids, fibrinolytic therapy

4. False lowering: at the time of administration of drugs with anti-thrombin action (e.g., dabigatran)

Prothrombin time prolongation

1. Vitamin K deficiency, oral warfarin

2. Liver failure, malnutrition

3. Deficiency or inhibitor of extrinsic coagulation factor

4. Ingestion of a direct oral anticoagulant

Table 3 Representative underlying diseases and pathologies that must be differentiated (Continued)

5. False prolongation: insufficient blood sample volume, addition of an anti-coagulant

Decreased antithrombin activity

1. Liver failure, malnutrition

2. Extravasation due to inflammation (e.g., sepsis)

3. Degradation by granulocyte elastase (e.g., sepsis)

4. Congenital antithrombin deficiency

5. Drug-induced: L-asparaginase

Elevated TAT, SF, or F_{1+2}

1. Thrombosis: deep vein thrombosis, pulmonary embolism

2. Some atrial fibrillation

Note: However, DIC may also occur with the above conditions and diseases

Representative underlying diseases and pathologies that must be differentiated

Table 3 shows the representative underlying diseases and pathologies that must be differentiated from DIC.

DIC diagnostic criteria

The first step is to confirm, according to the algorithm (Fig. 1), which diagnostic criteria can be applied to the patient in question, and then proceed to the diagnosis of DIC using Table 4. For the basic type, scoring should be performed using the data for the platelet count, FDP, fibrinogen, PT ratio, AT activity, and coagulation activation-associated molecular markers (elevation of TAT, SF, or F_{1+2}). The total score should be calculated, and a diagnosis of DIC should be made for the basic type and the infectious type if the total is 6 points or more and for the hematopoietic disorder type if the total is four points or more. The point for diagnosis of DIC in infectious type is more than 6 points though there is one less item to check with the infectious type as compared to the basic type. This reason is that depression in fibrinogen is hardly observed in DIC caused by infection. However, the point for diagnosis of DIC in infectious type might be modified from 6 points to 5 points after validation of the new DIC diagnostic criteria. Table 4 shows that 3 points are subtracted for liver failure. Scoring for underlying diseases and clinical symptoms was included in the JMHW criteria [22] but omitted from the new criteria.

Depending on the value for the platelet count, the score covered a range of 0 to 3 points (the same range as in the JMHW criteria), adding another 1 point if a decrease of ≥30 % is seen within 24 h. However, for a platelet count of ≤5 × 10^4/μL, no extra point is added even if there is a decrease of ≥30 % within 24 h, so the maximum score for the platelet count is 3 points.

Table 4 JSTH's provisional draft DIC diagnostic criteria

Classification of type	Basic		Hematopoietic disorder		Infectious	
Platelet count (×10⁴/µl)	>12	0 p			>12	0 p
	8< – ≤12	1 p			8< – ≤12	1 p
	5< – ≤8	2 p			5< – ≤8	2 p
	≤5	3 p			≤5	3 p
	≥30 % decrease w/in 24 h (*1)	+1 p			≥30 % decrease w/in 24 h (*1)	+1 p
FDP (µg/ml)	<10	0 p	<10	0 p	<10	0 p
	10≤ – <20	1 p	10≤ – <20	1 p	10 ≤ – <20	1 p
	20≤ – <40	2 p	20≤ -<40	2 p	20≤ – <40	2 p
	≥40	3 p	≥40	3 p	≥40	3 p
Fibrinogen (mg/dl)	>150	0 p	>150	0 p		
	100< – ≤150	1 p	100< – ≤150	1 p		
	≤100	2 p	≤100	2 p		
Prothrombin time ratio	<1.25	0 p	<1.25	0 p	<1.25	0 p
	1.25≤ – <1.67	1 p	1.25≤ – <1.67	1 p	1.25≤ – <1.67	1 p
	≥1.67	2 p	≥1.67	2 p	≥1.67	2 p
Antithrombin (%)	>70	0 p	>70	0 p	>70	0 p
	≤70	1 p	≤70	1 p	≤70	1 p
TAT, SF or F$_{1+2}$	<2-fold of normal upper limit	0 p	<2-fold of normal upper limit	0 p	<2-fold of normal upper limit	0 p
	≥2-fold of normal upper limit	1 p	≥2-fold of normal upper limit	1 p	≥2-fold of normal upper limit	1 p
Liver failure (*2)	No	0 p	No	0 p	No	0 p
	Yes	-3 p	Yes	-3 p	Yes	-3 p
DIC diagnosis	≥6 p		≥4 p		≥6 p	

p: points
• (*1): For a platelet count of >5 × 10⁴/µL, points will be added if the time-course conditions of decrease are met (no points will be added for a platelet count of ≤5 × 10⁴). The maximum score for the platelet count is 3 points
• For institutions that do not measure FDP (institutions that measure only D-dimer), 1 point will be added if D-dimer increases ≥2-fold the normal upper limit. However, in principle, FDP should also be measured and re-evaluation performed after the results are in hand
• Prothrombin time ratio: If ISI is close to 1.0, INR will also be acceptable (However, there is no evidence supporting recommendation of the use of PT-INR for diagnosis of DIC.)
• Thrombin-antithrombin complex (TAT), soluble fibrin (SF), prothrombin fragment 1+2 (F$_{1+2}$): For blood sampling in difficult cases and route blood sampling, false-high values may increase. Thus, in comparison with elevation of FDP and/or D-dimer, re-testing should be done if TAT and/or SF is markedly elevated. Confirmation is needed even if the results on the same day are not in time
• Regardless of the presence or absence of DIC immediately after surgery, changes in DIC-like markers such as elevation of TAT, SF, FDP, or D-dimer or a decrease in AT, may be observed, and judgment should be made with care
• (*2) Liver failure: Corresponds to "a prothrombin time activity of ≤40 % or an INR value of ≥1.5 due to severe liver dysfunction seen within eight weeks of onset of initial symptoms following liver impairment that develops in a normal liver or a liver that is thought to exhibit normal liver function" (acute liver failure) or "cirrhosis with a Child-Pugh classification of B or C (≥7 points)" (chronic liver failure) that may be viral or autoimmune in origin, drug-induced, or caused by circulatory failure"
Even when DIC is strongly suspected but these diagnostic criteria are not met, there should be no interference with anti-coagulation therapy based on the physician's judgment, but repeated evaluation is necessary

For FDP, fibrinogen, and the PT ratio, the ranges and point scoring methods were the same as those in the JMHW criteria.

The AT activity was not included as a test item in the JMHW criteria, but it has been adopted in the new criteria. A score of 1 point is assigned for an AT activity of ≤70 %.

The coagulation-fibrinolysis system molecular markers were also not used as test items in the JMHW criteria, but they have been adopted in the new criteria. One point is given if these values are ≥2-fold the respective upper limit of the standard range. In the cases of blood

sampling being difficult and route blood sampling, values may be increased due to false high values [64], and re-testing should be performed if the TAT and SF data are markedly higher than the degrees of elevation of FDP and D-dimer.

Liver failure includes acute liver failure and chronic liver failure. For acute liver failure, we adopted the terminology used in the diagnostic criteria created by the Ministry of Health, Labour and Welfare's Intractable Hepato-Biliary Diseases Study Group, which uses the new "acute liver failure" in place of "fulminant hepatitis" [98]. That is, acute liver failure was defined as being caused by viral infection or autoimmune, drug, or circulatory failure, and "liver failure develops in a liver that is normal or is thought to exhibit normal function, and within eight weeks from the initial appearance of symptoms the prothrombin time activity is ≤40 % or the INR value is ≥1.5 due to a high degree of liver dysfunction". Chronic liver failure was defined as "Child-Pugh classification B or C cirrhosis (≥7 points)" [99].

Other tests relating to DIC diagnosis, and their significance

Following diagnosis of DIC, testing should be performed for the markers listed in Table 5, which are useful for disease type classification and pathological assessment.

Points of difference between the JMHW criteria and the new criteria

The new criteria make it clear that the algorithm should be used, and the diagnostic criteria should be selected based on the underlying pathology. Even in the JMHW criteria, the scoring method is different for the leukemia and non-leukemia groups, whereas the new criteria make it clear that the diagnostic criteria should be selectively used not only for the hematopoietic disorder type but also the infectious type.

Regarding elimination of the platelet count from the score for the hematopoietic disorder type, the JMHW criteria did the same for the leukemia group, while the new criteria also eliminate fibrinogen from the score for the infectious type.

Although scoring was performed for the clinical symptoms and underlying disease in the JMHW criteria, it was omitted from the new criteria for the above-mentioned reasons.

Table 5 Other tests relating to DIC diagnosis, and their significance

Test	Significance
Plasmin-α_2 plasmin inhibitor complex (PIC)	The higher the values, the greater the fibrinolytic activation
α_2 plasmin inhibitor (α_2PI)	This is consumed and decreases due to fibrinolytic activation. However, it is also decreased by liver failure alone, and it is elevated in acute inflammatory diseases.
Protein C (PC)	Low values correlate with a poor prognosis. However, it is also decreased by vitamin K deficiency and/or liver failure alone.
Plasminogen activator inhibitor-1 (PAI-1)	High values in infectious-type DIC correlate with a poor prognosis.
HMGB-1	High values correlate with a poor prognosis.
e-XDP	Both low and markedly elevated values in infectious-type DIC correlate with a poor prognosis.

Points were not added for a temporal decrease in the platelet count in the JMHW criteria, but this was made a 1-point item in the new criteria.

At present, AT activity was tentatively included in the new criteria, and it was decided that validation will be performed at multiple institutions. However, even if AT activity is <70 %, the criteria do not recommend that administration of an AT preparation always be carried out. The overall decision to administer an AT preparation always resides with the attending physician.

Verification must be performed as to which coagulation-fibrinolysis molecular markers are good, but diagnostic criteria that incorporate molecular markers are completely novel.

In the JMHW criteria, as well, 3 points are supposed to be subtracted for liver cirrhosis and chronic hepatitis whose pathology approaches that of liver cirrhosis. However, this has not necessarily been carried out properly in clinical practice, and it had been one of the causes of DIC misdiagnosis. For the new criteria, we took into account that, on that background, the criteria had not conventionally been applied to cases of fulminant hepatitis, and we incorporated a 3-point reduction for liver failure in the table in the new criteria.

Conclusion

DIC, based on the presence of underlying disease, has a common pathology in that systemic, persistent, marked coagulation activation is caused. However, there are many points of difference in terms of the degree of fibrinolytic activation, the way in which clinical symptoms manifest, and the degree of formation of pathological blood clots. In regard to diagnosis of DIC, it also makes sense to apply diagnostic criteria selectively depending on the pathology.

DIC diagnostic criteria have great significance in regard to patients' treatment and prognosis. The JMHW criteria have been extensively used in Japan, but it has been pointed out that they have many problems, such as their poor sensitivity in diagnosing DIC due to infections. Meanwhile, the JAAM criteria are effective for diagnosing DIC due to infection, but they are not applicable to all underlying diseases.

In this paper, we have presented the provisional draft DIC diagnostic criteria of the Japanese Society on Thrombosis and Hemostasis. These new criteria have many laudable aspects, including selective use of diagnostic criteria depending on the underlying disease, incorporation of molecular markers and antithrombin, and measures to reduce misdiagnoses. We look forward to further refinement and improvement of these new criteria in the future.

Abbreviations

DIC: Disseminated intravascular coagulation; ISTH: International Society on Thrombosis and Haemostasis; SSC: Scientific Standardization Committee; PAI-1: Plasminogen activator inhibitor-1; LPS: Lipopolysaccharide; TAT: Thrombin-antithrombin complex; SF: Soluble fibrin; F_{1+2}: Prothrombin fragment 1 + 2; PIC: Plasmin-α_2 plasmin inhibitor complex; FDP: Fibrin/fibrinogen degradation products; α_2 PI: α_2 plasmin inhibitor; APL: Acute promyelocytic leukemia; TF: Tissue factor; JMHW: Japanese Ministry of Health and Welfare; JAAM: Japanese Association for Acute Medicine; JSTH: Japanese Society on Thrombosis and Hemostasis; AT: Antithrombin

Acknowledgement

None.

Funding

Meeting expenses were funded by Japanese Society on Thrombosis and Hemostasis.

Authors' contributions

HA, HT, TU, YE, KO, KK, SM and HW made substantial contributions to the conception of the manuscript, revised the manuscript critically for important intellectual content, provided final approval of the version to be submitted. All authors read and approved the final manuscript.

Competing interests

The authors declare that they have no competing interests with this article. They neither benefited from any source of funding nor sponsorship.

Author details

[1]Department of Internal Medicine (III), Kanazawa University School of Medicine, 13-1, Takaramachi, Kanazawa 920-8641, Japan. [2]Department of Internal Medicine, Niigata Prefectural Kamo Hospital, 1-9-1 Aomicho, Kamo, Niigata 959-1397, Japan. [3]Department of Laboratory Medicine, National Hospital Organization Takasaki General Medical Center, 36 Takamatsu-Cho, Takasaki, Gunma 370-0829, Japan. [4]Department of Critical and Intensive Care Medicine, Shiga University of Medical Science, Seta Tsukinowa-cho, Otsu, Shiga 520-2192, Japan. [5]Gastroenterology and Hepatology Center, Kitakyushu City Yahata Hospital, 4-18-1, Nishihon-machi, Yahatahigashi-ku, Kitakyushu, Fukuoka 805-8534, Japan. [6]Department of Hematology, Teikyo University School of Medicine, 2-11-1 Kaga Itabashi-Ku, Tokyo 173-8605, Japan. [7]Department of Clinical and Laboratory Medicine, Tokyo Saiseikai Central Hospital, 1-4-17, Mita, Minato-ku, Tokyo 108-0073, Japan. [8]Department of Molecular and Laboratory Medicine, Mie University Graduate School of Medicine, Tsu, Mie 514-8507, Japan.

References

1. Levi M, Ten Cate H. Disseminated intravascular coagulation. N Engl J Med. 1999;341:586–92.
2. Franchini M, Lippi G, Manzato F. Recent acquisitions in the pathophysiology, diagnosis and treatment of disseminated intravascular coagulation. Thromb J. 2006;4:4.
3. Gando S. Microvascular thrombosis and multiple organ dysfunction syndrome. Crit Care Med. 2010;38(2 Suppl):S35–42.
4. Hunt BJ. Bleeding and coagulopathies in critical care. N Engl J Med. 2014; 370:847–59.
5. Wada H, Asakura H, Okamoto K, Iba T, Uchiyama T, et al. Expert consensus for the treatment of disseminated intravascular coagulation in Japan. Thromb Res. 2010;125:6–11.
6. Taylor Jr FB, Toh CH, Hoots WK, Wada H, Levi M, Scientific Subcommittee on Disseminated Intravascular Coagulation (DIC) of the International Society on Thrombosis and Haemostasis (ISTH). Towards definition, clinical and laboratory criteria, and a scoring system for disseminated intravascular coagulation. Thromb Haemost. 2001;86:1327–30.
7. Matsuda T. Clinical aspects of DIC–disseminated intravascular coagulation. Pol J Pharmacol. 1996;48:73–5.
8. Asakura H, Ontachi Y, Mizutani T, Kato M, Saito M, Kumabashiri I, et al. An enhanced fibrinolysis prevents the development of multiple organ failure in disseminated intravascular coagulation in spite of much activation of blood coagulation. Crit Care Med. 2001;29:1164–8.
9. Asakura H. Classifying types of disseminated intravascular coagulation: clinical and animal models. J Intensive Care. 2014;2(1):20.
10. Takahashi H, Tatewaki W, Wada K, Hanano M, Shibata A. Thrombin vs. plasmin generation in disseminated intravascular coagulation associated with various underlying disorders. Am J Hematol. 1990;33:90–5.
11. Asakura H, Jokaji H, Saito M, Uotani C, Kumabashiri I, Morishita E, Yamazaki M, Aoshima K, Matsuda T. Study of the balance between coagulation and fibrinolysis in disseminated intravascular coagulation using molecular markers. Blood Coagul Fibrinolysis. 1994;5:829–32.
12. Menell JS, Cesarman GM, Jacovina AT, McLaughlin MA, Lev EA, Hajjar KA. Annexin II and bleeding in acute promyelocytic leukemia. N Engl J Med. 1999;340:994–1004.
13. Madoiwa S, Someya T, Hironaka M, Kobayashi H, Ohmori T, Mimuro J, et al. Annexin 2 and hemorrhagic disorder in vascular intimal carcinomatosis. Thromb Res. 2007;119:229–40.
14. Yamamoto K, Ito H, Hiraiwa T, Tanaka K. Effects of nafamostat mesilate on coagulopathy with chronic aortic dissection. Ann Thorac Surg. 2009;88:1331–3.
15. Takahashi T, Suzukawa M, Akiyama M, Hatao K, Nakamura Y. Systemic AL amyloidosis with disseminated intravascular coagulation associated with hyperfibrinolysis. Int J Hematol. 2008;87:371–4.
16. Ontachi Y, Asakura H, Arahata M, Kadohira Y, Maekawa M, Hayashi T, et al. Effect of combined therapy of danaparoid sodium and tranexamic acid on chronic disseminated intravascular coagulation associated with abdominal aortic aneurysm. Circ J. 2005;69:1150–3.
17. Koseki M, Asada N, Uryu H, Takeuchi M, Asakura H, Matsue K. Successful combined use of tranexamic acid and unfractionated heparin for life-threatening bleeding associated with intravascular coagulation in a patient with chronic myelogenous leukemia in blast crisis. Int J Hematol. 2007;86:403–6.
18. Gando S, Wada H, Thachil J, Scientific and Standardization Committee on DIC of the International Society on Thrombosis and Haemostasis (ISTH). Differentiating disseminated intravascular coagulation (DIC) with the fibrinolytic phenotype from coagulopathy of trauma and acute coagulopathy of trauma-shock (COT/ACOTS). J Thromb Haemost. 2013;11:826–35.
19. Gando S, Hayakawa M. Pathophysiology of trauma-induced coagulopathy and management of critical bleeding requiring massive transfusion. Semin Thromb Hemost. 2016;42:155–65.
20. Asakura H, Suga Y, Yoshida T, Ontachi Y, Mizutani T, Kato M, et al. Pathophysiology of disseminated intravascular coagulation (DIC) progresses at a different rate in tissue factor-induced and lipopolysaccharide-induced DIC models in rats. Blood Coagul Fibrinolysis. 2003;14:221–8.
21. Hayakawa M, Gando S, Ieko M, Honma Y, Homma T, Yanagida Y, et al. Massive amounts of tissue factor induce fibrinogenolysis without tissue hypoperfusion in rats. Shock. 2013;39:514–9.
22. Kobayashi N, Maekawa T, Takada M, Tanaka H, Gonmori H. Criteria for diagnosis of DIC based on the analysis of clinical and laboratory findings in 345 DIC patients collected by the research committee on DIC in Japan. Bibl Haematol. 1983;49:265–75.
23. Wada H, Gabazza EC, Asakura H, Koike K, Okamoto K, Maruyama I, et al. Comparison of diagnostic criteria for disseminated intravascular coagulation (DIC): diagnostic criteria of the International Society of Thrombosis and Hemostasis and of the Japanese Ministry of Health and Welfare for overt DIC. Am J Hematol. 2003;74:17–22.
24. Japanese Society on Thrombosis and Hemostasis/DIC subcommittee. Diagnostic criteria for disseminated intravascular coagulation by the

Japanese Society on Thrombosis and Hemostasis —tentative criteria—. Jpn J Thromb Hemost. 2014;25:629–46. in Japanese.

25. Kienast J, Juers M, Wiedermann CJ, Hoffmann JN, Ostermann H, Strauss R, et al. Treatment effects of high-dose antithrombin without concomitant heparin in patients with severe sepsis with or without disseminated intravascular coagulation. J Thromb Haemost. 2006;4:90–7.

26. Dhainaut JF, Yan SB, Joyce DE, Pettilä V, Basson B, Brandt JT, et al. Treatment effects of drotrecogin alfa (activated) in patients with severe sepsis with or without overt disseminated intravascular coagulation. J Thromb Haemost. 2004;2:1924–33.

27. Takemitsu T, Wada H, Hatada T, Ohmori Y, Ishikura K, Takeda T, et al. Prospective evaluation of three different diagnostic criteria for disseminated intravascular coagulation. Thromb Haemost. 2011;105:40–4.

28. Wada H, Wakita Y, Nakase T, Shimura M, Hiyoyama K, Nagaya S, Mie DIC Study Group, et al. Outcome of disseminated intravascular coagulation in relation to the score when treatment was begun. Thromb Haemost. 1995;74:848–52.

29. Gando S, Iba T, Eguchi Y, Ohtomo Y, Okamoto K, Koseki K, Japanese Association for Acute Medicine Disseminated Intravascular Coagulation (JAAM DIC) Study Group, et al. A multicenter, prospective validation of disseminated intravascular coagulation diagnostic criteria for critically ill patients: comparing current criteria. Crit Care Med. 2006;34:625–31.

30. Gando S, Saitoh D, Ogura H, Mayumi T, Koseki K, Ikeda T, Japanese Association for Acute Medicine Disseminated Intravascular Coagulation (JAAM DIC) Study Group, et al. Natural history of disseminated intravascular coagulation diagnosed based on the newly established diagnostic criteria for critically ill patients: results of a multicenter, prospective survey. Crit Care Med. 2008;36:145–50.

31. Levi M, Toh CH, Thachil J, Watson HG. Guidelines for the diagnosis and management of disseminated intravascular coagulation. British Committee for Standards in Haematology. Br J Haematol. 2009;145:24–33.

32. Di Nisio M, Baudo F, Cosmi B, D'Angelo A, De Gasperi A, Malato A, Schiavoni M, Squizzato A. on behalf of the Italian Society for Thrombosis and Haemostasis: Diagnosis and treatment of disseminated intravascular coagulation: Guidelines of the Italian Society for Haemostasis and Thrombosis (SISET). Thromb Res. 2012;129:e177–184.

33. Wada H, Thachil J, Di Nisio M, Mathew P, Kurosawa S, Gando S, The Scientific Standardization Committee on DIC of the International Society on Thrombosis Haemostasis, et al. Guidance for diagnosis and treatment of DIC from harmonization of the recommendations from three guidelines. J Thromb Haemost. 2013;11:761–7.

34. Perrier A, Desmarais S, Miron MJ, de Moerloose P, Lepage R, Slosman D, et al. Non-invasive diagnosis of venous thromboembolism in outpatients. Lancet. 1999;353(9148):190–5.

35. Wells PS, Anderson DR, Rodger M, Forgie M, Kearon C, Dreyer J, et al. Evaluation of D-dimer in the diagnosis of suspected deep-vein thrombosis. N Engl J Med. 2003;349:1227–35.

36. Spadaro A, Tortorella V, Morace C, Fortiguerra A, Composto P, Bonfiglio C, et al. High circulating D-dimers are associated with ascites and hepatocellular carcinoma in liver cirrhosis. World J Gastroenterol. 2008;14:1549–52.

37. Takahashi H, Tatewaki W, Wada K, Niwano H, Shibata A. Fibrinolysis and fibrinogenolysis in disseminated intravascular coagulation. Thromb Haemost. 1990;63:340–4.

38. Sawamura A, Hayakawa M, Gando S, Kubota N, Sugano M, Wada T, et al. Disseminated intravascular coagulation with a fibrinolytic phenotype at an early phase of trauma predicts mortality. Thromb Res. 2009;124:608–13.

39. Madoiwa S, Kitajima I, Ohmori T, Sakata Y, Mimuro J. Distinct reactivity of the commercially available monoclonal antibodies of d-dimer and plasma FDP testing to the molecular variants of fibrin degradation products. Thromb Res. 2013;132:457–64.

40. Levi M, Opal SM. Coagulation abnormalities in critically ill patients. Crit Care. 2006;10:222.

41. Singh RK, Baronia AK, Sahoo JN, Sharma S, Naval R, Pandey CM, Poddar B, et al. Prospective comparison of new Japanese Association for Acute Medicine (JAAM) DIC and International Society of Thrombosis and Hemostasis (ISTH) DIC score in critically ill septic patients. Thromb Res. 2012;129:e119–25.

42. Gando S. The utility of a diagnostic scoring system for disseminated intravascular coagulation. Crit Care Clin. 2012;28:373–88.

43. Okamoto K, Wada H, Hatada T, Uchiyama T, Kawasugi K, Mayumi T, et al. Frequency and hemostatic abnormalities in pre-DIC patients. Thromb Res. 2010;126:74–8.

44. Wada H, Sakuragawa N, Mori Y, Takagi M, Nakasaki T, Shimura M, et al. Hemostatic molecular markers before the onset of disseminated intravascular coagulation. Am J Hematol. 1999;60:273–8.

45. Bakhtiari K, Meijers JC, de Jonge E, Levi M. Prospective validation of the international society of thrombosis and haemostasis scoring system for disseminated intravascular coagulation. Crit Care Med. 2004;32:2416–21.

46. Yu M, Nardella A, Pechet L. Screening tests of disseminated intravascular coagulation: guidelines for rapid and specific laboratory diagnosis. Crit Care Med. 2000;28:1777–80.

47. Hyman DM, Soff GA, Kampel LJ. Disseminated intravascular coagulation with excessive fibrinolysis in prostate cancer: a case series and review of the literature. Oncology. 2011;81:119–25.

48. Lee HJ, Park HJ, Kim HW, Park SG. Comparison of laboratory characteristics between acute promyelocytic leukemia and other subtypes of acute myeloid leukemia with disseminated intravascular coagulation. Blood Res. 2013;48:250–3.

49. Rattray DD, O'Connell CM, Baskett TF. Acute disseminated intravascular coagulation in obstetrics: a tertiary centre population review (1980 to 2009). J Obstet Gynaecol Can. 2012;34:341–7.

50. Scherer RU, Spangenberg P. Procoagulant activity in patients with isolated severe head trauma. Crit Care Med. 1998;26:149–56.

51. Jelenska MM, Szmidt J, Bojakowski K, Grzela T, Palester-Chlebowczyk M. Compensated activation of coagulation in patients with abdominal aortic aneurysm: effects of heparin treatment prior to elective surgery. Thromb Haemost. 2004;92:997–1002.

52. Kushimoto S, Gando S, Saitoh D, Ogura H, Mayumi T, Koseki K, et al. Clinical course and outcome of disseminated intravascular coagulation diagnosed by Japanese Association for Acute Medicine criteria: Comparison between sepais and trauma. Thromb Haemost. 2008;100:1099–105.

53. Pati HP, Saraya AK, Charan VD, Sundaram KR, Sharma MC, Choudhary VP. Prognostic role of screening tests of haemostasis and underlying diseases in acute disseminated intra-vascular coagulation in adults. Clin Lab Haematol. 1994;16:9–13.

54. Voves C, Wuillemin WA, Zeerleder S. International Society on Thrombosis and Haemostasis score for overt disseminated intravascular coagulation predicts organ dysfunction and fatality in sepsis patients. Blood Coagul Fibrinolysis. 2006;17.

55. Kinasewitz GT, Zein JG, Lee GL, Nazir SA, Taylor Jr FB. Prognostic value of a simple evolving disseminated intravascular coagulation score in patients with severe sepsis. Crit Care Med. 2005;33:2214–21.

56. Tripodi A, Chantarangkul V, Primignani M, Fabris F, Dell'Era A, Sei C, Mannucci PM. The international normalized ratio calibrated for cirrhosis (INR(liver)) normalizes prothrombin time results for model for end-stage liver disease calculation. Hepatology. 2007;46:520–7.

57. Tripodi A, Chantarangkul V, Primignani M, Dell'Era A, Clerici M, Iannuzzi F, et al. Point-of-care coagulation monitors calibrated for the international normalized ratio for cirrhosis (INRliver) can help to implement the INRliver for the calculation of the MELD score. J Hepatol. 2009;51:288–95.

58. Kawasugi K, Wada H, Hatada T, Okamoto K, Uchiyama T, Kushimoto S, et al. Evaluation of overt DIC in various underlying disease. Thromb Res. 2011;128:186–90.

59. Asakura H, Wada H, Okamoto K, Iba T, Uchiyama T, Eguchi Y, et al. Evaluation of haemostatic molecular markers for diagnosis of disseminated intravascular coagulation in patients with infections. Thromb Haemost. 2006;95:282–7.

60. Kushimoto S, Wada H, Kawasugi K, Okamoto K, Uchiyama T, Seki Y, et al. Increased ratio of soluble fibrin formation/thrombin generation in patients with DIC. Clin Appl Thromb Hemost. 2012;18:628–32.

61. Wada H, Kobayashi T, Abe Y, Hatada T, Yamada N, Sudo A, et al. Elevated levels of soluble fibrin or D-dimer indicate high risk of thrombosis. J Thromb Haemost. 2006;4:1253–8.

62. Dempfle CE, Wurst M, Smolinski M, Lorenz S, Osika A, Olenik D, et al. Use of soluble fibrin antigen instead of D-dimer as fibrin-related marker may enhance the prognostic power of the ISTH overt DIC score. Thromb Haemost. 2004;91:812–8.

63. Okamoto K, Takaki A, Takeda S, Katoh H, Ohsato K. Coagulopathy in disseminated intravascular coagulation due to abdominal sepsis: determination of prothrombin fragment 1 + 2 and other markers. Haemostasis. 1992;22:17–24.

64. Omote M, Asakura H, Takamichi S, Shibayama M, Yoshida T, Kadohira Y, et al. Changes in molecular markers of hemostatic and fibrinolytic activation

under various sampling conditions using vacuum tube samples from healthy volunteers. Thromb Res. 2008;123:390–5.

65. Dhainaut JF, Shorr AF, Macias WL, Kollef MJ, Levi M, Reinhart K, et al. Dynamic evolution of coagulopathy in the first day of severe sepsis: relationship with mortality and organ failure. Crit Care Med. 2005;33:341–8.

66. Lavrentieva A, Kontakiotis T, Bitzani M, Papaioannou-Gaki G, Parlapani A, Thomareis O, et al. Early coagulation disorders after severe burn injury: impact on mortality. Intensive Care Med. 2008;34:700–6.

67. Gando S, Sawamura A, Hayakawa M, Hoshino H, Kubota N, Oshiro A. First day dynamic changes in antithrombin III activity after supplementation have a predictive value in critically ill patients. Am J Hematol. 2006;81:907–14.

68. Maeda K, Hirota M, Ichihara A, Ohmuraya M, Hashimoto D, Sugita H, et al. Applicability of disseminated intravascular coagulation parameters in the assessment of the severity of acute pancreatitis. Pancreas. 2006;32:87–92.

69. Fourrier F, Chopin C, Goudemand J, Hendrycx S, Caron C, Rime A, et al. Septic shock, multiple organ failure, and disseminated intravascular coagulation. Compared patterns of antithrombin III, protein C, and protein S deficiencies. Chest. 1992;101:816–23.

70. Iba T, Saito D, Wada H, Asakura H. Efficacy and bleeding risk of antithrombin supplementation in septic disseminated intravascular coagulation: a prospective multicenter survey. Thromb Res. 2012;130:e129–33.

71. Egi M, Morimatsu H, Wiedermann CJ, Tani M, Kanazawa T, Suzuki S, et al. Non-overt disseminated intravascular coagulation scoring for critically ill patients: the impact of antithrombin levels. Thromb Haemost. 2009;101:696–705.

72. Sivula M, Tallgren M, Pettila V. Modified score for DIC in the critically ill. Intensive Care Med. 2005;31:1209–14.

73. Okabayashi K, Wada H, Ohta S, Shiku H, Nobori T, Maruyama K. Hemostatic markers and the sepsis-related organ failure assessment score in patients with DIC in an intensive care unit. Am J Hematol. 2004;76:225–9.

74. Gando S, Kameue T, Nanzaki S, Nakanishi Y. Disseminated intravascular coagulation is a frequent complication of systemic inflammatory response syndrome. Thromb Haemost. 1996;75:224–8.

75. Mesters RM, Mannucci PM, Coppola R, Keller T, Ostermann H, Kienast J. Factor VIIa and antithrombin III activity during severe sepsis and septic shock in neutropenic patients. Blood. 1996;88:881–6.

76. Dixit A, Kannan M, Mahapatra M, Choudhry VP, Saxena R. Roles of protein C, protein S, and antithrombin III in acute leukemia. Am J Hematol. 2006;81:171–4.

77. Kobayashi A, Matsuda Y, Mitani M, Makino Y, Ohta H. Assessment of the usefulness of antithrombin-III in the management of DIC in obstetrically ill patients. Clin Appl Thromb Hemost. 2010;16:688–93.

78. Aibiki M, Fukuoka N, Umakoshi K, Ohtsubo S, Kikuchi S. Serum albumin levels anticipate antithrombin III activities before and after antithrombin III agent in critical patients with DIC. Shock. 2007;27:139–44.

79. Asakura H, Ontachi Y, Mizutani T, Kato M, Ito T, Saito M, et al. Decreased plasma activity of antithrombin or protein C is not due to consumption coagulopathy in septic patients with disseminated intravascular coagulation. Eur J Haematol. 2001;67:170–5.

80. Rodeghiero F, Mannucci PM, Vigano S, Barbui T, Gugliotta L, Cortellaro M, et al. Liver dysfunction rather than intravascular coagulation as the main cause of low protein C and antithrombin III in acute leukemia. Blood. 1984;63:965–9.

81. Joly B, Barbay V, Borg JY, Le Cam-Duchez V. Comparison of markers of coagulation activation and thrombin generation test in uncomplicated pregnancies. Thromb Res. 2013;132:386–91.

82. Choi Q, Hong KH, Kim JE, Kim HK. Changes in plasma levels of natural anticoagulants in disseminated intravascular coagulation: high prognostic value of antithrombin and protein C in patients with underlying sepsis or severe infection. Ann Lab Med. 2014;34:85–91.

83. Ishikura H, Nishida T, Murai A, Nakamura Y, Irie Y, Tanaka J, et al. New diagnostic strategy for sepsis-induced disseminated intravascular coagulation: a prospective single-center observational study. Crit Care. 2014;18:R19.

84. Koyama K, Madoiwa S, Tanaka S, Koinuma T, Wada M, Sakata A, et al. Evaluation of hemostatic biomarker abnormalities that precede platelet count decline in critically ill patients with sepsis. J Crit Care. 2013;28:556–63.

85. Fukao H, Ueshima S, Okada K, Yamamoto K, Matsuo T, Matsuo O. Tissue-type plasminogen activator, type 1 plasminogen activator inhibitor and their complex in plasma with disseminated intravascular coagulation. Thromb Res. 1992;68:57–65.

86. Garcia-Frade LJ, Lorente JA, Garcia-Avello A, de Pablo R, Landín L. Plasminogen activator inhibitor-1 levels determine the profibrinolytic response in disseminated intravascular coagulation. Am J Hematol. 1992;41:303–4.

87. Gando S, Nakanishi Y, Tedo I. Cytokines and plasminogen activator inhibitor-1 posttrauma disseminated intravascular coagulation: Relationship to multiorgan dysfunction syndrome. Crit Care Med. 1995;23:1835–42.

88. Watanabe R, Wada H, Miura Y, Murata Y, Watanabe Y, Sakakura M, et al. Plasma levels of total plasminogen activator inhibitor-1(PAI-1) and tPA/PAI-1 complex in patients with disseminated intravascular coagulation and thrombotic thrombocytopenic purpura. Clin Appl Thromb Haemost. 2001;7:229–33.

89. Madoiwa S, Nunomiya S, Ono T, Shintani Y, Ohmori T, Mimuro J, et al. Plasminogen activator inhibitor 1 promotes a poor prognosis in sepsis-induced disseminated intravascular coagulation. Int J Hematol. 2006;84:398–405.

90. Hatada T, Wada H, Nobori T, Okabayashi K, Maruyama K, Abe Y, et al. Plasma concentrations and importance of High Mobility Group Box protein in the prognosis of organ failure in patients with disseminated intravascular coagulation. Thromb Haemost. 2005;94:975–9.

91. Semeraro N, Ammollo CT, Semeraro F, Colucci M. Sepsis, thrombosis and organ dysfunction. Thromb Res. 2012;129:290–5.

92. Madoiwa S, Tanaka H, Nagahama Y, Dokai M, Kashiwakura Y, Ishiwata A, et al. Degradation of cross-linked fibrin by leukocyte elastase as alternative pathway for plasmin-mediated fibrinolysis in sepsis-induced disseminated intravascular coagulation. Thromb Res. 2011;127:349–55.

93. Hayakawa M, Sawamura A, Gando S, Kubota N, Uegaki S, Shimojima H, et al. Disseminated intravascular coagulation at an early phase of trauma is associated with consumption coagulopathy and excessive fibrinolysis both by plasmin and neutrophil elastase. Surgery. 2011;149:221–30.

94. Gando S, Hayakawa M, Sawamura A, Hoshino H, Oshiro A, Kubota N, et al. The activation of neutrophil elastase-mediated fibrinolysis is not sufficient to overcome the fibrinolytic shutdown of disseminated intravascular coagulation associated with systemic inflammation. Thromb Res. 2007;121:67–73.

95. Ono T, Mimuro J, Madoiwa S, Soejima K, Kashiwakura Y, Ishiwata A, et al. Severe secondary deficiency of von Willebrand factor-cleaving protease (ADAMTS13) in patients with sepsis-induced disseminated intravascular coagulation: its correlation with development of renal failure. Blood. 2006;107:528–34.

96. Matsumoto T, Wada H, Nobori T, Nakatani K, Onishi K, Nishikawa M, et al. Elevated plasma levels of fibrin degradation products by granulocyte-derived elastase in patients with disseminated intravascular coagulation. Clin Appl Thromb Hemost. 2005;11:391–400.

97. Kohno I, Inuzuka K, Itoh Y, Nakahara K, Eguchi Y, Sugo T, et al. A monoclonal antibody specific to the granulocyte-derived elastase-fragment D species of human fibrinogen and fibrin: its application to the measurement of granulocyte-derived elastase digests in plasma. Blood. 2000;95:1721–8.

98. Mochida S, Takikawa Y, Nakayama N, Oketani M, Naiki T, Yamagishi Y, et al. Diagnostic criteria of acute liver failure: A report by the Intractable Hepato-Biliary Diseases Study Group of Japan. Hepatol Res. 2011;41:805–12.

99. Pugh RN, Murray-Lyon IM, Dawson JL, Pietroni MC, Williams R. Transection of the oesophagus for bleeding oesophageal varices. Br J Surg. 1973;60:646–9.

6

Aspirin plus tirofiban inhibit the thrombosis induced by Russell's viper venom

Ren-Chieh Wu[1], Ping-Tse Chou[2] and Li-Kuang Chen[1,2,3]*

From The 9th Congress of the Asian-Pacific Society on Thrombosis and Hemostasis
Taipei, Taiwan.

Abstract

Background: Thrombosis and coagulopathy are the commonest hematological manifestations of envenomation of Russell's viper venom (RVV). Factor X is activated by a factor X-activating enzyme from Russell's viper venom (RVV-X) to start the coagulation cascade. We established an animal model with local ischemic effects induced by RVV. We tried to treat RVV envenomation with antiplatelets and anticoagulants without recourse to antivenom.

Methods: RVV was injected into the foot pad of mice. We observed the effects at different intervals and compared local changes in ischemia with drug treatment after 30 min.

Results: A combination of aspirin plus tirofiban could prevent the ischemic change induced by RVV. The antithrombotic effects of single-use of aspirin or tirofiban were better than single-use of heparin or clopidogrel.

Conclusion: The aspirin + tirofiban group had a better outcome with respect to prevention of tissue ischemia and gangrene. This indicates that the activation and aggregation of platelets is the major cause of thrombosis induced by RVV.

Keywords: Russell's viper venom, Mouse model, Thrombosis, Antiplatelet

Background

Daboia russelli ("Russell's viper") is distributed throughout ten South-East Asian countries, including Taiwan [1]. The effects of Russell's viper venom (RVV) can lead to many different severe conditions such as coagulopathy, thrombotic microangiopathy [2], stroke [3], renal failure [4], generalized increase in capillary permeability, and rhabdomyolysis and neurotoxicity. However, these effects can vary among the different subspecies [5, 6]. Incoagulable blood caused by consumption coagulopathy (including disseminated intravascular coagulation (DIC) and thrombocytopenia) is one of the commonest features and the leading cause of death due to RVV across the entire geographical distribution of the species [5–7]. DIC induced by RVV can lead to massive occlusion of

the renal microvasculature with fibrin deposition and parenchymal ischemia [8] and may be a predisposing factor of acute renal failure. Disseminated thrombus formation has been shown to develop in the large vessels of small animals bitten by Russell's viper [7, 9]. DIC with coagulation factors activated by an activator of factor X from the RVV can eventually lead to the production of stabilized fibrin, which could be the reason for vessel obstruction [7]. Systemic thrombosis was reported in 15 % of patients with systemic envenoming from *Daboia russelli formosensis* (Formosan Russell's viper) [10]. From our experience, the severity of DIC, renal failure, and thrombocytopenia caused by Formosan Russell's viper venom is associated with clinical outcome (Wu et al. unpublished data). We wanted to create an animal model for the hemorrhagic property of Formosan Russell's viper venom. Anticoagulation agents or antiplatelet agents could then be tested to see if they could prevent venom-induced thrombosis and sub sequent organ damage.

* Correspondence: lkc@tzuchi.com.tw
[1]Department of Emergency Medicine, Tzu Chi Medical Center, Hualien, Taiwan
[2]Department of Laboratory Diagnosis, School of Medicine, Tzu Chi University, Hualien, Taiwan
Full list of author information is available at the end of the article

Thrombosis occludes vessels, which then leads to local tissue ischemia; the subsequent tissue necrosis is suspected to be the leading cause of multiple-organ damage. An animal model of RVV-induced thrombosis has not been reported. We constructed an animal model with measurement of local changes in cyanosis, gangrene, mummification, and tissue necrosis after injection of a sub-lethal dose of RVV into the foot pad of mice to mimic the thrombosis caused by RVV. We then used the model to test aspirin, clopidogrel, tirofiban and heparin for the prevention of venom-induced vessel occlusion and tissue necrosis.

Methods
Materials
All snakes were obtained in eastern Taiwan. The venom of *Daboia russelli formosensis* was collected directly from the snakebite through parafilm in a test-tube every month. Each batch of venom was pooled from a one-year collection of more than eight Formosan Russell's vipers. We tested the LD50 of RVV in 25-gmice via the intraperitoneal route.

Animal model
Female NMRI mice from the National Animal Center (age, 6–8 weeks; 25 ± 3 g) were used. Aspirin, tirofiban, clopidogrel and heparin were the anticoagulant drugs used.

Prior to anticoagulant agent injections, sub-lethal doses of RVV (0.05 μL) were injected into the left foot pads of each experimental mice. This dosage was chosen because the LD_{50} through this inject route was demonstrated in literature, in tested mice, to be 0.1 μL. Subsequently, anticoagulant agents were injected via the intraperitoneal route 30 min after envenomation. The degree of local ischemic change and the change in kinetics at different time intervals were compared with the drugs treated 30 min after envenomation.

Drugs
Aspirin (brand name, Stin; manufactured by China Chemical & Pharmaceutical Company Limited, Taiwan), tirofiban (Aggrastat; MSD, USA), clopidogrel (Plavix; Sanofi Aventis, France) and heparin (Agglutex; China Chemical & Pharmaceutical) were used.

Effects of aspirin
Eighteen mice were divided into three groups of six. All mice were injected with 0.05μLvenom in the left foot pad. Group 1 was treated once with aspirin (10 mg/kg, i.p.). Group 2 was treated with aspirin once (40 mg/kg, i.p.). Group 3 was the control group and had no treatment. The observation time intervals were day-1, day-2, and day-7.

Effects of tirofiban plus another drug
Thirty mice were divided into five groups of six mice were injected with 0.05μLvenom into their left foot pad. Except for the control group, all other mice were injected with tirofiban (12 mg/kg) initially and every 8 h until the experiment was complete. Group 1 was the control group and agents were not administered. Mice in group 2 were injected with tirofiban only. Group 3 contained mice that were additionally injected once with aspirin (10 mg/kg, i.p.). Group 4 contained mice that were additionally injected once with clopidogrel (1 mg, i.p.). Group 5 contained mice that were additionally injected with heparin (5 units, i.p.). The observation time interval was 16 h and 48 h after injection.

Effects of clopidogrel and heparin
In addition to the control group, two groups of six mice were also studied. Group 1 was administered clopidogrel (1 mg/25 g weight, i.p.) and group 2 was given heparin (5 units, i.p.). Changes were observed at 8, 16, and 48 h.

Results
The thrombogenic mouse foot model
The degree and kinetics of ischemia in local tissue was constant among the six mice in each group (Tables 1 and 2). The natural course of envenoming in mice feet is shown in Fig. 1. We observed changes in mice feet at 15 min, 16 h, 48 h and 7 days after envenoming. Fifteen minutes after envenoming, local tissue cyanosis was noted. A gangrenous change in mice feet was observed 16 h after envenoming. Mummification of mice feet was observed after 48 h. Foot necrosis was observed on day7 (Fig. 1). The distinction of mummification (dry gangrene) and gangrene was made because gangrene, when properly treated, is reversible.

Table 1 Preventative effects of antiplatelets and anticoagulants against tissue ischemia induced by RVV

Treatment	Percentage of ischemic change (%)			
	Cyanosis	Gangrene	Mummification	Necrosis
Negative (venom only)	100 % (6/6)	100 % (6/6)	100 % (6/6)	100 % (6/6)
Aspirin (As) low	100 % (6/6)	100 % (6/6)	100 % (6/6)	100 % (6/6)
Aspirin high	100 % (6/6)	100 % (6/6)	0 % (0/6)	0 % (0/6)
Tirofiban(T)	100 % (6/6)	100 % (6/6)	0 % (0/6)	0 % (0/6)
Heparin (H)	100 % (6/6)	100 % (6/6)	100 % (6/6)	100 % (6/6)
Clopidogrel (C)	100 % (6/6)	100 % (6/6)	100 % (6/6)	100 % (6/6)
Ag and C	100 % (6/6)	100 % (6/6)	0 % (0/6)	0 % (0/6)
Ag and H	100 % (6/6)	100 % (6/6)	0 % (0/6)	0 % (0/6)
Ag and As	0 % (0/6)	0 % (0/6)	0 % (0/6)	0 % (0/6)

Table 2 Effects and distribution of tissue damage induced by RVV envenomation reacted with treatment of antiplatelets and anticoagulants

Treatment	Degree of ischemic change			
	Cyanosis	Gangrene	Mummification	Necrosis
Negative (venom only)[a]	All plantar	All plantar	All plantar	All plantar
Aspirin (As) low	All plantar	All plantar	3/4 plantar	1/2 plantar
Aspirin high	All plantar	1/2 plantar	none	none
Tirofiban (T)[b]	Half plantar	Digits	none	none
Heparin (H)	All plantar	1/2 plantar	1/2 plantar	1/2 plantar
Clopidogrel (C)	All plantar	1/2 plantar	1/2 plantar	1/2 plantar
Ag and C[c]	All plantar	3/4 plantar	none	none
Ag and H[c]	Digits	Digits	none	none
Ag and As[b]	none	none	none	none

[a]Reference to Fig. 1
[b]Reference to Fig. 4
[c]Reference to Fig. 5

However tissue mummification is irreversible and will ultimately lead to tissue necrosis.

Effects of aspirin at different doses

A high dose of aspirin (40 mg/kg) was better than a lower dose (10 mg/kg) (Figs. 2 and 3). Aspirin showed no obvious effects on early ischemic change in mice feet, but prevented subsequent progression to gangrene (Fig. 3). The lower-dose aspirin group showed gangrenous change 24 h after envenomation, and mummification at day7. The higher-dose aspirin group showed ischemic changes and gangrene at 24 h and 48 h; the condition of foot recovered at day7, but local swelling persisted. Overall, all mice did not completely recover,

but outcome in the treated group was better than that in the control group at identical observation points.

Combined use of tirofiban with aspirin/clopidogrel/heparin

The difference in outcome between the groups is shown in Fig. 4 and Fig. 5. The best result occurred in the tirofiban + aspirin group: the ischemia was completely prevented. Necrosis was noted at the tip of the digits in the tirofiban + heparin group. The tip of the digits and some plantar necrosis was noted in the single-use tirofiban group. Severe plantar necrosis was noted in the tirofiban + clopidogrel group. The outcome in all treated groups was better than that in the control group.

Single use of clopidogrel and heparin

The clopidogrel group was slightly better than the heparin group, but the single-use clopidogrel group and single-use heparin group had virtually no effect on the prevention of tissue necrosis and gangrene (Fig. 6 and Fig. 7). Necrosis was noted and distal digits amputated in the heparin group. The clopidogrel group showed tissue necrosis, but amputation was not necessary. The difference between the treatment group and control group was not so clear. The tirofiban group showed a better outcome than that in the heparin group and clopidogrel group at identical observation points.

Discussion

Formosan Russell's viper is the sixth most frequent cause of poisonous snakebites in Taiwan [11]. As a result of urbanization, Formosan Russell's vipers have gradually moved towards undeveloped regions. The time interval between snakebite and administration of antivenom is

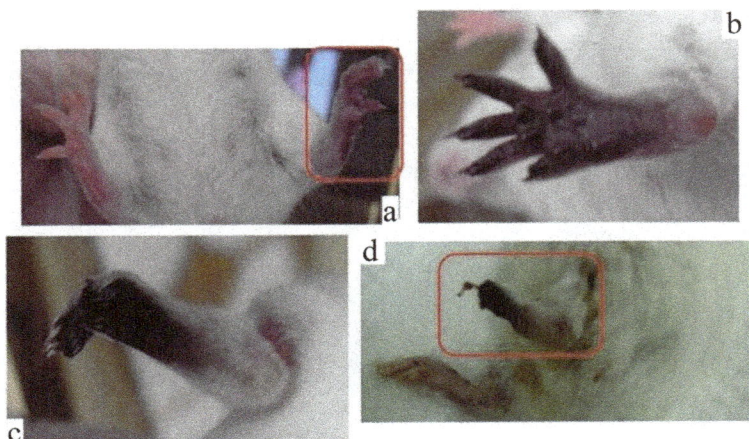

Fig. 1 The natural course of venom, injected at foot of mice. **a** venom injected 15 min later. **b** venom injected 1 day later. **c** venom injected 2 days later. **d** venom injected 7 days later

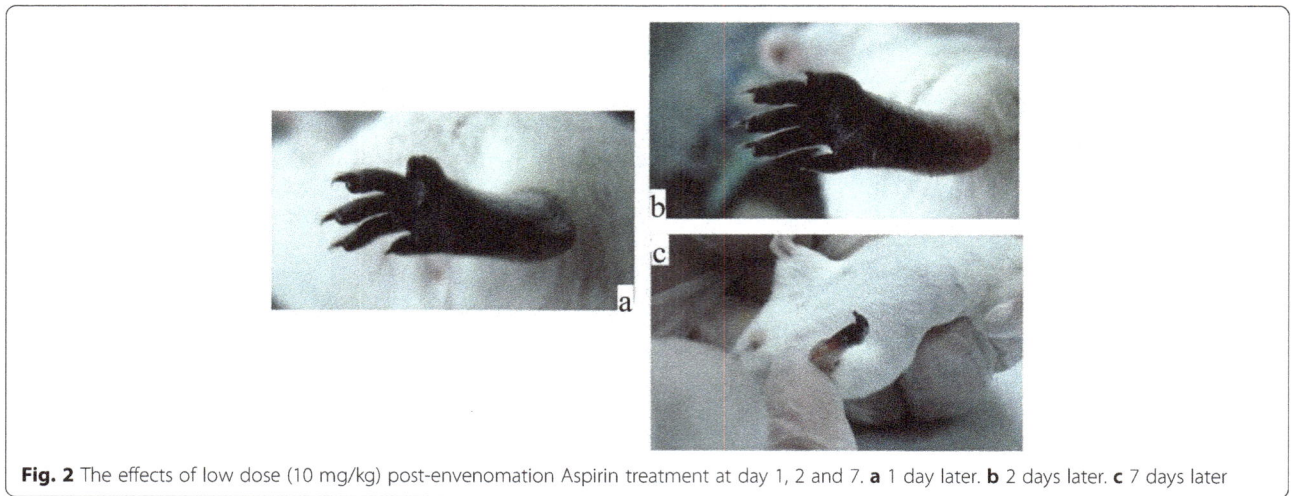

Fig. 2 The effects of low dose (10 mg/kg) post-envenomation Aspirin treatment at day 1, 2 and 7. **a** 1 day later. **b** 2 days later. **c** 7 days later

the major factor of successful treatment [12, 13]. Patients bitten by Formosan Russell's viper (particularly in southern and eastern Taiwan) are usually far away from hospitals that have this antivenom, so replacing the antivenom with another medical treatment is crucial. Coagulopathy is the major effect of RVV envenomation [3, 14]. We tested various antiplatelets and anticoagulants to control the effect of coagulopathy to improve the outcome of RVV envenomation.

The component RVV-X in RVV acts on factor X to increase the amount of thrombin. An increased concentration of thrombin activates platelets and enhances clot formation. Platelet-rich clots are resistant to fibrinolysis [15]. Antiplatelet agents may help to prevent further activation and aggregation of platelets, and reduce the ratio of platelets compared with other components in clots.

Aspirin alone at a high dose showed obvious protection from venom-induced ischemia and necrosis of

tissue (Fig. 3). The effect of aspirin was dose-dependent, but the adverse effects of high-dose aspirin are internal bleeding and bleeding tendency, and the dose is relatively high in humans. The recommended maximum dose of aspirin for anti-inflammatory purposes is 4500 mg/day [16]. Aspirin is relatively inexpensive and readily available in pharmacies. It has been used for decades as an analgesic and for the prevention of thrombosis. Aspirin can be used via the oral route and is very convenient for using outside the hospital setting. For reducing aspirin dosage, we tried to combine it with other drugs.

From the results of combined use of dual antiplatelet agents, tirofiban + aspirin produced a better outcome than that in the other groups (Fig. 4 and Table 1). All mice feet fully protected without the use of antivenom. The aspirin dose was reduced from 40 mg/kg to 10 mg/kg, an acceptably low analgesic dose [16]. The effect of tirofiban + heparinon outcome was moderate. However,

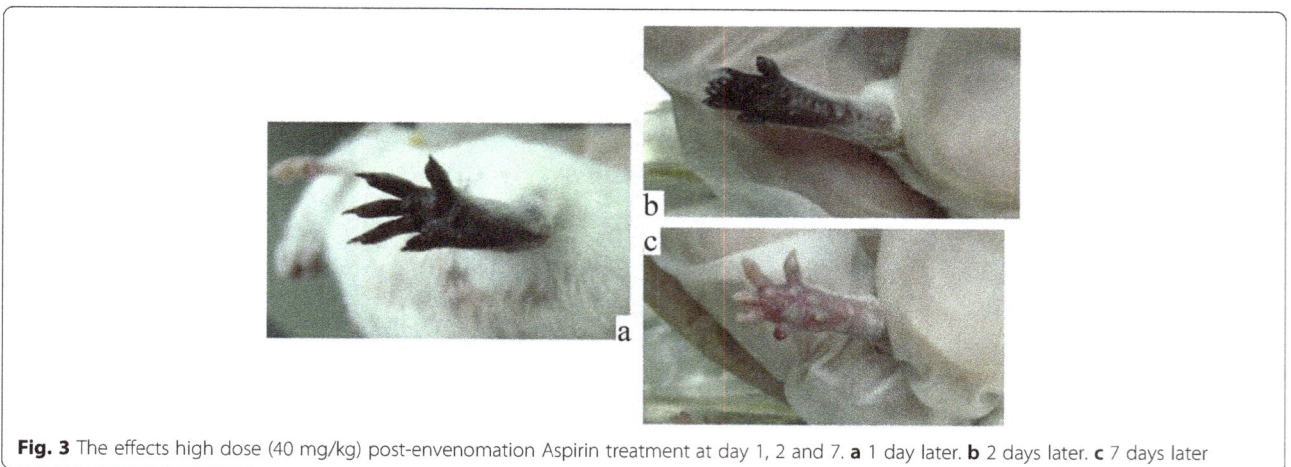

Fig. 3 The effects high dose (40 mg/kg) post-envenomation Aspirin treatment at day 1, 2 and 7. **a** 1 day later. **b** 2 days later. **c** 7 days later

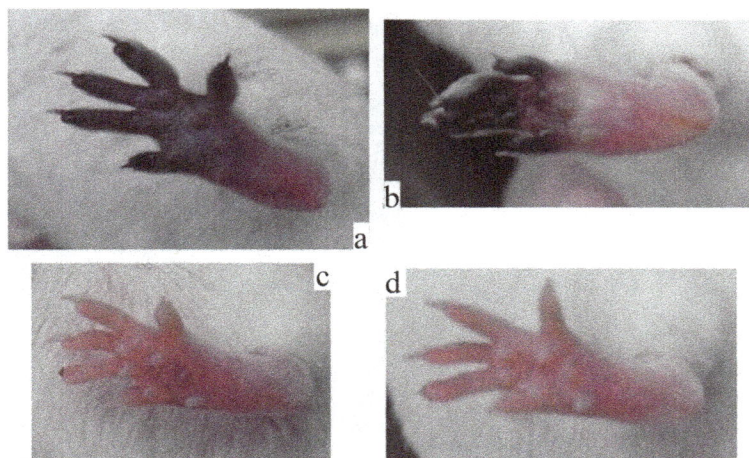

Fig. 4 The effects of post-envenomation treatment with tirofiban and aspirin. **a** One day after tirofiban treatment. **b** Two days after tirofiban treatment. **c** One day after tirofiban + aspirin treatment. **d** Two days after tirofiban + aspirin treatment

the recovery in mice feet was partial, and the toe tips were necrotized, but outcome was better than in the single-use tirofiban group. The tirofiban + clopidogrel group showed no difference from the control group. Tirofiban + aspirin could completely reverse the thrombotic effects induced by the venom toxin of Formosan Russell's viper without the use of antivenom.

Aspirin is well known for its antiplatelet properties, and is used to treat ischemic stroke, angina and acute myocardial infarction [17]. Aspirin irreversibly inactivates cyclooxygenase and then blocks thromboxane formation [18]. Thromboxane acts as a strong signal to amplify platelet activation by inducing irreversible platelet aggregation [19]. Thromboxane inhibits the activity of adenyl cyclase, leading to intraplatelet activation signals [20]. A decreased level of thromboxane inhibits the aggregation of platelets at injured endothelium, and blocks clot formation [21].

Heparin is used in stroke [22], acute coronary syndrome [23], deep-vein thrombosis [24–27], pulmonary embolism [24–27] and in cardiopulmonary bypass due to its anticoagulation effects. Heparin combined with antithrombin then inactivates thrombin, but has no effects on thrombin already adhered to fibrin [28]. The heparin–antithrombin complex can inhibit activation of factor X with high specificity [29], but heparin has little effect on already formed clots [30].

ADP binds to the Gq-protein-linked P2Y1 receptor on platelets, causing a change in cell shape, calcium mobilization, and initiation of reversible aggregation [31]. ADP also binds to the Gi-linked P2Y12 receptor on platelets to amplify aggregation via adenylylcyclase-mediated production of cyclic AMP [32]. Several studies reported the important role of the P2Y12 receptor in platelet thrombus formation and stabilization of collagen-coated

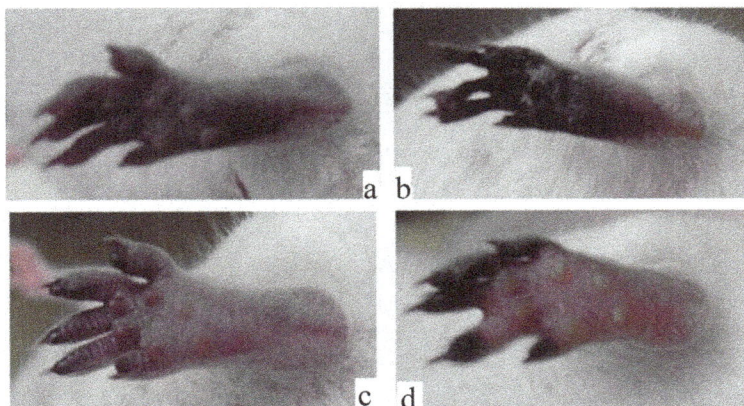

Fig. 5 The effects of post-envenomation treatment with tirofiban, and clopidogrel or heparin. **a** One day after tirofiban + clopidogrel treatment. **b** Two days after tirofiban + clopidogrel treatment. **c** One day after tirofiban + heparin treatment. **d** Two days after tirofiban + heparin treatment

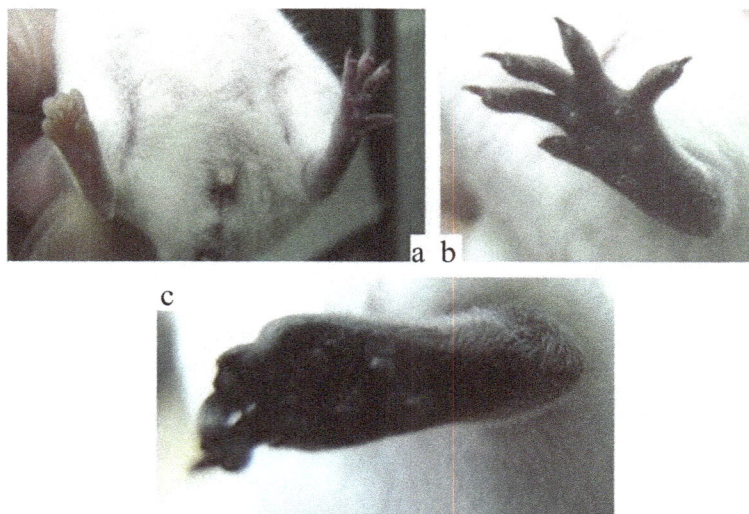

Fig. 6 The effects of post-envenomation treatment with a single dose of clopidogrel. **a** clopidogrel (1 mg/BW 25 g) 8 h later. **b** clopidogrel (1 mg/BW 25 g) 1 day later. **c** clopidogrel (1 mg/BW 25 g) 2 days later

surfaces under flow conditions [33–35]. The resulting platelet activation triggers a conformational change in glycoprotein IIb/IIIa receptors, which increases their affinity for fibrinogen. Clopidogrel acts on the ADP receptor on the platelet surface and inhibits platelet activation [36, 37], but has no effects on collagen-mediated activation and aggregation of platelets. We hypothesize that the observed endothelial damages were results of the exposure of collagen fibers to zinc metalloproteinase haemorrhagins that are present in RVV. This hypothesis may explain the lack of platelet inhibition by clopidogrel in this study.

Tirofiban is non-peptide small molecule that acts as an inhibitor of the glycoprotein IIb/IIIa receptor complex on the surface of platelets. It is used with aspirin or heparin in the treatment of angina and non-Q myocardial infarction [23]. The surface glycoproteins of platelets can combine with exposed collagen fibers in the vessel wall. Inhibition of platelet adherence to collagen fibers can prevent platelets from activation and aggregation, thereby stopping clot formation.

Aspirin inhibits the aggregation of platelets and stabilizes platelets, preventing activation then blocking clot formation. The inhibition is irreversible until new platelets are produced. Combined use of a glycoprotein IIb/IIIa inhibitor and aspirin stabilized platelets from activation and stopped clot formation. Platelet phospholipids

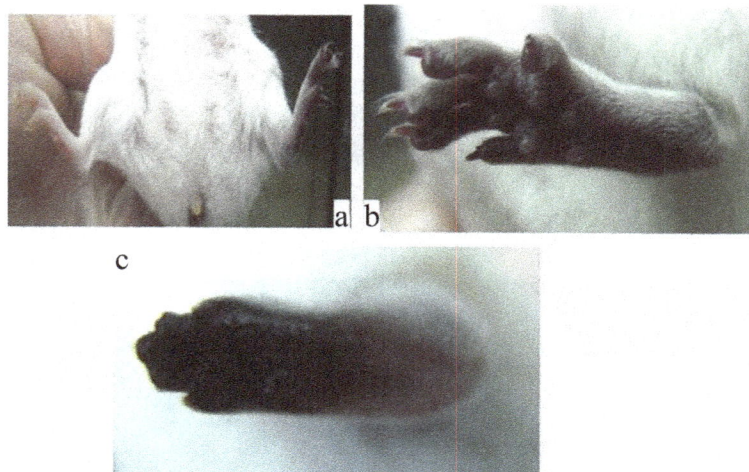

Fig. 7 The effects of post-envenomation treatment with a single dose of heparin. **a** heparin(5U/BW 25 g) 8 h later. **b** heparin(5U/BW 25 g) 1 day later. **c** heparin(5U/BW 25 g) 2 days later

help to activate factor X in the intrinsic pathway, and the formation of thrombin from prothrombin in extrinsic and intrinsic pathways. Platelet stabilization therefore prevents prothrombin being formed from thrombin. McFarlane was the first to identify activation off actor X in RVV [38–40]. RVV-X (the factor X-activating enzyme from RVV) has been well characterized as a proteinase [41, 42]. Irrespective of the rapidity of treatment for RVV envenomation, the RVV-X in venom will act as factor X before treatment to start to coagulation cascade. RVV-X acts before heparin in almost all conditions of envenoming, and coagulation started immediately after envenoming, Heparin works as an anticoagulant to prevent further clotting but cannot inhibit the action of platelets, and has no effect on clotting that has already occurred. Heparin therefore cannot reverse the effects of RVV for tissue ischemia and gangrene. Outcome in the aspirin plus tirofiban group with respect to prevention of tissue ischemia and gangrene was better than that in the heparin group. This indicated that the activation and aggregation of platelets was the major reason for thrombosis induced by RVV.

Conclusion

Polyvalent antivenom is the "gold-standard" treatment for envenomation of Formosan Russell's viper. However, antivenom just neutralizes the snake toxin to block the subsequent coagulation cascade, but there is no evidence that it affects already formed fibrin (or even thrombosis). The reversal and prevention of toxin-induced DIC and renal failure of antivenom is effective only if administered early. From the present study, aspirin + tirofiban showed an excellent outcome without the need for antivenom. We suggest the use of aspirin plus tirofiban should be used for envenomation by Russell's viper irrespective of whether specific antivenom is available or not. Antivenom is reserved and prescribed only in specific hospitals in Taiwan, but aspirin and tirofiban are available in most hospitals. The accessibility of aspirin is much higher than antivenom, particularly for mountaineers and villagers far from such specialist hospitals. For victims of snakebites far away from such hospitals, we tried to afford effective and safe first-aid to prevent the adverse effects of RVV.

Authors' contribution
R-CW was a graduate student, had prepared the medicines for experiments and first manuscript of this article. P-T C was a research assistant, had performed the foot pad injections and measurements in mice. L-K C was principle investigator of this project had completed the experiment design, supervises and final manuscript of this article. All authors read and approved the final manuscript.

Competing interests
The authors declare that they have no competing interest.

Author details
[1]Department of Emergency Medicine, Tzu Chi Medical Center, Hualien, Taiwan. [2]Department of Laboratory Diagnosis, School of Medicine, Tzu Chi University, Hualien, Taiwan. [3]Branch of Clinical Pathology, Department of Laboratory Medicine, Tzu Chi Medical Center, Hualien, Taiwan.

References
1. Wüster W, Golay P, Warrell DA. Synopsis of recent development in venomous snake systematic. Toxicon. 1997;35(3):319–40.
2. Isbister GK. Snake bite Does't Cause Disseminated Intravascular Coagulation: Coagulopathy and Thrombotic Microangiopathy in Snake Envenoming. Semin Thromb Hemost. 2010;36(4):444–51.
3. Gawarammana I, Menchs S, Jeganathan K. Acute Ischemic Stroke due to bites by Daboiarusselli in Sri Lanka – First authenticated case series. Toxicon. 2009;54(4):421–8.
4. Suntravat M, Yusuksawad M, Sereemaspun A, Pérez JC, Nuchprayoon I. Effect of purified Russell's viper venom-factor X activator (RVV-X) on renal hemodynamics, renal functions, and coagulopathy in rats. Toxicon. 2011;58(3):230–8.
5. Warrell DA. Snake venoms in science and clinical medicine. 1. Russell's viper: biology, venom and treatment of bites. Trans R Soc Trop Med Hyg. 1989;83(6):732–40.
6. Myint-Lwin, Warrell DA, Phillips RE, Tin-Nu-Swe, Tun-Pe, Maung-Maung-Lay. Bites by Russell's viper (Viper russelli siamensis) in Burma: hemostatic, vascular and renal disturbance and response to treatment. Lancet. 1985; 2 (8467): 1259-64
7. Phillips RE, Theakston RDG, Warrell DA, Galigedara Y, Abeysekera DT, Dissanayaka P, Huton RA, Aloysius DJ. Paralysis, rhabdomyolysis and hemolysis cause by bites of Russell's viper (Viper russelli pulchella) in Sri Lanka: failure of Indian (Haffkine) antivenom. Q J Med. 1988;68(257):691–716.
8. Than-Than, Francis N, Tin-Nu-Swe, Myint-Lwin, Tun-Pe, Soe-Soe, Maung-Maung O, Phillips RE, Warrell DA. Contribution of focal hemorrhage and microvascular fibrin deposition to fatal envenoming by Russell's viper (Viper russelli siamensis) in Bruma. Acta Tropica.1989; 46 (1): 23-38
9. Lee CY. Toxicological studies on the venom of Viper russelli formosensis. Part 1. Toxicity and pharmacological properties. J Formos Med Assoc. 1948;47:65–98.
10. Hung DZ. Taiwan's venomous snakebite: epidemiological, evolution and geographic differences. Trans R Soc Trop Med Hyg. 2004;98(2):96–101.
11. Hung DZ, Wu ML, Deng JF, Lin-Shiau SY. Russell's viper snakebites in Taiwan: differences from other Asian countries. Toxicon. 2002a; 40(9): 1291-8.
12. Hung DZ, et al. Antivenom treatment and renal dysfunction in Russell's viper snakebite in Taiwan: a case series. Trans R Soc Trop Med Hyg. 2006; 100(5):489–94.
13. Maduwage K, Isbister GK. Current Treatment for Venom-Induced Consumption Coagulopathy Resulting from Snakebite. PLoS Negl Trop Dis. 2014;8(10):e3220. doi:10.1371/journal.pntd.0003220.
14. Narang SK, Paleti S, Asad MA, Samina T. Acute ischemic infarct in the middle cerebral artery territory following a Russell's viper bite. Neurol India. 2009;57(4):479–80.
15. Collet JP, Montalesco G, Lesty C, Weisel JW. A structural and dynamic investigation of the facilitating effect of glycoprotein IIb/IIIa inhibitors in dissolving platelet-rich clots. Circ Res. 2002;90(4):428–34.

16. Katzung BG. Basic and Clinical Pharmacology, 10th edition. International edition. New York, NY: McGraw-Hill; 2007a; pp. 576 Table 36-1.

17. Antithrombotic Trialists's Collaboration. Collaborative meta-analysis of randomized trials of antiplatelet therapy for prevention of death, myocardial infarction, and stroke in high risk patients. BMJ. 2002;324(7329):71–86.

18. Katzung BG. Basic and Clinical Pharmacology, 10th edition. International edition. New York, NY: McGraw-Hill; 2007b; pp. 300.

19. Quinn M, Fitzgerald D. Platelet function. New Jersey U.S.A.: Human Press; 2005. p. 270.

20. Raychowdhury MK, Yukawa M, Collins LJ, et al. Alternative splicing produces a divergent cytoplasmic tail in the human endothelial thromboxane A2 receptor. J Biol Chem. 1994;269(30):19256–61.

21. Katzung BG. Basic and Clinical Pharmacology, 10th edition. International edition. New York, NY: McGraw-Hill; 2007c; pp. 295 and 299.

22. Adams Jr HP, del Zoppo G, Alberts MJ, et al. Guidelines for the early management of adults with ischemic stroke: a guideline from the American Heart Association/American Stroke Association Stroke Council, Clinical cardiology Council, Cardiovascular Radiology and Interventional Council, and the Atherosclerotic Peripheral Vascular Disease and Quality of Care Outcomes in Research Interdisciplinary Working Groups: the American Academy of Neurology affirms the value of this guideline as an educational tool for neurologists. Stoke. 2007;38(5):1655–711.

23. Anderson JL, Adams CD, Antman EM, et al. ACC/AHA guidelines for the management of patients with unstable/angina/non-ST-Elevation myocardial infarction; a report of the American College of Cardiology/American Heart Association Task Force on Practice Guidelines (Writing Committee to Revise the 2002 Guidelines for the Management of Patients With Unstable Anginal/Non-ST-Elevation Myocardial infarction) developed in collaboration with the American College of Emergency Physicians, the Society for Cardiovascular Angiography and Interventions, and the Society of Thoracic Surgeons endorsed by the American Association of Cardiovascular and Pulmonary Rehabilitation and the Society for Academic Emergency Medicine. J Am Coll Cardiol. 2007;50(7):e1–e157.

24. Barritt DW, Jordon PM. Anticoagulant drugs in the treatment of pulmonary embolism: a controlled trial. Lancet. 1960;1(7138):1309–12.

25. Theroux P, Ouimet H, McCans J, Latour JG, Joly P, Levy G, et al. Aspirin, heparin, or both to treat acute unstable angina? N Engl J Med. 1988;319(17):1105–11.

26. Hull RD, Raskob GE, Hirsh J, Jay RM, Leclerc JR, Geerts WH, et al. Continuous intravenous heparin compared with intermittent subcutaneous heparin in the initial treatment of proximal-vein thrombosis. N Engl J Med. 1986; 315(18):1109–14.

27. Turpie AG, Robinson JG, Doyle DJ, Mulji AS, Mishkel GJ, Sealey BJ, et al. Comparison of high-dose with low-dose subcutaneous heparin to prevent left ventricular mural thrombosis in patients with acute transmural anterior myocardial infarction. N Engl J Med. 1989;320(6):352–7.

28. Katzung BG. Basic and Clinical Pharmacology, 10th edition. International edition. New York, NY: McGraw-Hill; 2007d; pp. 546.

29. Katzung BG. Basic and Clinical Pharmacology, 10th edition. International edition. New York, NY: McGraw-Hill; 2007e; pp. 543 Figure 34-1.

30. Hirsh J. Heparin. N Engl J Med. 1991;324(22):1565–74.

31. Hechler B, Leon C, Vial C, Vigne P, Frelin C, Cazenave JP, Gachet C. The P2Y1 receptor is necessary for adenosine 5'-diphosphate-induced platelet aggregation. Blood. 1998;92(1):152–9.

32. Communi D, Janssens R, Suarez-Huerta N, Robaye B, Boeynaems JM. Advances in signaling by extracellular nucleotides, the role and transduction mechanisms of P2Y receptors. Cell Signal. 2000;12(6):351–60.

33. Cattaneo M, Savage B, Ruggeri Z. Effects of pharmacological inhibition of the P2Y1 and P2Y12 ADP receptors on shear-induced platelet aggregation and platelet thrombus formation on a collagen-coated surface under flow condition. Blood. 2001;98:239a.

34. Turner NA, Moake JL, McIntire LV. Blockade of adenosine diphosphate receptors P2Y12 and P2Y1 is required to inhibit platelet aggregation in whole blood under flow. Blood. 2001;98(12):3340–5.

35. Goto S, Tamura N, Eto K, Ikeda Y, Handa S. Functional significance of adenosine 5'-diphosphage receptor (P2Y12) in platelet activation initiated by binding of von Willebrand factor to platelet GP Ibalpha induced by conditions of high shear rate. Circulation. 2002;105(21):2531–6.

36. Hung DZ, Wu ML, Deng JF, Yang DY, Lin-Shiau. Multiple thrombotic occlusions of vessel after Russell's viper envenoming. Pharmacol Toxicol. 2002b; 91(3): 106-10

37. Schrör K. Clinical pharmacology of the adenosine diphosphate (ADP) receptor antagonist, clopidogrel. Vascular Med. 1998;3(3):247–51.

38. Tans G, Rosing J. Snake Venom Activators of Factor X: An overview. Haemostasis. 2001;31(3-6):225–33.

39. Yamada D, Sekiy F. Prothrombin and factor X activator activities in the venoms of Viperidae snakes. Toxicon. 1997;35(11):1581–9.

40. MacFarlane RG. The coagulant action of Russell's viper venom: the use of antivenom in defining its reaction with a serum factor. Br J Haematol. 1961;7:496–511.

41. Furie BC, Furie B. Coagulant protein of Russell's viper venom. Methods Enzymol. 1976;45:191–205.

42. Takeya H, Nishida S, Miyata T, et al. Coagulation factor X activating enzyme from Russell's viper venom (RVV-X). A novel metalloproteinase with disintegrin (platelet aggregation inhibitor)-like and C-type lectin-like domains. J Biol Chem. 1992;267(20):14109–17.

7

The reversal effect of prothrombin complex concentrate (PCC), activated PCC and recombinant activated factor VII against anticoagulation of Xa inhibitor

Nina Haagenrud Schultz[1,2,3,4*], Hoa Thi Tuyet Tran[1,3], Stine Bjørnsen[1], Carola Elisabeth Henriksson[5], Per Morten Sandset[1,2,4] and Pål Andre Holme[1,2,4]

Abstract

Background: An increasing number of patients are treated with direct-acting oral anticoagulants (DOACs), but the optimal way to reverse the anticoagulant effect is not known. Specific antidotes are not available and prothrombin complex concentrate (PCC), activated PCC (aPCC) and recombinant factor VIIa (rFVIIa) are variously used as reversal agents in case of a major bleeding. We aimed to determine the most effective haemostatic agent and dose to reverse the effect of rivaroxaban in blood samples from patients taking rivaroxaban for therapeutic reasons.

Methods: Blood samples from rivaroxaban-treated patients ($n = 50$) were spiked with PCC, aPCC and rFVIIa at concentrations imitating 80%, 100% and 125% of suggested therapeutic doses. The reversal effect was assessed by thromboelastometry in whole blood and a thrombin generation assay (TGA) in platelet-poor plasma. Samples from healthy subjects ($n = 40$) were included as controls.

Results: In thromboelastometry measurements, aPCC and rFVIIa had a superior effect to PCC in reversing the rivaroxaban-induced lenghtening of clotting time (CT). aPCC was the only haemostatic agent that shortened the CT down to below the control level. Compared to healthy controls, patients on rivaroxaban also had a prolonged lag time and decreased peak concentration, velocity index and endogenous thrombin potential (ETP) in platelet-poor plasma. aPCC reversed these parameters more effectively than rFVIIa and PCC. There were no differences in efficacy between 80%, 100% and 125% doses of aPCC.

Conclusions: aPCC seems to reverse the anticoagulant effect of rivaroxaban more effectively than rFVIIa and PCC by evaluation with thromboelastometry and TGA in vitro.

Keywords: Rivaroxaban, Reversal, Prothrombin complex concentrate, Activated prothrombin complex concentrate, Recombinant aFVIIa

Background

The efficacy and safety of direct-acting oral anticoagulants (DOACs), including the factor Xa inhibitor rivaroxaban, in the prevention and treatment of thromboembolic disorders have been demonstrated in a number of clinical studies [1, 2]. It is documented that the associated bleeding risk is lower for rivaroxaban than for warfarin [3]. Spontaneous and trauma-induced bleeding episodes do, however, still occur in patients on DOACs [4, 5]. Large phase 3 studies have shown that the relative risk of major bleeding is 1.1% for patients taking DOACs compared to 1.8% in patients taking warfarin. Real-world data from observational studies confirm these results [6–8]. Guidelines for treatment of major bleedings on rivaroxaban are inconsistent [9, 10]. Although routines for supportive treatment, such as fluid replacement and blood transfusions, topical haemostatic measures and charcoal administration in case

* Correspondence: schultzj@online.no
[1]Research Institute of Internal Medicine, Oslo University Hospital, Box 4950 Nydalen, N-0424 Oslo, Norway
[2]Department of Haematology, Oslo University Hospital, Box 4950 Nydalen, N-0424 Oslo, Norway
Full list of author information is available at the end of the article

of recent tablet intake have been established, there is not a consensus on how to reverse the anticoagulant effect of rivaroxaban in case of major or life-threatening bleeding. A generic reversal agent of factor Xa inhibitors, andexanet alpha, has shown promising results [11], but no antidote is yet commercially available.

Three haemostatic agents have been suggested as surrogate antidotes, but the documentation on the effect and optimal dosage is limited and divergent. Four-factor prothrombin complex concentrate (PCC) is used as an antidote to warfarin, replacing coagulation factors II, VII, IX, and X in their zymogen or inactive forms. Haemophiliacs with inhibitors are treated with recombinant activated factor VII (rFVIIa) and/or activated PCC (aPCC) containing coagulation factors II, IX, and X, and FVIIa. Several studies have evaluated the reversing effect of these surrogate antidotes on haemostatic parameters in animals [12, 13] and by using blood from healthy subjects taking rivaroxaban or blood spiked with rivaroxaban ex vivo [14–20]. It has been shown that different PCCs incompletely reverse the anticoagulation effect of rivaroxaban on the thrombin generation assay (TGA) parameter endogenous thrombin potential (ETP) [21], and there is increasing evidence suggesting that aPCC and rFVIIa have a better effect [14, 17, 19]. To our knowledge, the reversing effect of those agents has not yet been studied on patients taking rivaroxaban for therapeutic reasons.

The aims of the present study were to compare PCC, aPCC and rFVIIa as surrogate antidotes in 50 patients on therapeutic rivaroxaban doses, and to find the most effective dose to reverse the anticoagulant effect of rivaroxaban in these patients.

Methods
Study design
This is an in vitro study where the ability of PCC, aPCC and rFVIIa to reverse the effect of rivaroxaban was tested in blood collected from patients treated with rivaroxaban.

Participants
Fifty patients treated with therapeutic doses of rivaroxaban for various approved indications and 40 healthy controls, without previous history of vascular disease, were recruited in the study. Patients between 18 and 85 years of age who had taken rivaroxaban for more than two months were eligible. Controls were recruited from the same age group. Ongoing treatment with antiplatelet drug(s) and/or non-steroidal antiinflammatory drug(s) was an exclusion criterium for both patients and controls. All participants gave written informed consent, and the study was approved by the Norwegian regional committee for medical and health research ethics.

Haemostatic agents and doses
We evaluated the following reversal agents in this study: 4-PCC (Cofact®, Sanquin, Amsterdam, the Netherlands), aPCC (FEIBA®, Baxter AG, Vienna, Austria) and rFVIIa (Novoseven®, NovoNordisk, Copenhagen, Denmark). The concentrations included in this study were chosen to imitate 80%, 100% and 125% of the doses suggested for clinical use in case of a major bleeding in a patient treated with a DOAC according to existing guidelines. For PCC the suggested 100% dose is 40 IU/kg, aPCC 50 IU/kg and rFVIIa 90 µg/kg [22]. The drugs were dissolved in sterile water to stock solutions of 34 IU/mL PCC, 34 IU/mL aPCC and 68 µg/mL rFVIIa. Doses of the spiked haemostatic agents were calculated assuming that an adult had 65 mL blood/kg.

Blood collection
Blood was collected from an antecubital vein of the patients through a 21Gx19 mm butterfly needle (Vacuette® Greiner Bio-One GmbH, Kremsmunster, Austria) with minimal use of stasis. The first 2-4 mL of blood was discarded. The blood collection tubes for the measurements of thrombin generation and thromboelastometry (0,109 M citrate Monovette®, Sarstedt, Nümbrecht, Germany) were manually prefilled with Corn Trypsin Inhibitor (CTI) (Haematologic Tecnologies Incorporates, Essex Junction, VT, USA) at a final concentration of 20 µg/mL. Test tubes that were not filled completely were discarded. For anti-FXa activity measurements we used 4.5 mL Vacutainer® tubes (Becton-Dickinson, Franklin Lakes, NJ, USA) containing 0.5 mL 0.109 M buffered citrate without CTI. The blood sampling was performed at the time of presumed peak concentration of rivaroxaban in the patients, about 2 h after the drug intake.

Preparations
For measurements of rivaroxaban concentration by an anti-FXa activity assay, citrated plasma was obtained after centrifugation for 15 min at 2000 g in RT. The supernatant was carefully collected and stored at -80 °C for 2–3 months before measurements of anti-FXa activity were performed.

Whole blood containing CTI for measurements of thromboelastometry and thrombin generation from each patient was pooled and divided into 10 aliquots of 5 mL. Haemostatic agents were added in the doses mentioned above, and one aliquot was always left untreated to represent the baseline value.

Aliquots of whole blood spiked with three different haemostatic agents at increasing concentrations and the untreated aliquot were incubated at 37 °C for 30 min. Then the samples were further subdivided. Platelet-poor plasma (PPP) was obtained by centrifugation for 13 min at 12000 g in RT, and the supernatant was carefully collected. PPP was immediately frozen and stored at -80 °C for 1–3 months before measurement of thrombin generation. The remaining whole blood was incubated at 37 °C for another 30–90 min before measurements by thromboelastometry were performed.

Anti-FXa activity measurements
To measure rivaroxaban concentration in citrated plasma, an anti-FXa activity method calibrated for rivaroxaban was performed on STA-R Evolution® coagulometer (Diagnostica Stago S.A.S., Asnières sur Seine, France) [23] according to the manufacturer's instructions.

Thrombin generation assay
Thrombin generation was measured in PPP using the Calibrated Automated Thrombogram (CAT) (Diagnostica Stago, Asnière, France) with the Thrombinoscope software (Thrombinoscope BV®, Maastricht, The Netherlands) [24, 25]. PPP, supplemented with the three different reversal agents in three different concentrations, were run in triplicates. The thrombin generation parameters lag time, peak of maximum thrombin concentration, velocity index and the total amount of thrombin generated, i.e. endogenous thrombin potential (ETP), were recorded. The PPP reagent containing 5 pM TF and 4 µM phospholipids was used to initiate thrombin generation.

Thromboelastometry
CTI-containing whole blood (with reversal agents in three different concentrations) were run in duplicates and the clotting time (CT; seconds), clot formation time (CFT; seconds), maximum velocity (MaxV; mm/s), area under curve (AUC) and maximum clot firmness (MCF; mm) were measured by ROTEM® (TEM Innovations, Munich, Germany) with low tissue factor activated ROTEM [26]. Prior to measurements, the plastic test cups were prepared with 40 µL buffer (a mixture of equal parts of buffer 1: 20 mM Hepes, 150 mM NaCl, pH 7.4 and buffer 2: 20 mM Hepes, 150 mM NaCl, 200 mM $CaCl_2$, pH 7.4). Recombinant relipidated TF (Innovin®, Dade Behring, Liederbach, Germany) diluted in a total volume of 20 µL of buffer 1 was also added. To initiate the reaction, whole blood (280 µL) was added and the total volume of reagents and whole blood in each cup was 340 µL. The final TF dilution was 1:70 000, corresponding to a theoretical concentration of 0.35 pM.

Statistical analysis
The analysis of variance (ANOVA-test) was used followed by the post-hoc test Tukey multiple comparison. Statistical calculations were performed by using SPSS version 21 (SPSS, Inc, Chicago, USA) and statistical significance was set to $p < 0.05$.

The Spearman's rank correlation coefficient was used when assessing the relationship between rivaroxaban concentration and coagulation parameters. The data are expressed as mean value with a 95% confidence interval (CI 95%) or one standard deviation (SD).

Results
Between October 2014 and May 2015, 50 patients treated with therapeutic doses of rivaroxaban were enrolled in the study at Akershus University Hospital. In the same time period 40 controls were included. All 50 patients used 20 mg of rivaroxaban once daily. The indications for rivaroxaban treatment were deep vein thrombosis, pulmonary embolism and atrial fibrillation. The main characteristics of patients and controls are displayed in Table 1.

Anti-FXa activity measurements
The mean rivaroxaban concentration in the patient group was 216.7 ng/mL (95% CI 188.2–245.3). Rivaroxaban concentrations were compared to thromboelastometry parameters in whole blood and to TGA parameters in PPP. Only data for CT and ETP are shown. The Spearman's correlation coefficient between rivaroxaban concentration and CT was 0,68 ($p < 0.005$) (Fig. 1a). There was also a linear negative correlation between rivaroxaban levels and ETP in PPP ($r = -0.72$; $p < 0.005$) (Fig. 1b).

Thrombin generation
Rivaroxaban affected all thrombin generation parameters in PPP. Mean lag time was prolonged more than 3-fold relative to untreated controls (mean difference 6.5 min, 95% CI 5.7–7.3). Peak concentration was reduced by almost 90% (mean difference 167.1 nM, 95% CI

Table 1 Characteristics of patients and controls

	Patients (n = 50)	Controls (n = 40)
Age – years	53.1 (14.9)	50.3 (12.8)
Weight – kg	87.1 (16.5)	-
Time after intake – minutes	130.1 (14.9)	-
Platelet count – x 10^9/L	142.6 (54.7)	171.8 (54.3)
Platelet count in PRP – x 10^9/L	146.3 (44.5)	152.4 (26.0)
Rivaroxaban dose (mg od)	20	0
Sex (female)	26 (52%)	24 (60%)
Deep vein thrombosis	21 (42%)	-
Pulmonary embolism	28 (56%)	-
Atrial fibrillation	1 (2%)	-

Values are given in mean (SD) or n (%)

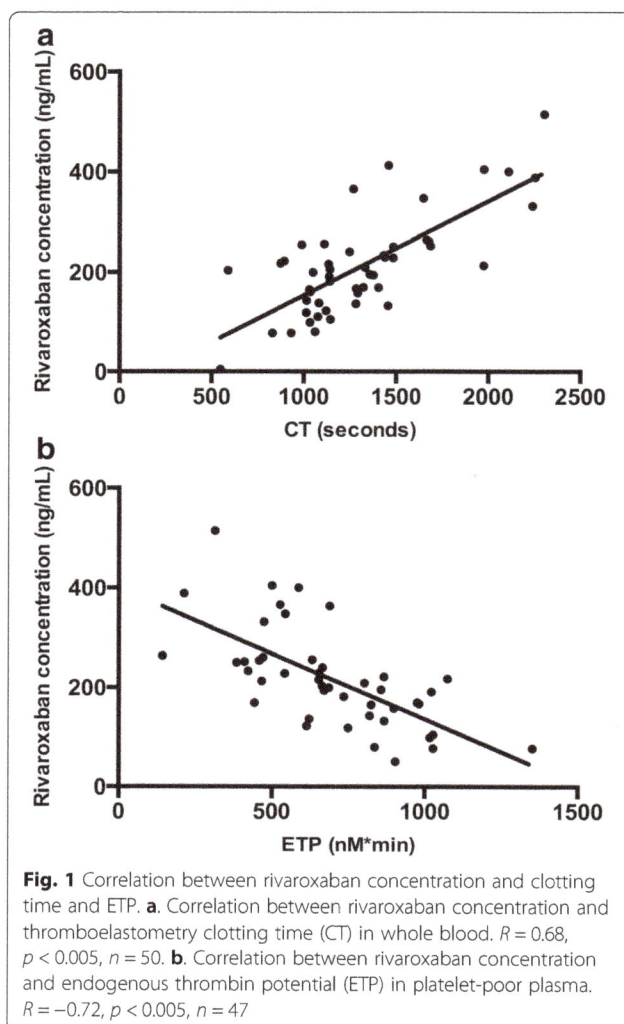

Fig. 1 Correlation between rivaroxaban concentration and clotting time and ETP. **a**. Correlation between rivaroxaban concentration and thromboelastometry clotting time (CT) in whole blood. $R = 0.68$, $p < 0.005$, $n = 50$. **b**. Correlation between rivaroxaban concentration and endogenous thrombin potential (ETP) in platelet-poor plasma. $R = -0.72$, $p < 0.005$, $n = 47$

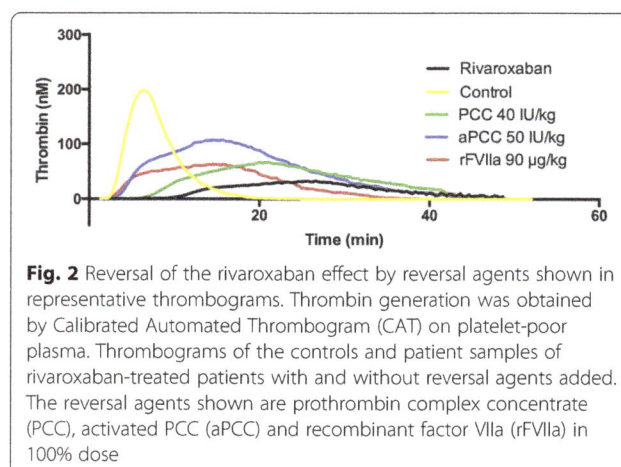

Fig. 2 Reversal of the rivaroxaban effect by reversal agents shown in representative thrombograms. Thrombin generation was obtained by Calibrated Automated Thrombogram (CAT) on platelet-poor plasma. Thrombograms of the controls and patient samples of rivaroxaban-treated patients with and without reversal agents added. The reversal agents shown are prothrombin complex concentrate (PCC), activated PCC (aPCC) and recombinant factor VIIa (rFVIIa) in 100% dose

161.6–172.7), Velocity Index (VI) by approximately 97% (mean difference 58.2 nM/min, 95% CI 57.8–58.6) and ETP by approximately 40% (mean difference 532.9 nM*min, 95% CI 416.0–649.8) (Fig. 2).

The haemostatic agents improved the thrombin generation parameters at varying degrees. PCC in a 100% dose did not cause a significant shortening of the lag time (mean difference 1.6 min, 95% CI 1.1–2.2). rFVIIa in 100% dose (90 μg/kg) was more effective than PCC in shortening the lag time (mean difference 6.6 min, 95% CI 5.7–7.4) but this effect was not significantly different from aPCC 100% dose which shortened lag time by 50% (mean reduction 5.5 min, 95% CI 4.7–6.3) (Fig. 3a). PCC in a 100% dose almost doubled peak concentration (mean difference 37.7 nM, 95% CI 29.5–45.9), and so did the 100% dose of rFVIIa (mean difference 36.1 nM, 95% CI 30.2–42.0). However, both those agents were less effective than aPCC 100% which caused an increase in peak concentration by 400% (mean difference 83.9 nM,

95% CI 71.4–96.4) (Fig. 3b). The velocity index (VI) was increased by 240% by PCC 100% (mean difference 3.0 nM/min, 95% CI 2.3–3.8), and by 400% by rFVIIa 100% (mean difference 6.2 nM/min, 95% CI 4.6–7.9). aPCC in the 100% dose had a significantly better reversal effect increasing VI than PCC and rFVIIa and increased VI by 800% (mean difference 12.9 nM/min, 95% CI 9.6–14.6) (Fig. 3c). The total amount of thrombin generated, ETP, was increased by the 100% dose of PCC by 130% (mean difference 802.5 nM*min, 95% CI 649.2–955.8), and by the 100% dose of rFVIIa by 80% (mean difference 452.7 nM*min, 95% CI 365.7–539.7). The 100% dose of aPCC had a more pronounced effect than PCC and rFVIIa and increased ETP by 235% (mean difference 1382.5 nM*min, 95% CI 1203.1–1561.9) (Fig. 3d).

There was not a dose–response relationship for any of the reversal agents on any of the TGA parameters. aPCC 125% of the suggested dose in clinical use reversed the TGA parameters in a similar manner to the 80% dose aPCC (lag time: $p = 0.99$, peak concentration: $p = 1.0$, velocity index: $p = 0.99$, ETP: $p = 0.6$). Furthermore the reversing effect of the lowest dose aPCC (80%) was more pronounced than the highest dose of PCC (125%) in all TGA parameters ($p < 0.005$) (Fig. 3a-d).

Thromboelastometry

Compared to controls, rivaroxaban doubled the CT (mean difference 674.4 s, 95% CI 527.8–820.9) (Table 2). PCC shortened the rivaroxaban-induced prolongation of CT by 25% (mean difference 386.9 s, 95% CI 263.0–510.8) and there was not a significant difference between the 80%, 100% and 125% doses (32 IU/kg, 40 IU/kg or 50 IU/kg). Adding rFVIIa caused a shortening of the CT by approximately 40% (mean difference 636.6 s, 95% CI 523.4–747.7) and aPCC shortened CT by 60% (mean difference 892.1 s, 95% CI 762.2–1022.1). There was not a significant difference between rFVIIa and aPCC in a 100%

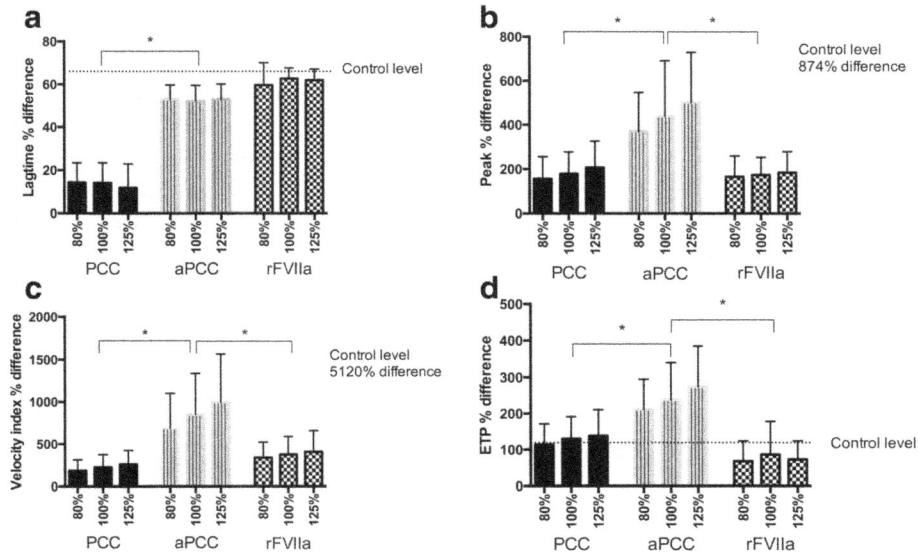

Fig. 3 Difference in thrombin generation parameters after adding reversal agents in different doses. Differences in thrombin generation parameters are expressed as per cent difference from baseline (rivaroxaban with no haemostatic agent added). The doses of the haemostatic agents are 80%, 100% and 125% of the suggested doses, as described under study design. **a**. Lag time obtained by Calibrated Automated Thrombogram (CAT) on platelet-poor plasma (minutes); **b**. Peak height of thrombin obtained by CAT on platelet-poor plasma (nM); **c**. Velocity index obtained by CAT on platelet-poor plasma (nM/min); **d**. Endogenous Thrombin Potential (ETP) obtained by CAT on platelet-poor plasma (nM*min). Control level, the difference between the mean control value and the patient baseline values, is illustrated by the dotted line. *$p < 0.005$. PCC: prothrombin complex concentrate, aPCC: activated PCC, rFVIIa: recombinant factor VIIa

dose nor between the highest doses of these haemostatic agents. However, aPCC was the only haemostatic agent that shortened CT down below the level of the controls, and the 80% dose of aPCC was more effective than the highest dose (125%) of PCC ($p < 0.005$) (Fig. 4a)th=tlb=

Treatment with rivaroxaban (Table 2) and addition of haemostatic agents (data not shown) influenced CFT in the same manner as CT. However, neither rivaroxaban (Table 2) nor the haemostatic agents (data not shown) affected the thromboelastometry parameters MCF, maxV and AUC.

Subgroup analysis - patients with a high rivaroxaban concentration

A subgroup analysis was performed on the patients with the highest rivaroxaban concentrations, defined by a

Table 2 Thromboelastometry results before adding haemostatic agents

	Patients	Controls	p-value
Clotting time (CT) - sec	1379.4 (510.2)	705.8 (198.1)	<0.001
Clot formation time – sec	278.6 (157.0)	187.6 (40.1)	<0.001
Maximum clot firmness – mm	57.4 (9.7)	56.0 (5.2)	0.12
Maximum velocity – mm/s	7.0 (5.5-9.0)[a]	8.0 (7.0-10.0)[a]	0.83
Area under the curve –mm x sec	5695.3 (1103.5)	5620.4 (498.1)	0.11

Numbers are given as mean (SD) if not otherwise specified
[a]Median (interquartile range)

rivaroxaban concentration >300 ng/L (mean 400.6 ng/mL, 95% CI 335.3–466.0) ($n = 6$). Those patients had the longest CT in WB (mean clotting time 2425.6 s, 95% CI 1774.8–3076.3) and lowest ETP in PPP (mean ETP 531.1 nM/min, 95% CI-187.7–1249.9). We found the same pattern as in the main analysis, i.e. that aPCC increased ETP more than PCC ($p < 0.001$) and rFVIIa ($p < 0.001$). All three haemostatic agents reduced the CT in the subgroup analysis, but there was not a significant difference between the three drugs ($p = 1.0$) (Fig. 4b).

Discussion

In the present study we evaluated the ability of three different non-specific reversal agents, PCC, aPCC, and rFVIIa, to reverse the anticoagulant effect of rivaroxaban. The TGA and thromboelastometry parameters affected by rivaroxaban were improved by all three haemostatic agents, but at various degrees. In summary, aPCC reversed rivaroxaban-induced changes in TGA (velocity index, peak height and ETP) more efficiently than PCC and rFVIIa. Also, the rivaroxaban-induced prolongation of CT in whole blood was shortened more efficiently by aPCC and rFVIIa than PCC. Adding aPCC even brought the CT to below the level of the controls, and also increased the ETP to above the control level. Furthermore, we did not find an additional effect by increasing the dose of aPCC from 80% to 125% in the

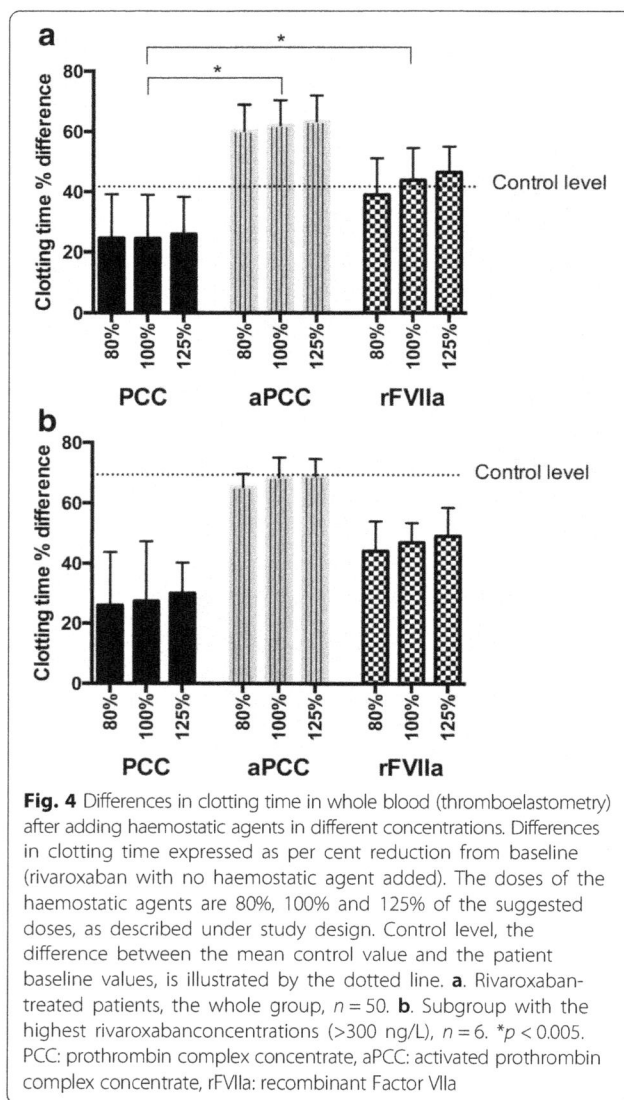

Fig. 4 Differences in clotting time in whole blood (thromboelastometry) after adding haemostatic agents in different concentrations. Differences in clotting time expressed as per cent reduction from baseline (rivaroxaban with no haemostatic agent added). The doses of the haemostatic agents are 80%, 100% and 125% of the suggested doses, as described under study design. Control level, the difference between the mean control value and the patient baseline values, is illustrated by the dotted line. **a**. Rivaroxaban-treated patients, the whole group, n = 50. **b**. Subgroup with the highest rivaroxabanconcentrations (>300 ng/L), n = 6. *p < 0.005. PCC: prothrombin complex concentrate, aPCC: activated prothrombin complex concentrate, rFVIIa: recombinant Factor VIIa

all components of the coagulation cascade in physiologic concentrations, mostly in inactive forms, and is traditionally used to reverse the effect of Warfarin. Because rivaroxaban specifically inhibits FXa, replacing all factors in an inactive form is not considered as an effective treatment of a major bleeding.

The fact that PCC is widely used as a reversal agent in rivaroxaban-treated patients is partly based on findings in the study performed by Eerenberg et al. [16] where the effect of PCC as an effective reversal agent was demonstrated. In another study, Zhou et al. [13] found that PCC 50 IU/kg had effect impairing increase of cererebral haematoma induced by rivaroxaban in mice. In these studies, aPCC was not evaluated and thereafter, several studies have shown that PCC has an insufficient effect in reversing the coagulation parameters (ETP and prothrombin time in PPP) altered by rivaroxaban [21]. Furthermore, Escolar et al. and Perzborn et al. have shown that aPCC and rFVIIa had a superior effect compared to PCC in shortening the CT in whole blood (thromboelastometry) and aPCC had a better effect in improving TGA parameters in rivaroxaban-spiked samples [17, 19].

Our results were also partly in line with a study performed by Herrmann and colleagues where 15 patients treated prohylactically with a low dose of rivaroxaban before orthopaedic surgery were included [27]. Here PCC and aPCC proved to be more effective reversal agents than rFVIIa, but, in contrast to our study rivaroxaban did not affect the thromboelastometry parameters CT and CFT. However, Herrmann and coauthors included patients with lower doses of rivaroxaban and a lower mean concentrations of rivaroxaban may therefore be a reasonable explanation for this difference. Another possible explanation may be different sampling conditions of whole blood (without CTI) and the use of different initiating reagents.

In our study, there was not a significant difference in efficacy between the different doses of aPCC. One explanation for the lack of dose-dependency might be that the amount of TF used to initiate the thrombin generation was too high to detect minor dose–response relationships for the reversal agents. Another reason for the lack of dose–response relationship may be that the maximum effect has already been reached at a dose of 80% aPCC. Whether this is the case in vivo, is not known. We did not test higher doses because this information in clinical practice is not considered useful. To test lower doses, however, could have given us interesting information.

There are concerns about the thrombogenicity of the haemostatic agents we have studied [28–30] and clinical data about thromboembolic complications associated with reversal of DOACs are limited. Cases have been reported where aPCC has been administrated to patients

assays used in this study. Our finding, i.e. that aPCC was the most effective drug, is in accordance with previous studies performed on healthy volunteers [14, 17, 19].

In this study we used the 4-factor PCC, Cofact®, which does not contain any heparin. However, to exert an antithrombotic effect, protein C and S are present in Cofact®, but this is not the case for aPCC or rFVIIa which are pure factor concentrates. How protein C and S influence the results is not known, and it is possible that their presence is the reason for the inferior effect of PCC to reverse the anticoagulant effect of rivaroxaban in this study. One possible way to find this out would be to use a 4-factor PCC which does not contain any natural anticoagulants, for example PPSB-S.D (Solvent Detergent)®(CAF-DCF, Belgium). The effect of fresh frozen plasma (FFP) has not been investigated in this study. FFP is derived from whole blood and contains

under DOAC treatment with an intracranial bleeding, and an increased risk of thrombosis was not observed [31–34]. One of the questions we asked in our study was whether a lower dose of a haemostatic agent than the guidelines recommend would be sufficient to reverse the anticoagulation effect of rivaroxaban. Because the lowest dose of aPCC (80%) was significantly more effective in reversing rivaroxaban-induced alterations in the coagulation assays than the highest doses PCC and rFVIIa, and because aPCC reversed ETP and CT to beyond the levels of the controls, one might speculate that even a lower dose of aPCC than 80% could be sufficient for reversing the rivaroxaban-induced changes. A lower dose might also reduce the risk of thromboembolic events.

Different doses of rivaroxaban to imitate an overdose situation were not included in this study. We did, however, a subgroup analysis ($n = 6$) of the patients with the highest rivaroxaban concentrations (>300 ng/mL). Those six patients also had the longest clotting time in whole blood. and the lowest ETP in PPP. Like in the main patient group we found that the reversing effect of aPCC was superior to the other reversal agents measured by ETP in PPP but we did not see a difference between the reversal agents in shortening of the CT. However, the lack of statistical difference of the post-hoc test might be due to the low number of cases in the subgroup.

A limitation of our study is that it was an in vitro study and will therefore not completely reflect the in vivo situation. In contrast to previous studies, we recruited patients taking rivaroxaban for therapeutic reasons which may have given us results closer to a real life situation. A positive impact of aPCC on the clinical outcome of an actively bleeding patient receiving rivaroxaban has been reported in several cases. This is, however, not studied in clinical trials [31–34]. It is also a general issue whether coagulation assays are predictive to assess the risk of bleeding. Only randomized clinical trials may be able to give such information.

Conclusions

The haemostatic agent aPCC reversed rivaroxaban-induced changes in TGA parameters more efficiently than PCC and rFVIIa, and thromboelastometry parameters more efficiently than PCC in vitro. We studied three different concentrations of PCC, aPCC and rFVIIa and did not find a dose–response relationship in any of these drugs. Given the potential prothrombotic effect of these drugs, doses beyond suggestions in guidelines should be avoided.

We found a strong correlation between ETP and CT and the rivaroxaban concentration. However, future studies are needed to evaluate if these parameters can be used to identify a clinically relevant hypocoagulability or non-compliance in rivaroxaban-treated patients.

Abbreviations

aPCC: Acivated prothrombin complex concentrate; CAT: Calibrated automated thrombogram; CFT: Clot formation time; CT: Clotting time; CTI: Corn trypsin inhibitor; DOAC: Direct-acting oral anticoagulant; ETP: Endogenous thrombin potential; MCF: Maximum clot firmness; PCC: Prothrombin complex concentrate; PPP: Platelet-poor plasma; rFVIIa: Recombinant activated Factor VII; ROTEM: Rotational Thromboelastometry; RT: Room temperature; TGA: Thrombin generation assay; VI: Velocity Index

Acknowledgements

The authors would like to thank Marissa LeBlanc and Richard Lee for statistical assistance and the Department of Medical Biochemistry at Oslo University Hospital for performing the anti-Xa assays.

Funding

The study was financially supported by an unrestricted research grant from Bayer, Germany.

Authors' contributions

NHS performed the experiments, interpreted the data and drafted the manuscript. HTTT designed and planned the study and contributed to the manuscript. SB performed the experiments, supervised in the laboratory work and contributed to the manuscript. PMS and CEH added useful information in the research process and revised and made relevant additions to the manuscript. PAH planned the study, analysed the data and revised the manuscript. All authors read and approved the final manuscript.

Competing interests

The study was financially supported by an unrestricted research grant from Bayer, Germany to author Pål Andre Holme. The other authors declare that they have no competing interests.

Author details

[1]Research Institute of Internal Medicine, Oslo University Hospital, Box 4950 Nydalen, N-0424 Oslo, Norway. [2]Department of Haematology, Oslo University Hospital, Box 4950 Nydalen, N-0424 Oslo, Norway. [3]Department of Haematology, Akershus University Hospital, N-1478 Lørenskog, Norway. [4]Institute of Clinical Medicine, Faculty of Medicine, University of Oslo, Box 1171 Blindern, N-0318 Oslo, Norway. [5]Department of Medical Biochemistry, Oslo University Hospital, Box 4950 Nydalen, N-0424 Oslo, Norway.

References

1. van Es N, Coppens M, Schulman S, Middeldorp S, Büller HR. Direct oral anticoagulants compared with vitamin K antagonists for acute venous thromboembolism: evidence from phase 3 trials. Blood. 2014;124:1968–75.
2. Yeh CH, Hogg K, Weitz JI. Overview of the new oral anticoagulants: opportunities and challenges. Arterioscler Thromb Vasc Biol. 2015;35:1056–65.
3. Coleman CI, Antz M, Bowrin K, Evers T, Simard EP, Bonnemeier H, et al. Real-world evidence on stroke prevention in patients with atrial fibrillation in the United States: the REVISIT-US study. Curr Med Res Opin. 2016;32:2047–53.
4. Patel MR, Mahaffey KW, Garg J, Pan G, Singer DE, Hacke W, et al. Rivaroxaban versus warfarin in nonvalvular atrial fibrillation. N Engl J Med. 2011;365(10):883–91.

5. Eerenberg ES, Middeldorp S, Levi M, Lensing AW, Büller HR. Clinical impact and course of major bleeding with rivaroxaban and vitamin K antagonists. J Thromb Haemost. 2015;13:1590–6.

6. Fontaine GV, Mathews KD, Woller SC, Stevens SM, Lloyd JF, Evans RS. Major bleeding with dabigatran and rivaroxaban in patients with atrial fibrillation: a real-world setting. Clin Appl Thromb Hemost. 2014;20:665–72.

7. Larsen TB, Rasmussen LH, Skjøth F, Lip GY. Efficacy and safety of dabigatran etexilate and warfarin in "real-world" patients with atrial fibrillation: a prospective nationwide cohort study. J Am Coll Cardiol. 2013;61:2264–73.

8. Kucher N, Aujesky D, Beer JH, Mazzolai L, Baldi T, Banyai M, et al. Rivaroxaban for the treatment of venous thromboembolism. The SWIss Venous ThromboEmbolism Registry(SWIVTER). Thromb Haemost. 2016;116:472–9.

9. Pernod G, Albaladejo P, Godier A, Samama CM, Susen S, Gruel Y, et al. Management of major bleeding complications and emergency surgery in patients on long-term treatment with direct oral anticoagulants, thrombin or factor-Xa inhibitors: proposals of the working group on perioperative haemostasis (GIHP) - March 2013. Arch Cardiovasc Dis. 2013;106:382–93.

10. Kaatz S, Kouides PA, Garcia DA, Spyropolous AC, Crowther M, Douketis JD, et al. Guidance on the emergent reversal of oral thrombin and factor Xa inhibitors. Am J Hematol. 2012;87:S141–5.

11. Siegal DM, Curnutte JT, Connolly SJ, Lu G, Conley PB, Wiens BL, et al. Andexanet Alfa for the Reversal of Factor Xa Inhibitor Activity. N Engl J Med. 2015;373:2413–24.

12. Perzborn E, Gruber A, Tinel H, Marzec UM, Buetehorn U, Buchmueller A, et al. Reversal of rivaroxaban anticoagulation by haemostatic agents in rats and primates. Thromb Haemost. 2013;110:162–72.

13. Zhou W, Zorn M, Nawroth P, Bütehorn U, Perzborn E, Heitmeier S, et al. Hemostatic therapy in experimental intracerebral hemorrhage associated with rivaroxaban. Stroke. 2013;44:771–8.

14. Arellano-Rodrigo E, Lopez-Vilchez I, Galan AM, Molina P, Reverter JC, Carné X, et al. Coagulation Factor Concentrates Fail to Restore Alterations in Fibrin Formation Caused by Rivaroxaban or Dabigatran in Studies With Flowing Blood From Treated Healthy Volunteers. Transfus Med Rev. 2015;29:242–9.

15. Dinkelaar J, Molenaar PJ, Ninivaggi M, de Laat B, Brinkman HJ, Leyte A. In vitro assessment, using thrombin generation, of the applicability of prothrombin complex concentrate as an antidote for Rivaroxaban. J Thromb Haemost. 2013;11:1111–8.

16. Eerenberg ES, Kamphuisen PW, Sijpkens MK, Meijers JC, Buller HR, Levi M. Reversal of rivaroxaban and dabigatran by prothrombin complex concentrate: a randomized, placebo-controlled, crossover study in healthy subjects. Circulation. 2011;124:1573–9.

17. Escolar G, Arellano-Rodrigo E, Lopez-Vilchez I, Molina P, Sanchis J, Reverter JC, et al. Reversal of rivaroxaban-induced alterations on hemostasis by different coagulation factor concentrates - in vitro studies with steady and circulating human blood. Circ J. 2015;79:331–8.

18. Marlu R, Hodaj E, Paris A, Albaladejo P, Cracowski JL, Pernod G. Effect of non-specific reversal agents on anticoagulant activity of dabigatran and rivaroxaban: a randomised crossover ex vivo study in healthy volunteers. Thromb Haemost. 2012;108:217–24.

19. Perzborn E, Heitmeier S, Laux V, Buchmüller A. Reversal of rivaroxaban-induced anticoagulation with prothrombin complex concentrate, activated prothrombin complex concentrate and recombinant activated factor VII in vitro. Thromb Res. 2014;133:671–81.

20. Korber MK, Langer E, Ziemer S, Perzborn E, Gericke C, Heymann C. Measurement and reversal of prophylactic and therapeutic peak levels of rivaroxaban: an in vitro study. Clin Appl Thromb Hemost. 2014;20:735–40.

21. Dzik WH. Reversal of oral factor Xa inhibitors by prothrombin complex concentrates: a re-appraisal. J Thromb Haemost. 2015;13:S187–94.

22. Weitz JI, Quinlan DJ, Eikelboom JW. Periprocedural management and approach to bleeding in patients taking dabigatran. Circulation. 2012;126:2428–32.

23. Samama MM, Contant G, Spiro TE, Perzborn E, Flem LL, Guinet C, et al. Evaluation of the anti-factor Xa chromogenic assay for the measurement of rivaroxaban plasma concentrations using calibrators and controls. Thromb Haemost. 2012;107:379–87.

24. Hemker HC, Giesen P, Al Dieri R, Regnault V, de Smedt E, Wagenvoord R, et al. Calibrated automated thrombin generation measurement in clotting plasma. Pathophysiol Haemost Thromb. 2003;33:4–15.

25. Hemker HC, Al Dieri R, de Smedt E, Béguin S. Thrombin generation, a function test of the haemostatic-thrombotic system. Thromb Haemost. 2006;96:553–61.

26. Sørensen B, Johansen P, Christiansen K, Woelke M, Ingerslev J. Whole blood coagulation thrombelastographic profiles employing minimal tissue factor activation. J Thromb Haemost. 2003;1:551–8.

27. Herrmann R, Thom J, Wood A, Phillips M, Muhammad S, Baker R. Thrombin generation using the calibrated automated thrombinoscope to assess reversibility of dabigatran and rivaroxaban. Thromb Haemost. 2014;111:989–95.

28. Kohler M, Hellstern P, Lechler E, Uberfuhr P, Müller-Berghaus G. Thromboembolic complications associated with the use of prothrombin complex and factor IX concentrates. Thromb Haemost. 1998;80:399–402.

29. Aledort LM. Factor VIII inhibitor bypassing activity (FEIBA) - addressing safety issues. Haemophilia. 2008;14:39–43.

30. O'Connell KA, Wood JJ, Wise RP, Lozier JN, Braun MM. Thromboembolic adverse events after use of recombinant human coagulation factor VIIa. JAMA. 2006;295:293–8.

31. Messana E, Wilson SS. Activated Pcc (Feiba) for Reversal of Rivaroxaban-Induced Life-Threatening Bleeding-a Case Series. Crit Care Med. 2015;43:303.

32. Maurice-Szamburski A, Graillon T, Bruder N. Favorable outcome after a subdural hematoma treated with feiba in a 77-year old patient treated with rivaroxaban. J Neurosurg Anesthesiol. 2014;26:183.

33. Kiraly A, Lyden A, Periyanayagam U, Chan J, Pang PS. Management of hemorrhage complicated by novel oral anticoagulantsin the emergency department: case report from the northwestern emergency medicine residency. Am J Ther. 2013;20:300–6.

34. Dibu JR, Weimer JM, Ahrens C, Manno E, Frontera JA. The role of FEIBA in reversing Novel Oral Anticoagulants in Intracerebral Hemorrhage. Neurocrit Care. 2016;24:413–9.

8

Clinical evaluation of thrombotic microangiopathy: identification of patients with suspected atypical hemolytic uremic syndrome

Yu-Min Shen

From The 9th Congress of the Asian-Pacific Society on Thrombosis and Hemostasis
Taipei, Taiwan.

Abstract

Atypical hemolytic uremic syndrome (aHUS) is a rare genetic disorder caused by defective complement regulation resulting in thrombotic microangiopathy (TMA). Patients can present as children or adults. The syndrome consists of hemolytic anemia with schistocytosis, thrombocytopenia, significant renal damage, and/or other organ system dysfunction(s). Patients with aHUS may succumb to the complications of the disease with the very first manifestation; surviving patients often suffer from progressive organ dysfunction with significant morbidity and mortality despite plasma infusion or plasma exchange. Eculizumab, a humanized monoclonal antibody to C5, was approved for treatment of aHUS in 2011. This is an expensive but highly effective therapy changing the lives and improving the outcome of patients with aHUS. Making timely and accurate diagnosis of aHUS can be life-saving if eculizumab treatment is begun promptly. Finding a genetic mutation in a complement regulatory protein is diagnostic with the appropriate clinical syndrome, but at least 30 % of patients do not have defined or reported mutations. Thus the diagnosis rests on the clinical acumen of the physician. However, the clinical manifestations of aHUS are shared by other etiologies of thrombotic microangiopathy. While laboratory finding of undetectable ADAMTS13 activity defines TTP, distinguishing aHUS from the other causes of TMA remains an art. In addition, aHUS can be unmasked by conditions with enhanced complement activation, such as systemic lupus erythematosus, pregnancy, malignant hypertension, and hematopoietic stem cell transplantation. Thus if TMA occurs in the setting of enhanced complement activation, one must consider aHUS as an underlying etiology, especially if treatment of the condition does not resolve the TMA.

Keywords: Thrombotic microangiopathy, Atypical hemolytic uremic syndrome, Thrombotic thrombocytopenic purpura, Complement dysregulation

Abbreviations: ADAMTS13, A dysintegrin and metalloproteinase with thrombospondin type 1 motif, member 13; AFLP, Acute fatty liver of pregnancy; aHUS, Atypical hemolytic uremic syndrome; APS, Antiphospholipid syndrome; CFH, Complement factor H; CFI, Complement factor I; DAT, Direct antiglobulin test; DIC, Disseminated intravascular coagulation; GvHD, Graft versus host disease; HELLP, Hemolysis elevated liver enzymes and low platelets; HSCT, Hematopoietic stem cell transplantation; HTN, Hypertension; LDH, Lactate dehydrogenase; MAHA, Microangiopathic hemolytic anemia; MCP, Membrane cofactor protein; SLE, Systemic lupus erythematosus; TM, Thrombomodulin; TMA, Thrombotic microangiopathy; TTP, Thrombotic thrombocytopenic purpura

Correspondence: yu-min.shen@utsouthwestern.edu
Department of Internal Medicine, University of Texas Southwestern Medical
Center, Dallas, TX 75390-8852, USA

Background

The clinical syndrome of organ dysfunction, microangiopathy hemolytic anemia and thrombocytopenia, most often caused by various forms of thrombotic microangiopathy, is a diagnostic enigma for the clinicians at the frontlines evaluating the critically ill. Historically, with poor understanding of pathophysiologic mechanisms, and plasma exchange being the only accepted therapy, recognition of the clinical syndrome was all that was needed to manage such patients. The precise understanding of the diagnostic entities within this syndrome in the last two decades, and availability of a specific therapeutic option, are forcing clinicians to retool their knowledge base in order to better serve their patients. This article reviews the distinction between atypical hemolytic uremic syndrome and other causes of thrombotic microangiopathy, especially thrombotic thrombocytopenic purpura, and proposes a diagnostic/management algorithm.

Review

What is thrombotic microangiopathy?

Thrombotic microangiopathy (TMA) is a pathologic condition with abnormalities in the blood vessel walls of arterioles and capillaries resulting in microvascular thrombosis [1]. There are several disease states that can lead to TMA (Table 1) [2, 3]. Clinically TMA is nearly always accompanied by microangiopathic hemolytic anemia (MAHA), a non-immune hemolytic anemia resulting from intravascular red cell fragmentation with schistocytosis and thrombocytopenia due to consumption. The direct antiglobulin test (DAT) is negative, and lactate dehydrogenase (LDH) is typically markedly elevated; bilirubin is modestly increased, while haptoglobin is undetectable. MAHA is most often caused by TMA, but intravascular devices such as prosthetic heart valve or left ventricular assist devices may also cause MAHA. In addition, many systemic disorders can be associated with MAHA with or without TMA (Table 2) [2, 3]. Rarely paroxysmal nocturnal hemoglobinuria and heparin-induced thrombocytopenia can present with MAHA and thrombocytopenia. It takes an astute clinician with the proper laboratory acumen to decipher the underlying cause of TMA/MAHA in a given patient.

Hemolytic uremic syndromes and TTP

Hemolytic uremic syndrome (HUS) affects children and adults, and is characterized by MAHA, thrombocytopenia, and significant renal dysfunction. In most cases HUS is caused by Shiga-toxin bearing E coli; rarely pneumococcal infection can also lead to HUS [4]. However, in a small minority of patients, with so-called atypical hemolytic uremic syndrome (aHUS), no infectious agent is found. aHUS is a rare genetic disorder characterized by complement-mediated TMA resulting from mutations affecting the regulation of the alternative complement pathway. Numerous loss of function mutations in factor H, factor I, membrane cofactor protein, thrombomodulin, as well as gain of function mutations in C3 and factor B, have been discovered [5]. Patients present at all stages of life despite the genetic nature of the disease, and it is poorly understood what protects the patients from having disease manifestations until later in life. Historically, HUS and aHUS are discussed in the setting of thrombotic thrombocytopenic purpura (TTP), as the pathophysiology underlying these disorders were not known, and the clinical presentations are often indistinguishable. Since the reports of absolute ADAMTS13 deficiency (von Willebrand factor-cleaving metalloprotease) in TTP caused by autoimmune antibody to ADAMTS13 in 1998 by Tsai [6] and Furlan [7], TTP is now recognized as a distinct disorder

Table 1 Causes of TMA

Thrombotic thrombocytopenic purpura (TTP)	Absence of ADAMTS13, the von Willebrand factor cleaving metalloprotease. Acquired due to autoimmune antibody to ADAMTS13, or hereditary (Upshaw-Schulman syndrome).
Infectious hemolytic uremic syndrome (ST-HUS)	Shiga toxins produced by Shigella dysenteriae and some serotypes of Escherichia coli (O157:H7 and O104:H4), cause direct damage to kidney epithelial and mesangial cells, and vascular endothelial cells. Rarely pneumococcus or other infectious agents with neuraminidase can expose the Thomsen-Friedenreich antigen on cell surfaces to result in hemolysis and direct endothelial injury.
Atypical or complement-mediated HUS	Hereditary deficiency of complement regulatory proteins (factor H, factor H related proteins, factor I, membrane cofactor protein, thrombomodulin) that normally regulate and restrict the activation of the alternative complement pathway, or hereditary abnormalities (factor B, C3) that accelerate the activation of the alternative complement pathway, leading to complement-mediated damage to vascular endothelium and kidneys. Acquired deficiency of complement factor H or factor I can be caused by autoimmune antibodies. Recessive mutations in diacylglycerol kinase epsilon (DGKE) is thought to result in a prothrombotic state with TMA in infancy (distinct from DGKE nephropathy). Plasminogen mutation was suggested to be the cause of aHUS in one case report.
Drug-induced TMA	Immune-mediated caused by drug-dependent antibodies that damage platelets, neutrophils and endothelial cells (quinine, gemcitabine, oxaliplatin and quetiapine). Dose-dependent toxicity-mediated caused by direct endothelial damage (gemcitabine, mitomycin, cyclosporine, tacrolimus, sirolimus, bevacizumab, oxymorphone).
Metabolism-mediated TMA	Disorders of intracellular vitamin B12 metabolism due to mutations in the MMACHC gene. Associated with elevated homocysteine and low methionine levels in plasma, with methylmalonic aciduria.

Table 2 Systemic disorders associated with TMA/MAHA (conditions with augmented or enhanced complement activation)

Pregnancy complications
Severe hypertension
Systemic infections (viremia, fungemia)
Systemic malignancies (chemotherapy, tumor cell embolism)
Systemic rheumatologic disorders (systemic lupus, scleroderma, catastrophic antiphospholipid syndrome)
Hematopoietic stem cell transplantation (myeloablative drugs, immunosuppression, viremia/fungemia)
Intravenous radiologic contrast media or exposures to biomaterials during vascular procedures

with absence of detectable levels of ADAMTS13 activity as the defining feature of TTP [8]. Thus infectious HUS, atypical or complement-mediated HUS, and TTP have distinct pathophysiological mechanisms, and should no longer be regarded and treated as the same disease.

Previously, there was no utility in making a diagnostic distinction between HUS, aHUS and TTP as all patients were treated with plasma exchange. Plasma exchange remains the mainstay of therapy for TTP to remove the autoimmune antibody and to replenish the absent enzyme. Prognosis of TTP is excellent with early recognition of disease and prompt institution of plasma exchange [9]. Proper antibiotic therapy and supportive care is now considered the treatment of choice for infectious HUS. Since September 2011, eculizumab, a humanized monoclonal antibody against C5, was approved by the FDA for treatment of patients with TMA secondary to aHUS. With the high response rates of eculizumab and potential for renal recovery in aHUS patients [10], separating the rare patient with aHUS from infectious HUS and TTP is now a clinical urgency.

Diagnostic approach to aHUS

When a critically ill patient with MAHA and thrombocytopenia is encountered, the differential diagnoses listed in Tables 1 and 2 should be considered [2, 3]. Several entities should be easily ruled out on clinical grounds, such as drugs, malignancy, pregnancy, hypertension and hematopoietic stem cell transplantation. Laboratory studies can identify rheumatologic disorders, B12 deficiency, antiphospholipid syndrome, and DIC. Therefore, the main differential consideration is TTP versus infectious HUS or atypical HUS. Infectious HUS can be identified with diarrheal illness with positive testing for the Shiga toxin; TTP now has a diagnostic test with ADAMTS13 activity [11–15]. However, testing with rapid

turn-around time is not available at most institutions. Clinical findings and laboratory data may be helpful. TTP is not known to involve the lungs, and rarely results in liver dysfunction. Renal disease is typically mild in TTP patients (creatinine <1.7–2.3 mg/dL), while thrombocytopenia is more severe (<30 × 10^9/L) compared to aHUS patients [16, 17], but overlap is considerable (unpublished data); the most recent patient diagnosed to have TTP at our institution had a creatinine of 5 mg/dL and platelet count of 47 × 10^9/L. For atypical or complement-mediated HUS, while finding a pathologic mutation in the regulatory proteins of the alternative complement pathway is diagnostic, only a few reference laboratories offer the genetic analysis, and registry data show that at least 30 % of patients with aHUS do not have currently known mutations. Genetic testing is also expensive and time consuming; with the exception of Machaon Diagnostics, the results are not available for at least 3–4 weeks. Having a negative genetic analysis certainly does not rule out aHUS, and not all laboratories offer whole exome sequencing. Thus the diagnosis of aHUS remains clinical. The recommended approach is to initiate plasma exchange therapy while waiting for diagnostic tests (such as ADAMTS13 activity) [18]. If ADAMT13 activity is below the level of detection, TTP is diagnosed and plasma exchange is continued until resolution of the MAHA and thrombocytopenia. If ADAMTS13 is detectable, and there is no diarrheal illness, then atypical HUS is the most likely diagnosis; keep in mind that atypical HUS especially in adults may present with a diarrheal illness without Shiga-toxin, due to involvement of the gastrointestinal tract. Response to plasma exchange can be helpful, with TTP patients responding in 3–5 days, while the response in aHUS patients is at best partial with improvement of hematologic parameters while organ functions continue to worsen [18].

In summary, when a patient with MAHA, thrombocytopenia and organ dysfunction, a detectable level of ADAMTS13 activity and absence of Shiga-toxin induced diarrheal illness should raise the clinical suspicion for atypical or complement-mediated HUS. Empiric plasma exchange should be initiated while waiting for results of the ADAMTS13 activity and Shiga toxin testing. Less than optimal response in 5 days to empiric plasma exchange should heighten the suspicion that the patient does not have TTP and treatment for aHUS should be considered.

Conditions with augmented or enhanced complement activation and aHUS

As mentioned in Table 2, there are several systemic conditions or disorders that can present with MAHA, thrombocytopenia, and organ dysfunction [2, 3]. These are in fact conditions with enhanced complement activation that can potentially unmask patients with mutations associated with aHUS. Registry data suggest that aHUS presents with conditions with enhanced complement activation nearly 70 % of the time [19]. When MAHA, thrombocytopenia, and organ dysfunction occur in patients with such a condition, care must be taken to monitor for prompt resolution of the hematologic abnormalities and organ dysfunction once the condition is resolved. Persistence of the hematologic abnormalities and/or organ dysfunction despite resolution of the condition with enhanced complement activation should lead to investigations for ADAMTS13 activity and/or Shiga toxin depending on the clinical situation, and consideration of empiric therapy with plasma exchange or initiation of eculizumab. It should be noted that whether the complement system is in fact enhanced or amplified is difficult to determine. Blood complement levels and detection of increased deposition of complement components in microvasculature remain investigational.

Pregnancy

Fakhouri et al. conducted a retrospective analysis of 100 adult female patients with aHUS. 21 had pregnancy-associated aHUS, and 79 % were post-partum. Mutations associated with aHUS were detected in 18 of the 21 patients. The risk for pregnancy associated aHUS was highest during a second pregnancy. Women with aHUS and documented genetic defects were more likely to have fetal loss and pre-eclampsia compared to those with aHUS but no genetic abnormalities [20].

Similar to non-pregnancy-associated aHUS, differentiating pregnancy-associated aHUS from other TMA is difficult due to clinical resemblance with other disorders including HELLP (hemolysis, elevated liver enzymes and low platelets), AFLP (acute fatty liver of pregnancy), and TTP. It is suggested that DIC picture and significant liver dysfunction would point towards HELLP or AFLP, and the absence of DIC and relatively normal liver enzymes are consistent with TTP or aHUS [21]. Pregnancy-associated TTP occurs in the late second or third trimester, with a median time at 23 weeks. This is thought to be related to the gradual rise of von Willebrand factor concentration with advancing gestation while ADAMTS13 activity decreases. In contrast, pregnancy-associated aHUS occurs mostly in the post-partum period, when effective control of the alternative complement pathway in the fluid phase is required [20].

The PROMISSE study is a multi-institutional observation study designed to identify predictors of pregnancy outcome in patients with systemic lupus erythematosus or positive antiphospholipid antibodies. Patients were screened for mutations in membrane cofactor protein (MCP), complement factor I (CFI), and complement factor H (CFH). Forty out of 250 patients (17 %) enrolled had pre-eclampsia. Seven patients were found to have mutations, and all 7 were amongst the 40 who had pre-eclampsia. None of the 34 without pre-eclampsia screened had a mutation documented. Thus in this study 17.5 % of patients with history of pre-eclampsia in the setting of systemic lupus erythematosus or positive antiphospholipid antibodies had mutations associated with aHUS. It is likely that mutations associated with aHUS contributed to the development of pre-eclampsia in patients with lupus and/or antiphospholipid antibodies (Fig. 1) [22].

To illustrate these points, the first patient at our institution treated with eculizumab for aHUS presented during her third pregnancy at 20 weeks of gestation with marked hypertension, and edema. She was admitted to the obstetric service and treatment for presumed pre-eclampsia was begun. However, despite lowering her blood pressure to the near normal range and delivery of the nonviable fetus, her creatinine increased to 4 mg/dL, while her hemoglobin decreased to 6 g/dL and platelet count to 20×10^9/L. She had modest amount of schistocytes on the blood smear, and ADAMTS13 activity was found to be normal on two separate occasions. She did not have diarrhea. She was empirically treated with 7 days of plasma exchange with minimal change in her clinical parameters. At that point presumptive diagnosis of pregnancy-associated aHUS was made, and she was initiated on eculizumab. By the second week of eculizuamb her hematologic abnormalities and serum creatinine began to normalize, with complete resolution of the disease manifestations by the fourth week. She has remained in remission as long as she is receiving eculizumab on schedule.

Malignant hypertension

While severe hypertension enhancing complement activity is not established, both infectious and atypical HUS, are often associated with significant hypertension. In contrast, TTP is not associated with malignant hypertension. This observed difference could be explained by a lower incidence and lesser degree of renal disease in TTP compared to HUS. Endothelial dysfunction is likely the common mechanism linking malignant hypertension and TMA. Endothelial dysfunction can result from either complement dysregulation, as seen in aHUS, or sheer stress in malignant hypertension [23]. Thus it is possible that endothelial injury from malignant hypertension can induce MAHA in a patient with underlying complement dysregulation (Fig. 1). An illustrative case is reported by Totina et al. A 10-month old child presenting with malignant hypertension and MAHA, but normal platelet count and normal renal function. Renal function and platelet count deteriorated during the hospital course, and renal biopsy demonstrated pathologic evidence of TMA. Molecular

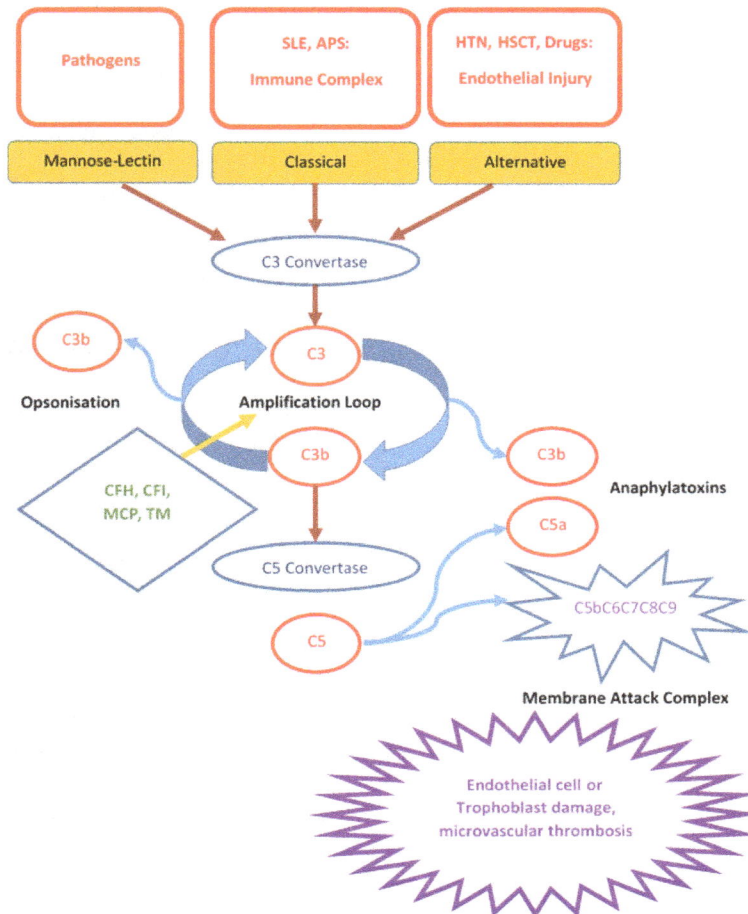

Fig. 1 Complement system in the pathogenesis of thrombotic microangiopathies. SLE: systemic lupus erythematosus; APS: antiphospholipid syndrome; HTN: hypertension; HSCT: hematopoietic stem cell transplantation; CFH: complement factor H; CFI: complement factor I; MCP: membrane cofactor protein; TM: thrombomodulin

analysis showed a complement factor H mutation of unknown significance [24].

The distinction between malignant hypertension-associated TMA and TMA causing malignant hypertension is an important one as TMA causing malignant hypertension may well represent aHUS and respond to eculizumab. Absence of retinal changes (cotton-wool spots, flame hemorrhages, or retinal arteriolar narrowing) is consistent with TMA causing malignant hypertension, but not exclusively [23].

Systemic rheumatologic disorders

As mentioned above, complement dysregulation contributes to endothelial injury via the alternative pathway leading to TMA. In rheumatologic disorders such as lupus erythematosus and antiphospholipid syndrome, autoimmune antibodies form immune complexes, and activate the complement system via the classical pathway [25]. Active lupus is considered to be a risk factor for developing TMA in a Korean study [26]. Thus patients with genetic mutations associated with aHUS are particularly susceptible to TMA when there is tissue damage from uncontrolled rheumatologic disorders (Fig. 1). Specifically, for the integrity of the renal cells and glomerular basement membane, complement regulation is of particular importance [25]. Therefore, patients with rheumatologic disorders such as lupus erythematosus and genetic mutations associated with aHUS are particularly at risk for TMA.

Given the frequent occurrence of hemolytic anemia and thrombocytopenia in lupus patients, recognizing TMA in a lupus patient can be challenging. A Taiwanese retrospective analysis of lupus patients with TMA showed that while it is a rare occurrence at 1 % (consistent with other reports), a high mortality rate of 52 % is noted (prior to availability of eculizumab, despite plasma exchange in the majority of patients) [27]. TTP again is the main differential diagnosis when evaluating patients with TMA in the setting of lupus, occurring in 1–4 % of lupus patients with a high mortality [28]. Thus it is absolutely important to obtain ADAMTS13 testing in a lupus patient with TMA, and if ADAMTS13 activity is not absent, consider aHUS.

El-Husseini et al. reported a 24 year old female patient with lupus and lupus nephritis who developed MAHA, thrombocytopenia and worsening renal function despite intensification of treatment for lupus nephritis. Repeat kidney biopsy demonstrated both lupus nephritis and TMA. While genetic testing was not performed, patient's clinical condition did not improve until eculizumab therapy was instituted, and thus patient is presumed to have developed aHUS in the setting of lupus and lupus nephritis [29]. This case again illustrates the importance of recognizing possible aHUS as a cause of persistent TMA when the underlying conditions with enhanced complement activation have been adequately treated. Investigations to identify risk features and determine the incidence of aHUS amongst lupus patients with TMA are vital.

Stem cell transplant

Transplant-associated TMA is a frequently encountered (~30 %) but poorly understood complication in recipients of hematopoietic stem cell transplantation (HSCT) [30]. It is noted to be more frequent in older patients and recipients of unrelated donor transplants, both of which are risk factors for acute graft versus host disease.

It is more frequent in females, recipients of grafts with a major or bidirectional ABO blood group mismatch. The frequency of transplant-associated TMA correlated with GvHD severity [31]. With the current knowledge that endothelial cells are targets of acute GvHD (Fig. 1) [32], patients with genetic defects affecting complement regulation are thought to be more prone to develop transplant-associated TMA. Jodele et al. studied the genetic fingerprint of susceptibility for transplant-associated TMA, and found that HSCT recipients with multiple complement gene variants (≥3) are at high risk for severe transplant-associated TMA [33]. Thus transplant-associated TMA is likely a form of aHUS unmasked by the endothelial dysfunction resulting from the conditioning regimen, GvHD, and possibly the use of calcineurin inhibitors. In this particular type of TMA, absence of ADAMTS13 activity is generally not observed, and treatment with plasma exchange is rarely helpful [34]. Eculizumab not surprisingly is found to be effective in high risk transplant-associated TMA patients [30].

Conclusion

Atypical or complement-mediated HUS is a TMA caused by mutations affecting the regulation of alternative complement pathway. Clinical presentation with MAHA, thrombocytopenia, and significant organ dysfunction can mimic other TMA-causing entities. Absent

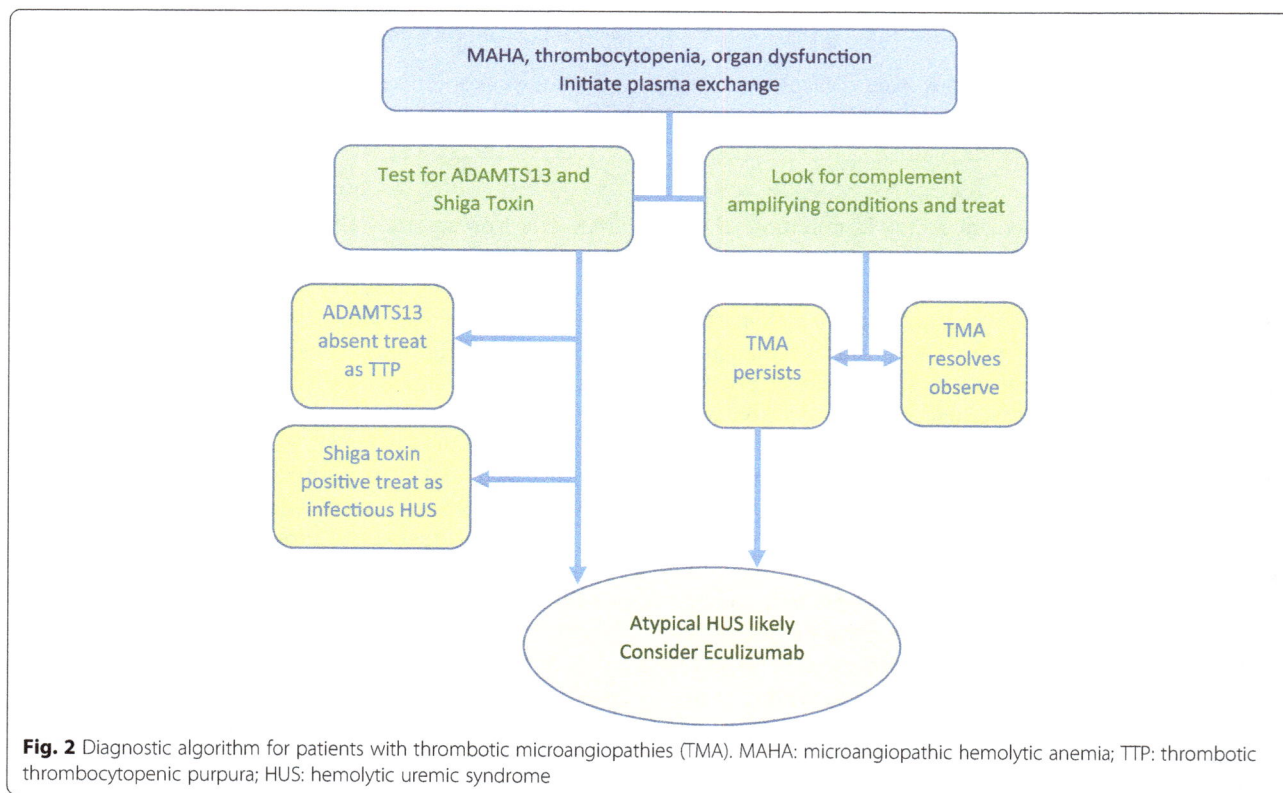

Fig. 2 Diagnostic algorithm for patients with thrombotic microangiopathies (TMA). MAHA: microangiopathic hemolytic anemia; TTP: thrombotic thrombocytopenic purpura; HUS: hemolytic uremic syndrome

ADAMTS13 activity rules in TTP, while diarrheal illness with Shiga-toxin producing bacteria points toward infectious HUS. When TMA occurs in the setting of conditions with enhanced complement activity such as pregnancy, rheumatic disorders, malignant hypertension, and HSCT, persistence or worsening TMA despite treatment of the associated conditions should raise the clinical suspicion for aHUS (Fig. 2). If aHUS is reasonably suspected, early intervention with anti-complement therapy should be considered especially when extra-renal complications are present; such patients are at increased risk of sudden death due to brain ischemia or cardiac complications.

Acknowledgements
None.

Author's contributions
Yu-Min Shen fully contributed to the manuscript.

Competing interests
Yu-Min Shen serves on the speakers' bureau and advisory boards of Alexion Pharmaceuticals Inc.

References

1. Tsai HM. A mechanistic approach to the diagnosis and management of atypical hemolytic uremic syndrome. Transfus Med Rev. 2014;28(4): 187–97.
2. George JN, Charania RS. Evaluation of patients with microangiopathic hemolytic anemia and thrombocytopenia. Semin Thromb Hemost. 2013; 39(2):153–60.
3. George JN, Nester CM. Syndromes of thrombotic microangiopathy. N Engl J Med. 2014;371(19):1847–8.
4. Spinale JM, Ruebner RL, Kaplan BS, Copelovitch L. Update on Streptococcus pneumoniae associated hemolytic uremic syndrome. Curr Opin Pediatr. 2013;25(2):203–8.
5. Noris M, Remuzzi G. Atypical hemolytic-uremic syndrome. N Engl J Med. 2009;361(17):1676–87.
6. Tsai HM, Lian EC. Antibodies to von Willebrand factor-cleaving protease in acute thrombotic thrombocytopenic purpura. N Engl J Med. 1998;339(22):1585–94.
7. Furlan M, Robles R, Galbusera M, Remuzzi G, Kyrle PA, Brenner B, et al. von Willebrand factor-cleaving protease in thrombotic thrombocytopenic purpura and the hemolytic-uremic syndrome. N Engl J Med. 1998;339(22):1578–84.
8. Sarode R, Bandarenko N, Brecher ME, Kiss JE, Marques MB, Szczepiorkowski ZM, et al. Thrombotic thrombocytopenic purpura: 2012 American Society for Apheresis (ASFA) consensus conference on classification, diagnosis, management, and future research. J Clin Apher. 2014;29(3):148–67.
9. George JN. How I, treat patients with thrombotic thrombocytopenic purpura: 2010. Blood. 2010;116(20):4060–9.
10. Legendre CM, Licht C, Muus P, Greenbaum LA, Babu S, Bedrosian C, et al. Terminal complement inhibitor eculizumab in atypical hemolytic-uremic syndrome. N Engl J Med. 2013;368(23):2169–81.
11. Barbot J, Costa E, Guerra M, Barreirinho MS, Isvarlal P, Robles R, et al. Ten years of prophylactic treatment with fresh-frozen plasma in a child with chronic relapsing thrombotic thrombocytopenic purpura as a result of a congenital deficiency of von Willebrand factor-cleaving protease. Br J Haematol. 2001;113(3):649–51.
12. Bianchi V, Robles R, Alberio L, Furlan M, Lammle B. Von Willebrand factor-cleaving protease (ADAMTS13) in thrombocytopenic disorders: a severely deficient activity is specific for thrombotic thrombocytopenic purpura. Blood. 2002;100(2):710–3.
13. Bitzan M, Schaefer F, Reymond D. Treatment of typical (enteropathic) hemolytic uremic syndrome. Semin Thromb Hemost. 2010;36(6):594–610.
14. Sadler JE. Von Willebrand factor, ADAMTS13, and thrombotic thrombocytopenic purpura. Blood. 2008;112(1):11–8.
15. Tsai HM. Pathophysiology of thrombotic thrombocytopenic purpura. Int J Hematol. 2010;91(1):1–19.
16. Coppo P, Schwarzinger M, Buffet M, Wynckel A, Clabault K, Presne C, et al. Predictive features of severe acquired ADAMTS13 deficiency in idiopathic thrombotic microangiopathies: the French TMA reference center experience. PLoS One. 2010;5(4):e10208.
17. Zuber J, Fakhouri F, Roumenina LT, Loirat C, Fremeaux-Bacchi V, French Study Group for a HCG. Use of eculizumab for atypical haemolytic uraemic syndrome and C3 glomerulopathies. Nat Rev Nephrol. 2012; 8(11):643–57.
18. Laurence J. Atypical hemolytic uremic syndrome (aHUS): making the diagnosis. Clin Adv Hematol Oncol. 2012;10(10 Suppl 17):1–12.
19. Noris M, Caprioli J, Bresin E, Mossali C, Pianetti G, Gamba S, et al. Relative role of genetic complement abnormalities in sporadic and familial aHUS and their impact on clinical phenotype. Clin J Am Soc Nephrol. 2010;5(10): 1844–59.
20. Fakhouri F, Roumenina L, Provot F, Sallee M, Caillard S, Couzi L, et al. Pregnancy-associated hemolytic uremic syndrome revisited in the era of complement gene mutations. J Am Soc Nephrol. 2010;21(5):859–67.
21. Pourrat O, Coudroy R, Pierre F. Differentiation between severe HELLP syndrome and thrombotic microangiopathy, thrombotic thrombocytopenic purpura and other imitators. Eur J Obstet Gynecol Reprod Biol. 2015;189:68–72.
22. Salmon JE, Heuser C, Triebwasser M, Liszewski MK, Kavanagh D, Roumenina L, et al. Mutations in complement regulatory proteins predispose to preeclampsia: a genetic analysis of the PROMISSE cohort. PLoS Med. 2011; 8(3):e1001013.
23. Mathew RO, Nayer A, Asif A. The endothelium as the common denominator in malignant hypertension and thrombotic microangiopathy. J Am Soc Hypertens. 2016;10(4):352–9.
24. Totina A, Iorember F, El-Dahr SS, Yosypiv IV. Atypical hemolytic-uremic syndrome in a child presenting with malignant hypertension. Clin Pediatr (Phila). 2013;52(2):183–6.
25. Java A, Atkinson J, Salmon J. Defective complement inhibitory function predisposes to renal disease. Annu Rev Med. 2013;64:307–24.
26. Kwok SK, Ju JH, Cho CS, Kim HY, Park SH. Thrombotic thrombocytopenic purpura in systemic lupus erythematosus: risk factors and clinical outcome: a single centre study. Lupus. 2009;18(1):16–21.
27. Chen MH, Chen MH, Chen WS, Mu-Hsin Chang P, Lee HT, Lin HY, et al. Thrombotic microangiopathy in systemic lupus erythematosus: a cohort study in North Taiwan. Rheumatology (Oxford). 2011;50(4):768–75.
28. Vaidya S, Abul-ezz S, Lipsmeyer E. Thrombotic thrombocytopenic purpura and systemic lupus erythematosus. Scand J Rheumatol. 2001; 30(5):308–10.
29. El-Husseini A, Hannan S, Awad A, Jennings S, Cornea V, Sawaya BP. Thrombotic microangiopathy in systemic lupus erythematosus: efficacy of eculizumab. Am J Kidney Dis. 2015;65(1):127–30.
30. Jodele S, Dandoy CE, Myers KC, El-Bietar J, Nelson A, Wallace G, et al. New approaches in the diagnosis, pathophysiology, and treatment of pediatric hematopoietic stem cell transplantation-associated thrombotic microangiopathy. Transfus Apher Sci. 2016;54(2):181–90.
31. Martinez MT, Bucher C, Stussi G, Heim D, Buser A, Tsakiris DA, et al. Transplant-associated microangiopathy (TAM) in recipients of allogeneic

hematopoietic stem cell transplants. Bone Marrow Transplant. 2005;
36(11):993–1000.

32. Biedermann BC, Sahner S, Gregor M, Tsakiris DA, Jeanneret C, Pober JS, et al.
Endothelial injury mediated by cytotoxic T lymphocytes and loss of
microvessels in chronic graft versus host disease. Lancet. 2002;359(9323):
2078–83.

33. Jodele S, Zhang K, Zou F, Laskin B, Dandoy CE, Myers KC, et al. The genetic
fingerprint of susceptibility for transplant-associated thrombotic
microangiopathy. Blood. 2016;127(8):989–96.

34. van der Plas RM, Schiphorst ME, Huizinga EG, Hene RJ, Verdonck LF, Sixma
JJ, et al. von Willebrand factor proteolysis is deficient in classic, but not in
bone marrow transplantation-associated, thrombotic thrombocytopenic
purpura. Blood. 1999;93(11):3798–802.

Oligonucleotides targeting coagulation factor mRNAs: use in thrombosis and hemophilia research and therapy

Marco Heestermans[1,2]* (iD) and Bart J.M. van Vlijmen[1,2]

Abstract

Small interfering (si) RNAs and antisense oligonucleotides (ASOs; here for simplicity reasons, both referred to as oligonucleotides) are small synthetic RNA or DNA molecules with a sequence complementary to a (pre)mRNA. Although the basic mechanisms of action between siRNAs and ASO are distinct, a sequence-specific interaction of the both oligonucleotides with the target (pre)mRNA alters the target's fate, which includes highly effective sequence-specific blockade of translation and consequently depletion of the corresponding protein. For a number of years, these oligonucleotides have been used as a tool in biological research to study gene function in vitro. More recently, safe and specific delivery of these oligonucleotides to the liver of mammals has been achieved and optimized. This not only allowed their use for in vivo gene studies in physiology and disease, but also opened the opportunity for the development of a new generation of RNA-specific drugs for therapeutic purposes. In 2013, the first oligonucleotide product targeting RNA from the hepatic cholesterol pathway was approved. For blood coagulation, a large portion of key proteins are produced in the liver, and thereby siRNAs and ASOs can also be used as appropriate tools to target these proteins in vivo. In this review, we describe the first use of oligonucleotides for this purpose from zebrafish to primates. As the use of oligonucleotides allows avoidance of early lethality associated with full deficiency of several coagulation factors, it has proved to be of value for studying these proteins in physiology and disease. Currently, oligonucleotides are tested as therapeutics, with the ultimate goal to beneficially modulate the hemostatic balance in thrombosis and hemophilia patients. We discuss both the preclinical and clinical studies of a number of siRNAs and ASOs with the potential to be introduced as drugs for prophylactic and/or treatment of thrombosis or hemophilia. We conclude that for the coagulation field, oligonucleotides are of value for research purposes, and now the moment has come to fulfill their promise as therapeutics.

Keywords: siRNA, Antisense oligonucleotides, RNA, Therapy, Liver, Coagulation

Background

Small interfering (si) RNAs and antisense oligonucleotides (ASOs; here for simplicity reasons, both referred to as oligonucleotides) are small synthetic RNA or DNA molecules with a sequence complementary to a (pre)mRNA. Sequence-specific interaction of the siRNA or ASO with the target (pre)mRNA alters the target's fate, which includes sequence-specific blockade of translation and consequently depletion of the corresponding protein.

siRNAs and ASOs have potential in research and therapy; design of sequence-specific oligonucleotides and testing their efficacy in vitro can be relatively easily achieved, and off-target effects are limited. Moreover, siRNAs and ASOs have a relatively simple chemistry, malleability, and delivery (at least in vitro), allowing the oligonucleotides to become a frequently used tool in biological research for studying gene function in a variety of eukaryotic cell types. The major differences between siRNAs and ASOs comprise differences regarding their chemical structure and their mode of action, but considering their primary biological impact i.e., silencing the target (pre)mRNAs target, both are highly effective [1–3].

* Correspondence: m.heestermans@lumc.nl
[1]Einthoven Laboratory for Experimental Vascular Medicine, Leiden University Medical Center, Leiden, The Netherlands
[2]Department of Internal Medicine, Division of Thrombosis and Hemostasis, Leiden University Medical Center, Leiden, The Netherlands

Already in 1978, it was shown that ASOs proved successful in targeting (pre)mRNAs in vivo in experimental animals [4]. More recently, in 2003, also siRNAs showed strong in vivo potency [5], and delivering siRNAs to the liver proved feasible and successful [6, 7]. siRNAs and ASOs both successfully escape degradation in both the blood circulation and intracellular lysosomes, and effectively reach the appropriate cellular compartment to find their complementary (pre)mRNA. Hepatic delivery allowed the use of oligonucleotides for in vivo gene function studies in normal (hepatic) physiology or for disease analogues to the in vitro approach. Moreover, siRNAs and ASOs allow validation of therapeutic targets in pre-clinical trials forming the stepping stone towards clinical application [8–10]. As blood coagulation factors are predominantly expressed in the liver, venous thrombosis and hemophilia are diseases that may particularly benefit from the oligonucleotide approach; both when it comes to use as a research tool in preclinical research as well as an approach for therapy.

In this review, we will discuss the possibilities for using oligonucleotides in venous thrombosis and hemophilia research and therapy. First, we will outline the chemical and cellular differences between siRNAs and ASOs. Next, we will discuss their usefulness to study coagulation physiology and pathophysiology (i.e., thrombosis and hemophilia) in animal models. Finally, we will examine the current status of the exciting first clinical applications of oligonucleotide approach in venous thrombosis and hemophilia, and the potentials that come along with this novel treatment modality.

siRNA and ASO biology and delivery

Although the target of siRNAs and ASOs is the same i.e., the (pre)mRNA of the gene of interest, their mechanism of action is different. In short, siRNAs are synthetic RNA duplexes consisting of two unmodified annealed 21-mer oligonucleotides. When siRNAs enter the cytosol, the antisense strand i.e., the strand which specifically targets an mRNA, forms a complex with an endoribonuclease enzyme called Dicer for loading into RNA-induced silencing complex (RISC), which enables their stabilization. A single RISC, with the RNase Argonaute-2 (for which siRNA competes with microRNAs, as discussed in [11]) as its functional unit for accommodating RNA breakdown and the antisense strand for the specificity, can target and break down multiple mRNAs in the cytosol. This process is also known as RNA interference [1, 12]. Whereas siRNAs enter the cell as a duplex, ASOs are single stranded antisense nucleic acids (DNA, RNA, or an chemical analogue), typically 8–50 nucleotides long. ASOs are not recognized by Dicer and not built into RISC upon entering the cytosol; depending on their chemical modification, they directly

recognize their (pre)mRNA target in the cytosol or nucleus, due to their complementarity [13]. ASOs can block, break down (after recruitment of RNase H), or induce exon skipping of the mRNA [2]. In contrast to siRNAs, where a single RISC can degrade multiple mRNAs, ASOs typically interact with a single (pre)mRNA.

With the desire to use oligonucleotides in vivo, the delivery to the correct cell and cellular compartment without being degraded has been an important issue. Thus far, the delivery of oligonucleotides to the liver in mammals is an area where significant progress has been made: siRNAs can be packaged in liposomes with a high tropism for the liver, and they can be conjugated to specific ligands (the so called- N-acetylgalactosamine (GalNAC) ligands, which allows the uptake via hepatocyte-specific asialoglycoprotein receptors) which mediate receptor-mediated take-up by hepatocytes [14–17]. A liposome-based formulation and hepatic delivery has also been described for other oligonucleotides [18]. Upon systemic delivery, the biodistribution of ASOs is broad, and the highest concentrations are typically found in the liver and the kidneys [19–21]. This delivery is an aspecific process and works via a yet unknown mechanism, however it is likely that the relative amphipathic nature of molecules contribute to this cell-specific distribution. Differences in the delivery of the compound (packaging versus an aspecific process) and the later discovery of (the functioning of) siRNAs are probably the main reasons why ASOs are ahead for entering into (pre)clinical trials. More recently, it has been reported recently that ASOs can alsobe GalNAc conjugated, and that they are (successfully) tested in (pre)clinical trials [22, 23].

Because the liver appears to be the most successfully targeted organ thus far - although there are interesting reports showing e.g., successful delivery of siRNAs to endothelium and leukocytes [24, 25] - we will focus in this review on targeting mRNA encoded by genes expressed in hepatocytes. This successful hepatic delivery of oligonucleotides makes an mRNA-targeting approach specifically interesting for studies and eventually therapies where a liver-produced protein is a major contributor to the physiology and/or pathophysiology of a certain disease, such as hepatitis, hypercholesterolemia, hemophilia, and thrombosis [26]. For this review, we will focus solely on the use of oligonucleotides for targeting liver-produced coagulation proteins, to study their role in biology and modulate their activity in hemophilia and thrombosis with the ultimate goal to fight or prevent the disease.

siRNAs and ASOs to study coagulation gene function in physiology and disease

A conventional approach to study gene function in vivo is by generating genetically modified animals. Recently, the developments leading to CRISPR/cas9-mediated genome editing have allowed generation of mutant and/ or knockout within a period of months [27]. Nevertheless, extensive breeding programs, also for the generation of proper (littermate) controls, remain expensive, and gene deletion may preclude detailed study of gene function due to perinatal lethality or gene redundancy. Regarding coagulation, most genes from the extrinsic, common, or anticoagulant pathways have been deleted in mice, which often resulted in early lethality, mostly as a result of coagulopathy [28, 29].

As an alternative to the genetic modification approach, oligonucleotides can be used to transiently silence a gene of interest. Using oligonucleotides is simple, fast, cheap, and there are no issues with generating the appropriate controls, because a group of identical mice can be injected with a scrambled control sequence, which is structurally comparable. Moreover, because of the acute silencing of oligonucleotides, analyses can be performed before potential compensatory pathways have become active, and results can be easy translated to other species (including human), as long as the genome has been sequenced.

siRNAs and ASOs in animal models for coagulation - zebrafish

A relatively new animal model for the study of blood coagulation and related processes is the zebrafish (*Danio rerio*). These fish possess a conserved and sophisticated coagulation system, which in essence follows the same principles as the system in mammals [30, 31]. Moreover, the low cost of maintenance and their low turnover time between subsequent generations make them appealing for (bio)medical research.

The oligonucleotide of choice in this animal are the so-called morpholinos, a subclass of ASOs which got their name because their backbone consists of methylenemorpholine rings [32]. These oligonucleotides do not degrade the targeted mRNA, but rather block translation by making the target mRNA inaccessible for ribosomes. The coagulation factors fibrinogen, prothrombin, and factor VII have been silenced in vivo using morpholinos.

For fibrinogen, zebrafish produce orthologues for the three chains of the mature protein, and it has an in vivo expression pattern comparable to mammals. Moreover, fibrinogen strands are incorporated in the (experimental) thrombus of a zebrafish, and upon morpholino-mediated downregulation of either of the three orthologues, larvae suffer from intracranial and intramuscular hemorrhages [33].

Morpholino-mediated downregulation of prothrombin causes two distinct phenotypes in zebrafish larvae. Some larvae suffer from serious developmental issues causing premature death (even before blood flow has developed), while others develop a bleeding phenotype during a later

stage of embryonic development [34]. These results recapitulate the hemophilic phenotype that is seen in experimental mammalian animals with deficiencies of these factors. Moreover, a microarray analysis was performed on mRNA from zebrafish treated which were with prothrombin-morpholinos [35]. A total of 63 upregulated or downregulated genes were identified, although their exact function remains to be determined.

Using coagulation factor VII-specific morpholinos, it was shown in zebrafish that hepsin plays a crucial role in activating factor VII [36]. Besides fibrinogen, prothrombin, and factor VII, more genes involved in hemostasis, such as von Willebrand factor and genes involved in thrombocyte production and function, have been targeted in zebrafish using morpholinos [37–39].

Although translating results from zebrafish to humans remains difficult due to a wide evolutionary gap between both species, the presented data imply that using zebrafish-specific advantages can contribute in unraveling processes of hemostasis, with a clear role for the use of oligonucleotides as a tool.

siRNAs and ASOs in animal models for coagulation - mammals

In order to study processes involving coagulation factors, mammalian animal models, such as mice, rats, and rabbits, are genetically closer related to humans. In these mammals it has been shown that siRNAs and ASOs can be delivered to the liver in vivo to silence (pre)mRNAs of proteins produced in hepatocytes [26, 40–42]. Several genes involved in the extrinsic, common, or anticoagulant pathway of coagulation have been targeted.

Antithrombin, protein C, and protein S are important natural anticoagulants, and individuals with partial deficiencies in either of these factors have an increased risk to develop venous thrombosis, while full deficiency is rare and very severe or incompatible with life [43]. Genetically modified mice missing either of these anticoagulants die *in utero* because of thrombotic complications. However, using siRNAs, the anticoagulants antithrombin or protein C can be silenced transiently in adult mice to study them in a less anticoagulant environment. When both natural anticoagulants are silenced simultaneously mice develop spontaneous venous thrombosis, a phenotype which is characterized by the formation of fibrin-rich thrombi in the head and rapid consumption of coagulation factors [44].

This mouse model allowed studying factors involved in (experimental) venous thrombosis pathophysiology. Platelets appeared to be crucial for spontaneous venous thrombosis to occur, whereas neutrophils were not rate limiting, and lowering of plasma coagulation factor XII surprisingly seemed to aggravate rather than rescue the thrombotic phenotype [45].

Oligonucleotides can be used as a tool to study the effect of transiently silencing a certain gene, to bypass early lethality. An interesting example of such an approach has been described for studying the role of (pro)thrombin in Sickle cell disease (SCD) [46]. Genetically modified mice missing prothrombin are not viable due to fatal prenatal bleeding complications, so the authors were forced to choose another approach. Using prothrombin-specific designed gapmers (a class of ASOs where the internal sequence block is protected from nuclease degradation by artificially modified ribonucleotide monomers) prothrombin was transiently silenced SCD mice. It was shown that in SCD mice reduced levels of prothrombin lowered inflammation and endothelial cell dysfunction, and improved multiple SCD-associated organ pathologies and overall survival. These data imply that targeting a single coagulation factor i.e., prothrombin can ameliorate SCD pathology.

Using a comparable approach, the transcription factors hepatocyte nuclear factor 4α and CCAAT/enhancer-binding protein α were silenced using siRNAs, to study their regulatory role in the transcription of coagulation genes, demonstrating that by means of siRNAs the role of a gene in a certain process can be simply and rapidly unraveled [47].

Oligonucleotides as therapeutics – animal studies

Besides using oligonucleotides as a tool for the study of gene function, they are also candidate therapeutics in the field of blood coagulation. All key proteins (with the exception of tissue factor and membrane bound receptors such as thrombomodulin, endothelial protein C receptor, and protease-activated receptors) are predominantly expressed in the liver. Moreover, a major advantage of using oligonucleotide drugs over other more conventional therapeutic strategies lies in the drugs' target: (pre)mRNAs. Targeting proteins is complex due to their three-dimensional structure and small conformational differences which can cause complete loss of function of a drug, while (pre)mRNAs just differ in their gene-specific sequence. This means that conventional ("protein-based") drugs have to undergo an elaborate screening process for compounds that inhibit the protein of interest in both experimental animals (during preclinical studies) and humans (actual trials), while for RNA-based drugs solely the oligonucleotide sequence needs to be adjusted. Moreover, oligonucleotide drugs can stably repress protein levels over the course of several weeks. In addition, oligonucleotides are not expected to become subject to an immunogenic response, inhibitors, or resistance during therapy.

The fundamental process of blood coagulation and the disease of venous thrombosis can be effectively inhibited in humans by using agents such as vitamin K antagonists, heparins, and the new generation of direct oral anticoagulants [48, 49]. All these therapeutics target components of the common pathway of coagulation. Outside the common pathway, coagulation factor IX might be an interesting candidate to target for the prevention of thrombosis. With an siRNA against this coagulation factor, it has been shown in rats that protein activity can be reduced with 50-99%. This reduced activity prevented experimental thrombosis without causing a bleeding phenotype. Over 99% inhibition of factor IX activity resulted in a bleeding phenotype, similar to factor IX deficient rats [50]. This observation makes an "intermediate" dose of siRNAs against factor IX (resulting in 50–99% reduction of activity) potentially interesting for therapeutic purposes.

Although targeting individual components from the coagulation cascade proved effective in preventing thrombosis, bleeding often remains a clinically relevant side effect. To circumvent this problem, coagulation factors XI and XII, both involved in the intrinsic, or contact-activation, pathway of coagulation have been introduced to target for preventing venous thrombosis [51–53]. Based on data derived from mouse studies, deficiency or transient lowering of factor XI and XII prevents thrombosis without (severe) bleeding as a side effect, unlike any other traditional coagulation factor. These reports coincide with human data, where individuals with a factor XII deficiency do not have a bleeding tendency, and factor XI deficient patients (although occasionally suffering from mild and injury-related events, hemophilia C) even seem to be protected from developing thrombotic events [54–56]. Moreover, both plasma proteins are exclusively produced in the liver, making them accessible for oligonucleotide therapy.

Coagulation factor XII is a plasma protease which upon activation initiates the intrinsic pathway of coagulation. When rats deficient in factor XII were compared with rats treated with a specific siRNA against factor XII (99% reduction in plasma factor XII), both showed protection in arterial as well as in venous thrombosis models [57]. In rabbits, a factor XII-specific ASO prolonged the time to occlusion in a catheter thrombosis model by 2.2 fold [58]. Comparable thromboprotective effects were obtained in mouse studies. Specific lowering of factor XII or (pre)kallikrein (an activator of the zymogen factor XII) using an ASO, resulted in reduced thrombus formation models for arterial and venous thrombosis, without a significant effect on normal hemostasis [59].

Coagulation factor XII is not only involved in (experimental) hemostasis, but also in release of bradykinin from high molecular weight kininogen, an inflammatory component mediating the dilation of blood vessels. Specific gain-of-function mutations in factor XII causing increased contact-mediated auto activation, which causes enhanced release of bradykinin and massive swelling, underlies hereditary angioedema type III [60]. Interestingly, experimental data in mice show that upon lowering factor XII or (pre)kallikrein using a specific oligonucleotide, certain characteristics associated with this disease can be prevented, which opens perspectives for treatment [61–63].

Coagulation factor XI is activated by factor XII towards activated factor XI. In mice, ASO-mediated specific and dose-dependent reduction of plasma factor XI showed an antithrombotic effect in various arterial and venous thrombosis models [40]. In parallel groups, mice were treated with either warfarin or enoxaparin, a commonly used vitamin K antagonist and low molecular weight heparin, respectively. Although the antithrombotic effect was considered equally effective in all groups, factor XI ASO-treated mice performed significantly better in a hepatectomy surgical bleeding model. In rabbits, lowering of factor XI prolonged the time to occlusion in a catheter thrombosis model, in a similar fashion as factor XII [58]. After these promising results, the role of factor XI and its therapeutic antithrombotic potential was tested in non-human primates. Again using mRNA-specific ASOs, it was first shown that plasma factor XI can be lowered in a dose-dependent manner without increasing the risk of bleeding [64]. In a second study, the antithrombotic potential of FXI-ASO was tested in non-human primates. In an arteriovenous shunt thrombosis model protection from thrombosis was reported, which coincided with a decreased thrombin generation [65]. These studies formed solid proof to continue with using an ASO against factor XI in clinical trials. Interestingly, silencing coagulation factors XI and XII also attenuated atherothrombosis in mice [66, 67], which implies that silencing these factors also might be useful in treating atherothrombotic complications.

Besides targeting procoagulant proteins to prevent venous thrombosis, targeting anticoagulants might also be useful in preventing disease, in a situation where the hemostatic balance has shifted towards bleeding i.e., hemophilia. Current therapies to treat hemophilia are based on administering plasma derived or recombinant proteins to replace the missing coagulation factors. The need for developing alternative treatment strategies is high, since a large portion of treated hemophilia patients develops inhibitory antibodies against these administered proteins. A promising approach which likely circumvents this problem is by silencing an anticoagulant using oligonucleotides, which can cause a shift towards a renewed hemostatic equilibrium. This hypothesis was tested by targeting antithrombin [68]. When factor VIII-deficient hemophilic mice were treated with an siRNA against antithrombin, the hemophilic phenotype disappeared in a dose-dependent manner without thrombotic complications. In the next animal model of choice, non-

human primates (cynomolgus monkeys) with antibody induced FVIII deficiency, a dose-dependent silencing of antithrombin was again observed. Moreover, thrombin generation were restored to normal levels when treating the monkeys with the siRNA, which opened the perspective to test this drug in humans.

Oligonucleotides as therapeutics – human studies

Recently, the first oligonucleotide drug targeting specifically the liver has been approved by the United States' Food and Drug Administration. This therapeutic, an ASO called mipomersen (Kynamro®), directly targets the pre-mRNA of apolipoprotein B, which causes a significant downregulation of the corresponding plasma protein. This specific downregulation allows more release of very low density lipoprotein (VLDL) from the liver to the bloodstream, which will cause a drop of LDL-cholestorol levels in plasma [69, 70]. This is in line with the concept of the oligonucleotide drugs, which has been outlined previously. Mipomersen has been approved to treat homozygous familial hypercholesterolemia, and the availability of mipomersen is currently being investigated for more risk groups with high cholesterol levels to protect them from cardiovascular disease (http://www.fda.gov/NewsEvents/Newsroom/PressAnnouncements/ucm337195.htm).

The approval of mipomersen might cause a domino effect for the use of oligonucleotides which target mRNA in the liver for treating other human diseases: The first hurdle of safely delivering oligonucleotides to the liver has been overcome, so by using the same chemical formulation many more hepatic mRNAs can be targeted, which is an appealing prospect. Two oligonucleotide drugs are currently being tested in the field of coagulation, one for venous thrombosis treatment and one for hemophilia.

Coagulation factor XI has been investigated extensively in animal models for its role in coagulation, and whether it can be a therapeutic target to prevent venous thrombosis without introducing bleeding as a side effect [71]. Recently, the results of a clinical trial were reported, where an ASO against factor XI (FXI-ASO) was used for the prevention of deep-vein thrombosis after knee arthroplasty [72]. Previously, FXI-ASO was considered safe to use in humans since no side effects (including bleeding) were observed in a prior study [73]. When comparing a high and low dose FXI-ASO with conventional enoxaparin treatment, the bleeding risk was not significantly different (although less bleeding events were scored for FXI-ASO patients). Interestingly, treatment of patients with the low dose of FXI-ASO appeared safe considering the risk of deep-vein thrombosis, where the high dose was even considered superior to enoxaparin. Currently, a phase 2 clinical trial has been completed in which the efficacy of FXI-ASO in patients with end-stage renal disease was evaluated, with the primary goal to monitor the safety and tolerability of the ASO (ISIS 416858, Ionis pharmaceuticals). Significant and dose-dependent reductions in FXI activity were observed upon treatment (http://ir.ionispharma.com/phoenix.zhtml?c=222170&p=irol-news Article&ID=2217775).

As outlined previously, on the other side of the spectrum hemophilia can be treated by transient lowering of antithrombin, to restore the hemostatic balance. Currently, a human-specific antithrombin siRNA named *Fitusiran* is being tested in phase 1 clinical trials. This siRNA, amongst others candidate siRNAs which are tested in clinical trials, is chemically modified to improve its systemic stability and is conjugated to a GalNAc-ligand, which allows hepatocyte-specific uptake [17]. The phase 1 clinical trial is done in a diverse group of individuals, including healthy volunteers, patients with hemophilia A or B, and with or without inhibitors against supplemented recombinant proteins [74]. The goal of this trial is to evaluate the safety and tolerability of multiple doses of subcutaneously administered *Fitusiran*. Moreover, thrombin generation assays in plasma derived from hemophilia patients are performed to test whether they recover towards levels of healthy individuals. Preliminary data show that hemophilia patients did not develop any serious (thromboembolic) complications because of the drug. Considering functionality of the drug, when antithrombin levels were lowered to >75% thrombin generation peaks were increased in a dose-dependent manner with 289%. Positive interim results of two clinical trials (phase 1 and phase 2) for *Fiturisan* have been reported late 2016 (ALN-AT3SC, Alnylam pharmaceuticals, http://www.alnylam.com/capella/presentations/fitusiran-data-ash-2016/).

Conclusions

Hepatic in vivo gene silencing using oligonucleotides has shown to be specific and rapidly applicable in multiple animal models. The approach can not only serve as an alternative for using genetically modified animals (although restricted to the liver), it can also help unraveling biological processes which cannot be studied otherwise. Moreover, promising preclinical trials for the development of new oligonucleotide drugs to treat thrombosis and hemophilia have been reported.

Since the introduction of mipomersen in 2013, the first oligonucleotide drugs are slowly finding their way towards the clinic (currently, three ASOs and no siRNAs yet). Together with all the preclinical data, it has been shown that the process of delivering oligonucleotides to the liver can be achieved in a safe way (thus far, no specific toxicities have been observed). Currently, preventing adverse events (at the injection site or from infusions) of oligonucleotide drugs remains an important

issue, which means that reducing the dosage of the drugs is crucial. The dosages can be lowered by, for instance, the conjugation of GalNAc-ligands to oligonucleotides to improve cell-specific delivery [22]. When these delivery and dosage issues can be solved, more clinical situations will present where using oligonucleotides will be regarded advantageous over using classical therapies.

Thrombosis and hemophilia are two diseases where the current treatment can be improved, and the two drugs which are currently investigated in clinical trials show promise. An important advantage compared to current therapies for hemophilia is that the effect of oligonucleotides remains for a longer time period, in contrast to the low-interval dosing of conventional treatment. This would mean that patients will go from daily to monthly treatment. Moreover, hemophilia patients who develop inhibitors against supplemented factor VIII or IX will benefit from this novel treatment option, since oligonucleotides will likely not provoke this immune response.

Although the mode of action of oligonucleotides in humans compared to current therapies can be regarded as a great benefit, it can be a problem in situations when rapid reversal of the silenced protein is necessary. In some cases, singular treatment with recombinant proteins will be a solution, although correct dosing would be crucial. A more elegant solution would be to use an oligonucleotide antidote. Recently, it was shown in mice that upon prothrombin-specific ASO treatment, complementary sense oligonucleotide antidote (SOAs) reversed the antithrombotic phenotype by specifically binding of ASOs intracellularly [75]. Even though these data are promising, therapeutic usefulness has to be proven for individual ASOs. Moreover, it has been shown that reversal of siRNA therapy is feasible using complementary high affinity oligonucleotides as a "synthetic target" or decoy to abrogate silencing activity of antisense-loaded RISC (Reversir™, http://www.alnylam.com/web/assets/Reversir_OTS_101315.pdf). Currently, the strategy has been reported to be functional for reversal of the effect of an siRNA against coagulation factor IX. The major disadvantage of this oligonucleotide-specific approach is that it may take too long for the antidote to restore original levels of the initially silenced protein. For this reason, in the case of a sudden event such as a surgical intervention, an oligonucleotide-specific antidote may not be adequate and recombinant proteins or fresh frozen plasma treatment are still necessary.

In conclusion, in fundamental research oligonucleotides targeting coagulation factors in the liver can serve multiple purposes, and can improve our understanding about coagulation biology, in physiology and disease. Considering oligonucleotide-based silencing of coagulation factors to treat thrombosis or hemophilia, for the short term, validation studies focused on the safety and efficacy of the products for clinical applications look promising. For the long term, a whole new class of drugs might enter the market, where oligonucleotides might have the potency to be delivered to other organs than the liver, or allow allele-specific silencing. Moreover, an entire panel of genes could be silenced by including multiple oligonucleotides in a single treatment. Time will tell whether the new generation of RNA-targeting therapeutics can fulfill its promise.

Acknowledgements
The authors would like to thank Prof. dr. Pieter H. Reitsma for critical reading and helpful discussion of the manuscript.

Funding
Not applicable.

Authors' contributions
MH and BJMvV wrote the manuscript. Both authors read and approved the final manuscript.

Competing interests
The authors declare that they have no competing interests.

References
1. Sharp PA. RNA interference–2001. Genes Dev. 2001;15(5):485–90.
2. Dias N, Stein CA. Antisense oligonucleotides: basic concepts and mechanisms. Mol Cancer Ther. 2002;1(5):347–55.
3. Watts JK, Corey DR. Silencing disease genes in the laboratory and the clinic. J Pathol. 2012;226(2):365–79.
4. Stephenson ML, Zamecnik PC. Inhibition of Rous sarcoma viral RNA translation by a specific oligodeoxyribonucleotide. Proc Natl Acad Sci U S A. 1978;75(1):285–8.
5. Song E, et al. RNA interference targeting Fas protects mice from fulminant hepatitis. Nat Med. 2003;9(3):347–51.
6. Schroeder A, et al. Lipid-based nanotherapeutics for siRNA delivery. J Intern Med. 2010;267(1):9–21.
7. Kastelein JJ, et al. Potent reduction of apolipoprotein B and low-density lipoprotein cholesterol by short-term administration of an antisense inhibitor of apolipoprotein B. Circulation. 2006;114(16):1729–35.
8. Goodchild J. Therapeutic oligonucleotides. Methods Mol Biol. 2011;764:1–15.
9. de Fougerolles A, et al. Interfering with disease: a progress report on siRNA-based therapeutics. Nat Rev Drug Discov. 2007;6(6):443–53.
10. Bennett CF, Swayze EE. RNA targeting therapeutics: molecular mechanisms of antisense oligonucleotides as a therapeutic platform. Annu Rev Pharmacol Toxicol. 2010;50:259–93.
11. Loinger A, et al. Competition between small RNAs: a quantitative view. Biophys J. 2012;102(8):1712–21.
12. Novina CD, Sharp PA. The RNAi revolution. Nature. 2004;430(6996):161–4.
13. Gooding M, et al. Oligonucleotide conjugates - Candidates for gene silencing therapeutics. Eur J Pharm Biopharm. 2016;107:321–40.
14. Akinc A, et al. A combinatorial library of lipid-like materials for delivery of RNAi therapeutics. Nat Biotechnol. 2008;26(5):561–9.
15. John M, et al. Effective RNAi-mediated gene silencing without interruption of the endogenous microRNA pathway. Nature. 2007;449(7163):745–7.
16. Maier MA, et al. Biodegradable lipids enabling rapidly eliminated lipid nanoparticles for systemic delivery of RNAi therapeutics. Mol Ther. 2013;21(8):1570–8.
17. Parmar R, et al. 5'-(E)-vinylphosphonate: a stable phosphate mimic can improve the RNAi activity of siRNA-GalNAc conjugates. Chembiochem. 2016;17(11):985–9.
18. Mathew E, et al. Cytosolic delivery of antisense oligonucleotides by listeriolysin O-containing liposomes. Gene Ther. 2003;10(13):1105–15.
19. Zhang H, et al. Reduction of liver Fas expression by an antisense oligonucleotide protects mice from fulminant hepatitis. Nat Biotechnol. 2000;18(8):862–7.
20. Prakash TP, et al. Targeted delivery of antisense oligonucleotides to hepatocytes using triantennary N-acetyl galactosamine improves potency 10-fold in mice. Nucleic Acids Res. 2014;42(13):8796–807.
21. Geary RS, et al. Pharmacokinetics, biodistribution and cell uptake of antisense oligonucleotides. Adv Drug Deliv Rev. 2015;87:46–51.
22. Viney NJ, et al. Antisense oligonucleotides targeting apolipoprotein(a) in people with raised lipoprotein(a): two randomised, double-blind, placebo-controlled, dose-ranging trials. Lancet. 2016;388(10057):2239–53.
23. Yu RZ, et al. Disposition and Pharmacokinetics of a GalNAc3-Conjugated Antisense Oligonucleotide Targeting Human Lipoprotein (a) in Monkeys. Nucleic Acid Ther. 2016;26(6):372–80.
24. Dahlman JE, et al. In vivo endothelial siRNA delivery using polymeric nanoparticles with low molecular weight. Nat Nanotechnol. 2014;9(8):648–55.
25. Novobrantseva TI, et al. Systemic RNAi-mediated gene silencing in nonhuman primate and rodent myeloid cells. Mol Ther Nucleic Acids. 2012;1:e4.
26. Sehgal A, Vaishnaw A, Fitzgerald K. Liver as a target for oligonucleotide therapeutics. J Hepatol. 2013;59(6):1354–9.
27. Ledford H. CRISPR, the disruptor. Nature. 2015;522(7554):20–4.
28. Leadley Jr RJ, et al. Contribution of in vivo models of thrombosis to the discovery and development of novel antithrombotic agents. J Pharmacol Toxicol Methods. 2000;43(2):101–16.
29. Cleuren AC, van Vlijmen BJ, Reitsma PH. Transgenic mouse models of venous thrombosis: fulfilling the expectations? Semin Thromb Hemost. 2007;33(6):610–6.
30. Kretz CA, Weyand AC, Shavit JA. Modeling disorders of blood coagulation in the Zebrafish. Curr Pathobiol Rep. 2015;3(2):155–61.
31. Weyand AC, Shavit JA. Zebrafish as a model system for the study of hemostasis and thrombosis. Curr Opin Hematol. 2014;21(5):418–22.
32. Bill BR, et al. A primer for morpholino use in Zebrafish. Zebrafish. 2009;6(1):69–77.
33. Vo AH, et al. Loss of fibrinogen in zebrafish results in symptoms consistent with human hypofibrinogenemia. PLoS One. 2013;8(9):e74682.
34. Day K, Krishnegowda N, Jagadeeswaran P. Knockdown of prothrombin in zebrafish. Blood Cells Mol Dis. 2004;32(1):191–8.
35. Day KR, Jagadeeswaran P. Microarray analysis of prothrombin knockdown in zebrafish. Blood Cells Mol Dis. 2009;43(2):202–10.
36. Khandekar G, Jagadeeswaran P. Role of hepsin in factor VII activation in zebrafish. Blood Cells Mol Dis. 2014;52(1):76–81.
37. Sundaramoorthi H, et al. Knockdown of alphaIIb by RNA degradation by delivering deoxyoligonucleotides piggybacked with control vivo-morpholinos into zebrafish thrombocytes. Blood Cells Mol Dis. 2015;54(1):78–83.
38. Carrillo M, et al. Zebrafish von Willebrand factor. Blood Cells Mol Dis. 2010;45(4):326–33.
39. Kim S, et al. Vivo-Morpholino knockdown of alphaIIb: a novel approach to inhibit thrombocyte function in adult zebrafish. Blood Cells Mol Dis. 2010;44(3):169–74.
40. Zhang H, et al. Inhibition of the intrinsic coagulation pathway factor XI by antisense oligonucleotides: a novel antithrombotic strategy with lowered bleeding risk. Blood. 2010;116(22):4684–92.
41. Chen Z, et al. Proof-of-concept studies for siRNA-mediated gene silencing for coagulation factors in rat and rabbit. Mol Ther Nucleic Acids. 2015;4:e224.
42. Ankrom W, et al. Preclinical and translational evaluation of coagulation factor IXa as a novel therapeutic target. Pharmacol Res Perspect. 2016;4(1):e00207.
43. Di Minno MN, et al. Natural anticoagulants deficiency and the risk of venous thromboembolism: a meta-analysis of observational studies. Thromb Res. 2015;135(5):923–32.

44. Safdar H, et al. Acute and severe coagulopathy in adult mice following silencing of hepatic antithrombin and protein C production. Blood. 2013;121(21):4413–6.

45. Heestermans M, et al. Role of platelets, neutrophils, and factor XII in spontaneous venous thrombosis in mice. Blood. 2016;127(21):2630–7.

46. Arumugam PI, et al. Genetic diminution of circulating prothrombin ameliorates multiorgan pathologies in sickle cell disease mice. Blood. 2015;126(15):1844–55.

47. Safdar H, et al. Modulation of mouse coagulation gene transcription following acute in vivo delivery of synthetic small interfering RNAs targeting HNF4alpha and C/EBPalpha. PLoS One. 2012;7(6):e38104.

48. Becattini C, Agnelli G. Treatment of venous Thromboembolism with new anticoagulant agents. J Am Coll Cardiol. 2016;67(16):1941–55.

49. van Es N, et al. Direct oral anticoagulants compared with vitamin K antagonists for acute venous thromboembolism: evidence from phase 3 trials. Blood. 2014;124(12):1968–75.

50. Metzger JM, et al. Titrating haemophilia B phenotypes using siRNA strategy: evidence that antithrombotic activity is separated from bleeding liability. Thromb Haemost. 2015;113(6):1300–11.

51. Muller F, Gailani D, Renne T. Factor XI and XII as antithrombotic targets. Curr Opin Hematol. 2011;18(5):349–55.

52. Weitz JI. Factor XI and factor XII as targets for new anticoagulants. Thromb Res. 2016;141 Suppl 2:S40–5.

53. Kenne E, et al. Factor XII: a novel target for safe prevention of thrombosis and inflammation. J Intern Med. 2015;278(6):571–85.

54. Meijers JC, et al. High levels of coagulation factor XI as a risk factor for venous thrombosis. N Engl J Med. 2000;342(10):696–701.

55. Salomon O, et al. Reduced incidence of ischemic stroke in patients with severe factor XI deficiency. Blood. 2008;111(8):4113–7.

56. Cushman M, et al. Coagulation factors IX through XIII and the risk of future venous thrombosis: the Longitudinal Investigation of Thromboembolism Etiology. Blood. 2009;114(14):2878–83.

57. Cai TQ, et al. Factor XII full and partial null in rat confers robust antithrombotic efficacy with no bleeding. Blood Coagul Fibrinolysis. 2015; 26(8):893–902.

58. Yau JW, et al. Selective depletion of factor XI or factor XII with antisense oligonucleotides attenuates catheter thrombosis in rabbits. Blood. 2014;123(13):2102–7.

59. Revenko AS, et al. Selective depletion of plasma prekallikrein or coagulation factor XII inhibits thrombosis in mice without increased risk of bleeding. Blood. 2011;118(19):5302–11.

60. Bjorkqvist J, et al. Defective glycosylation of coagulation factor XII underlies hereditary angioedema type III. J Clin Invest. 2015;125(8):3132–46.

61. Bhattacharjee G, et al. Inhibition of vascular permeability by antisense-mediated inhibition of plasma kallikrein and coagulation factor 12. Nucleic Acid Ther. 2013;23(3):175–87.

62. Akinc A, et al. An investigational RNAi therapeutic targeting factor XII (ALN-F12) for the treatment of hereditary Angioedema. J Allergy Clin Immunol. 2016;137(2):Ab254.

63. Melquist S, et al. Targeting Factor 12 (F12) with a novel RNAi delivery platform as a prophylactic treatment for Hereditary Angioedema (HAE). J Allergy Clin Immunol. 2016. Conference(var.pagings): p. AB251.

64. Younis HS, et al. Antisense inhibition of coagulation factor XI prolongs APTT without increased bleeding risk in cynomolgus monkeys. Blood. 2012;119(10):2401–8.

65. Crosby JR, et al. Antithrombotic effect of antisense factor XI oligonucleotide treatment in primates. Arterioscler Thromb Vasc Biol. 2013;33(7):1670–8.

66. van Montfoort ML, et al. Factor XI regulates pathological thrombus formation on acutely ruptured atherosclerotic plaques. Arterioscler Thromb Vasc Biol. 2014;34(8):1668–73.

67. Vu TT, et al. Arterial thrombosis is accelerated in mice deficient in histidine-rich glycoprotein. Blood. 2015;125(17):2712–9.

68. Sehgal A, et al. An RNAi therapeutic targeting antithrombin to rebalance the coagulation system and promote hemostasis in hemophilia. Nat Med. 2015;21(5):492–7.

69. Li N, et al. Mipomersen is a promising therapy in the management of hypercholesterolemia: a meta-analysis of randomized controlled trials. Am J Cardiovasc Drugs. 2014;14(5):367–76.

70. Duell PB, et al. Long-term mipomersen treatment is associated with a reduction in cardiovascular events in patients with familial hypercholesterolemia. J Clin Lipidol. 2016;10(4):1011–21.

71. Lowenberg EC, et al. Coagulation factor XI as a novel target for antithrombotic treatment. J Thromb Haemost. 2010;8(11):2349–57.

72. Buller HR, et al. Factor XI antisense oligonucleotide for prevention of venous thrombosis. N Engl J Med. 2015;372(3):232–40.

73. Liu Q, et al. ISIS-FXIRx, a novel and specific antisense inhibitor of factor XI, caused significant reduction in FXI antigen and activity and increased aPTT without causing bleeding in healthy volunteers. Blood. 2011;118(21):97–8.

74. Pasi KJ, et al. A subcutaneously administered investigational RNAi therapeutic (ALN-AT3) targeting antithrombin for treatment of hemophilia: interim weekly and monthly dosing results in patients with hemophilia A or B. Blood. 2015;126(23).

75. Crosby JR, et al. Reversing antisense oligonucleotide activity with a sense oligonucleotide antidote: proof of concept targeting prothrombin. Nucleic Acid Ther. 2015;25(6):297–305.

10

Hemophilia A gene therapy via intraosseous delivery of factor VIII-lentiviral vectors

Carol H. Miao[1,2]

From The 9th Congress of the Asian-Pacific Society on Thrombosis and Hemostasis
Taipei, Taiwan.

Abstract

Current treatment of hemophilia A (HemA) patients with repeated infusions of factor VIII (FVIII; abbreviated as *F8* in constructs) is costly, inconvenient, and incompletely effective. In addition, approximately 25 % of treated patients develop anti-factor VIII immune responses. Gene therapy that can achieve long-term phenotypic correction without the complication of anti-factor VIII antibody formation is highly desired. Lentiviral vector (LV)-mediated gene transfer into hematopoietic stem cells (HSCs) results in stable integration of FVIII gene into the host genome, leading to persistent therapeutic effect. However, ex vivo HSC gene therapy requires pre-conditioning which is highly undesirable for hemophilia patients. The recently developed novel methodology of direct intraosseous (IO) delivery of LVs can efficiently transduce bone marrow cells, generating high levels of transgene expression in HSCs. IO delivery of E-F8-LV utilizing a ubiquitous EF1α promoter generated initially therapeutic levels of FVIII, however, robust anti-FVIII antibody responses ensued neutralized functional FVIII activity in the circulation. In contrast, a single IO delivery of G-FVIII-LV utilizing a megakaryocytic-specific GP1bα promoter achieved platelet-specific FVIII expression, leading to persistent, partial correction of HemA in treated animals. Most interestingly, comparable therapeutic benefit with G-F8-LV was obtained in HemA mice with pre-existing anti-FVIII inhibitors. Platelets is an ideal IO delivery vehicle since FVIII stored in α-granules of platelets is protected from high-titer anti-FVIII antibodies; and that even relatively small numbers of activated platelets that locally excrete FVIII may be sufficient to promote efficient clot formation during bleeding. Additionally, combination of pharmacological agents improved transduction of LVs and persistence of transduced cells and transgene expression. Overall, a single IO infusion of G-F8-LV can generate long-term stable expression of hFVIII in platelets and correct hemophilia phenotype for long term. This approach has high potential to permanently treat FVIII deficiency with and without pre-existing anti-FVIII antibodies.

Keywords: Hemophilia A, Factor VIII, Gene therapy, Intraosseous delivery, Lentiviral vectors, Megakaryocyte-specific gene expression, Anti-FVIII inhibitory antibodies, Stem cell gene therapy

Abbreviations: FVIII (F8 in constructs), Factor VIII; HemA, Hemophilia A; HSC, Hematopoietic stem cells; BM, Bone marrow; IO, Intraosseous; LV, Lentiviral vector; EF1α, Human elongation factor 1 alpha; Gp1bα, Glycoprotein 1b alpha; WAS, Wiskott-Aldrich syndrome; MLD, Metachromatic leukodystrophy

Correspondence: carol.miao@seattlechildrens.org
[1]Seattle Children's Research Institute, Seattle, WA, USA
[2]Department of Pediatrics, University of Washington, Seattle, WA, USA

Background

Deficiency of blood clotting factor VIII (FVIII) results in hemophilia A (HemA), a serious bleeding disorder. Current treatment of HemA patients with repeated infusions of FVIII is costly, inconvenient, and incompletely effective [1]. In addition, approximately 25 % of treated patients develop anti-FVIII immune responses. Gene therapy that can achieve long-term phenotypic correction without the complication of anti-FVIII antibody formation represents a highly desirable approach to treat HemA patients.

Previous phase I gene therapy clinical trials [2–4], however, produced only transient, low-level FVIII expression due to inefficient gene delivery and induction of immune responses to FVIII and/or gene therapy vectors. The hematopoietic stem cells (HSCs) in bone marrow (BM) can serve as a significant target for stable integration of therapeutic genes into the genome. Therapeutic levels of FVIII have been obtained by ex vivo gene therapy using HSCs transduced by retroviral vectors carrying porcine FVIII combined with immune suppression and busulfan [5, 6]. However, it is highly undesirable to perform pre-conditioning for hemophilia patients.

It is demonstrated recently that in vivo gene transfer can be successfully carried out by direct intraosseous (IO) injection using several different vectors including adeno-, retro-, and lenti-viral vectors (LVs) [7–10]. HSCs can be efficiently transduced by these vectors and the transgene expression was detected in both progenitors and differentiated cell lineages [7, 8, 11]. This in vivo protocol corrected BM defects for long-term in diseased animals with Fanconi anemia [11]. Many drawbacks of ex vivo gene therapy, including maintenance of stem cell properties, low levels of engraftment, and side effects of cytokine stimulation can be evaded [9, 10, 12]. Most importantly, no pre-conditioning of the subject is required for this approach, thus providing a novel strategy for treating HemA.

In this concise review, we will discuss the recently developed novel approach of IO delivery of LVs to correct hemA [10]. The benefit and limitations of using LVs driven by ubiquitous and megakaryocyte-specific promoters will be compared. The potential of the development of this novel in vivo technology into clinically feasible gene transfer protocol to treat hemA patients, especially the clinically challenging patients with pre-existing inhibitory antibodies will be discussed.

Review

Gene therapy vs. protein replacement therapy and other therapies

Current treatment of hemophilia involves repeated infusions of FVIII protein either as regular prophylaxis or treatment during bleeding episodes. For severe patients, the standard treatment consists of intravenous infusion of factor VIII concentrates three times per week or every other day [6, 7]. In addition, 25 % of the patients develop inhibitory antibodies to FVIII following repeated infusions of FVIII. In recent years, efforts have been made to improve the efficacy of protein replacement therapy. One of the major successes is to prolong the half-life of FVIII in circulation [13]. This is recently achieved by either attaching polyethylene glycol (PEG) to FVIII (PEGylated FVIII) [14, 15] or fusing a monomeric Fc fragment of immunoglobulin G [16] or albumin [17] to FVIII. Less frequent infusions of FVIII can be administered to patients with these long lasting FVIII proteins. Another successful approach is the development of a humanized bispecific antibody (emicizumab; ACE910) that binds to activated factor IX and factor X and mimics the cofactor function of FVIII [18, 19]. In the first clinical trial, the patients were given subcutaneous emicizumab weekly for 12 weeks. The bleeding rate decreased significantly in hemophilia patients with and without inhibitory antibodies. Nonetheless, these therapies still need frequent infusions of costly reagent and the long-term side effects such as formation of antibodies against the products themselves still need to be evaluated over time. Compared to drug or protein therapy, gene therapy can achieve a prolonged therapeutic effect with only one or a few treatment for the lifetime.

Comparison between different viral vector-mediated gene therapies for hemophilia

Recently, clinical trials of gene delivery of factor IX mediated by adenovirus-associated viral (AAV) vectors into the liver generated encouraging results in hemophilia B patients [20–22]. Furthermore, AAV-mediated, liver-directed gene transfer of FVIII produced therapeutic levels of gene expression in mice, dogs or macaques [23–25]. Most recently, Biomarin reported encouraging results of phase I/II clinical trial in a small number of patients using AAV5-mediated gene transfer. Five out of six high dose patients showed FVIII levels ranging between 4 and 60 % [26]. However it was noted there was elevation of ALT liver enzyme levels and a prophylactic corticosteroid therapy was given. The duration of clinical benefit in the treated patients remains to be determined. Furthermore, AAVs persist as episomal, concatemerized vectors following in vivo gene transfer, whereas transgene expression cassettes integrate into the host genome following LV transduction, leading to long-term therapeutic effect. If successful, a single treatment of LV-mediated gene therapy will be sufficient for life-long effect. Additionally, one key advantage of LV over traditional integrating gamma retroviral vectors is that it can transduce both non-dividing and dividing cells, leading to significantly increased efficiency targeting primitive stem cells. Furthermore, addition of SIN

LTR elements in self-inactivating (SIN)-LVs provided improved safety by reducing transactivation capacity [27], thus permitting inclusion of enhancer-less internal promoters in the transgene expression cassettes [28]. In two recent clinical trials of ex vivo gene therapy for Wiskott-Aldrich Syndrome (WAS) [29] and Metachromatic leukodystrophy (MLD) [30], dramatic clinical improvement was obtained without adverse effects or aberrant clonal expansion. These results are very encouraging, suggesting that LV may be a safer gene therapy vector compared with traditional retroviral vector.

In vivo HSC gene therapy mediates sustained transduction of HSCs in HemA mice

Although ex vivo HSC transduction/transplantation protocols can successfully deliver FVIII into HemA mice [6, 31], the procedure requires pre-conditioning using potentially toxic, myelosuppressive agents. On the contrary, IO delivery to transduce HSCs in vivo can bypass this step, which is more desirable for treating hemophilia patients. Furthermore, no significant thrombocytopenia potentially induced by preconditioning regimens is expected with the IO delivery protocol. Additionally, compared with intravenous infusion of LVs into the circulation, IO delivery directly introduced LVs into the BM microenvironment, thus significantly enhancing the transduction efficiency of HSCs. In our recent report, a syringe pump was used to slowly infuse VSV-G pseudotyped SIN-LV vectors into the BM so that more vectors can be in better contact with the resident cells to achieve high levels

of transduction [10] (Fig. 1a). When the BM cells were examined 7 days post infusion of M-GFP-LV driven by a ubiquitous MND promoter, a significant GFP signal was observed in HSCs of the treated mice (Fig. 1b). Furthermore, GFP expression persisted in 10–50 % HSCs up to 160 days (Fig. 1c&d), indicating that IO delivery of LVs has achieved efficient transduction of primitive progenitor cells in BM. Moreover, lower numbers of transduced cells were initially found in the untreated leg compared to the treated leg (Fig. 1b), whereas at later times, similar numbers of transduced cells were obtained at both sites (Fig. 1c), indicating that the transduced HSCs were transferred from treated to untreated BM sites over time. These results clearly demonstrated that IO LV delivery mediates sustained transduction of hematopoietic stem/progenitor cells [10, 32].

Comparison between IO deliveries of F8-LVs driven by two different promoters

As mentioned in the introduction, one of the major complications of hemophilia treatment is the formation of anti-FVIII inhibitory antibodies. For achieving successful gene therapy, it is essential to prevent or evade anti-FVIII immune responses. For this purpose, platelet has been considered as a potential gene transfer vehicle to ectopically express FVIII because: (1) FVIII can be released to promote clot formation when the circulating platelets are recruited to and activated at the injury sites, (2) when needed, ectopic FVIII can be provided by circulating platelets that are produced daily from megakaryocytes in BM, (3) in

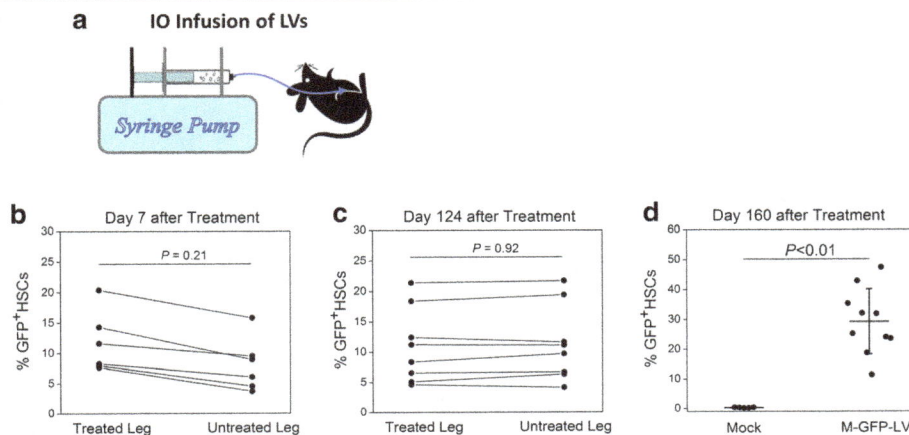

Fig. 1 GFP expression in BM cells following IO infusion of M-GFP-LV. **a** Schematic of IO infusion of vectors into the mice with an infusion speed of 10 µl/min, which was precisely controlled by a programmable microfluidics syringe pump. **b** C57BL/6 mice were intraosseously delivered with M-GFP-LV (1.1×10^8 ifu/animal, $n = 6$) on day 0. BM cells were isolated from treated or untreated legs and GFP expression in Lin$^-$Sca1$^+$c-Kit$^+$ HSCs were examined on day 7 by flow cytometry. **c** C57BL/6 mice were given IO infusion of M-GFP-LV (1.1×10^8 ifu; $n = 8$) on day 0. GFP expression in Lin$^-$Sca1$^+$c-Kit$^+$ HSCs of treated and untreated legs was evaluated on day 124. **d** C57BL/6 mice were given IO infusion of M-GFP-LV (8.8×10^8 ifu/animal; $n = 10$) or PBS (20 µl/animal, mock; $n = 5$) on day 0. Long-term GFP expression in Lin$^-$Sca1$^+$c-Kit$^+$ HSCs was detected on day 160. This figure is reproduced from Ref [10]

particular, platelet FVIII stored in α-granules is not neutralized by anti-FVIII antibodies in the circulation [33, 34]. Previous reports showed that platelet-restricted expression of FVIII using megakaryocyte-specific promoters (glycoprotein (Gp) αIIb [31, 33, 34], Gp1bα [35] and platelet factor 4 [36]) can partially correct hemophilia phenotype in transgenic mice or in lethally irradiated HemA mice treated with ex vivo gene therapy. Ectopic expression of FVIII in platelets locally delivers protein and concomitantly evades anti-FVIII immune responses in treating HemA.

In our recent study [10], it was found that IO delivery of E-F8-LV using a ubiquitous human elongation factor-1α (EF1α) promoter into BMs of hemA mice efficiently transduced HSCs and produced initial high-levels of FVIII. However, a robust immune response to FVIII was induced, eliminating functional FVIII in the circulation (Fig. 2a). In contrast, a single IO delivery of G-F8-LV using a human megakaryocytic-specific GP1bα promoter produced persistent platelet-specific expression of FVIII (Fig. 2b), leading to persistent, partial correction of HemA phenotype (Fig. 2c). Interestingly, we did not detect hFVIII activity or anti-hFVIII antibody in plasma up to 160 days post treatment (Fig. 2d), implying that little or no hFVIII expression was secreted into the circulation. These results are consistent with previous work using the Gp1bα promoter to direct FVIII expression in platelets [35, 37]. It was shown that FVIII co-localized with VWF and stored in α-granules of platelets via a regulated secretory pathway [34].

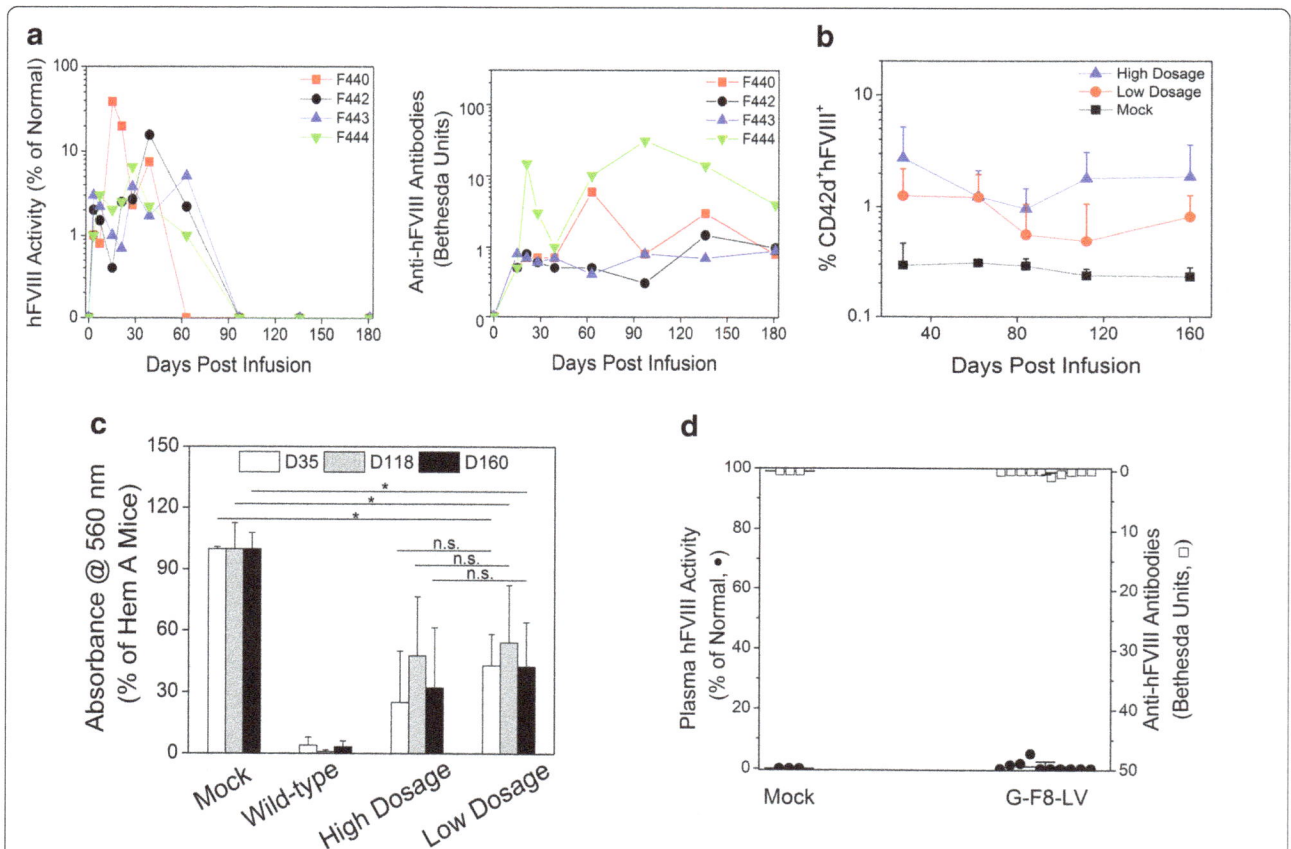

Fig. 2 Comparison of hFVIII levels in plasma and/or platelets after a single IO infusion of E-F8-LVs and G-F8-LVs. **a** HemA mice were intraosseously infused with E-F8-LV (5×10^7 ifu/animal, $n = 4$) or PBS (20 μl/animal, mock, $n = 3$) on day 0. Plasma samples were collected and hFVIII activity and anti-FVIII antibodies were measured by aPTT and Bethesda assay, respectively. No FVIII activity or anti-FVIII antibody was detected in the PBS treated control mice (data not shown). **b-d** HemA mice were given IO infusion of G-F8-LV (2.2×10^7 ifu/animal or 2.2×10^6 ifu/animal) or PBS (20 μl/animal, mock) on day 0. **b** Platelets were isolated from peripheral blood of high ($n = 8$) or low ($n = 5$) titer G-F8-LV treated or mock ($n = 3$) mice. hFVIII expression levels in CD42d⁺ platelets were evaluated by flow cytometry on day 27, 62, 84, 112 and 160. **c** HemA phenotype correction of G-F8-LV treated mice was monitored by tail clip assay on day 35, 118, and 160 ($n = 4-7$/group). The average blood loss of untreated HemA mice was set as 100 %. Wild-type C57BL/6 mice were used as positive controls. * $P < 0.05$. **d** Plasma samples were collected from high titer G-F8-LV treated ($n = 10$) or mock ($n = 3$) mice, and hFVIII activity and anti-FVIII antibodies were measured by aPTT and Bethesda assay, respectively. This figure is reproduced from Ref [10]

A single IO infusion of G-F8-LV produced persistent expression of FVIII in platelets

Following IO delivery, up to 3 % of platelets expressed FVIII driven by platelet-specific promoters [10] (Fig. 3a). The average hFVIII antigen level evaluated by ELISA was 1 mU per 1×10^8 platelets, a level comparable to previously described transgenic animals expressing platelet FVIII by chromogenic assay [35]. Our results clearly showed that Gp1bα specifically drives FVIII expression in platelets following IO infusion and that FVIII stored in platelets corrects the HemA phenotype. It should be noted that platelet delivered FVIII may produce different kinetics of clot formation temporally and spatially from plasma FVIII as see in the laser injury mouse model [38]. However, enhancement of clot formation with platelet-targeted gene therapy has been demonstrated previously using a range of injury models including tail bleeding assay, survival assay, digital cuticular bleeding assay, and ferric chloride-induced arterial injury model [31, 33–35]. Our recent results [10] clearly showed that even low levels of FVIII released from platelets could partially correct the HemA phenotype. Incorporation of variant FVIII cDNAs with higher expression levels including codon optimized

FVIII [24, 25, 39] may further increases the therapeutic effect of IO delivery targeting platelets. Additionally, although platelet-stored FVIII is proven to restore hemostasis, the mouse models have their limitations. Human clinical trials will be the ultimate demonstration that a reduction in incidence of spontaneous bleeds (such as joint bleeds) can be achieved.

FVIII ectopically expressed and stored in platelets corrects HemA mice with pre-existing high-titer inhibitor antibodies

Much effort has been devoted to investigate effective means to overcome the complication of inhibitory antibody formation to FVIII, including the development of immune modulation protocols (see recent Review [40]) or generation of tissue-specific vectors (including promoter and envelope) or delivery of vectors via specific route [41, 42] to induce tolerance to FVIII. Shi and colleagues [33, 43] reported that pre-conditioning and ex vivo gene transfer of HSCs expressing platelet FVIII improved hemostasis in HemA mice with pre-existing inhibitory antibodies. Our investigation [10] demonstrates that a single IO delivery of G-F8-LV generated significant functional FVIII activity (Fig. 3b). Most importantly,

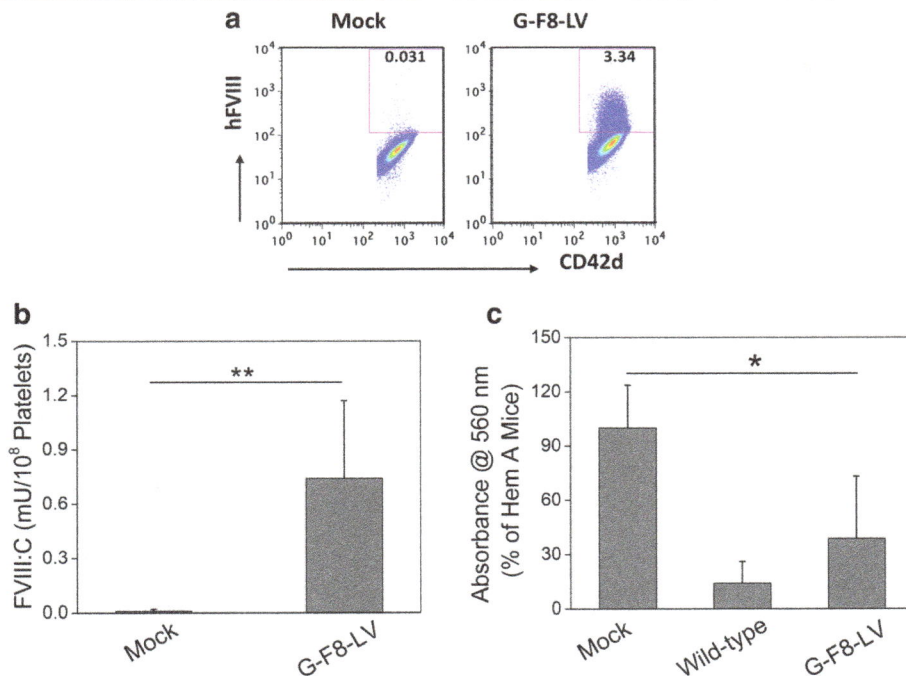

Fig. 3 hFVIII expression in platelets of G-F8-LV treated inhibitor HemA mice corrected their hemophilia A phenotype. Inhibitor HemA mice were established by repeated intraperitoneal injection (3x/week for 2 weeks) of 3U rhFVIII into 10- to 12-week-old HemA mice. These inhibitor HemA mice were then intraosseously infused with G-F8-LV (2.2×10^7 ifu/animal) or PBS (20 μl/animal, mock) on day 0. **a** Platelets were isolated from peripheral blood and marked with CD42d+, and their GFP expression levels at 5 months post infusion. **b** Platelets from LV-treated ($n = 5$) and mock ($n = 3$) mice and lysed. The resulting lysate was examined for hFVIII expression level by ELISA on day 27 post infusion. **c** The phenotypic correction of G-F8-LV treated HemA inhibitor mice ($n = 7$) was examined by tail clip assays on day 160 post infusion. The average blood loss of untreated HemA ($n = 10$) mice was set as 100 %. Wild-type C57BL/6 mice ($n = 8$) were used as positive controls. * $P < 0.05$, ** $P < 0.005$. This figure is reproduced from Ref [10]

persistent, partial therapeutic effect was obtained despite of the presence of pre-existing high-titer anti-FVIII antibodies (Fig. 3c). These results indicate that FVIII ectopically expressed and stored in α-granules of the platelets and released at the injury sites represents a promising strategy to HemA patients with high-titer inhibitors, including individuals who were previously excluded from gene therapy clinical trials.

Use pharmacological approaches to enhance in situ transduction efficiency of HSCs following IO delivery of LVs into the BM

Furthermore, following IO delivery of LVs in immune-competent mice, we found lymphocyte infiltrates in BM and gradual decreases of transduced cells, which are similar to the innate and adaptive responses observed from LV transduction in hepatocytes [44–46]. By administering a short course of combination drug treatment with Dexamethasone (Dex) and AntiCD8α antibody, we were able to achieve better initial transduction and reduce the potential of generating CTLs and other adaptive immune responses [47]. These agents in combination synergistically augmented LV transduction.

Conclusions

Although long-lasting factor concentrates have improved efficacy of protein replacement therapy, and FVIII-mimetic bispecific antibody is promising as an alternative treatment especially for patients with inhibitory antibodies, these therapies require frequent, at least weekly dosing of costly reagents. With the recent successes in clinical trials of AAV-mediated gene transfer, it is anticipated that gene therapy will be the next generation medicine for hemophilia treatment. The potential obstacles of AAV-mediated gene therapy include unpredictable events of transaminase elevation, potential requirement of repeated treatment that cannot be performed due to pre-existing anti-AAV immune responses, and the prohibitively high cost of high-titer vectors needed for hemA treatment. The recently developed novel strategy of IO delivery of F8-LVs [10] can efficiently transduce bone marrow cells and express FVIII in HSCs without the requirement of using potentially toxic, myelosuppressive pre-conditioning methods and the risk of inducing thrombocytopenia. Although ubiquitous expression of FVIII and secretion into the circulation induced high-titer inhibitory antibody production and eliminated functional FVIII activity, a single IO infusion of G-F8-LVs driven by a megakaryocyte-specific promoter produced long-term stable expression of hFVIII in platelets and corrected hemophilia phenotype

for long term. Most significantly, this strategy is proven successful in HemA mice with pre-existing inhibitory antibodies. Use of combination of pharmacological agents further enhanced the persistence of transduced cells and transgene expression. IO delivery is already a clinically proven method for drug delivery. IO LV delivery can be easily developed for human clinical trials for hemophilia patients with and without pre-existing inhibitory antibodies. This new simple novel protocol has the potential for a single treatment to achieve life-long therapeutic effect for hemophilia.

Authors' contributions
Review concept, design, drafting, and revision: CHM.

Competing interests
The author declares that she has no competing interests.

References
1. Gringeri A, Mantovani LG, Scalone L, Mannucci PM, Grp CS. Cost of care and quality of life for patients with hemophilia complicated by inhibitors: the COCIS Study Group. Blood. 2003;102:2358–63.
2. Roth DA, Tawa Jr NE, O'Brien JM, Treco DA, Selden RF. Nonviral transfer of the gene encoding coagulation factor VIII in patients with severe hemophilia A. N Engl J Med. 2001;344:1735–42.
3. Powell JS, Ragni MV, White 2nd GC, et al. Phase 1 trial of FVIII gene transfer for severe hemophilia A using a retroviral construct administered by peripheral intravenous infusion. Blood. 2003;102:2038–45.
4. White 2nd GC. Gene therapy in hemophilia: clinical trials update. Thromb Haemost. 2001;86:172–7.
5. Doering CB, Gangadharan B, Dukart HZ, Spencer HT. Hematopoietic stem cells encoding porcine factor VIII induce pro-coagulant activity in hemophilia A mice with pre-existing factor VIII immunity. Mol Ther. 2007;15:1093–9.
6. Ide LM, Gangadharan B, Chiang KY, Doering CB, Spencer HT. Hematopoietic stem-cell gene therapy of hemophilia A incorporating a porcine factor VIII transgene and nonmyeloablative conditioning regimens. Blood. 2007;110:2855–63.
7. McCauslin CS, Wine J, Cheng L, et al. In vivo retroviral gene transfer by direct intrafemoral injection results in correction of the SCID phenotype in Jak3 knock-out animals. Blood. 2003;102:843–8.
8. Worsham DN, Schuesler T, von Kalle C, Pan D. In vivo gene transfer into adult stem cells in unconditioned mice by in situ delivery of a lentiviral vector. Mol Ther. 2006;14:514–24.
9. Pan D, Gunther R, Duan WM, et al. Biodistribution and toxicity studies of VSVG-pseudotyped lentiviral vector after intravenous administration in mice with the observation of in vivo transduction of bone marrow. Mol Ther. 2002;6:19–29.
10. Wang X, Shin SC, Chiang AF, Khan I, Pan D, Rawlings DJ, Miao CH. Intraosseous delivery of lentiviral vectors targeting factor VIII expression in platelets corrects murine hemophilia A. Mol Ther. 2015;23:617–26.
11. Habi O, Girard J, Bourdages V, Delisle M-C, and Carreau M. Correction of Fanconi anemia group c hematopoietic stem cells following intrafemoral gene transfer. Anemia, 2010;2010.

12. Baum C, Dullmann J, Li ZX, Fehse B, Meyer J, Williams DA, von Kalle C. Side effects of retroviral gene transfer into hematopoietic stem cells. Blood. 2003; 101:2099–114.

13. Kaufman RJ, Powell JS. Molecular approaches for improved clotting factors for hemophilia. Hematol Am Soc Hematol Educ Program. 2013;2013:30–6.

14. Gu JM, Ramsey P, Evans V, et al. Evaluation of the activated partial thromboplastin time assay for clinical monitoring of PEGylated recombinant factor VIII (BAY 94–9027) for haemophilia A. Haemophilia. 2014;20:593–600.

15. Mei B, Pan C, Jiang H, et al. Rational design of a fully active, long-acting PEGylated factor VIII for hemophilia A treatment. Blood. 2010;116:270–9.

16. Nolan B, Mahlangu J, Perry D, et al. Long-term safety and efficacy of recombinant factor VIII Fc fusion protein (rFVIIIFc) in subjects with haemophilia A. Haemophilia. 2016;22:72–80.

17. Schulte S. Innovative coagulation factors: albumin fusion technology and recombinant single-chain factor VIII. Thromb Res. 2013;131 Suppl 2:S2–6.

18. Uchida N, Sambe T, Yoneyama K, Fukazawa N, Kawanishi T, Kobayashi S, Shima M. A first-in-human phase 1 study of ACE910, a novel factor VIII-mimetic bispecific antibody, in healthy subjects. Blood. 2016;127:1633–41.

19. Shima M, Hanabusa H, Taki M, et al. Factor VIII-Mimetic Function of Humanized Bispecific Antibody in Hemophilia A. N Engl J Med. 2016;374:2044–53.

20. Monahan PE. Gene therapy in an era of emerging treatment options for hemophilia B. J Thromb Haemost. 2015;13 Suppl 1:S151–60.

21. Nathwani AC, Reiss UM, Tuddenham EG, et al. Long-term safety and efficacy of factor IX gene therapy in hemophilia B. N Engl J Med. 2014;371:1994–2004.

22. Nathwani AC, Tuddenham EGD, Rangarajan S, et al. Adenovirus-associated virus vector-mediated gene transfer in hemophilia B. N Engl J Med. 2011; 365:2357–65.

23. Callan MB, Haskins ME, Wang P, Zhou S, High KA, Arruda VR. Successful phenotype improvement following gene therapy for severe hemophilia a in privately owned dogs. PLoS One. 2016;11:e0151800.

24. McIntosh J, Lenting PJ, Rosales C, et al. Therapeutic levels of FVIII following a single peripheral vein administration of rAAV vector encoding a novel human factor VIII variant. Blood. 2013;121:3335–44.

25. Siner JI, Iacobelli NP, Sabatino DE, et al. Minimal modification in the factor VIII B-domain sequence ameliorates the murine hemophilia A phenotype. Blood. 2013;121:4396–403.

26. Adams B. BioMarin says hemophilia A gene therapy data 'encouranging'. http://www.fiercebiotech.com/biotech/biomarin-says-hemophilia-a-gene-therapy-data-encouraging, 2016: April 20, 2016.

27. Zhou S, Mody D, DeRavin SS, et al. A self-inactivating lentiviral vector for SCID-X1 gene therapy that does not activate LMO2 expression in human T cells. Blood. 2010;116:900–8.

28. Knight S, Bokhoven M, Collins M, Takeuchi Y. Effect of the internal promoter on insertional gene activation by lentiviral vectors with an intact HIV long terminal repeat. J Virol. 2010;84:4856–9.

29. Aiuti A, Biasco L, Scaramuzza S, et al. Lentiviral hematopoietic stem cell gene therapy in patients with Wiskott-Aldrich syndrome. Science. 2013;341: 1233151.

30. Biffi A, Montini E, Lorioli L, et al. Lentiviral hematopoietic stem cell gene therapy benefits metachromatic leukodystrophy. Science. 2013;341:1233158.

31. Shi Q, Wilcox DA, Fahs SA, et al. Lentivirus-mediated platelet-derived factor VIII gene therapy in murine haemophilia A. J Thromb Haemost. 2007;5:352–61.

32. Wang CX, Sather BD, Wang X, et al. Rapamycin relieves lentiviral vector transduction resistance in human and mouse hematopoietic stem cells. Blood. 2014;124:913–23.

33. Kuether E, Schroeder J, Fahs S, et al. Lentivirus-mediated platelet gene therapy of murine hemophilia A with pre-existing ant-factor VIII immunity. J Thromb Haemost. 2012;10:1570–80.

34. Shi QZ, Wilcox DA, Fahs SA, et al. Factor VIII ectopically targeted to platelets is therapeutic in hemophilia A with high-titer inhibitory antibodies. J Clin Investig. 2006;116:1974–82.

35. Yarovoi HV, Kufrin D, Eslin DE, et al. Factor VIII ectopically expressed in platelets: efficacy in hemophilia A treatment. Blood. 2003;102:4006–13.

36. Damon AL, Scudder LE, Gnatenko DV, Sitaraman V, Hearing P, Jesty J, Bahou WF. Altered bioavailability of platelet-derived factor VIII during thrombocytosis reverses phenotypic efficacy in haemophilic mice. Thromb Haemost. 2008;100:1111–22.

37. Ohmori T, Mimuro J, Takano K, et al. Efficient expression of a transgene in platelets using simian immunodeficiency virus-based vector harboring glycoprotein Ib alpha promoter: in vivo model for platelet-targeting gene therapy. FASEB J. 2006;20:1522–4.

38. Neyman M, Gewirtz J, Poncz M. Analysis of the spatial and temporal characteristics of platelet-delivered factor VHI-based clots. Blood. 2008;112: 1101–8.

39. Ward NJ, Buckley SM, Waddington SN, et al. Codon optimization of human factor VIII cDNAs leads to high-level expression. Blood. 2011;117:798–807.

40. Scott DW, Pratt KP, Miao CH. Progress toward inducing immunologic tolerance to factor VIII. Blood. 2013;121:4449–56.

41. Matsui H, Shibata M, Brown B, et al. A murine model for induction of long-term immunologic tolerance to factor VIII does not require persistent detectable levels of plasma factor VIII and involves contributions from Foxp3(+) T regulatory cells. Blood. 2009;114:677–85.

42. Sack BK, Merchant S, Markusic DM, Nathwani AC, Davidoff AM, Byrne BJ, Herzog RW. Transient B cell depletion or improved transgene expression by codon optimization promote tolerance to factor VIII in gene therapy. PLoS One. 2012;7:e37671.

43. Shi Q, Fahs SA, Wilcox DA, et al. Syngeneic transplantation of hematopoietic stem cells that are genetically modified to express factor VIII in platelets restores hemostasis to hemophilia A mice with preexisting FVIII immunity. Blood. 2008;112:2713–21.

44. Brown BD, Sitia G, Annoni A, et al. In vivo administration of lentiviral vectors triggers a type I interferon response that restricts hepatocyte gene transfer and promotes vector clearance. Blood. 2007;109:2797–805.

45. Agudo J, Ruzo A, Kitur K, Sachidanandam R, Blander JM, Brown BD. A TLR and non-TLR mediated innate response to lentiviruses restricts hepatocyte entry and can be ameliorated by pharmacological blockade. Mol Ther. 2012; 20:2257–67.

46. Akira S, Uematsu S, Takeuchi O. Pathogen recognition and innate immunity. Cell. 2006;124:783–801.

47. Wang X, Lyle MJ, Fu R, Miao CH. Enhancing factor VIII expression in platelets of hemophilia A mice following intraosseous delivery of lentiviral vectors. New Orleans: American Society of Gene and Cell Therapy 18th Annual Meeting; 2015. p. 245.

11

Vitamin K antagonist use: evidence of the difficulty of achieving and maintaining target INR range and subsequent consequences

Jeff R. Schein[1], C. Michael White[2,3], Winnie W. Nelson[1], Jeffrey Kluger[3], Elizabeth S. Mearns[2] and Craig I. Coleman[2,3]*

Abstract

Vitamin K antagonists (VKAs) are effective oral anticoagulants that are titrated to a narrow therapeutic international normalized ratio (INR) range. We reviewed published literature assessing the impact of INR stability - getting into and staying in target INR range - on outcomes including thrombotic events, major bleeding, and treatment costs, as well as key factors that impact INR stability.

A time in therapeutic range (TTR) of ≥65 % is commonly accepted as the definition of INR stability. In the real-world setting, this is seldom achieved with standard-of-care management, thus increasing the patients' risks of thrombotic or major bleeding events. There are many factors associated with poor INR control. Being treated in community settings, newly initiated on a VKA, younger in age, or nonadherent to therapy, as well as having polymorphisms of CYP2C9 or VKORC1, or multiple physical or mental co-morbid disease states have been associated with lower TTR. Clinical prediction tools are available, though they can only explain <10 % of the variance behind poor INR control.

Clinicians caring for patients who require anticoagulation are encouraged to intensify diligence in INR management when using VKAs and to consider appropriate use of newer anticoagulants as a therapeutic option.

Keywords: Vitamin K antagonists, International normalized ratio, Anticoagulation, Atrial fibrillation, Venous thromboembolism

Background

Vitamin K antagonists (VKAs) such as warfarin inhibit the enzyme vitamin K epoxide reductase and consequently the recycling of inactive vitamin K epoxide back to its active, reduced form [1]. Vitamin K in its active form is required for the synthesis of various clotting factors (II, VII, IX and X) involved in the coagulation cascade (as well as the anti-clotting proteins C and S); and thus, VKAs result in the depletion of these factors (within 72–96 h after dosing) and an anticoagulated state.

VKAs are indicated for the prevention of thrombotic events in patients with atrial fibrillation (AF) and following venous thromboembolism (VTE) [2, 3]. For stroke prevention in AF patients, VKA therapy that is dose-adjusted to maintain an international normalized ratio (INR) range of 2.0 to 3.0 is associated with a 64 % reduction in the risk of stroke compared to placebo [4]. In patients suffering an acute VTE (either deep vein thrombosis (DVT) or pulmonary embolism (PE)), adjusted-dose VKA use (preceded by a parenteral anticoagulant) significantly reduces the risk of recurrence of thrombotic events [3, 5, 6]. Adjusted-dose VKAs are included in clinical guidelines for AF and VTE [2, 3, 7, 8] with a target INR range of 2.0–3.0.

* Correspondence: craig.coleman@hhchealth.org
[2]Department of Pharmacy Practice, University of Connecticut School of Pharmacy, 69 N. Eagleville Road, Storrs, CT 06269-3092, USA
[3]Hartford Hospital Division of Cardiology, 80 Seymour Street, Hartford, CT 06102-5037, USA
Full list of author information is available at the end of the article

The objective of this paper is to provide an assessment of "INR stability" with VKA use and patient outcomes in contemporary practice. INR stability refers to achieving and maintaining target INR range (typically 2–3, but not always). Therefore, if target INR range is not achieved or maintained this would be considered INR *in*stability.

We will determine: 1) to what extent INR instability can be anticipated, 2) whether INR instability is predictable, and 3) the consequences of INR instability.

Metrics of INR

Despite 60 years of clinical experience, the maintenance of stable INR in patients using VKA remains a challenging task. While numerous metrics have been used in clinical studies of VKAs to assess the quality of anticoagulation control [9, 10], time in therapeutic range (TTR) (most commonly calculated using Rosendaal's method of linear interpolation [11]) is the most frequently reported. Experts have suggested that the minimum target TTR should be no less than 65 % [12–15] but this goal is often not met [16–22] even in modern day RCTs [23–32] (Table 1). A large observational assessment of 40,404 patients in the VA population demonstrated that 42 % of patients had INR stability (defined as TTR > 70 %) while 34 % had moderate instability (TTR 50 to 70 %), and 23 % had high instability (TTR <50 %) [33]. A recently published retrospective analysis from the CoagClinic™ database assessed 9433 patients who met the inclusion criteria and had been using warfarin for over 6 months [34]. In these chronic warfarin patients, more than 90 % had at least one value below 2 and 82 % had at least one value above 3 (Fig. 1).

Using data from the multicenter ORBIT-AF (Outcomes Registry for Better Informed Treatment of Atrial Fibrillation) registry, the INR stability of 3749 patients on chronic warfarin therapy for 6 months was assessed [35]. Only 26 % (95%CI: 24 to 27 %) of patients had 80 % or more of their INRs between 2 and 3. Among this subgroup with INR stability, 92 % (95%CI: 90 to 94 %) had at least one value outside of the normal INR range while 36 % (95%CI: 33 to 39 %) had an INR below 1.5 or above 4 over the subsequent year. Thus, even the "cream of the crop" – those patients able to achieve most of their values within target range within a 6-month period – had at least occasional out-of-range values over longer-term follow-up.

Multiple meta-analyses of randomized and real-world studies have been performed in order to estimate the quality of INR control in AF and VTE populations receiving VKAs [16–20, 22]. These meta-analyses demonstrate poor INR control to be 'the rule rather than the exception' with TTRs and proportion of INR measurement in range typically falling near or below 60 % and nearly twice the amount of time being spent below versus above the therapeutic INR range (Table 2) [16–20, 22].

The literature from clinical trials and observational studies substantiate that INR stability is not readily attainable and when it occurs, is rarely sustainable over time.

Consequences of INR Instability
Outcomes
The consequences of INR instability are multifaceted. INR instability was associated with clinical events, higher level of medication non-persistence and discontinuation, utilization of more healthcare resources, and therefore, higher costs. According to meta-analyses of AF or mixed populations assessing INR control and associated events [18, 36–38], greater than half of all thromboembolic events occurred when patients have an INR < 2.0, while

Table 1 Mean time in the therapeutic range observed in recent atrial fibrillation and venous thromboembolism randomized controlled trials of novel target oral anticoagulants

Study	Disease state	Mean TTR	TTR in month 1[a]	TTR in later months[a]
ARISTOTLE	NVAF	62 %		
ENGAGE-TIMI-48 2013	NVAF	65 %		
RE-LY 2009	NVAF	64 %		
ROCKET-AF, 2010	NVAF	55 %		
AMPLIFY	VTE	61 %	NR	NR
EINSTEIN-DVT	DVT	58 %	54 %	66 % (month 10)
EINSTEIN-PE	PE	63 %	58 %	73 % (month 11)
Hokusai-VTE	VTE	64 %	NR	NR
RECOVER 1	VTE	60 %	53 %	66 % (month 6)
RECOVER 2	VTE	57 %	51 %	54–62 % (months 3–6)

DVT deep vein thrombosis, *NR* not reported, *NVAF* nonvalvular atrial fibrillation, *PE* pulmonary embolism, *TTR* time in the therapeutic range, *VTE* venous thromboembolism
[a]For venous thromboembolism studies only

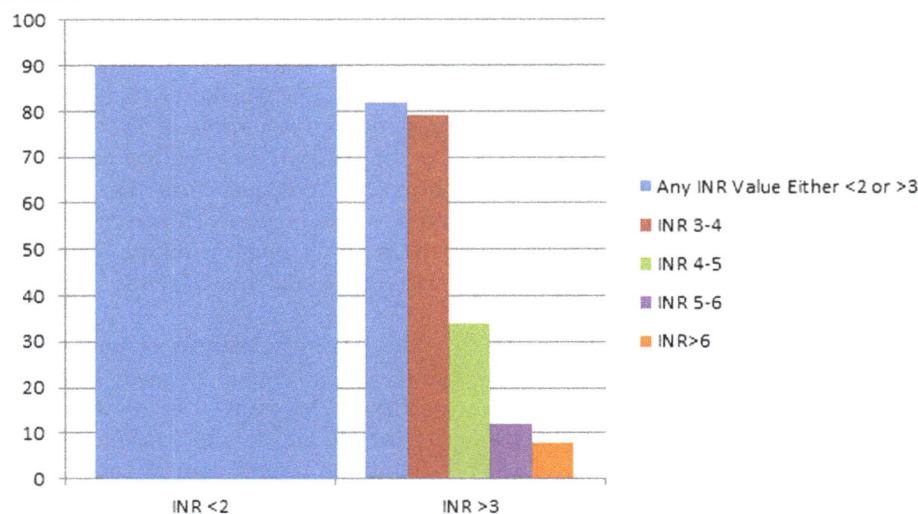

Fig. 1 Percent of patients with ≥1 INRs outside the normal therapeutic range. This figure displays the % of people in an analysis [34] of the CoagCheckTM database with at least one INR value outside of the normal therapeutic range with blue boxes showing the percent of patients who were either below 2.0 (90 %) or above 3.0 (82 %). The red, green, purple, and orange boxes display the percent of people who ever achieved a level of 3.0–4.0, 4.0–5.0, 5.0–6.0, and >6.0, respectively. The same individual could be represented in multiple categories given their INRs achieved over time including being below 2.0 and above 3.0

over 40 % of all hemorrhagic events occurred at an INR >3.0. In VTE patients, subtherapeutic INRs were found to be present during 58 % of recurrent VTEs [17].

An observational study by Nelson et al, [38] using the Veterans Health Administration (VHA) dataset, explored the relationship between out-of-range INRs and clinical outcomes in 34,346 patients with non-valvular AF (NVAF) who were newly initiated on warfarin therapy. When INR values were below range (<2), patients were much more likely to experience adverse thrombotic or embolic events (Fig. 2). Patients were at an increased risk of major

bleeding with both subtherapeutic INR values (RR = 2.58 95%CI: 2.19–3.03) as well as supratherapeutic INR values, (RR = 1.55, 95%CI: 1.21–1.97). All event rates were qualitatively the highest when patients had an INR < 2. While most of these events were stroke associated with sub-therapeutic values, increased bleeding events were also observed. While only speculative (and we could not identify supportive literature) it is possible the increased bleeding associated with sub-therapeutic INRs is due a lag in time between the actual event and the true INR value. This emphasizes the need for

Table 2 Results of meta-analyses evaluating the international normalized ratio stability in atrial fibrillation or venous thromboembolism patients

Meta-Analysis, Year	Population	TTR, % (95 % CI)	TBR, % (95 % CI)	TAR, % (95 % CI)	PINRR, % (95 % CI)	PINRBR, % (95 % CI)	PINRAR, % (95 % CI)
Mearns 2014	AF	61 (59 to 62)	25 (23 to 27)	14 (13 to 15)	59 (53 to 59)	26 (23 to 29)	13 (11 to 17)
Mearns 2014	VTE	61 (59 to 63)	25 (23 to 26)	15 (14 to 17)	59 (54 to 64)	26 (23 to 29)	13 (9 to 19)
Erkens 2012 (Month 1)	VTE	54 (NR)	42 (NR)	12 (NR)	NR	NR	NR
Erkens 2012 (Months 1–3)		56 (NR)	35 (NR)	19 (NR)	NR	NR	NR
Erkens 2012 (Month 1–6+)		60 (NR)	24 (NR)	17 (NR)	NR	NR	NR
Erkens 2012 (Month 4–12+)		75 (NR)	21 (NR)	12 (NR)	NR	NR	NR
Wan 2008 (RCT)	AF	67 (44 to 73)	20 (18 t to 40)	14 (9 to 17)	67 (48 to 84)	24 (14 to 32)	8 (2 to 24)
Wan 2008 (Prospective)		61 (56 to 66)	21 (14 to 29)	14 (13 to 30)	—	—	—
Wan 2008 (Retrospective)		59 (29 to 75)	25 (9 to 52)	14 (9 to 39)	53 (34 to 68)	26 (10 to 51)	17 (14 to 29)
Cios 2009	AF	59 (57 to 61)	NR	NR	NR	NR	NR
Reynolds 2004	AF	61 (NR)	26 (NR)	13 (NR)	61 (NR)	25 (NR)	14 (NR)

AF atrial fibrillation, *CI* confidence interval, *NR* not reported, *PINRAR* proportion of INRs above range, *PINRBR* proportion of INRs below range, *PINRR* proportion of INRs in range; *RCT* randomized controlled trial, *TAR* time above range, *TBR* time below range, *TTR* time in range, *VTE* venous thromboembolism
— = evaluated, but no data

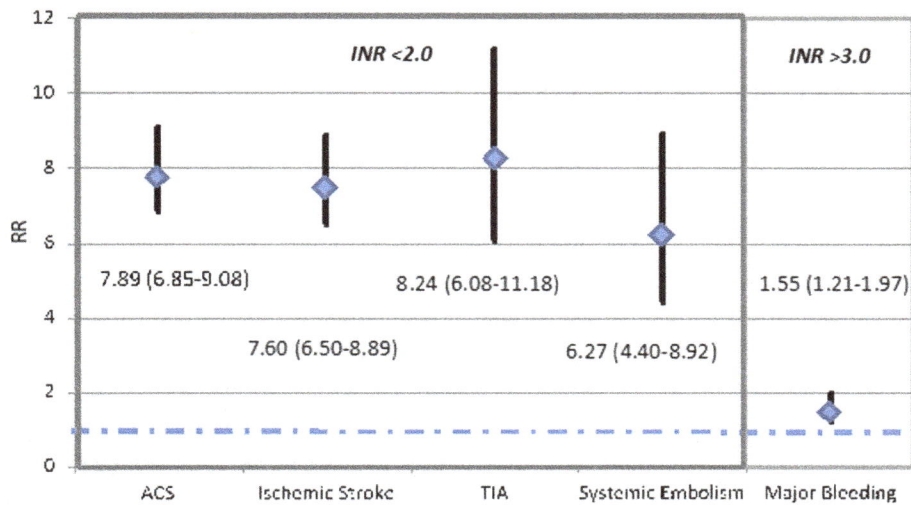

Fig. 2 Risks of adverse outcomes for people with INRs <2.0 or >3.0. Adapted from data from an observational study using the Veterans Health Administration dataset [38] showing the relative risk (RR) of adverse thrombotic or embolic events in patients with subtherapeutic INRs versus normal INRs and then major bleeding vents with supertherapeutic INRs versus normal INRs. The diamond represents the actual RR with the line representing the 95 % confidence interval and the blue dashed line representing a RR of 1.0, where the risk of outcomes would have been the same as those with normal INRs

close INR monitoring to prevent subtherapeutic warfarin dosing.

Further evidence showed the link between INR instability and clinical events. In meta-analyses that examine the relationship between TTR and the prediction of adverse events, a significant negative relationship has been observed [19]. In patients with AF, 1 thrombotic or major hemorrhagic event per 100 patient-years could be avoided by improving TTR by 7 % or 12 %, respectively [19]. Likewise in patients with VTE, for every 1 % increase in TTR, recurrent thromboembolic events may be reduced by 0.46 % per year and major hemorrhagic events reduced by 0.30 % [17]. Furthermore, in a nested case control analysis of the Atrial fibrillation Clopidogrel Trial with Irbesartan for prevention of Vascular Events (ACTIVE W) study, patients who experienced an ischemic stroke had a TTR 9.5 % lower than those without any ischemic event [39]. The TTR of patients with a major hemorrhage was 7.2 % lower when compared to those without an event, again, suggesting that TTR is a useful predictor for both hemorrhagic and thromboembolic events. Of note, ACTIVE W also found that patients spent a greater amount of time out of range in the 1–2 months preceding a major bleeding event or stroke which suggests even a temporary period out of range can lead to a bleeding event or stroke.

Inability to achieve high TTR in clinical practice is associated with non-persistence and medication discontinuation [40]. In an analysis of longitudinal anticoagulation management records from 15,276 US patients with NVAF, discontinuation of therapy occurred in less than 4 months among patients with unstable INR. Patients who achieved INR stabilization were 10 times more likely to remain on warfarin therapy beyond 1 year. In another observational study using the Symphony Health Solutions' Patient Transactional Database, patients who were prescribed rivaroxaban had a lower risk of treatment nonpersistence [HR 0.66 (95%CI: 0.60–0.72)] compared to patients who were prescribed warfarin [41]. A similar analysis of the Truven Health Market Scan Research Databases showed comparable findings, that NVAF patients who received rivaroxaban were 46 % less likely to discontinue therapy compared to those receiving warfarin [42]. Continued protection by anticoagulation is particularly important for patients with NVAF, since the risk of stroke is expected to increase with age and additional comorbidities [43].

Costs

INR instability was associated with higher healthcare utilization and costs. In an observational study using the Premier Perspective Comparative Hospital Database, hospital length of stay was 5.27 days vs. 4.46 days, leading to significant differences in hospitalization costs ($13,255 vs. $11,993, P < 0.001) [44, 45]. In another comprehensive cost analysis of 23,588 patients with NVAF who were on warfarin for at least 30 days from the US Veteran's Administration, investigators randomly selected an INR value from a patient and classified it as being below 2, 2–3, or above 3 and then evaluated total direct costs (i.e. inpatient, outpatient medical, and outpatient pharmacy costs) over the next 30 days. Mean direct costs over 30-days after exposure to an INR <2.0, between 2 and 3, and >3.0 were $5126, $2355 and $3419 (Fig. 3) [46]. These findings remained robust in a sensitivity analysis with a more stringent definition of the cohort. The substantial cost difference between in-range and out-of-range time is significant across a broad warfarin population with atrial fibrillation.

The literature suggests that INR instability has important clinical and financial consequences which underscore the need for greater vigilance on achieving INR stability or the use of a novel oral anticoagulant which provides more consistent pharmacologic effects.

Predicting INR Instability
Predictors
Based on data from adjusted meta-regression or multivariate analyses of large datasets, INR stability is known to vary greatly based upon various study- and patient-level factors (Table 3) [15–17, 21, 47, 48]. The use of anticoagulation clinics can positively impact higher TTR attainment but only ~1/3 of VKA patients have access to these advanced services [49]. Therefore, a broad understanding of factors predicting INR instability is beneficial for clinical practice.

Two of the most extensive studies were conducted by Apostolakis et al. (SAMe-TT2R2) [14] and Rose et al. (VARIA) [48] and provided insight into factors affecting anticoagulation control. Apostolakis and colleagues [14] used data from the 1061 patients in the Atrial Fibrillation Follow-up Investigation of Rhythm Management (AFFIRM) trial to identify clinical factors associated with TTR. Based upon these results, the SAMe-TT2R2 score was derived

(and eventually validated) whereby 1 or 2 points are assigned for important patient factors (Table 4). Scores ≥2 were found to be associated with decreased odds of achieving a TTR ≥65 % (previously described as the minimum target TTR) [14].

The Veterans AffaiRs study to Improve Anticoagulation (VARIA) [48] used data from over 124,000 veterans receiving warfarin for any indication (55 % AF, 35 % VTE, 10 % other) between 2006 and 2008; and evaluated the effect of various patient characteristics on TTR in those starting warfarin (first 6 months of therapy) and who were experienced (on therapy for >6 months). Like the SAMe-TT2R2 derivation/validation study, female gender, younger age, minority status and co-morbid physical conditions were also found to be associated with lower TTR in VARIA (in both the inception or experienced cohorts) but there were a large number of additional factors which were identified, such as alcohol abuse, number of hospitalizations, and various comorbidities, such as heart failure, diabetes, chronic kidney disease, and others. The VARIA investigators also created a clinical prediction tool but eliminated race because they did not wish to perpetuate disparities in care, eliminated poverty and distance to drive to receive care because they felt it was hard to assess, and eliminated other factors to simplify the model. Their model is available in a downloadable excel spreadsheet from Supplemental Appendix 3S at http://onlinelibrary.wiley.com/doi/10.1111/j.1538-7836.2010.03996.x/full. In addition to the factors in the SAMeTT2R2 score, this tool also assesses the indication for use, total number of chronic medications, substance abuse, mental illnesses, number

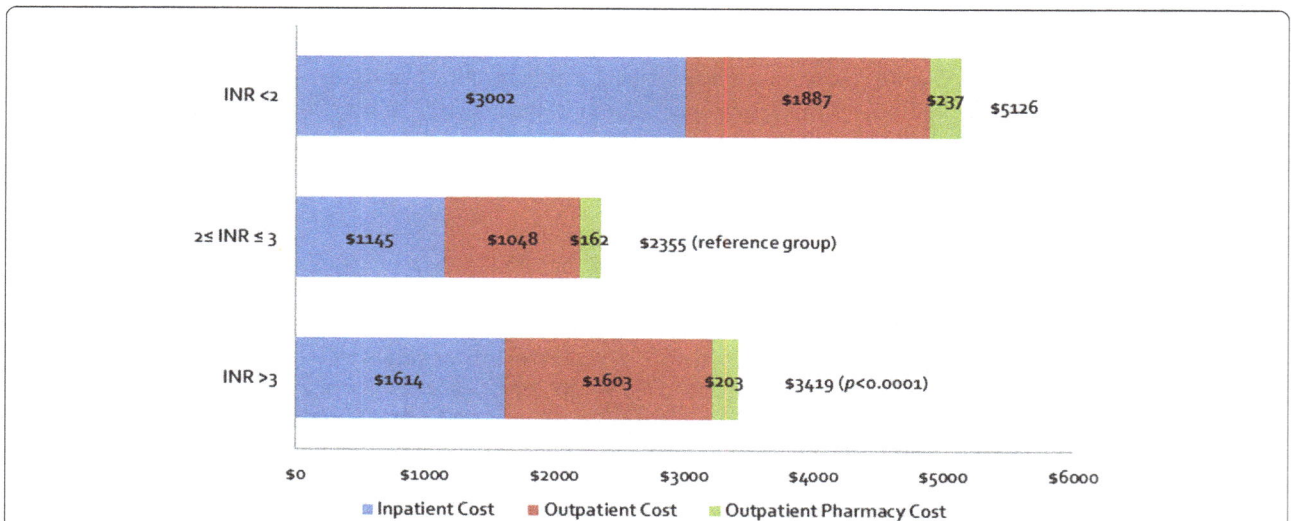

Fig. 3 Costs Associated with In Range and Out of Range INRs. Adapted from data from a US Veterans Administration dataset [46] where the total costs are displayed in blue and the constituent costs of inpatient, outpatient, and outpatient pharmacy costs are in red, green, and purple, respectively. The total costs in the therapeutic INR group is significantly lower than those with abnormally low or high INR groups. Note that the highest costs were associated with suboptimal INR values (i.e., INR <2.0)

Table 3 Summative assessment of factors shown to positively or negatively impact INR stability

Factor	Data source	Significant factors the impact INR stability
Poorer INR Stability		
VKA Use in Community Setting vs. Anticoagulation Clinic	Meta-Regression	↓ TTR by 7.1 to 7.2 %
VKA Naïve vs. VKA-Experienced	Meta-Regression	↓ TTR by 5.3 %
Heart Failure	Multivariate Analysis	OR 1.41 for TTR Instability
Diabetes Mellitus	Multivariate Analysis	OR 1.28 for TTR Instability
Stroke History	Multivariate Analysis	OR 1.15 for TTR Instability
Higher CHADS2 Score	Multivariate Analysis	↓ TTR by 7.6 % (SAMe-TT2R2)
Female Gender	Multivariate Analysis	↓ TTR by 6.0 % (SAMe-TT2R2)
Younger Age	Multivariate Analysis	↓ TTR by 20.3 % Age <50 (SAMe-TT2R2)
		↓ TTR by 7.7 % Age 50–60 (SAMe-TT2R2)
Minority Status	Multivariate Analysis	↓ TTR by 18.5 % (SAMe-TT2R2)
Smoking	Multivariate Analysis	↓ TTR by 10.8 % (SAMe-TT2R2)
Amiodarone Use	Multivariate Analysis	↓ TTR by 7.7 % (SAMe-TT2R2)
Better INR Stability		
VKA Self Management vs. No Self Management	Meta-Regression	↑ TTR by 7.0 %
European/United Kingdom Treatment vs. Elsewhere	Meta-Regression	↑ TTR by 9.7 %
Non-Warfarin VKAs vs. Warfarin	Meta-Regression	↑ TTR by 9.2 %
Male Gender	Multivariate Analysis	OR 0.78 for TTR Instability
Hypertension	Multivariate Analysis	OR 0.86 for TTR Instability
Beta-Blocker Use	Multivariate Analysis	↑TTR by 4.8 % (SAMe-TT2R2)
Verapamil Use	Multivariate Analysis	↑ TTR by 6.3 % (SAMe-TT2R2)

OR Odds Ratio, *TTR* Time in Therapeutic Range, *VKA* Vitamin K Antagonist

Table 4 SAMe-TT2R2 scoring system and implications

Criteria	One point	Two points	Points
Sex	Female gender		1
Age	Age < 60 years old		1
Medical history	Two or more co-morbidities: • Hypertension • Diabetes • Coronary disease • Peripheral artery disease • Heart failure • Prior stroke • Pulmonary disease • Renal disease • Liver disease		1
Treatment	Treatment with amiodarone		1
Tobacco		Tobacco use in the past 2 years	2
Race		Non-Caucasian race	2
Maximum points			8

The SAMe-TT2R2 score allows an initial patient assessment to discern who is unlikely to achieve a TTR ≥65 %. Patients that score ≥ 2 have reduces odds of achieving TTR ≥65 %. It does not include the risk associated with instability after initiation, only the ability to achieve longer term control [17]

of hospitalizations, and the general quality of TTR attainment in other patients within that healthcare setting. Even with all of these additional factors, the R-squared value only ranged from 3.2 to 6.8 % suggesting that the much of the variability in TTR is not explained by this model. Furthermore, while the study assessed TTR at therapy initiation and after chronic therapy, the authors stated that the prediction tool is not to be used as a means to assess long term control, and that clinical experience from past VKA therapy is the preferred method [48].

Factors that effect INR instability

Two reasons why the clinical prediction tools are inadequate may be related to genetics and adherence to therapy. Patient genotype plays an important role in INR stability [12, 50–52]. At least 30 genes contribute to the anticoagulant effects of VKAs, with one third of the variance in warfarin dosing related to mutations in genes leading to the synthesis of CYP2C9 and vitamin K epoxide reductase (VKORC1) [12, 50–52]. Patients with CYP2C9*2 and CYP2C9*3 polymorphisms have decreased enzymatic activity, metabolize warfarin (and to a lesser extent acenocoumarol) more slowly, have a 1.4- to 3.6-fold increased risk of supratherapeutic

INR, and often take longer to achieve stable dosing [53–55]. VKORC1 polymorphisms can result in either a heightened (group A haplotype) or reduced effect (group B haplotype) of warfarin which alters the risk of thromboembolism and bleeding accordingly [12]. Based on this data, the Food and Drug Administration altered the package insert recommending clinicians consider genetic testing before initiating warfarin therapy [56]. However, the cost-effectiveness of this approach is questionable; with economic models suggesting genotyping of patients would cost more than $170,000 per AF patient quality-adjusted life-year (QALY) gained (far above the commonly accepted willingness-to-pay threshold of $50,000 per QALY) [57].

Medication adherence was highlighted as an important variable in VKA INR stability in the American College of Chest Physicians (ACCP) guidelines [12]. Identified predictors of VKA nonadherence include not being married, not having a vehicle for transportation, education levels beyond high school, currently employed, lower levels of mental health functioning, poor cognitive functioning, and greater drug regimen complexity [58, 59]. In addition, studies have identified patient dissatisfaction with care as a cause of medication non-adherence in patients with cardiovascular disease states [60]. This is noteworthy since patient satisfaction with warfarin therapy has been shown to be poor in recent studies of AF [61] and VTE patients [62]. In the above-mentioned studies, poor patient satisfaction in either AF or VTE patients (measure by the Anti-Clot Treatment Scale) was related to the burden and frustration of taking VKAs resulting from fear of bleeding/bruising, diet and alcohol interactions and the perceived hassle of INR monitoring. One of the frequently cited studies evaluating the association between VKA non-adherence and INR control is the International Normalized Ratio Adherence and Genetics (IN-RANGE) Study [63]. IN-RANGE was a prospective cohort study conducted at 3 US anticoagulation clinics and assessed warfarin adherence using a medication electronic monitoring system (MEMS). The study followed 136 patients taking warfarin for a variety of reasons (but predominantly AF and VTE) for a mean of 32-weeks and found that missed warfarin doses (missed MEMS bottle openings) were common, with 92 % of patients missed at least 1 dose, and one-third missed more than 20 % of their doses. A total of 1490 INRs values were collected, with 40 % out of range and 26 % being below range. Upon multivariable regression analysis, researchers found that for every 10 % increase in missed warfarin doses (days without a dose), there was a 14 % increase in the adjusted odds of under-anticoagulation (having an INR < 2.0); and patients who missed >20 % of their doses (missed 20 days of warfarin therapy) had a 2.10-fold (95%CI: 1.48–2.96) increase in their odds of having an INR < 2.0 [63].

Existing research provided good understanding of the drivers behind poor INR control. The research findings indicate that many of the patient factors are not modifiable and are also not sufficiently reliable to predict whether VKA will perform well for a particular patient.

Modalities to optimize clinical management of VKAs

There are several modalities to improve the clinical management of patients on VKAs including computer assisted dosing and patient self-testing or management. In a randomized study of 13,219 patients conducted in 32 centers around the world, the impact of software program guided VKA therapy was compared with experienced clinician dosing [64]. Unadjusted INR time in range was 67 and 66 % with computer-assisted versus experienced clinician dosing. However, in order to elicit these comparable results, the experienced medical staff randomized to use the computer assisted program provided 11 % of the dosages because the computer failed to provide it and the dose was changed 11 % of the time because the results were felt inaccurate. In addition, the computer-advised appointment intervals were changed by experienced clinicians 34 % of the time. More data is needed to truly determine the impact of computer assisted dosing in less experienced clinicians versus very experienced clinicians/anticoagulation specialists.

Point of care testing by the patient or clinician allow rapid determination of the INR without the need for a centralized laboratory to acquire and analyze the samples. In a meta-analysis of 22 studies, including 4 studied deemed of high methodological quality, the precision and accuracy of the CoaguChek XS, INRatio, ProTime/ProTime3, and Smartcheck INR coagulameter systems were assessed [65]. The CoaguChek system was the most commonly assed and yielded a coefficient of variation that ranged from 1.4 to 5.9 and the concordance ranged between 93 to 100 % showing congruence. The other systems have coefficients of variation ranging from 3.7 to 8.4 and concordance values ranging from 81 to 97 % (with the exception of one trial of the ProTime system where the concordance was only 39 %. In general, point of care testing is accurate and can facilitate patient self-testing (where the patient self-tests the INR but clinician doses) or patient self-management (where the patient self-tests and self-adjusts VKA therapy based on the INR.

In an 8-month open label crossover trial conducted in Canadian primary care offices, patients ($n = 11$, 99 patient months, 122 INR determinations) underwent patient self-management or physician management for 4 months [66]. Patients were trained and given an algorithm to follow that specified the new dose and the timeframe for which to reassess the INR. The mean proportion of INR values in therapeutic range among subjects in the PSM and physician-management groups was 82 and 80 %, respectively ($p = 0.82$). Ten of the 11 patients preferred PSM to physician management and elected to continue with this strategy after study completion ($P = .001$). No calls or visits were made to the physician regarding dose adjustment during the patient self-management period. There were no episodes of major bleeding or thromboembolic events. Studies like this are promising but preliminary and it is unclear whether this is an effective therapy for highly motivated and intelligent patients or patients with health disparities or care barriers.

Conclusions

While experts recommend that patients spend at least 65 % of their TTR, this is seldom achieved or sustained over time. A more common pattern – based on the literature – is that there is high variability, and even the patients who achieve target INR range do not remain in this target range for long. Patients are more likely to have INR below the therapeutic range, exposing them to significant risk of adverse clinical events. Not achieving a high TTR can result in thrombotic and major bleeding events, inability to remain on therapy, and higher cost of care. To avoid the adverse consequences of unstable INR, careful evaluation of patients prior to initiating therapy is important. Clinical prediction tools are available, though they can only explain <10 % of the variance behind poor INR control because of the complex drivers of genetic variation and patient medication adherence. Clinicians caring for patients who require anticoagulation are encouraged to apply intensified diligence in INR management when using VKAs.

Abbreviations

ACCP, American College of Chest Physicians; ACTIVE W, Atrial fibrillation Clopidogrel Trial with Irbesartan for prevention of Vascular Events; AF, atrial fibrillation; CI, confidence interval; DVT, deep vein thrombosis; GARFIELD, Global Anticoagulant Registry in the FIELD; ICER, incremental cost-effectiveness ratio; ICH, intracerebral hemorrhage; INR, international normalized ratio; IN-RANGE, International Normalized Ratio Adherence and Genetics; MEMS, medication electronic monitoring system; NOAC, novel oral anticoagulant; PE, pulmonary embolism; PINRR, proportion of INR measurements in range; QALY, quality-adjusted life-year; RCT, randomized controlled trial; TTR, time in therapeutic range; UK, United Kingdom; VARIA, Veterans AffaiRs Study to Improve Anticoagulation; VKA, vitamin K antagonist; VKOR, vitamin K epoxide reductase

Acknowledgements
None.

Funding
This review was funded by Janssen Scientific Affairs, LLC, Raritan, NJ, USA. The authors maintained full control over the content of the review and preparation of the manuscript. Janssen reviewed the final manuscript prior to submission.

Authors' contributions
Review concept and design: CIC, JRS. Acquisition of data: CMW, ESM, JK, CIC. Analysis and interpretation of data: JRS, CMW, WWN, ESM, JK, CIC. Drafting of the manuscript: CMW, JRS, WWN, ESM, CIC. Critical revision of the manuscript for important intellectual content: CMW, JRS, WWN, CIC, JK. Administrative, technical, or material support: CIC. Study supervision: CIC, JRS. CIC and JRS had full access to all the data in the review and take responsibility for the integrity of the manuscript. All authors read and approved the final manuscript.

Competing interests
Dr. Coleman has received honoraria for participation on advisory boards and Speaker's bureaus and has received research funding from Janssen Scientific Affairs, LLC, Raritan, NJ. Drs. Schein and Nelson are employees of Janssen Scientific Affairs, LLC and are stockholders of Johnson & Johnson. Drs. Mearns, Kluger and White have no conflicts to report.

Author details
[1]Janssen Scientific Affairs, LLC, Health Economics & Outcomes Research, Raritan, NJ, USA. [2]Department of Pharmacy Practice, University of Connecticut School of Pharmacy, 69 N. Eagleville Road, Storrs, CT 06269-3092, USA. [3]Hartford Hospital Division of Cardiology, 80 Seymour Street, Hartford, CT 06102-5037, USA.

References

1. Coumadin (warfarin sodium) tablets prescribing information. Bristol-Myers Squibb, Princeton, NJ. Available at: http://packageinserts.bms.com/pi/pi_coumadin.pdf (last accessed on August 4, 2014).
2. You JJ, Singer DE, Howard PA, Lane DA, Eckman MH, Fang MC, Hylek EM, Schulman S, Go AS, Hughes M, Spencer FA, Manning WJ, Halperin JL, Lip GY. Antithrombotic therapy for atrial fibrillation: Antithrombotic Therapy and Prevention of Thrombosis, 9th ed: American College of Chest Physicians Evidence-Based Clinical Practice Guidelines. Chest. 2012;141(2 Suppl):e531S–75.
3. Kearon C, Akl EA, Ornelas J, Blaivas A, Jimenez D, Bounameaux H, Huisman M, King CS, Morris TA, Sood N, Stevens SM, Vintch JR, Wells P, Woller SC, Moores L. Antithrombotic Therapy for VTE Disease: CHEST Guideline and Expert Panel Report. Chest. 2016;149:315–52.
4. Hart RG, Pearce LA, Aguilar MI. Meta-Analysis: Antithrombotic therapy to prevent stroke in patients who have nonvalvular atrial fibrillation. Ann Intern Med. 2007;146:857–67.
5. Brandjes DP, Heijboer H, Büller HR, de Rijk M, Jagt H, ten Cate JW. Acenocoumarol and heparin compared with acenocoumarol alone in the initial treatment of proximal-vein thrombosis. N Engl J Med. 1992;327:1485–9.
6. Gallus A, Jackaman J, Tillett J, Mills W, Wycherley A. Safety and efficacy of warfarin started early after submassive venous thrombosis or pulmonary embolism. Lancet. 1986;2:1293–6.
7. January CT, Wann LS, Alpert JS, Calkins H, Cleveland JC Jr, Cigarroa JE, Conti JB, Ellinor PT, Ezekowitz MD, Field ME, Murray KT, Sacco RL, Stevenson WG, Tchou PJ, Tracy CM, Yancy CW. 2014 AHA/ACC/HRS Guideline for the Management of Patients With Atrial Fibrillation: Executive Summary: A Report of the American College of Cardiology/American Heart Association Task Force on Practice Guidelines and the Heart Rhythm Society. J Am Coll Cardiol. 2014. doi:10.1016/j.jacc.2014.03.021. [Epub ahead of print].
8. Association European Heart Rhythm, European Association for Cardio-Thoracic Surgery, Camm AJ, Kirchhof P, Lip GY, Schotten U, Savelieva I, et al. Guidelines for the management of atrial fibrillation: the Task Force for the Management of Atrial Fibrillation of the European Society of Cardiology (ESC). Europace. 2010;12(10):1360–420. doi:10.1093/europace/euq350.
9. Mearns ES, Hawthorne J, Song JS, Coleman CI. Measures of vitamin K antagonist control reported in atrial fibrillation and venous thromboembolism studies: a systematic review. BMJ Open. 2014;4(6): e005379. doi:10.1136/bmjopen-2014-005379.

10. Fitzmaurice DA, Kesteven P, Gee KM, Murray ET, McManus R. A systematic review of outcome measures reported for the therapeutic effectiveness of oral anticoagulation. J Clin Pathol. 2003;56:48–51.

11. Rosendaal FR, Cannegieter SC, van der Meer FJ, Briët E. A method to determine the optimal intensity of oral anticoagulant therapy. Thromb Haemost. 1993;69:236–9.

12. Ageno W, Gallus AS, Wittkowsky A, Crowther M, Hylek EM, Palareti G, American College of Chest Physicians. Oral anticoagulant therapy: Antithrombotic Therapy and Prevention of Thrombosis, 9th ed: American College of Chest Physicians Evidence-Based Clinical Practice Guidelines. Chest. 2012;141(2 Suppl):e44S–88.

13. Connolly SJ, Pogue J, Eikelboom J, Flaker G, Commerford P, Franzosi MG, Healey JS, Yusuf S; ACTIVE W Investigators. Benefit of oral anticoagulant over antiplatelet therapy in atrial fibrillation depends on the quality of international normalized ratio control achieved by centers and countries as measured by time in therapeutic range. Circulation. 2008;118:2029–37.

14. Apostolakis S, Sullivan RM, Olshansky B, Lip GY. Factors affecting quality of anticoagulation control among patients with atrial fibrillation on warfarin: the SAMe-TT$_2$R$_2$ score. Chest. 2013;144:1555–63.

15. Costa GL, Lamego RM, Colosimo EA, Valacio RA, Moreira MC. Identifying potential predictors of high-quality oral anticoagulation assessed by time in therapeutic international normalized ratio range: a prospective, long-term, single-center, observational study. Clin Ther. 2012;34:1511–20.

16. Mearns ES, White CM, Kohn CG, Hawthorne J, Song JS, Meng J, Schein JR, Raut MK, Coleman CI. Quality of vitamin K antagonist control and outcomes in atrial fibrillation patients: a meta-analysis and meta-regression. Thromb J. 2014;12:14.

17. Mearns ES, Kohn CG, Song JS, Hawthorne J, Meng J, White CM, Raut MK, Schein JR, Coleman CI. Meta-analysis to assess the quality of international normalized ratio control and associated outcomes in venous thromboembolism patients. Thromb Res. 2014;134:310–9.

18. Erkens PM, ten Cate H, Büller HR, Prins MH. Benchmark for time in therapeutic range in venous thromboembolism: a systematic review and meta-analysis. PLoS One. 2012;7(9):e42269.

19. Wan Y, Heneghan C, Perera R, Roberts N, Hollowell J, Glasziou P, Bankhead C, Xu Y. Anticoagulation control and prediction of adverse events in patients with atrial fibrillation: a systematic review. Circ Cardiovasc Qual Outcomes. 2008;1:84–91.

20. Cios DA, Baker WL, Sander SD, Phung OJ, Coleman CI. Evaluating the impact of study-level factors on warfarin control in U.S.-based primary studies: a meta-analysis. Am J Health Syst Pharm. 2009;66:916–25.

21. van Walraven C, Jennings A, Oake N, Fergusson D, Forster AJ. Effect of study setting on anticoagulation control: a systematic review and metaregression. Chest. 2006;129:1155–66.

22. Reynolds MW, Fahrbach K, Hauch O, Wygant G, Estok R, Cella C, Nalysnyk L. Warfarin anticoagulation and outcomes in patients with atrial fibrillation: a systematic review and metaanalysis. Chest. 2004;126:1938–45.

23. Patel MR, Mahaffey KW, Garg J, Pan G, Singer DE, Hacke W, Breithardt G, Halperin JL, Hankey GJ, Piccini JP, Becker RC, Nessel CC, Paolini JF, Berkowitz SD, Fox KA, Califf RM; ROCKET AF Investigators. Rivaroxaban versus warfarin in nonvalvular atrial fibrillation. N Engl J Med. 2011;365:883–91.

24. Connolly SJ, Ezekowitz MD, Yusuf S, Eikelboom J, Oldgren J, Parekh A, Pogue J, Reilly PA, Themeles E, Varrone J, Wang S, Alings M, Xavier D, Zhu J, Diaz R, Lewis BS, Darius H, Diener HC, Joyner CD, Wallentin L, RE-LY Steering Committee and Investigators. Dabigatran versus warfarin in patients with atrial fibrillation. N Engl J Med. 2009;361:1139–51.

25. Giugliano RP, Ruff CT, Braunwald E, Murphy SA, Wiviott SD, Halperin JL, Waldo AL, Ezekowitz MD, Weitz JI, Špinar J, Ruzyllo W, Ruda M, Koretsune Y, Betcher J, Shi M, Grip LT, Patel SP, Patel I, Hanyok JJ, Mercuri M, Antman EM; ENGAGE AF-TIMI 48 Investigators. Edoxaban versus warfarin in patients with atrial fibrillation. N Engl J Med. 2013;369:2093–104.

26. Granger CB, Alexander JH, McMurray JJ, Lopes RD, Hylek EM, Hanna M, Al-Khalidi HR, Ansell J, Atar D, Avezum A, Bahit MC, Diaz R, Easton JD, Ezekowitz JA, Flaker G, Garcia D, Geraldes M, Gersh BJ, Golitsyn S, Goto S, Hermosillo AG, Hohnloser SH, Horowitz J, Mohan P, Jansky P, Lewis BS, Lopez-Sendon JL, Pais P, Parkhomenko A, Verheugt FW, Zhu J, Wallentin L; ARISTOTLE Committees and Investigators. Apixaban versus warfarin in patients with atrial fibrillation. N Engl J Med. 2011;365:981–92.

27. Schulman S, Kearon C, Kakkar AK, Mismetti P, Schellong S, Eriksson H, et al. Dabigatran versus warfarin in the treatment of acute venous thromboembolism. N Engl J Med. 2009;361:2342–52.

28. Schulman S, Kakkar AK, Goldhaber SZ, Schellong S, Eriksson H, Mismetti P, Christiansen AV, Friedman J, Le Maulf F, Peter N, Kearon C; RE-COVER II Trial Investigators. Treatment of acute venous thromboembolism with dabigatran or warfarin and pooled analysis. Circulation. 2014;129:764–72.

29. EINSTEIN investigators. Oral rivaroxaban for symptomatic venous thromboembolism. N Engl J Med. 2010;363:2499–510.

30. EINSTEIN-PE investigators. Oral rivaroxaban for the treatment of symptomatic pulmonary embolism. N Engl J Med. 2012;366:1287–97.

31. Agnelli G, Buller HR, Cohen A, Curto M, Gallus AS, Johnson M, Masiukiewicz U, Pak R, Thompson J, Raskob GE, Weitz JI; AMPLIFY Investigators. Oral apixaban for the treatment of acute venous thromboembolism. N Engl J Med. 2013;369:799–808.

32. Hokusai-VTE Investigators, Büller HR, Décousus H, Grosso MA, Mercuri M, Middeldorp S, Prins MH, Raskob GE, Schellong SM, Schwocho L, Segers A, Shi M, Verhamme P, Wells P. Edoxaban versus warfarin for the treatment of symptomatic venous thromboembolism. N Engl J Med. 2013;369:1406–15.

33. Razouki Z, Ozonoff A, Zhao S, et al. Improving quality measurement for anticoagulation: adding international normalized ratio variability to percent time in therapeutic range. Circ Cardiovasc Qual Outcomes 2014;7:Doi:10.1161/circoutcomes.114.00804/-/DCI.

34. Nelson WW, Desai S, Damaraju CV, et al. International normalized ratio stability in warfarin-experiences patients with nonvalvular atrial fibrillation. Am J Cardiovasc Drugs. 2015;15:205–11.

35. Pokorney S, Simon DN, Thomas L, et al. The myth of the stable INR patient: results from ORBIT-AF. J Am Coll Cardiol. 2015;65(Suppl 10S):A344.

36. Oake N, Fergusson DA, Forster AJ, van Walraven C. Frequency of adverse events in patients with poor anticoagulation: a meta-analysis. CMAJ. 2007;176:1589–94.

37. Oake N, Jennings A, Forster AJ, Fergusson D, Doucette S, van Walraven C. Anticoagulation intensity and outcomes among patients prescribed oral anticoagulant therapy: a systematic review and meta-analysis. CMAJ. 2008;179:235–44.

38. Nelson WW, Wang L, Baser O, Damaraju CV, Schein JR. Out-of-range INR values and outcomes among new warfarin patients with non-valvular atrial fibrillation. Int J Clin Pharm. 2014. doi:10.1007/s11096-014-0038-3.

39. Nieuwlaat R, Connolly BJ, Hubers LM, Cuddy SM, Eikelboom JW, Yusuf S, Connolly SJ; ACTIVE Investigators. Quality of individual INR control and the risk of stroke and bleeding events in atrial fibrillation patients: a nested case control analysis of the ACTIVE W study. Thromb Res. 2012;129:715–9.

40. Nelson WW, Desai S, Damaraju CV, Lu L, Fields LE, Wildgoose P, Schein JR. International normalized ratio stabilization in newly initiated warfarin patients with nonvalvular atrial fibrillation. Curr Med Res Opin. 2014;30(12):2437–42.

41. Laliberte F, Cloutier M, Nelson WW, et al. Real-world comparative effectiveness and safety of rivaroxaban and warfarin in nonvalvular atrial fibrillation patients. Curr Med Res Opin. 2014;1:1–9. doi:10.1.1185/03007995.2014.907140.

42. Nelson WW, Song X, Thomson E, Coleman CI, Damaraju CV, Schein JR. Medication Persistence and Discontinuation of Rivaroxaban and Warfarin Therapy among Patients with Non-valvular Atrial Fibrillation. Curr Med Res Opin. 2014;30:2461–9.

43. Lip GY, Nieuwlaat R, Pisters R, Lane DA, Crijns HJ. Refining clinical risk stratification for predicting stroke and thromboembolism in atrial fibrillation using a novel risk factor-based approach: the euro heart survey on atrial fibrillation. Chest. 2010;137(2):263–72.

44. Laliberte F, Raut MK, Nelson WW, et al. Hospital length of stay: is rivaroxaban associated with shorter inpatient stay compared to warfarin among patient with non-vavlular atrial fibrillation? Curr Med Res Opin. 2014;30:645–53.

45. Laliberte F, Pilon D, Raut MK, et al. Is rivaroxaban associated with lower inpatient costs compared to warfarin among patients with non-valvular atrial fibrillation? Curr Med Res Opin. 2014;8:1521–8.

46. Nelson WW, Wang L, Baser O, Damaraju CV, Schein JR. Out-of-range international normalized ratio values and health care cost among new warfarin patients with non-valvular atrial fibrillation. J Med Econ. 2015;18:333–40.

47. Nelson WW, Choi JC, Vanderpoel J, Damaraju CV, Wildgoose P, Fields LE, Schein JR. Impact of co-morbidities and patient characteristics on international normalized ratio control over time in patient with nonvalvular atrial fibrillation. Am J Cardiol. 2013;112:509–12.

Vitamin K antagonist use: evidence of the difficulty of achieving and maintaining target INR...

93

48. Rose AJ, Hylek EM, Ozonoff A, Ash AS, Reisman JI, Berlowitz DR. Patient characteristics associated with oral anticoagulation control: results of the Veterans AffaiRs Study to Improve Anticoagulation (VARIA). J Thromb Haemost. 2010;8:2182–91.

49. Nutescu EA, Bathija S, Sharp LK, Gerber BS, Schumock GT, Fitzgibbon ML. Anticoagulation patient self-monitoring in the United States: considerations for clinical practice adoption. Pharmacotherapy. 2011;31:1161–74.

50. Wadelius M, Chen LY, Eriksson N, Bumpstead S, Ghori J, Wadelius C, Bentley D, McGinnis R, Deloukas P. Association of warfarin dose with genes involved in its action and metabolism. Hum Genet. 2007;121:23–34.

51. Krynetskiy E, McDonnell P. Building individualized medicine: prevention of adverse reactions to warfarin therapy. J Pharmacol Exp Ther. 2007;322:427–34.

52. Rieder MJ, Reiner AP, Gage BF, Nickerson DA, Eby CS, McLeod HL, Blough DK, Thummel KE, Veenstra DL, Rettie AE. Effect of VKORC1 haplotypes on transcriptional regulation and warfarin dose. N Engl J Med. 2005;352:2285–93.

53. Muszkat M, Blotnik S, Elami A, Krasilnikov I, Caraco Y. Warfarin metabolism and anticoagulant effect: a prospective, observational study of the impact of CYP2C9 genetic polymorphism in the presence of drug-disease and drug-drug interactions. Clin Ther. 2007;29:427–37.

54. Aithal GP, Day CP, Kesteven PJ, Daly AK. Association of polymorphisms in the cytochrome P450 CYP2C9 with warfarin dose requirement and risk of bleeding complications. Lancet. 1999;353:717–9.

55. Higashi MK, Veenstra DL, Kondo LM, Wittkowsky AK, Srinouanprachanh SL, Farin FM, Rettie AE. Association between CYP2C9 genetic variants and anticoagulation-related outcomes during warfarin therapy. JAMA. 2002;287:1690–8.

56. Food and Drug Administration. FDA Approves Updated Warfarin (Coumadin) Prescribing Information. August 16, 2007. Available at : http://www.fda.gov/NewsEvents/Newsroom/PressAnnouncements/2007/ucm108967.htm (Last accessed on August 4, 2014).

57. Eckman MH, Rosand J, Greenberg SM, Gage BF. Cost-effectiveness of using pharmacogenetic information in warfarin dosing for patients with nonvalvular atrial fibrillation. Ann Intern Med. 2009;150:73–83.

58. Orensky IA, Holdford DA. Predictors of noncompliance with warfarin therapy in an outpatient anticoagulation clinic. Pharmacotherapy. 2005;25:1801–8.

59. Platt AB, Localio AR, Brensinger CM, Cruess DG, Christie JD, Gross R, Parker CS, Price M, Metlay JP, Cohen A, Newcomb CW, Strom BL, Laskin MS, Kimmel SE. Risk factors for nonadherence to warfarin: results from the IN-RANGE study. Pharmacoepidemiol Drug Saf. 2008;17:853–60.

60. Morisky DE, Ang A, Krousel-Wood M, Ward HJ. Predictive validity of a medication adherence measure in an outpatient setting. J Clin Hypertens (Greenwich). 2008;10:348–54.

61. Coleman CI, Coleman SM, Vanderpoel J, Nelson W, Colby JA, Scholle JM, Kluger J. Patient satisfaction with warfarin- and non-warfarin-containing thromboprophylaxis regimens for atrial fibrillation. J Investig Med. 2013;61:878–81.

62. Bamber L, Wang MY, Prins MH, Ciniglio C, Bauersachs R, Lensing AW, Cano SJ. Patient-reported treatment satisfaction with oral rivaroxaban versus standard therapy in the treatment of acute symptomatic deep-vein thrombosis. Thromb Haemost. 2013;110:732–41.

63. Kimmel SE, Chen Z, Price M, Parker CS, Metlay JP, Christie JD, Brensinger CM, Newcomb CW, Samaha FF, Gross R. The influence of patient adherence on anticoagulation control with warfarin: results from the International Normalized Ratio Adherence and Genetics (IN-RANGE) Study. Arch Intern Med. 2007;167:229–35.

64. Poller L, Keown M, Ibrahim S, et al. An international multicenter randomized study of computer-assisted oral anticoagulant dosage vs. medical staff dosage. J Thromb Haemost. 2008;6:935–43.

65. Christensen TD, Larsen TB. Precision and accuracy of point of care testing coagulometers used for self-testing and self management of oral anticoagulation therapy. J Thromb Haemost. 2011;10:251–60.

66. Grunau BE, Wiens MO, Harder KK. Patient self-management of warfarin therapy: pragmatic feasibility study in Canadian primary care. Can Fam Physician. 2011;57:e292–8.

12

Impact of blood hypercoagulability on in vitro fertilization outcomes: a prospective longitudinal observational study

Grigoris T. Gerotziafas[1,2]*, Patrick Van Dreden[3], Emmanuelle Mathieu d'Argent[4], Eleftheria Lefkou[1], Matthieu Grusse[3], Marjorie Comtet[4], Rabiatou Sangare[3], Hela Ketatni[2], Annette K. Larsen[1] and Ismail Elalamy[1,2]

Abstract

Background: Blood coagulation plays a crucial role in the blastocyst implantation process and its alteration may be related to in vitro fertilization (IVF) failure. We conducted a prospective observational longitudinal study in women eligible for IVF to explore the association between alterations of coagulation with the IVF outcome and to identify the biomarkers of hypercoagulability which are related with this outcome.

Methods: Thirty-eight women eligible for IVF (IVF-group) and 30 healthy, age-matched women (control group) were included. In the IVF-group, blood was collected at baseline, 5–8 days after administration of gonadotropin-releasing hormone agonist (GnRH), before and two weeks after administration of human follicular stimulating hormone (FSH). Pregnancy was monitored by measurement of βHCG performed 15 days after embryo transfer. Thrombin generation (TG), minimal tissue factor-triggered whole blood thromboelastometry (ROTEM®), procoagulant phospholipid clotting time (Procoag-PPL®), thrombomodulin (TMa), tissue factor activity (TFa), factor VIII (FVIII), factor von Willebrand (FvW), D-Dimers and fibrinogen were assessed at each time point.

Results: Positive IVF occurred in 15 women (40%). At baseline, the IVF-group showed significantly increased TG, TFa and TMa and significantly shorter Procoag-PPL versus the control group. After initiation of hormone treatment TG was significantly higher in the IVF-positive as compared to the IVF-negative group. At all studied points, the Procoag-PPL was significantly shorter and the levels of TFa were significantly higher in the IVF-negative group compared to the IVF-positive one. The D-Dimers were higher in the IVF negative as compared to IVF positive group. Multivariate analysis retained the Procoag-PPL and TG as predictors for the IVF outcome.

Conclusions: Diagnosis of women with hypercoagulability and their stratification to risk of IVF failure using a model based on the Procoag-PPL and TG is a feasible strategy for the optimization of IVF efficiency that needs to be validated in prospective trials.

Keywords: Tissue factor, Blood coagulation tests, Thrombin generation, In vitro fertilization, Hypercoagulability

* Correspondence: grigorios.gerotziafas@aphp.fr
[1]Cancer Biology and Therapeutics, Centre de Recherche Saint-Antoine, Institut National de la Santé et de la Recherche Médicale (INSERM) U938 and Université Pierre et Marie Curie (UPMC), Sorbonne Universities, Paris, France
[2]Service d'Hématologie Biologique, Hôpital Tenon, Hôpitaux Universitaires Est Parisien, Assistance Publique Hôpitaux de Paris, 4, rue de la Chine, Paris Cedex 20, France
Full list of author information is available at the end of the article

Background

The link between blood hypercoagulability and infertility or in vitro fertilization (IVF) failure is a puzzling issue. Hypercoagulability could be intrinsic or caused by the hormone treatment preceding the IVF procedure [1–6]. Tissue factor is the major trigger of blood coagulation and thrombin generation is the ultimate step that leads to fibrin formation. The activation of coagulation induced by tissue factor (TF) expressed by perivascular decidualized human endometrial stromal cells is an essential part of the mechanism that favors blastocyst implantation and prevents peri-implantational hemorrhage during endovascular trophoblast invasion. Thrombin generation is required for cell proliferation, neoangiogenesis, trophoblast invasion and remodeling of the spiral arteries and arterioles [7–9]. Thus, the shift of blood coagulation equilibrium towards locally enhancement of thrombin generation may have some beneficial effects for a positive outcome of IVF. On the other hand, in infertile women activation or dysfunction of platelets, endothelial cells and monocytes has been observed [10, 11].

Newer laboratory assays allow the assessment of global blood coagulation and clot formation process. Among them, the Calibrated Automated Thrombogram® and the minimal TF-triggered whole blood thromboelastometry allow the evaluation of thrombin generation and clot formation processes [12–14]. The measurement of the procoagulant phospholipid dependent clotting time (Procoag-PPL®) reflects the plasma concentration of procoagulant membrane vesicles of cellular origin [15, 16]. Biomarkers of endothelial cell activation such as thrombomodulin activity (TMa) and TF activity (TFa) measured in plasma offer information on the status of the endothelial cells at the vasculature.

The aim of the present prospective, observational longitudinal study was to identify biomarkers of hypercoagulability which could have some predictive value for the IVF outcome. Thrombin generation, clot formation kinetics and molecular biomarkers of cellular hypercoagulability were assessed at women eligible for IVF at baseline (before any hormone treatment administration), at the down-regulation phase of the menstrual cycle and after ovarian stimulation. Biochemical diagnosis of pregnancy was the end-point of the study.

Methods

Study design and participants

A monocentric prospective, non-interventional cohort study was designed. From June 2014 to June 2015 blood samples were obtained from 38 women eligible for IVF (IVF-group). Women were recruited at the baseline consultation and then they were followed until pregnancy test was performed. Biochemical diagnosis of pregnancy was the end-point of the study. According to the levels of

β-chorionic gonadotropin (βHCG) women were stratified into two subgroups: IVF-positive if βHCG levels were higher than 100 IU/L and IVF-negative if (βHCG) levels were equal or lower than 100 IU/L. The evolution of the pregnancy was not recorded.

The control group consisted of 30 healthy, age-matched women, without any known hereditary or acquired thrombophilic alteration or personal history of thrombotic or bleeding disorder who had undergone at least one uneventful physically conceived pregnancy and without any personal history of miscarriage. The protocol of the study was in accordance with the commitment of the Helsinki declaration and was approved by the institutional ethics committee. All subjects provided informed written consent before inclusion in the study.

Inclusion criteria

Women were eligible for IVF according to established selection criteria applied in our institution. All women had full blood count, platelet count, prothrombin time, activated partial thromboplastin time, fibrinogen, renal and liver function within the normal range.

Exclusion criteria

Women younger than 18 years or older than 45 years, weight less than 50 kg or more than 100 kg, with a personal or family history of venous thromboembolism (VTE) or hemorrhagic syndromes, known hereditary or acquired thrombophilia, active anticoagulant or antiplatelet treatment or use of these agents during the last 30 days before inclusion, hospitalization for any reason within the previous 3 months, abnormal full blood count or platelet count and ongoing cardiovascular, renal or liver disease, malignancy, or arterial hypertension, known systematic or chronic disease (autoimmune syndrome, heart disease, severe or uncontrolled thyroid disease or HIV infection), treatment with non-steroid anti-inflammatory drugs within the last 10 days before inclusion, ovarian insufficiency (FSH > 9 IU/ml and/or number of antral follicles <8) or polycystic ovary syndrome (defined according to the Rotterdam criteria).

Hormone treatment for the artificial reproductive technique

Estrogen production was first down-regulated to induce controlled ovarian stimulation. Three different protocols of down regulation were used: a long gonadotropin-releasing hormone (GnRH) agonist or a short agonist or an antagonist. Ovarian stimulation was done with recombinant human follicular stimulating hormone (FSH) at doses ranging from 75 IU to 450 IU per day depending on age, body mass index (BMI), antral follicle count, size and number of follicles and estradiol levels (E2). This stimulation was initiated once pituitary desensitization had been achieved (E2 level <50 pg/mL). The response was followed by E2 measurement six days later and by ultrasound scanning of the ovarian follicles at days 9–10 after the first FSH injection, and repeated when necessary. Transvaginal oocyte retrieval was scheduled 35 to 36 h after human recombinant chorion gonadotrophin (hCG) injection and embryo transfer was performed 2–3 days later. On day 2, individually cultured embryos were evaluated on the basis of the number of blastomeres, blastomere size, fragmentation rate and presence of multinucleated blastomeres. Therefore, the ovocytes were retrieved 10 to 14 days after starting the stimulation with the FSH.

Outcomes

Achievement of biochemical pregnancy was the outcome of the study. Pregnancy was controlled by quantitative measurement of βHCG 15 days after embryo transfer.

Blood sampling

Blood samples were collected before the administration of any hormone treatment (T0) and during the IVF procedure as follows: at the maximal down-regulation of the menstrual cycle; between the 5th and 8th day from the administration of the GnRH agonist (T1); at maximal stimulation after treatment by FSH and before hCG injection (T2) and two weeks after gonadotropin-releasing hormone (GnRH) injection (T3). Blood samples were obtained by atraumatic puncture of the antecubital vein, using a 20-gauge needle without tourniquet, into siliconized vacutainer tubes containing 0.105 mol/L trisodium citrate; 1/9 v/v (Becton and Dickinson, France). Platelet-poor plasma (PPP) was obtained by double centrifugation at 2000 g for 20 min at room temperature and plasma aliquots were stored at −80 °C until assayed. Samples were assessed within two weeks after collection. Thromboelastometry was carried out with fresh whole blood.

Molecular and functional analysis

Thrombin generation assay. Thrombin generation in plasma was assessed using the Calibrated Automated Thrombogram assay (CAT®, Diagnostica Stago, Asnières France) according to manufacturers' instructions, in the presence of optimal concentrations of TF (5 pM) and procoagulant phospholipids (4 µM) using the PPP-Reagent®. Assay's performance has been published elsewhere [12, 17].

Minimal TF-triggered whole blood thromboelastometry (min TF-WB TEM) was assessed in citrated whole blood, on the ROTEM® instrument (TEM®, Munich, Germany). Thromboelastometry was performed at 37 °C in citrated fresh whole blood within 30 min after veinipuncture using 5 pM of TF as described elsewhere [18]. The following parameters of the thromboelastometric trace were analyzed: (a) *Clotting time* (CT, in sec): time from the start

of the sample run to the point of first significant clot appearance corresponding to an amplitude of 2 mm, (b) *Clot formation time* (CFT, in sec): time from CT until the level of clot firmness reaches an arbitrary value of 20 mm, (c) *α-angle* (degree): measurement of clot development kinetics, (d) *Maximum clot firmness* (MCF in mm): the maximum vertical amplitude of the thromboelastogram.

Procoagulant phospholipid-dependent clotting time (Proag-PPL) was measured with STA®Procoag-PPL, (Diagnostica Stago, Asnières, France) according to the manufacturer's instructions as described elsewhere. The inter- and intra-assay coefficients of variation were 3 and 4% respectively.

Thrombomodulin activity. Plasma levels of thrombomodulin activity (TMa) were measured with a functional test on the STA-R analyzer (Diagnostica Stago, Asnières, France) as described elsewhere [19]. The inter- and intra-assay coefficients of variation were 5 and 6% respectively.

Specific TF activity. Tissue Factor activity (TFa) in PPP was measured with a clotting-based assay as previously described [20, 21]. The inter- and intra-assay coefficients of variation were 7% and 5% respectively. The levels of, FVIII, FvW, D-Dimers and fibrinogen were measured with conventional assays according to the manufacturer's instructions (Diagnostica Stago, Asnières, France).

Statistical analysis

The calculation of the sample size was based on the minimum number of patients required for a significant power for the detection of differences (a) between the IVF and control group, (b) at the IVF at the studied time points, (c) between IVF positive and IVF negative groups. The minimum sample size of 27 individuals for each group (IVF and control as well as IVF at each time point) was defined to warrant a two-tail significance at the limit of 5% and a prediction power of 95% with a two-sided α level of 0.05. Regarding the sub-group analysis (IVF positive and IVF negative) the minimum size of 15 patients for each group warrants two-tail significance at the limit of 5% and a prediction power of 85% with a two-sided α level of 0.05.

Special effort and attention was given to avoid missing values. The data are presented as mean ± sd. The Mann–Whitney test for independent samples was used for the comparisons of the studied parameters between the IVF and the control group and between the IVF-positive and IVF-negative group. Non-parametric Wilcoxon test for related samples and ANOVA test were applied to compare changes in variables at the studied time points during the observation period. Pearsons' test was applied to control correlation between thrombogram parameters and studied blood coagulation variables. Dichotomous variables were compared with χ^2 test. The Upper Normal Limit (UNL) and the Lower Normal Limit (LNL) for each parameter of the studied variables were defined in the control group as follows: UNL = mean + 2 SD, and LNL: = mean − 2 SD. The UNL and LNL of the studied biomarkers were defined in the control group and were compared to the corresponding normal reference range used by our laboratory. The normal ranges have been established according to the requirements for the good quality of laboratory practice by performing the tests in healthy individuals representative of the general population regarding age, sex, ethnicity, BMI. Two-sided values of $p < 0.05$ were considered as statistically significant.

The model development started by defining the positive diagnosis of pregnancy (if βHCG levels were equal or lower than 100 IU/L) as the dependent variable. The first step consisted of the univariate analysis in order to identify the variables associated with positive pregnancy. The selection of independent variables (which are the biomarkers of hypercoagulability) was done at the level of 5% using the stepwise procedure. The multivariable linear regression model was used to explore the effect of the independent variables on pregnancy outcome. The variables, found to be significant in the univariate analysis ($p < 0.05$) were included in the multivariate analysis. The variable with the highest p value was excluded from the model. The discrimination capacity of the model was tested with receiver operating characteristics (ROC) analysis and the area under the curve (AUC) was calculated for the quantification of the discrimination capacity of the model. The SPSS statistical software package (Chicago inc 6.1) was used for statistical analysis. Values are mean ± standard deviation.

Results

In total 38 women were eligible for the study and completed the follow up. The clinical and demographic characteristics of the studied groups are shown in Table 1. Positive IVF occurred in 15 women (40%) and negative in 23 (60%). The demographic characteristics and the indication for IVF were similar in the IVF-positive and IVF-negative group. None of the women included in the IVF and the control group had hypertension, hyperlipidemia or diabetes. None of the women suffered thromboembolic complication.

The UNL and LNL of the studied biomarkers in the control group were not significantly different as compared to the respective normal reference ranges used in our laboratory (Table 2).

Baseline profile

At T0, the IVF-group showed significantly increased thrombin generation (marked by shorter lag-time and ttPeak and higher ETP, Peak and MRI), and significantly shorter Procoag-PPL as compared to the control group. At least one thrombogram parameter was higher than

Table 1 Demographic and clinical characteristics of women eligible for IVF and in subgroups stratified according to the IVF outcome

Characteristics	IVF group (n = 38)	IVF-positive (n = 15)	IVF-negative (n = 23)	Control group (n = 30)
Demographics				
Age (years)	33.7 ± 3.5	33.7 ± 3.5	33.7 ± 3.5	32.2 ± 2.2
BMI	22.8 ± 2.9	22.8 ± 2.9	22.8 ± 2.9	23.8 ± 2.1
Indication for IVF				
endometriosis	2	1	1	–
idiopathic	17	17	14	–
ovarian insufficiency	1	1		–
tubal	4	2	2	–
male origin	14	7	7	–
Previous pregnancy				
0	31	15	16	–
1	4	3	1	10
2	3	1	2	20
Previous miscarriages				
0	36	17	19	30
1	2	1	1	0
Cardiovascular risk factors				
Current smokers	7 (18%)	3 (10%)	4 (13%)	8 (27%)

the UNL in 50% of women and lower than the LNL in 14%. The IVF group also had significantly higher levels of TFa, TMa. The levels of FVIII, FvW, D-Dimers and fibrinogen were not significantly different between the IVF-group and the control group (Table 2).

Effect of down-regulation of the menstrual cycle

At T1, thrombin generation, Procoag-PPL, TFa, TMa, FVIII, fibrinogen and D-Dimers were not significantly different as compared to T0. The levels of FvW significantly increased as compared to T0 (Table 2). Women with ETP, Peak or MRI above the UNL at T0 did not show any significant differences at T1.

Effect of ovarian stimulation

At T2, Peak, MRI and the levels of FVIII and D-Dimers were significantly increased as compared to T1 (Table 2). In contrast the Procoag-PPL and the levels of TFa, TMa and FvW did not vary significantly as compared to T1.

Effect of GnRH treatment

At T3, thrombin generation was not significantly different as compared to T2. The Procoag-PPL, TFa and TMa, FvW, and fibrinogen remained at the same levels

Table 2 Baseline profile of hypercoagulability in women eligible for IVF and dynamic changes of the global coagulation tests and molecular biomarkers of hypercoagulability during hormone treatment in the cohort of women eligible for IVF and according to the IVF outcome

	Normal reference range	Control (n=30)	IVF T0			IVF T1			IVF T2			IVF T3		
			All women (n=38)	IVF-positive (n=15)	IVF-negative (n=23)	All women (n=38)	IVF-positive (n=15)	IVF-negative (n=23)	All women (n=38)	IVF-positive (n=15)	IVF-negative (n=23)	All women (n=38)	IVF-positive (n=15)	IVF-negative (n=23)
Lag time (min)	2.1–3.8	3.41 ± 0.24 UNL: 3.89 LNL: 2.93	2.88 ± 0.59***	2.94 ± 0.59	2.84 ± 0.59	2.64 ± 0.58°°°	2.60 ± 0.62	2.65 ± 0.58	2.64 ± 0.67°°°	2.68 ± 0.86	2.62 ± 0.56	2.51 ± 0.56+++	2.87 ± 0.66	2.39 ± 0.53
ttPeak (min)	4.0–6.6	6.48 ± 0.32 UNL: 7.12 LNL: 5.84	5.58 ± 1.06***	5.68 ± 1.07	5.51 ± 1.07	5.23 ± 0.9°°°	4.97 ± 0.80	5.35 ± 0.93	5.03 ± 0.99 °°°§	4.95 ± 1.24	5.08 ± 0.85	4.79 ± 1.03+++	5.54 ± 1.6	4.54 ± 0.81
ETP (nM.min)	1178–1600	1408 ± 80 UNL: 1568 LNL: 1248	1939.65 ± 646***	1992.10 ± 736.60	1903.89 ± 592.17	1744.52 ± 549.19°°°	2006.95 ± 569.74	1615.55 ± 505.49§	1950.54 ± 551.03 °°°§	2172.95 ± 539.59	1819.71 ± 529.65*	1536.38 ± 371.53+	1931 ± 388.91	1471.5 ± 315.68§
Peak (nM)	222–330	262 ± 25 UNL: 312 LNL: 212	352.3 ± 100***	359.55 ± 109.08	347.35 ± 95.34	330.32 ± 99.07°°°	399.89 ± 96.32	297.19 ± 83.51§	372.79 ± 82.11 °°°§L	415.89 ± 73.08	347.44 ± 78.16*	317.69 ± 80.33+++	355.69 ± 56	305.02 ± 58.28§
MRI (nM/min)	60–120	86.59 ± 14.10 UNL: 115 LNL: 58	135.27 ± 44***	135.76 ± 47.86	134.93 ± 42.66	132.62 ± 50.3°°°	173.17 ± 50.21	113.31 ± 38.03§	159.77 ± 44.53 °°°§L	188.83 ± 48.09	142.67 ± 32.90*	146.31 ± 49.47+++	152.66 ± 98	144.2 ± 29.95§
CT (sec)	140–307	245.57 ± 45.61 UNL: 335 LNL: 155	269.53 ± 74.47	251.53 ± 78.8	281.26 ± 70.79	233.78 ± 65.71	206.07 ± 41.44	251.41 ± 72.77§	236.40 ± 62.41	209.07 ± 42.35	254.62 ± 67.70§	204.43 ± 23.65+++	216.8 ± 7.66	197.56 ± 27.03§
CFT (sec)	6–155	80.46 ± 37.26 UNL: 155 LNL: 6	92.82 ± 28.43	93.2 ± 37.25	92.57 ± 21.82	89.94 ± 26.60	88.43 ± 26.73	90.91 ± 27.1	88.14 ± 21.68	88.43 ± 16.79	89.05 ± 24.78	79.79 ± 23.51	64.8 ± 13.08	88.11 ± 24.38§
α angle (°)	55–92	72.86 ± 7.35 UNL: 88 LNL: 57	71.76 ± 5.02	71.60 ± 6.25	71.87 ± 4.18	72.78 ± 4.29	72.86 ± 4.13	72.73 ± 4.48	72.89 ± 3.83	73.57 ± 3.03	72.43 ± 4.28	74.14 ± 4.35	76.8 ± 2.59	72.67 ± 4.53
MCF (mm)	54–74	65.86 ± 4.31 UNL: 75 LNL: 57	64.63 ± 7.59	60.67 ± 10.22	63.91 ± 5.1	64.47 ± 4.48	64.50 ± 4.69	64.45 ± 4.45	64.31 ± 5.02	64.03 ± 5.5	64.29 ± 4.82	66.64 ± 5.39	69 ± 3.81	65.33 ± 5.87
Procoag-PPL (sec)	42–85	60.21 ± 9.3 UNL: 79 LNL: 42	33.0 ± 5.36***	36.45 ± 5.83	30.53 ± 3.34§	35.5 ± 7.04°°°	41.37 ± 7.55	32.27 ± 4.18§	34.14 ± 4.71 °°°	37.45 ± 4.51	32.12 ± 3.63*	39.4 ± 6.45+++	41.09 ± 5.79	38.32 ± 6.88
TFa (pM)	0.02–0.25	0.24 ± 0.11 UNL: 0.46 LNL: 0.02	0.47 ± 0.31***	0.32 ± 0.23	0.59 ± 0.31§	0.40 ± 0.32°°	0.21 ± 0.19	0.51 ± 0.32§	0.42 ± 0.27 °°°	0.22 ± 0.15	0.55 ± 0.26*	0.4 ± 0.14+++	0.41 ± 0.18	0.45 ± 0.12

Table 2 Baseline profile of hypercoagulability in women eligible for IVF and dynamic changes of the global coagulation tests and molecular biomarkers of hypercoagulability during hormone treatment in the cohort of women eligible for IVF and according to the IVF outcome (Continued)

	Range	UNL/LNL												
TMa (%)	50–126	UNL: 126 LNL: 54	127.56 ± 61.54***	121.60 ± 38.38	131.81 ± 74.50	131 ± 50.54°°°	113.17 ± 54.49	133.86 ± 44.96	119.90 ± 39.26°°°	103.55 ± 34.07	129.89 ± 39.72§	126.9 ± 34.27++	122.43 ± 7.74	129.82 ± 44.01
FVIII (%)	50–150	UNL: 143 LNL: 67	101.31 ± 29.22	98.73 ± 27.50	103.14 ± 30.92	117 ± 40.45	115.25 ± 34.90	113.73 ± 28.86	140.10 ± 28.30°°°L	152.73 ± 24.71	132.39 ± 28.17*	117.7 ± 22.97+LL	133.57 ± 14.08	107.55 ± 22.10§
vWF (%)	50–150	UNL: 147 LNL: 63	99.44 ± 20.08	95.53 ± 14.31	102.24 ± 23.30	125.17 ± 23.11°°°£	116.08 ± 18.73	108.23 ± 21.50	129.14 ± 21.37°°°	137.09 ± 24.77	124.28 ± 18.03	113.4 ± 16.79		
F g (g/l)	1.8–4.0	UNL: 3.7 LNL: 2.1	3.18 ± 0.8	3.01 ± 0.7	3.28 ± 0.86	2.98 ± 0.64	3.02 ± 0.9	2.96 ± 0.48	3.02 ± 0.65	3.10 ± 0.9	2.98 ± 0.51	2.9 ± 0.57	3.17 ± 0.64	2.71 ± 0.47
D-Dimers (µg/ml)	<0.50	UNL: 0.49 LNL: 0.01	0.29 ± 0.12	0.29 ± 0.11	0.31 ± 0.13	0.30 ± 0.09	0.30 ± 0.09	0.3 ± 0.11	0.56 ± 0.28°°°L	0.39 ± 0.11	0.68 ± 0.31*	0.7 ± 0.4+++LL	0.49 ± 0.15	0.85 ± 0.45*

UNL upper normal limits, LNL lower normal limits, ETP the endogenous thrombin generation, CT clotting time, CFT clot formation time, TMa thrombomodulin activity, D-Di D-Dimer, FVIII factor VIII, Peak the peak concentration of thrombin, ttPeak time to reach the peak concentration of thrombin, MRI mean rate index of thrombin generation, AUC area under curve, a angle reflecting the fibrin polymerization rate, Procoag-PPL procoagulant phospholipid dependent clotting time, MCF maximum clot firmness, vWF von Willebrand factor activity, TFa tissue factor activity, Fg fibrinogen

*p < 0.05; **p < 0.01; ***p < 0.001, T0 versus control
°p < 0.05; °° p < 0.01; °°°p < 0.001, T1 versus control
θp < 0.05; θθ p < 0.01; θθθp < 0.001, T2 versus control
+p < 0.05; ++p < 0.01; +++p < 0.001, T3 versus control
£p < %0.05 T1 versus T0
Lp < 0.05 T2 versus T1
LLp < 0.05 T3 versus T2
§p < 0.05; IVF-negative versus IVF-positive

as in T2. The levels of FVIII significantly decreased at T3 as compare to T2. The levels of D-Dimers significantly increased as compared to T2 (Table 2).

At all studied time points the parameters of thromboelastometry were not significantly different between the IVF-group and the control group (Table 2).

Blood hypercoagulability and IVF outcome

At T2 and T3 the ETP, Peak and MRI were significantly higher in the IVF-positive as compared to the IVF-negative group. At T0, T1 and T2 the Procoag-PPL was significantly shorter in the IVF-negative group compared to the IVF-positive group. At all time points except T3, the levels of TFa were significantly higher in the IVF-negative group as compared to the IVF-positive group. The levels of TMa were significantly higher in the IVF-negative group as compared to the IVF-positive group only at T2. At T2 and T3 FVIII levels were significantly lower in IVF negative as compared to IVF positive. At T2 and T3, D-Dimers were significantly higher in the IVF-negative as compared to the IVF-positive group. At T1 and T2, the CT was significantly shorter in the IVF-positive group as compared to the IVF-negative. (Table 2).

The Procoag-PPL was inversely correlated with the lagtime ($r = -0.304$; $p = 0.013$), ETP ($r = -0,4$; $p = 0.001$) and MRI ($r = -0.380$; $p = 0.002$) as well as with the TFa ($r = -0.399$; $p = 0.001$). Thrombomodulin was inversely correlated with ETP ($r = -0.346$; $p = 0.019$).

Univariate analysis showed the following biomarkers to have a significant correlation with the positive outcome of IVF: at T0, the FvW; at T1 the ETP, Peak, MRI, Procoag-PPL and TFa; at T2, the ETP, Peak, MRI, Procoag-PPL, TFa and D-Dimers (Table 3).

There was a strong association between IVF-positive outcome and Procoag-PPL longer than 31.1 sec. Women who had Procoag-PPL between 31.1 and 54.9 sec had 24-fold higher probability for pregnancy than the women with Procoag-PPL values lower than 31.1 sec.

Multivariate analysis for the identification of biomarkers which are correlated with a positive outcome of IVF retained the Procoag-PPL and MRI of thrombin generation. Multivariate analysis applied at the T1 led to the construction of a prediction model including the Procoag-PPL and the MRI according to the equation:

$$Y = (0.043*MRI)*(0.45*Procoag\text{-}PPL)$$

The ROC curve showed a very good specificity and sensitivity of the model for the prediction of pregnancy since the area under the curve was 0.99 (Fig. 1).

Discussion

The present prospective longitudinal observational study demonstrates that at baseline, women eligible for IVF present blood hypercoagulability which is characterized by significant increase of platelet and endothelial cell activation biomarkers. The baseline state of cellular hypercoagulability, which persisted practically unchanged during the period of hormone treatment administration for IVF, was consisted of significantly shortening of Procoag-PPL clotting time. This test is correlated with increased concentration of procoagulant microparticles derived from platelets or other cells [22, 23]. The levels of TFa and TMa, at baseline and during hormone treatment, were also significantly increased as compared to age-matched women with naturally occurring uneventful pregnancies. The TFa and TMa are biomarkers of endothelial cell or platelet activation [24–26]. In addition, increased TFa levels in plasma is a marker of monocyte activation [27]. The Procoag-PPL, TFa and TMa levels were not significantly modified during treatment for estrogen down-regulation and ovarian stimulation indicating that the shift towards cellular hypercoagulability observed at baseline was not correlated with hormone variations. The data from the present study are in accordance with those recently published by Olausson et al. which demonstrate that platelet, endothelial and monocyte-derived microparticles and inflammation biomarkers are significantly increased in women undergoing IVF [28]. Thrombin generation was also significantly enhanced but the baseline levels of FVIII, FvW, D-Dimers and fibrinogen were similar to those observed in the control group, confirming previous studies [4]. To the best of our knowledge, this is the first study showing that infertility is linked to a systemic cell activation that offers procoagulant substances, mainly endothelial cells and platelets. This concept is supported by recent studies reporting that increased levels of plasminogen activator inhibitor 1 (PAI-1), thrombin activatable fibrinolysis inhibitor (TAFI) or tissue factor pathway inhibitor (TFPI), which are synthesized and secreted by activated endothelial cells are related with infertility and IVF failure [29–32].

Furthermore, the present study showed that short Procoag-PPL clotting time as well as increased TFa and TMa levels are independent risk factors for IVF failure. The implication of high levels of TF and procoagulant microparticles in the pathogenesis of infertility, IVF failure and vascular complications during pregnancy, such as recurrent first trimester miscarriage, fetal loss, stillbirth, early and severe pre-eclampsia or prematurity has already been reported by others (reviewed in [33, 34]). Herein, we demonstrate for a first time that the shortened Procoag-PPL associated with the mean rate index (MRI) of the propagation phase of thrombin generation assessed at the maximal down-regulation of the menstrual cycle (between the 5th and 8th day from the administration of the GnRH agonist) are predictors of IVF outcome. These tests could be used in the construction of a risk assessment model for IVF issue. The design of

Table 3 Univariate analysis and odds ratio of thrombin generation test and the biomarkers of hypercoagulability for the positive IVF outcome

Variables	T0		T1		T2		T3	
	odds ratio (95% Conf. Interval)	p	odds ratio (95% Conf. Interval)	p	odds ratio [95% Conf. Interval]	p	odds ratio (95% Conf. Interval)	p
lag-time (min)	1.288 (0.39–4.17)	0.672	0.855 (1.96–3.71)	0.835	1.583 (0.54–4.64)	0.403	2.564 (0.11–54.54)	0.56
ETP (nM.min)	0.999 (0.99–1.00)	0.936	1.002 (1.00–1.00)	0.047*	1.002 (1.00–1.003)	0.016*	1.000 (0.99–1.00)	0.625
Peak (nM)	0.999 (0.6–2.2)	0.974	1.013 (1.00–1.02)	0.006*	1.018 (1.01–1.03)	0.004*	1.001 (0.98–1.02)	0.952
ttPeak (min)	1.148 (0.59–2.23)	0.684	0.529 (0.13–2.16)	0.375	1.034 (0.40–2.66)	0.945	1.944 (0.42–8.93)	0.394
MRI (nM/min)	0.997 (0.98–1.01)	0.792	1.032 (1.01–1.05)	0.003*	1.037 (1.01–1.06)	0.005*	0.993 (0.96–1.02)	0.715
Procoag-PPL (sec)	1.009 (0.88–1.15)	0.895	1.399 (1.07–1.82)	0.013*	1.421 (1.08–1.86)	0.011*	1.112 (0.91–1.33)	0.32
TFa (pM)	0.329 (0.04–2.96)	0.322	0.0022 (0–0.21)	0.009*	4.60e−08 (2.14e−13.00)	0.007*	1.141 (1.03–1.27)	0.009
TMa (%)	0.997 (0.99–1.00)	0.598	0.987 (0.96–1.01)	0.223	0.977 (0.95–1.00)	0.107	0.993 (0.96–1.01)	0.368
FVIII (%)	1.003 (0.97–1.02)		1.004 (0.97–1.03)	0.799	1.028 (0.99–1.06)	0.137	1.143 (0.97–1.34)	0.119
VWF (%)	1.052 (1.01–1.08)	0.004*	1.009 (0.98–1.04)	0.578	1.012 (0.07–1.05)	0.581	1.062 (0.97–1.16)	0.166
Fibrinogen (g/L)	1.228 (0.48–3.16)	0.67	0.979 (0.18–5.16)	0.981	2.014 (0.31–13)	0.465	6.346 (0.63–63.38)	0.116
D-Dimers (µg/ml)	0.997 (0.99–1.00)	0.408	1 (0.99–1.00)	0.951	0.992 (0.98–0.99)	0.016*	1.243 (0.82–1.45)	0.234

the present study does not allow the identification of the underlying causes that lead to cellular activation and hypercoagulability which is observed at baseline. This investigation appears to be attractive for the elucidation of the link with hypercoagulability in women eligible for IVF. The association between hypercoagulablity and negative IVF outcome has recently been reported by Di Nisio et al., who proposed that the increase of D-Dimers levels in plasma is a predictor for IVF failure [35]. The implication of increased D-Dimers in the sterility is further supported by the data presented by Di Micco et al. [36]. The univariate analysis of the data reported herein confirms that the increase of D-Dimers during hormone treatment is a negative prognostic factor for IVF outcome. However, the impact of D-Dimers disappeared in the multivariate analysis indicating that high concentrations of procoagulant phospholipids, detected by the short Procoag-PPL, have a dominant role in negative IVF outcome.

Interestingly, increased thrombin generation was found to be a positive predictor for IVF outcome. This finding is in accordance with the concept that thrombin generation is necessary for blastocyst implantation, remodeling of decidualized human endometrial stromal cells and subsequent trophoblast invasion and remodeling of the spiral arteries and arterioles; a process driven by TF expression in the endometrial microenvironment which is in contact with mother's blood [7–10]. The concept that the non-suffering of endothelial cells, platelets or other cells that potentially release procoagulant phospholipids, is determinant for a positive IVF outcome is supported by our study. Indeed, the presence of high levels of procoagulant phospholipids

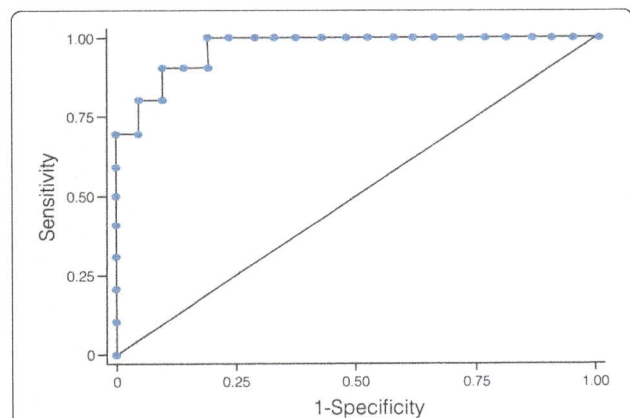

Fig. 1 The ROC analysis of the prediction model of the IVF outcome based on the MRI and Procoag-PPL. The AUC is 0.9667

in plasma, as expressed by shortened Procoag-PPL was the dominant parameter related with IVF failure while the decrease of thrombin generation was found to be a complementary factor. Control measurements showed that factor V and factor II levels were within the normal range (data not shown) ruling out clotting factors' consumption. The reasons for which thrombin generation is decreased in women with IVF failure have to be investigated.

At all studied time points the parameters of thromboelastometry were not significantly different between the IVF-group and the control group. Fibrinogen levels, platelet count and hematocrit are variables with a major impact on thromboelastometric profile. Both IVF-group and the control group had these variables within the normal ranges.

We found that when the ovarian stimulation was maximal, thrombin generation, FVIII, FvW and D-Dimers levels were significantly increased, in agreement with older studies [5, 37–41]. However, these changes were not reflected on the kinetics of clot formation and its qualitative characteristics when coagulation was triggered by a low TF concentration. In women undergoing hormone treatment for IVF preparation thromboelastographic analysis performed after triggering contact system showed a slight but significant acceleration of the kinetics of clot formation following GnRH treatment indicating that peak concentrations of estrogens are associated with a possible enhancement of FXII activation [42]. Women who had baseline thrombin generation above the UNL remained at the same levels during the down-regulation and the stimulation phase of the treatment (data not shown). Therefore, our data, in agreement with previous studies [43] and support the concept that hormone treatment for IVF represents a mild procoagulant stimulus, which has a minor effect on the global haemostatic balance, the kinetics of clot formation or its qualitative characteristics. Two weeks after hCG injection and embryo transfer, thrombin generation, TMa, TFa and Procoag-PPL remained without any significant modifications as compared to the phase of ovarian hyperstimulation. In contrast, the D-Dimers tended to increase and this finding is in agreement with others [2]. De Nisio et al., found that one week after the administration of gonadotropin, D-Dimers levels increased considerably [35]. We also found that even two weeks after GnRH injection D-Dimers levels are still increased, reflecting enhanced fibrin formation or fibrinolysis following r-hCG, as described by Biron et al. [2].

The present study has some limitations. The number of the enrolled women, although it provides sufficient statistical power to identify the most relevant biomarkers related with IVF outcome, does not allow generalizability of the model. The group of IVF women was heterogeneous regarding the IVF indication. In some women the indication

of the IVF was of male origin. Although the elimination of these cases did not significantly influence the final results, this does not warrant that the presence of this subpopulation had no impact on the results. A new prospective study in a larger population is planned to corroborate these findings. Women enrolled in the study were treated with three different protocols for estrogen down-regulation. The subgroup analysis according to the therapeutic protocol did not demonstrate any significant difference on the studied biomarkers among the subgroups (data not shown). Several different hormone treatments and protocols are applied for IVF preparation by the different IVF centers. Whether this protocol variability influences the kinetics of the studied biomarkers has to be investigated. However, the major findings of our study, which are (a) the presence of cell derived hypercoagulable state at the baseline, before any treatment administration and (b) the predictive value of the Procoag-PPL clotting time associated with the MRI of thrombin generation on IVF outcome are not influenced by the subsequent hormone treatments for ovarian stimulation. Although this study fulfils the criteria for the statistical power in the selection of the most clinically relevant biomarkers, a new prospective independent validation of this model is required in a larger multicenter study.

It has been suggested that heparin may improve the intrauterine environment in sub-fertile women, by enhancing growth factors to improve attachment of the embryo to the lining of the womb [44]. Thus low molecular weight heparin (LMWH) is often offered to women eligible for IVF as an adjunct treatment in an attempt to improve the probability for a positive outcome. However, a recent meta-analysis showed that it is unclear whether peri-implantation heparin administration in assisted reproduction treatment cycles improves clinical pregnancy rates in sub-fertile women [45]. The elaboration of a risk assessment model with the clinically relevant biomarkers of hypercoagulability proposed by the present study is of clinical interest in order to identify women who could benefit from the peri-implantation administration of antithrombotic treatment.

Conclusions

The data presented herein show that hypercoagulability of cellular origin is the dominant biological process related with IVF failure. Hypercoagulabilty of cellular origin appears at the baseline, before any hormone treatment administration and it is not modified by this treatment. The administration of hormone treatment during the IVF preparation does not lead to substantial alteration of global coagulation process. Among the large variety of the studied biomarkers, the evaluation of both Procoag-PPL and MRI of thrombin generation after down-regulation of the menstrual cycle appear to be the most clinically relevant biomarkers for the identification of the women at risk of IVF failure.

Abbreviations

AUC: Area under the curve; BMI: Body mass index; CAT: Calibrated Automated Thrombogram; CFT: Clot formation time; CT: Clotting time; E2: Estradiol; ETP: Endogenous thrombin potential; FSH: Follicular stimulating hormone; FVIII: Factor VIII; FvW: Factor von Willebrand; GnRH: Gonadotropin-releasing hormone agonist; hCG: Human recombinant chorion gonadotropin; IVF: In vitro fertilization; LNL: Lower Normal Limit; MCF: Maximum clot firmness; min TF-WB TEM: Minimal TF-triggered whole blood thromboelastometry; MRI: Mean rate index; PA1-1: Plasminogen activator inhibitor 1; PPP: Platelet poor plasma; Procoag-PPL: Procoagulant phospholipid clotting time; ROC: Receiver operating characteristics; TAFI: Thrombin activatable fibrinolysis inhibitor; TFa: Tissue factor activity; TFPI: Tissue factor pathway inhibitor; TG: Thrombin generation; TMa: Thrombomodulin activity; ttPeak: Time to Peak; UNL: Upper Normal Limit; VTE: Venous thromboembolism

Acknowledgements

The authors acknowledge the nurses from the Department of Obstetrics and Gynecology for their efforts to collect blood samples. The authors wish to thank the skilful technical assistance of the technicians of the Laboratory of Haemostasis, Service d'Hématologie Biologique, Hôpital Tenon and particularly Mme Marie Paule Roman and Severine Bouffard.

Funding

The study was supported by the Association de Recherche sur la Thrombose et l'Évaluation de son Risque (ARTER) and by an unrestricted grant by Diagnostica Stago.

Authors' contributions

GTG has made substantial contributions to conception and design of the study, analysis and interpretation of data, has been involved in drafting the manuscript has given final approval of the version to be published, agreed to be accountable for all aspects of the work in ensuring that questions related to the accuracy or integrity of any part of the work are appropriately investigated and resolved. PVD has made substantial contributions to study design and organization, acquisition, analysis and interpretation of data, has been involved in drafting the manuscript. EMD has made substantial contribution to the design of the study, the selection of the patients and the interpretation of the data, EL has made substantial contribution in the interpretation of the data, the writing and editing of the paper. MG: was responsible for the technical party. MC: was responsible for patients' recruitment. RS: was responsible of statistical analysis, interpretation of the data. HK: was responsible for data collection. AKL was responsible for critical revision of the article for important intellectual content. IE critically reviewed the manuscript. All authors read and approved the final manuscript.

Competing interests

The authors declare that they have no competing interests.

Capsule

Women eligible for IVF at baseline show hypercoagulability related with IVF failure. Hormone treatment does not enhance hypercoagulability. Shortened procoagulant phospholipid clotting time and mean rate index of thrombin generation are predictors for IVF failure.

Author details

[1]Cancer Biology and Therapeutics, Centre de Recherche Saint-Antoine, Institut National de la Santé et de la Recherche Médicale (INSERM) U938 and Université Pierre et Marie Curie (UPMC), Sorbonne Universities, Paris, France.

[2]Service d'Hématologie Biologique, Hôpital Tenon, Hôpitaux Universitaires Est Parisien, Assistance Publique Hôpitaux de Paris, 4, rue de la Chine, Paris Cedex 20, France. [3]Clinical Research Department, Diagnostica Stago, Gennevilliers, France. [4]Department of Obstetrics and Gynecology, Hôpital Tenon, Hôpitaux Universitaires Est Parisien, Assistance Publique Hôpitaux de Paris, Paris, France.

References

1. Andersson O, Blomback M, Bremme K, et al. Prediction of changes in levels of haemostatic variables during natural menstrual cycle and ovarian hyperstimulation. Thromb Haemost. 1997;77:901–4.
2. Biron C, Galtier-Dereure F, Rabesandratana H, et al. Hemostasis parameters during ovarian stimulation for in vitro fertilization: results of a prospective study. Fertil Steril. 1997;67:104–9.
3. Aune B, Høie KE, Oian P, Holst N, Osterud B. Does ovarian stimulation for in-vitro fertilization induce a hypercoagulable state? Hum Reprod. 1991;6:925–7.
4. Brummel-Ziedins KE, Gissel M, Francis C, et al. The effect of high circulating estradiol levels on thrombin generation during in vitro fertilization. Thromb Res. 2009;124:505–7.
5. Westerlund E, Henriksson P, Wallén H, et al. Detection of a procoagulable state during controlled ovarian hyperstimulation for in vitro fertilization with global assays of haemostasis. Thromb Res. 2012;130:649–53.
6. Chighizola CB, de Jesus GR. Antiphospholipid antibodies and infertility. Lupus. 2014;23:1232–8.
7. Girardi G. Role of tissue factor in feto-maternal development: a xiphos. J Thromb Haemost. 2011;9:250–6.
8. Lockwood CJ, Paidas M, Murk WK, et al. Involvement of human decidual cell-expressed tissue factor in uterine hemostasis and abruption. Thromb Res. 2009;124:516–20.
9. Krikun G, Lockwood CJ, Paidas MJ. Tissue factor and the endometrium: from physiology to pathology. Thromb Res. 2009;124:393–6.
10. Lockwood CJ, Krikun G, Caze R, et al. Decidual cell-expressed tissue factor in human pregnancy and its involvement in hemostasis and preeclampsia-related angiogenesis. Ann N Y Acad Sci. 2008;1127:67–72.
11. Gupta S, Agarwal A, Sharma RK. The role of placental oxidative stress and lipid peroxidation in preeclampsia. Obstet Gynecol Surv. 2005;60:807–16.
12. Spronk HM, Dielis AW, De Smedt E, et al. Assessment of thrombin generation II: validation of the calibrated automated thrombogram in platelet-poor plasma in a clinical laboratory. Thromb Haemost. 2008;100:362–4.
13. Hemker HC, Willems GM, Beguin S. A computer assisted method to obtain the propthrombin activation velocity in whole plasma independent of thrombin decay processes. Thromb Haemost. 1986;56:9–17.
14. Chakroun T, Gerotziafas GT, Seghatchian J, et al. The influence of fibrin polymerization and platelet-mediated contractile forces on citrated whole blood thromboelastography profile. Thromb Haemost. 2006;95:822–8.
15. Chaari M, Ayadi I, Rousseau A, et al. Impact of breast cancer stage, time from diagnosis and chemotherapy on plasma and cellular biomarkers of hypercoagulability. BMC Cancer. 2014;22(14):991–1004.
16. Gerotziafas GT, Van Dreden P, Chaari M, et al. The acceleration of the propagation phase of thrombin generation in patients with sickle cell disease is associated with circulating erythrocyte-derived microparticles. Thromb Haemost. 2012;107:1044–52.
17. Gerotziafas GT, Depasse F, Busson J, et al. Towards a standardization of thrombin generation assessment: the influence of tissue factor, platelets and phospholipids concentration on the normal values of Thrombogram-Thrombinoscope assay. Thromb J. 2005;3:16–27.
18. Konstantinidis K, Gerasimidis T, Verdy E, et al. Inhibition of clot formation process by treatment with the low-molecular-weight heparin nadroparin in patients with carotid artery disease undergoing angioplasty and stenting. A thromboelastography study on whole blood. Thromb Haemost. 2007;97:109–18.
19. Rousseau A, Favier R, Van Dreden P. Elevated circulating soluble thrombomodulin activity, tissue factor activity and circulating procoagulant phospholipids: new and useful markers for pre-eclampsia? Eur J Obstet Gynecol Reprod Biol. 2009;146:46–9.

20. Van Dreden P, Rousseau A, Savoure A, et al. Plasma thrombomodulin activity, tissue factor activity and high levels of circulating procoagulant phospholipid as prognostic factors for acute myocardial infarction. Blood Coagul Fibrinolysis. 2009;220:635–41.

21. Schneider P, Van Dreden P, Rousseau A, et al. M. Increased levels of tissue factor activity and procoagulant phospholipids during treatment of children with acute lymphoblastic leukaemia. Br J Haematol. 2010;148:582–92.

22. Patil R, Ghosh K, Satoskar P, et al. Elevated procoagulant endothelial and tissue factor expressing microparticles in women with recurrent pregnancy loss. PLoS One. 2013;8:e81407.

23. Patil R, Ghosh K, Shetty S. A simple clot based assay for the detection of procoagulant cell-derived microparticles. Clin Chem Lab Med. 2016;54:799–803.

24. Ohlin AK, Larsson K, Hansson M. Soluble thrombomodulin activity and soluble thrombomodulin antigen in plasma. J Thromb Haemost. 2005;3:976–82.

25. Boffa MC. Considering cellular thrombomodulin distribution and its modulating factors can facilitate the use of plasma thrombomodulin as a reliable endothelial marker. Haemostasis. 1996;26:233–43.

26. Iann A, Seigneur M. Soluble markers of endothelial cell function. Clin Hemorheol Microcirc. 1997;17:3.

27. Slavik L, Novak M, Ulehlova J, Prochazka M, Prochazkova J, Lattova V, Polak P, Pilka R. Possibility of coagulation system activation determination with tissue factor in pregnancy complications. Clin Lab. 2016;62:1851–6.

28. Olausson N, Mobarrez F, Wallen H, Westerlund E, Hovatta O, Henriksson P. Microparticles reveal cell activation during IVF - a possible early marker of a prothrombotic state during the first trimester. Thromb Haemost. 2016;116:517–23.

29. Martínez-Zamora MA, Creus M, Tassies D, Reverter JC, Civico S, Carmona F, et al. Reduced plasma fibrinolytic potential in patients with recurrent implantation failure after IVF and embryo transfer. Hum Reprod. 2011;26:510–6.

30. Sarto A, Rocha M, Martínez M, Sergio Pasqualini R. Hypofibrinolysis and other hemostatic defects in women with antecedents of early reproductive failure. Medicina (B Aires). 2000;60:441–7.

31. Romagnuolo I, Sticchi E, Fedi S, Cellai AP, Lami D, Alessandrello Liotta A, Rogolino A, Cioni G, Noci I, Abbate R, Fatini C. Is tissue factor pathway inhibitor a marker of procoagulable status in healthy infertile women undergoing ovarian stimulation for assisted reproduction? Blood Coagul Fibrinolysis. 2014;25:254–8.

32. Altmäe S, Salumets A, Bjuresten K, Kallak TK, Wånggren K, Landgren BM, Hovatta O, Stavreus-Evers A. Tissue factor and tissue factor pathway inhibitors TFPI and TFPI2 in human secretory endometrium–possible link to female infertility. Reprod Sci. 2011;18:666–78.

33. Alijotas-Reig J, Ferrer-Oliveras R, Ruffatti A, Tincani A, Lefkou E, Bertero MT, Coloma-Bazan E, de Carolis S, Espinosa G, Rovere-Querini P, Kuzenko A, Valverde EE, Robles A, Cervera R, Canti V, Fredi M, Gil-Aguado A, Lundelin K, Llurba E, Melnychuk T, Nalli C, Picardo E, Silvestro E, del Ross T, Farran-Codina I, EUROAPS Study Group Collaborators. Autoimmun Rev. 2015;14:387–9.

34. La Farina F, Raparelli V, Napoleone L, Guadagni F, Basili S, Ferroni P. Inflammation and thrombophilia in pregnancy complications: implications for risk assessment and clinical management. Cardiovasc Hematol Disord Drug Targets. 2016;15:187–203.

35. Di Nisio M, Porreca E, Di Donato V, et al. Plasma concentrations of D-dimer and outcome of in vitro fertilization. J Ovarian Res. 2014;22:58–62.

36. Di Micco P, D'Uva M, Strina I, Mollo A, Amato V, Niglio A, De Placido G. The role of d-dimer as first marker of thrombophilia in women affected by sterility: implications in pathophysiology and diagnosis of thrombophilia induced sterility. J Transl Med. 2004;2:38.

37. Lox C, Cañez M, Deleon F, et al. Hyperestrogenism induced by menotropins alone or in conjunction with luprolide acetate in in vitro fertilization cycles: the impact on hemostasis. Fertil Steril. 1995;63:566–70.

38. Harnett MJ, Bhavani-Shankar K, Datta S, et al. In vitro fertilization-induced alterations in coagulation and fibrinolysis as measured by thromboelastography. Anesth Analg. 2002;95:1063–6.

39. Winkler U, Bühler K, Koslowski S, et al. Plasmatic haemostasis in gonadotrophin-releasing hormone analogue therapy: effects of leuprorelin acetate depot on coagulatory and fibrinolytic activities. Clin Ther. 1992;14(Suppl A):114–20.

40. Westerlund E, Antovic A, Hovatta O, et al. Changes in von Willebrand factor and ADAMTS13 during IVF. Blood Coagul Fibrinolysis. 2011;22:127–31.

41. Richard-Davis G, Montgomery-Rice V, Mammen EF, Alshameeri RS, Morgan D, Moghissi KS. In vitro platelet function in controlled ovarian hyperstimulation cycles. Fertil Steril. 1997;67:923–7.

42. Orbach-Zinger S, Eidelman LA, Lutsker A, Oron G, Fisch B, Ben-Haroush A. The effect of in vitro fertilization on coagulation parameters as measured by thromboelastogram. Eur J Obstet Gynecol Reprod Biol. 2016;201:118–20.

43. Curvers J, Nap AW, Thomassen MC, Nienhuis SJ, Hamulyák K, Evers JL, Tans G, Rosing J. Effect of in vitro fertilization treatment and subsequent pregnancy on the protein C pathway. Br J Haematol. 2001;115:400–7.

44. Fluhr H, Spratte J, Ehrhardt J, et al. Heparin and low-molecular-weight heparins modulate the decidualization of human endometrial stromal cells. Fertil Steril. 2010;93:2581–7.

45. Akhtar MA, Sur S, Raine-Fenning N, et al. Heparin for assisted reproduction. Cochrane Database Syst Rev. 2013;8, CD009452. doi:10.1002/14651858. CD009452.

13

Management of venous thromboembolism: an update

Siavash Piran and Sam Schulman[*]

From The 9th Congress of the Asian-Pacific Society on Thrombosis and Hemostasis
Taipei, Taiwan.

Abstract

Venous thromboembolism (VTE), which constitutes pulmonary embolism and deep vein thrombosis, is a common disorder associated with significant morbidity and mortality. Landmark trials have shown that direct oral anticoagulants (DOACs) are as effective as conventional anticoagulation with vitamin K antagonists (VKA) in prevention of VTE recurrence and associated with less bleeding. This has paved the way for the recently published guidelines to change their recommendations in favor of DOACs in acute and long-term treatment of VTE in patients without cancer. The recommended treatment of VTE in cancer patients remains low-molecular-weight heparin. The initial management of pulmonary embolism (PE) should be directed based on established risk stratification scores. Thrombolysis is an available option for patients with hemodynamically significant PE. Recent data suggests that low-risk patients with acute PE can safely be treated as outpatients if home circumstances are adequate. There is lack of support for use of inferior vena cava filters in patients on anticoagulation. This review describes the acute, long-term, and extended treatment of VTE and recent evidence on the management of sub-segmental PE.

Keywords: Venous thromboembolism, Anticoagulation, Direct oral anticoagulants, Vitamin K antagonists

Abbreviations: ACCP, American College of Chest Physicians; CI, Confidence interval; CRNM, Clinically relevant non-major; CTEPH, Chronic thromboembolic pulmonary hypertension; CTPA, Computed tomography of the pulmonary angiography; DOAC, Direct oral anticoagulant; DVT, Deep vein thrombosis; IVC, Inferior vena cava; LMWH, Low-molecular weight heparin; PE, Pulmonary embolism; PESI, Pulmonary embolism severity index; SSPE, Sub-segmental pulmonary embolism; VKA, Vitamin K antagonists; VTE, Venous thromboembolism

Background

Venous thromboembolism (VTE), which includes deep vein thrombosis (DVT) and pulmonary embolism (PE), is one of the most common cardiovascular diseases occurring for the first time in about 1 in 1000 people [1, 2]. Its incidence rises with increasing age, for example to about 5 per 1000 people among those over 70 years of age [3]. VTE is associated with significant morbidity and mortality with the 30-day mortality rate in the absence of treatment of about 3 % for DVT and 31 % for PE [4]. The long-term complications of VTE are post-thrombotic syndrome (PTS), which occurs in 20 to 50 % of patients with DVT [5], and chronic thromboembolic pulmonary hypertension (CTEPH), which occurs in 2 to 4 % of patients with PE [6]. Patients with CTEPH have progressive dyspnea and exercise intolerance and those with PTS have chronic leg pain and swelling, which in a minority of patients can progress to development of venous ulcers. These conditions can significantly reduce the patient's quality of life. Furthermore, the management VTE is associated with substantial health care costs for not only the initial hospitalization but also for hospital re-admissions [7, 8]. Therefore, VTE is associated with significant morbidity and mortality.

* Correspondence: schulms@mcmaster.ca
Department of Medicine, Division of Hematology and Thromboembolism, and Thrombosis and Atherosclerosis Research Institute, McMaster University, Hamilton, ON L8L 2X2, Canada

Initial management

The initial management of patients with a PE should be based on risk stratification of the patient into low, intermediate, or high risk for 30-day mortality based on established risk scores such as pulmonary embolism severity index (PESI) or its simplified version (simplified PESI) [9, 10]. Low risk patients, who are hemodynamically stable, can be treated as outpatients if home circumstances are adequate [11, 12]. At the other extreme, patients with acute PE and hypotension or patients with DVT-associated phlegmasia of the lower leg should be considered for treatment with thrombolytic agents [13, 14].

Oral anticoagulants

Anticoagulants are the mainstay treatment of VTE and are given in three phases of acute, long-term (in the first 3 months), and extended treatment [14]. For many years initial treatment was started with a parenteral anticoagulant, for example low-molecular-weight heparin (LMWH), overlapping with a vitamin K antagonist (VKA), such as warfarin. The combination was continued for at least 5 days until the achievement of therapeutic anticoagulation with international normalized ratio of 2 to 3 [14]. Although conventional therapy with VKAs is effective and safe, it has some limitations including delayed onset, need for parental daily injections, and interactions with dietary vitamin K and numerous drugs. Over the past 5 years, 4 direct oral anticoagulants (DOACs) have been approved for acute and long-term treatment of VTE [15–20]. The DOACs were compared with conventional therapy and found to be as effective in prevention of VTE recurrence and associated with less bleeding. The recently published American College of Chest Physicians (ACCP) guidelines have changed their recommendations in favor of DOACs in acute and long-term treatment of VTE in patients without cancer [21]. In patients with cancer associated VTE, the recommended anticoagulation remains LMWH over VKA [21].

The aim of this review is to (1) describe the initial management of patients with acute PE including the role of thrombolytic agents in hemodynamically unstable patients and at the other extreme outpatient management of low risk patients, (2) summarize the evidence on acute, long-term, and extended treatment of VTE comparing DOACs versus VKA, and (3) review the recent data on the management of sub-segmental PE and the lack of support for use of inferior vena cava filters in patients on anticoagulation.

Review

Acute and long-term treatment of venous thromboembolism

Thrombolytic and interventional treatment for acute venous thromboembolism

Anticoagulant therapy alone is recommended over thrombolysis for most patients with an acute DVT with exception for those with extensive iliofemoral or proximal DVT at high risk of limb ischemia [14, 21]. Thrombolytic therapy (systemic or catheter-directed) increase clot lysis and reduce the incidence of PTS compared to anticoagulation alone [22, 23]. However, this is at the expense of higher rate of major bleeding and no difference in rate of recurrent VTE or mortality [22–24]. Massive proximal DVT or iliofemoral thrombosis associated with limb-threatening ischemia or severe symptomatic swelling may be treated with thrombolysis. Thrombolysis can be considered only after objective diagnosis of the DVT and in a patient with low bleeding risk. The CaVenT trial randomized 209 patients with iliofemoral DVT to catheter directed therapy (CDT) versus anticoagulation. They found that the patients treated with CDT had significantly less PTS at 2 years compared with those treated with anticoagulation (41 versus 56 %) [22]. Another study randomized 32 patients with iliofemoral DVT to receive either CDT or systemic thrombolysis, followed by anticoagulation [25]. The patients who were treated with CDT had less reflux in both the deep and superficial veins and more patients had venous valvular competence preserved compared with patients who underwent systemic thrombolysis. A large, multicenter trial (the ATTRACT trial) is currently underway that randomizes patients to receive pharmaco-mechanical catheter-directed thrombolysis (PCDT) plus standard therapy with anticoagulation versus standard therapy alone [26]. It will investigate whether PCDT should be routinely utilized to prevent PTS in patients with symptomatic proximal DVT [26].

Systemic thrombolysis is a widely accepted treatment for PE in patients with persistent hypotension (e.g., systolic blood pressure <90 mmHg for 15 min) and not at high risk of bleeding [14, 21]. The use of thrombolytic therapy in intermediate risk patients with acute PE associated with right ventricle (RV) dysfunction is controversial. The RV dysfunction is confirmed by echocardiogram or computed tomography and a positive troponin I/T. The potential indication for thrombolysis in this group is based on evidence that patients with severe RV dysfunction have worse prognosis than those without RV dysfunction [27]. Three recently published trials have examined the role of systemic thrombolysis in intermediate risk patients [28–30]. In the Moderate Pulmonary Embolism Treated Thrombolysis (MOPETT) trial, 121 patients were randomly assigned to receive heparin (unfractionated or LMWH) alone or the combination of tissue type plasminogen activator (tPA) plus heparin [28]. Compared to the heparin group, treatment with tPA resulted in lower rates of pulmonary hypertension and significantly lower pulmonary artery systolic pressures at 28 months. The rates of bleeding, recurrent PE, and mortality was similar in both groups [28]. In another trial comparing the combination of LMWH plus an intravenous bolus of tenecteplase versus LMWH alone in intermediate risk PE patients, those treated with tenecteplase had fewer adverse outcomes and better functional capacity at 90 days [29]. In a large multicenter randomized trial (PEITHO), 1005 intermediate risk patients with PE were randomized to tenecteplase and heparin or to heparin therapy alone [30]. Thrombolysis therapy led to reduction in the primary composite outcome of death or cardiovascular collapse at seven days after randomization although it increased major bleeding (including intracranial bleeding) with no overall gained benefit from thrombolysis [30]. A meta-analysis of 16 trials comprising 2115 intermediate risk patients reported that 59 patients would need to be treated with thrombolysis to prevent one death, while a major bleeding occurs with every 18 patients treated [13]. Further studies are needed to identify subgroups of intermediate risk patients who will benefit from systemic thrombolytic therapy.

CDT may be used in patients with acute PE at increased risk of bleeding as a lower dose of a thrombolytic agent is infused directly into the pulmonary artery via a catheter [31]. CDT is also effective in lowering pulmonary arterial pressure and improving RV function [32]. In a randomized controlled trial of 59 patients with acute intermediate risk PE, ultrasound-assisted catheter-directed thrombolysis followed by heparin was compared to treatment with heparin alone [33]. At 24 h, CDT improved the hemodynamics compared to anticoagulation. At 90 days of follow-up, there was no difference in mortality or major bleeding between the two groups [33]. Most of the evidence is limited by small sample size and of low quality compared to the available evidence for systemic thrombolysis. Systemic thrombolysis is therefore currently recommended over CDT in patients with acute PE who are candidates for thrombolysis [21].

Outpatient treatment of venous thromboembolism

Home therapy is commonly employed for patients with an acute DVT in clinical practice with a few exceptions. Several randomized controlled trials and meta-analyses, which have compared home therapy with LMWH versus inpatient therapy with intravenous unfractionated heparin, suggest that outpatient therapy is safe and feasible in most patients with acute DVT [34–36]. Outpatient therapy should not be selected for those with massive symptomatic DVT, high risk of bleeding, or hemodynamic instability due to concurrent symptomatic PE [37].

The outpatient treatment of acute PE is suggested with grade 2B evidence in the most recent ACCP guidelines in low-risk patients with adequate home circumstances [21]. The decision for outpatient management should take into account the patient's clinical condition, bleeding risk, their preference, and the available home support. Risk

stratification scores such as PESI or simplified PESI may be utilized to identify low-risk patients without RV dysfunction who are potential candidates for short in-hospital stay or entirely outpatient management [11, 12, 38]. With the recent changed recommendations in favor of DOACs for acute and long-term VTE treatment, future research should focus on the safety and efficacy of DOACs in outpatient management of acute VTE.

Vitamin K antagonists versus direct oral anticoagulants

Four DOACs including dabigatran, rivaroxaban, apixaban, and edoxaban were compared with conventional therapy in the RE-COVER I and II, EINSTEIN-DVT and PE, AMPLIFY, and Hokusai-VTE trials, respectively [15–20]. The study design was double-blinded in all trials except for the ENSTEIN trials, which used a prospective, randomized, open-label, blinded end point evaluation design. The study designs and treat protocols are compared in Table 1. The study populations were similar in these trials. In the dabigatran and edoxaban trials, parental anticoagulation was added to both DOAC and conventional therapy arms, and after at least 5 days patients were switched to the DOAC. Therefore, in clinical practice, patients should be initiated on parenteral anticoagulation and either switched to dabigatran or edoxaban after 5 days or it should be overlapped with a vitamin K antagonist. In contrast, in the rivaroxaban and apixaban trials DOACs were started without the need for initial parental anticoagulation. The primary efficacy outcome was recurrent VTE or VTE-related mortality in all 6 trials. The primary safety outcome was either major bleeding or a composite of major and clinically relevant non-major bleeding (CRNMB). The efficacy and safety outcomes of these trials are listed in Table 2. All of the trials excluded patients with severe renal dysfunction, those with active bleeding or at high risk of bleeding, and patients already on therapeutic anticoagulation. A recent pooled analysis of these 6 trials reported that DOACs have similar efficacy as VKA in treatment of acute VTE and significantly lower risk of major bleeding than VKA [39]. Recurrent VTE occurred in 2 % of those given DOAC versus 2.2 % in patients that received VKA (relative risk [RR] 0.90; 95 % confidence interval [CI], 0.77 – 1.06) [39]. A 39 % reduction in risk of major bleeding was reported in DOAC recipients compared to those who received VKA therapy (RR 0.61; 95 % CI, 0.45 – 0.83). Compared with recipients of VKA therapy, intracranial bleeding, fatal bleeding, and CRNMB were significantly reduced in the DOAC group [39]. Given the better safety profile of DOACs with less major bleeding, similar efficacy in prevention of recurrent VTE, and the convenience of administration of DOACs, the recent ACCP guidelines suggested DOACs over VKA for the acute and long-term treatment of VTE in patients without cancer [21].

Table 1 Comparison of study design and treatment protocols of trials on DOACs Versus VKA for treatment of acute VTE

Trial name	RE-COVER	RE-COVER II	EINSTEIN-DVT	EINSTEIN-PE	AMPLIFY	Hokusai-VTE
Year of Publication [Ref]	2009 [15]	2014 [16]	2010 [17]	2012 [18]	2013 [19]	2013 [20]
Design	Double-blinded	Double-blinded	PROBE	PROBE	Double-blinded	Double-blinded
Number of Patients	2539	2589	3449	4832	5395	8292
Indication for Anticoagulation	Acute VTE	Acute VTE	Acute DVT	Acute PE	Acute VTE	Acute VTE
DOAC Treatment Protocol	Dabigatran 150 mg twice daily	Dabigatran 150 mg twice daily	Rivaroxaban 15 mg twice daily for 3 weeks; then 20 mg once daily	Rivaroxaban 15 mg twice daily for 3 weeks; then 20 mg once daily	Apixaban 10 mg twice daily for days; then 5 mg twice daily	Edoxaban 60 once daily; patients with CrCl 30–50 mL/min, body weight ≤60 kg, or receiving strong P-glycoprotein inhibitors: edoxaban 30 mg once daily
Non-inferiority Margin for Hazard Ratio	2.75	2.75	2.0	2.0	1.8	1.5
Need for initial Parenteral Anticoagulation	Yes	Yes	No	No	No	Yes
Duration of Therapy (months)	6	6	3, 6, or 12	3, 6, or 12	6	≤12
TTR (%)	60	57	58	63	61	64

DOAC direct oral anticoagulant, *DVT* deep vein thrombosis, *PE* pulmonary embolism, *PROBE* prospective, randomized, open-label, blinded end point, *TTR* time in therapeutic range for warfarin, *VKA* vitamin K antagonists, *VTE* venous thromboembolism, *CrCl* creatinine clearance

Table 2 Efficacy and safety outcomes for treatment of acute VTE: DOACs versus VKA

Trial Name [Ref]	RE-COVER [15]	RE-COVER II [16]	EINSTEIN-DVT [17]	EINSTEIN-PE [18]	AMPLIFY [19]	Hokusai-VTE [20]
Primary Efficacy Outcome DOAC vs VKA (%)	Recurrent symptomatic VTE or related death: 2.4 vs 2.1[a]	Recurrent symptomatic VTE or related mortality: 2.3 vs 2.2[a]	Recurrent symptomatic VTE: 2.1 vs 3.0[a]	Recurrent symptomatic VTE: 2.1 vs 1.8[a]	Recurrent symptomatic VTE or related mortality: 2.3 vs 2.7[a]	Recurrent symptomatic VTE or related mortality: 3.2 vs 3.5[a]
Primary Safety Outcome(s)	Major bleeding; Major or CRNM bleeding: Any bleeding	Major bleeding Major or CRNM bleeding: Any bleeding	Major or CRNM bleeding	Major or CRNM bleeding	Major bleeding	Major or CRNM bleeding
Major Bleeding DOAC vs VKA (%)	1.6 vs 1.9	1.2 vs 1.7	0.8 vs 1.2	1.1[a] vs 2.2	0.6[a] vs 1.8	1.4 vs 1.6
Major or CRNM Bleeding DOAC vs VKA (%)	5.6 vs 8.8	5.0 vs 7.9	8.1 vs 8.1	10.3 vs 11.4	4.3[a] vs 9.7	8.5[a] vs 10.3

DOAC direct oral anticoagulant, *CRNM* clinically relevant non-major, *DOAC* direct oral anticoagulants, *VKA* vitamin K antagonists, *VTE* venous thromboembolism
[a]Statistically significant difference between the two groups

Management of VTE in patients with cancer

The major society guidelines including the ACCP, American Society of Clinical Oncology, and the National Comprehensive Cancer Network recommend use of LMWH for treatment of VTE in cancer patients [21, 40, 41]. Treatment with LMWH is continued for the duration of active cancer given that the risk of recurrent VTE can reach an annual risk of 20 % [42]. Five randomized trials have compared therapy with LMWH versus warfarin in cancer patients [43–47]. The details of these trials are outlined in Table 3. Two trials showed a reduction in the rates of recurrent VTE using LMWH with no effect on mortality or bleeding [44, 45], two showed no difference in any outcome [43, 46], and the recently published CATCH trial demonstrated a non-significant

reduction in the rate of recurrent VTE and lower risk of CRNMB in those who received LMWH [47].

There are no published randomized trials that a priori have compared DOACs with VKA or LMWH for treatment of VTE in cancer patients. A meta-analysis of the subsets with DVT and cancer totaling 1132 patients in the six trials that compared DOACs versus VKA [15–20] has been published [48]. They found similar rates of VTE recurrence (3.9 versus 6 %; odds ratio [OR] 0.63; 95 % CI, 0.37 – 1.10) and major bleeding (3.2 versus 4.2%; OR 0.77; 95 % CI, 0.41-1.44). Although these trials included cancer patients [15–20], they were typically not receiving active chemotherapy or radiation. The cancer patients included in these trials had usually completed treatment or had a previous history of cancer and are not a true representative

Table 3 Comparison of trials on LMWH versus VKA for treatment of VTE in cancer patients

Trial Name	CANTHANOX	CLOT	MAIN-LITE	ONCENOX	CATCH
Year of Publication [Ref]	2002 [43]	2003 [44]	2006 [45]	2006 [46]	2015 [47]
Design	Open-label	Open-label	Open-label	Open-label	Open-label
Number of Patients	146	676	200	122	900
Treatment Protocol	Enoxaparin 1.5 mg/kg daily	Dalteparin 200 IU/kg once daily for the first month then 150 IU/kg for 5 months	Tinzaparin 175 IU/kg once daily	Enoxaparin 1 mg/kg every 12 h for 5 days then enoxaparin 1 mg/kg or 1.5 mg/kg daily	Tinzaparin 175 IU/kg once daily
Duration of Therapy (months)	3	6	3	6	6
Primary Efficacy Outcome LMWH vs VKA (%)	Combination of major bleeding or recurrent VTE: 10.5 vs 21.1	Recurrent symptomatic VTE: 9[a] vs 17	Recurrent symptomatic VTE: 7 vs 10	Recurrent symptomatic VTE: enoxaparin 1 mg vs. 1.5 mg vs VKA 6.8 vs 6.3 vs 10.0	Composite of recurrent symptomatic VTE, fatal PE, or incidental VTE: 7.2 vs 10.5
Safety Bleeding Outcomes LMWH vs VKA (%)	Major bleeding: 7 vs 16; Fatal bleeding: 0 vs 8[a]	Major bleeding: 6 vs 4; Any bleeding 14 vs 19	Major bleeding: 7 vs 7; Any bleeding: 27 vs 24	Major bleeding: enoxaparin 1 mg vs. 1.5 mg vs VKA : 6.5 vs 11.1 vs 2.9	Major bleeding: 2.7 vs 2.4 CRNM bleeding: 10.9[a] vs 15.3

CRNM clinically relevant non-major, *DOAC* direct oral anticoagulants, *LMWH* low-molecular weight heparin, *PE* pulmonary embolism, *VKA* vitamin K antagonists, *VTE* venous thromboembolism
[a]Statistically significant difference between the two groups

of all cancer patients. The Hokusai VTE-cancer randomized open label trial is currently underway and will examine whether edoxaban is non-inferior to LMWH for treatment of VTE in cancer patients [49].

Extended treatment of venous thromboembolism

Extended anticoagulation can be employed in patients with unprovoked VTE to reduce the risk of recurrent VTE if the benefit/risk ratio favors continuation of anticoagulation while taking into account patient's risk of bleeding. All DOACs except for edoxaban have been compared with placebo in randomized trials for extended secondary VTE prevention beyond the initial three months of anticoagulation [17, 50, 51]. The details of these trials are compared in Table 4. All trials showed marked superiority of the DOACs over placebo for the prevention of recurrent VTE without significant increase in major bleeding [17,50, 51]. However, compared to the placebo arms, all DOACs had higher rate of CRNMB [17, 50, 51]. Duration of extended anticoagulation was 6 to 12 months in the EINSTEIN [17] and AMPLIFY-Extension [50] studies and 6 months in the RE-SONATE trial [51]. Two doses of apixaban were evaluated in the AMPLIFY-Extension trial and the rate of bleeding was lower for apixaban 2.5 mg twice daily than 5 mg twice daily [50]. A single regimen of rivaroxban (20 mg once daily) and dabigatran (150 mg twice daily) was used in the EINSTEIN and RE-SONATE studies.

Dabigatran is the only DOAC that has been compared with warfarin for extended VTE prevention in the RE-MEDY trial [51]. Dabigatran was non-inferior to warfarin in prevention of recurrent VTE (1.8 versus 1.3 %, hazard ratio [HR] 1.44; 95 % CI, 0.78–2.64) and had a significantly lower rate of major bleeding or CRNMB (HR 0.54; 95 % CI, 0.41–0.71). These results demonstrated that DOACs are effective in secondary VTE prevention with no significant increase in major bleeding. The ACCP guidelines recommend no change in the choice of anticoagulant agent in patients who need extended anticoagulation after the first 3 months of therapy [21]. Given the observed lower bleeding risk, the dose of apixaban may be reduced to 2.5 mg twice daily after the initial treatment.

Aspirin has been also evaluated in secondary VTE prevention in patients with first unprovoked VTE who have completed anticoagulant treatment. In this setting, randomized trials and a meta-analysis reported a 30 % reduction in rates of recurrent VTE compared to placebo or observation [52–55]. The ACCP guidelines suggest that aspirin is an available option in patients with unprovoked VTE that are stopping anticoagulant therapy if there are no contraindications to use of aspirin [21]. However, aspirin is not recommended as an alternative to anticoagulant therapy [21].

Treatment of VTE in special situations
Management of sub-segmental pulmonary embolism

The increase in utilization of a highly sensitive computed tomography pulmonary angiography (CTPA) has led to detection of incidental asymptomatic PE or small sub-segmental PE [56]. Whether or not patients with sub-segmental pulmonary embolism (SSPE) should be anticoagulated is controversial. It is unclear whether the SSPE detected by CTPA are artifacts and therefore false positive [57]. Furthermore, an isolated SSPE likely does not have the same risk of progression or VTE recurrence as a single segmental or lobar PE [57]. There are currently no published randomized trials for treatment of patients with SSPE. Retrospective studies have reported VTE recurrence in only a small number of patients with SSPE and without DVT, who were not anticoagulated.

Table 4 Comparison of extended duration DOAC trials

Trial Name	EINSTEIN-EXTENSION	AMPLIFY-EXT	RE-MEDY	RE-SONATE
Year of Publication [Ref]	2010 [17]	2013 [50]	2013 [51]	2013 [51]
Design	Double-blinded	Double-blinded	Double-blinded	Double-blinded
Comparison Arm	Placebo	Placebo	Warfarin	Placebo
Number of Patients	1197	2486	2866	1353
Treatment Protocol	Rivaroxaban 20 mg once daily	Apixaban 5 mg or 2.5 twice daily	Dabigatran 150 mg twice daily	Dabigatran 150 mg twice daily
Duration of Therapy (months)	6 to12	12	6 to 36	6
Primary Efficacy Outcome DOAC vs VKA or Placebo (%)	Recurrent symptomatic VTE: 1.3[a] vs 7.1	Recurrent symptomatic VTE or all-cause mortality: 3.8[a] vs 4.2[a] vs 11.6	Recurrent symptomatic VTE or related mortality: 1.8[a] vs 1.3	Recurrent symptomatic VTE or related mortality: 0.4[a] vs 5.6
Major Bleeding DOAC vs VKA or Placebo (%)	0.7 vs 0	0.2 vs 0.1 vs 0.5	0.9 vs 1.8	0.3 vs 0
Major and CRNM Bleeding DOAC vs VKA or Placebo (%)	6.0[a] vs 1.2	3.2 vs 4.3 vs 2.7	5.6[a] vs 10.2	5.3[a] vs 1.8

DOAC direct oral anticoagulant, *CRNM* clinically relevant non-major, *DOAC* direct oral anticoagulants, *VKA* vitamin K antagonists, *VTE* venous thromboembolism
[a]Statistically significant difference between the two groups

Table 5 Summary of retrospective studies on 3-month follow-up of patients with sub-segmental pulmonary embolism

Study	Musset et al.	Eyer et al.	Donato et al.	Pena et al.	Mehta et al.	Goy et al.	Ghazvinian et al.
Year of Publication [Ref]	2002 [59]	2005 [60]	2010 [61]	2012 [62]	2014 [63]	2015 [64]	2016 [65]
Method of Detection	SDCT	MDCT	MDCT	MDCT	MDCT	MDCT	V/P SPECT
Number of Patient with Positive CTPA	360	499	1463	724	NA[b]	550	NA[b]
Number of Patients with SSPE n/N (%)	12 (3.3)	67 (13.4)	93 (6.4)	70 (9.6)	32 (100)	82 (15)	54 (100)
Number of Untreated SSPE (%)	9 (75)	25 (37.3)	22 (22.9)	18 (25.7)	12 (37.5)	39 (47.6)	54 (100)
VTE (%)	0	0	0	0	0	0	4[a]

CTPA computed tomography pulmonary angiography, *NA* not applicable, *MDCT* multi-detector computed tomography pulmonary angiography, *SDCT* single-detector computed tomography pulmonary angiography, *SSPE* sub-segmental pulmonary embolism, *V/P SPECT* ventilation/perfusion singe photon emission computed tomography, *VTE* venous thromboembolism
[a]Two patients were diagnosed with a DVT
[b]Only examined patients with SSPE

[57, 58]. Details of these retrospective studies are summarized in Table 5 [59–65]. However, another retrospective study showed that patients with SSPE have similar rate of VTE recurrence as patients with larger PE during 3 months of anticoagulation [66]. The ACCP guidelines suggest performing bilateral ultrasounds to exclude proximal DVT before a decision is made not to treat a patient with SSPE [21]. If a DVT is detected then the patient should receive anticoagulation. However, if no proximal DVT is detected the guidelines suggest that the clinician assesses risk factors for VTE recurrence or progression and considers anticoagulation for those with high risk of VTE recurrence (e.g., recent surgery, immobilization, active cancer, previous history of VTE) [21]. Future prospective studies are needed to determine the optimal management strategy for patients with SSPE and no detected proximal DVT.

Role of inferior vena cava filter in management of acute venous thromboembolism

Inferior vena cava (IVC) filters are typically used in patients with an acute VTE and an absolute contraindication to anticoagulation (e.g., concurrent active bleeding) [67]. The IVC filter is removed once the bleeding risk is low and anticoagulation is given [14]. In patients with acute VTE already on anticoagulation with no absolute contraindications, studies suggest that there is lack of benefit to use of IVC filters in addition to anticoagulation [68–72]. In the PREPIC 1 trial, 400 patients with proximal DVT were randomized to either anticoagulation alone or anticoagulation plus IVC filter placement [68]. The initial 2-year PREPIC 1 study and a subsequently published 8-year follow-up reported that IVC filter insertion was associated with a reduction in the initial rate of PE, increase in the rate of DVT, and no difference in mortality [68, 69]. The PREPIC 2 trial examined the adjuvant role of IVC filters in patients with PE who received either anticoagulation alone or anticoagulation plus an IVC filter [70]. The filter was

removed at 3 months. There was no difference in the rates of recurrent VTE or mortality between the two groups [70]. In addition to lack of benefit, IVC filters are associated with complications including IVC filter thrombosis, DVT, and guide wire entrapment [71, 72]. The ACCP guidelines recommend against the use of IVC filters in patients on anticoagulation for acute VTE [21].

Conclusions

VTE is a major cause of morbidity and mortality. DOACs are suggested over VKA for acute and long-term treatment of VTE in patients without cancer, as they have been shown to be as effective as VKA in reducing VTE recurrence and associated with significantly less major bleeding. Future studies are needed to assess their safety and efficacy in outpatient treatment of acute VTE. LMWH is the current standard of care for treatment of VTE in cancer patients. Randomized trials are ongoing to examine the noninferiority of DOACs versus LMWH in cancer patients. Lastly, it is currently unclear whether or not to treat patients with SSPE and no proximal DVT; future prospective studies are needed to examine different management strategies in this patient group.

Acknowledgements
None.

Authors' contributions
SP and SS are responsible for writing and editing of the manuscript. Both authors read and approved the final manuscript.

Competing interests
Siavash Piran–nothing to disclose; Sam Schulman reports receiving consulting fees from Boehringer Ingelheim, Bristol-Myer-Squibb, Bayer and Daichii and grant support from Boehringer Ingelheim, Baxter and Octapharma.

References

1. White RH. The epidemiology of venous thromboembolism. Circulation. 2003;107(23 Suppl 1):14–8.
2. Martinez C, Cohen AT, Bamber L, Rietbrock S. Epidemiology of first and recurrent venous thromboembolism: a population-based cohort study in patients without active cancer. Thromb Haemost. 2014;112:255–63.
3. ISTH Steering Committee for World Thrombosis Day. Thrombosis: a major contributor to global disease burden. Thromb Res. 2014;134:931–8.
4. Søgaard KK, Schmidt M, Pedersen L, Horváth-Puhó E, Sørensen HT. 30-year mortality after venous thromboembolism: a population-based cohort study. Circulation. 2014;130:829–36.
5. Prandoni P, Lensing AW, Cogo A, Cuppini S, Villalta S, Carta M, et al. The long-term clinical course of acute deep venous thrombosis. Ann Intern Med. 1996;125:1–7.
6. Pengo V, Lensing AW, Prins MH, Marchiori A, Davidson BL, Tiozzo F, et al. Incidence of chronic thromboembolic pulmonary hypertension after pulmonary embolism. N Engl J Med. 2004;350:2257–64.
7. LaMori JC, Shohieber O, Mody SH, Bookhart BK. Inpatient resource use and cost burden of deep vein thrombosis and pulmonary embolism in the United States. Clin Ther. 2015;37:62–70.
8. Spyropoulos AC, Lin J. Direct medical costs of venous thromboembolism and subsequent hospital readmission rates: an administrative claims analysis from 30 managed care organizations. J Manag Care Pharm. 2007;13:475–86.
9. Donzé J, Le Gal G, Fine MJ, Roy PM, Sanchez O, Verschuren F, et al. Prospective validation of the Pulmonary Embolism Severity Index. A clinical prognostic model for pulmonary embolism. Thromb Haemost. 2008;100:943–8.
10. Jiménez D, Aujesky D, Moores L, Gómez V, Lobo JL, Uresandi F, et al. Simplification of the pulmonary embolism severity index for prognostication in patients with acute symptomatic pulmonary embolism. Arch Intern Med. 2010;170:1383–9.
11. Zondag W, Kooiman J, Klok FA, Dekkers OM, Huisman MV. Outpatient versus inpatient treatment in patients with pulmonary embolism: a meta-analysis. Eur Respir J. 2013;42:134–44.
12. Piran S, Le Gal G, Wells PS, Gandara E, Righini M, Rodger MA, et al. Outpatient treatment of symptomatic pulmonary embolism: a systematic review and meta-analysis. Thromb Res. 2013;132:515–9.
13. Chatterjee S, Chakraborty A, Weinberg I, Kadakia M, Wilensky RL, Sardar P, et al. Thrombolysis for pulmonary embolism and risk of all-cause mortality, major bleeding, and intracranial hemorrhage: a meta-analysis. JAMA. 2014;311:2414–21.
14. Kearon C, Akl EA, Comerota AJ, Prandoni P, Bounameaux H, Goldhaber SZ, et al. Antithrombotic therapy for VTE disease: Antithrombotic therapy and prevention of thrombosis, 9th ed: American College of Chest Physicians evidence-based clinical practice guidelines. Chest. 2012;141(2 Suppl):e419S–94.
15. Schulman S, Kearon C, Kakkar AK, Mismetti P, Schellong S, Eriksson H, et al. Dabigatran versus warfarin in the treatment of acute venous thromboembolism. N Engl J Med. 2009;361:2342–52.
16. Schulman S, Kakkar AK, Goldhaber SZ, Schellong S, Eriksson H, Mismetti P, et al. Treatment of acute venous thromboembolism with dabigatran or warfarin and pooled analysis. Circulation. 2014;129:764–72.
17. EINSTEIN Investigators, Bauersachs R, Berkowitz SD, Brenner B, Buller HR, Decousus H, et al. Oral rivaroxaban for symptomatic venous thromboembolism. N Engl J Med. 2010;363:2499–510.
18. EINSTEIN-PE Investigators, Büller HR, Prins MH, Lensin AW, Decousus H, Jacobson BF, et al. Oral rivaroxaban for the treatment of symptomatic pulmonary embolism. N Engl J Med. 2012;366:1287–97.
19. Agnelli G, Buller HR, Cohen A, Curto M, Gallus AS, Johnson M, et al. Oral apixaban for the treatment of acute venous thromboembolism. N Engl J Med. 2013;369:799–808.
20. Hokusai-VTE Investigators, Büller HR, Décousus H, Grosso MA, Mercuri M, Middeldorp S, et al. Edoxaban versus warfarin for the treatment of symptomatic venous thromboembolism. N Engl J Med. 2013;369:1406–15.
21. Kearon C, Akl EA, Ornelas J, Blaivas A, Jimenez D, Bounameaux H, et al. Antithrombotic therapy for VTE disease: CHEST guideline and expert panel Report. Chest. 2016;149:315–52.
22. Enden T, Haig Y, Kløw NE, Slagsvold CE, Sandvik L, Ghanima W, et al. Long-term outcome after additional catheter-directed thrombolysis versus

23. standard treatment for acute iliofemoral deep vein thrombosis (the CaVenT study): a randomised controlled trial. Lancet. 2012;379:31–8.
23. Watson L, Broderick C, Armon MP. Thrombolysis for acute deep vein thrombosis. Cochrane Database Syst Rev. 2014;1, CD002783.
24. Bashir R, Zack CJ, Zhao H, Comerota AJ, Bove AA. Comparative outcomes of catheter-directed thrombolysis plus anticoagulation vs anticoagulation alone to treat lower-extremity proximal deep vein thrombosis. JAMA Intern Med. 2014;174:1494.
25. Laiho MK, Oinonen A, Sugano N, Harjola VP, Lehtola AL, Roth WD, et al. Preservation of venous valve function after catheter-directed and systemic thrombolysis for deep venous thrombosis. Eur J Vasc Endovasc Surg. 2004;28:391.
26. Vedantham S, Goldhaber SZ, Kahn SR, Julian J, Magnuson E, Jaff MR, et al. Rationale and design of the ATTRACT Study: a multicenter randomized trial to evaluate pharmacomechanical catheter-directed thrombolysis for the prevention of postthrombotic syndrome in patients with proximal deep vein thrombosis. Am Heart J. 2013;165:523–30.e3.
27. Grifoni S, Olivotto I, Cecchini P, Pieralli F, Camaiti A, Santoro G, et al. Short-term clinical outcome of patients with acute pulmonary embolism, normal blood pressure, and echocardiographic right ventricular dysfunction. Circulation. 2000;101:2817–22.
28. Sharifi M, Bay C, Skrocki L, Rahimi F, Mehdipour M. Moderate pulmonary embolism treated With thrombolysis (from the "MOPETT" Trial). Am J Cardiol. 2013;111:273–7.
29. Kline JA, Nordenholz KE, Courtney DM, Kabrhel C, Jones AE, Rondina MT, et al. Treatment of submassive pulmonary embolism with tenecteplase or placebo: cardiopulmonary outcomes at 3 months: multicenter double-blind, placebo-controlled randomized trial. J Thromb Haemost. 2014;12:459–68.
30. Meyer G, Vicaut E, Danays T, Agnelli G, Becattini C, Beyer-Westendorf J, et al. Fibrinolysis for patients with intermediate-risk pulmonary embolism. N Engl J Med. 2014;370:1402–11.
31. McCabe JM, Huang PH, Riedl L, Eisenhauer AC, Sobieszczyk P. Usefulness and safety of ultrasound-assisted catheter-directed thrombolysis for submassive pulmonary emboli. Am J Cardiol. 2015;115:821–4.
32. Kuo WT, Banerjee A, Kim PS, DeMarco Jr FJ, Levy JR, Facchini FR, et al. Pulmonary embolism response to fragmentation, embolectomy, and catheter thrombolysis (PERFECT): initial results from a prospective multicenter registry. Chest. 2015;148:667–73.
33. Kucher N, Boekstegers P, Müller OJ, Kupatt C, Beyer-Westendorf J, Heitzer T, et al. Randomized, controlled trial of ultrasound-assisted catheter-directed thrombolysis for acute intermediate-risk pulmonary embolism. Circulation. 2014;129:479–86.
34. Koopman MM, Prandoni P, Piovella F, Ockelford PA, Brandjes DP, van der Meer J, et al. Treatment of venous thrombosis with intravenous unfractionated heparin administered in the hospital as compared with subcutaneous low-molecular-weight heparin administered at home. The Tasman Study Group. N Engl J Med. 1996;334:682–7.
35. Levine M, Gent M, Hirsh J, Leclerc J, Anderson D, Weitz J, et al. Comparison of low-molecular-weight heparin administered primarily at home with unfractionated heparin administered in the hospital for proximal deep-vein thrombosis. N Engl J Med. 1996;334:677–81.
36. Segal JB, Bolger DT, Jenckes MW, Krishnan JA, Streiff MB, Eng J, et al. Outpatient therapy with low molecular weight heparin for the treatment of venous thromboembolism: a review of efficacy, safety, and costs. Am J Med. 2003;115:298–308.
37. Douketis JD. Treatment of deep vein thrombosis: what factors determine appropriate treatment? Can Fam Physician. 2005;51:217–23.
38. Aujesky D, Roy PM, Verschuren F, Righini M, Osterwalder J, Egloff M, et al. Outpatient versus inpatient treatment for patients with acute pulmonary embolism: an international, open-label, randomised, non-inferiority trial. Lancet. 2011;378:41–8.
39. van Es N, Coppens M, Schulman S, Middeldorp S, Büller HR. Direct oral anticoagulants compared with vitamin K antagonists for acute venous thromboembolism: evidence from phase 3 trials. Blood. 2014;124:1968–75.
40. Lyman GH, Khorana AA, Kuderer NM, Lee AY, Arcelus JI, Balaban EP, et al. Venous thromboembolism prophylaxis and treatment in patients with

cancer: American Society of Clinical Oncology clinical practice guideline update. J Clin Oncol. 2013;31:2189–204.

41. Engman CA, Zacharski LR. Low molecular weight heparins as extended prophylaxis against recurrent thrombosis in cancer patients. J Natl Compr Canc Netw. 2008;6:637–45.

42. Prandoni P, Lensing AW, Piccioli A, Bernardi E, Simioni P, Girolami B, et al. Recurrent venous thromboembolism and bleeding complications during anticoagulant treatment in patients with cancer and venous thrombosis. Blood. 2002;100:3484–8.

43. Meyer G, Marjanovic Z, Valcke J, Lorcerie B, Gruel Y, Solal-Celigny P, et al. Comparison of low-molecular-weight heparin and warfarin for the secondary prevention of venous thromboembolism in patients with cancer: a randomized controlled study. Arch Intern Med. 2002;162:1729–35.

44. Lee AY, Levine MN, Baker RI, Bowden C, Kakkar AK, Prins M, et al. Low-molecular-weight heparin versus a coumarin for the prevention of recurrent venous thromboembolism in patients with cancer. N Engl J Med. 2003;349:146–53.

45. Hull RD, Pineo GF, Brant RF, Mah AF, Burke N, Dear R, et al. Long-term low-molecular-weight heparin versus usual care in proximal-vein thrombosis patients with cancer. Am J Med. 2006;119:1062–72.

46. Deitcher SR, Kessler CM, Merli G, Rigas JR, Lyons RM, Fareed J, et al. Secondary prevention of venous thromboembolic events in patients with active cancer: enoxaparin alone versus initial enoxaparin followed by warfarin for a 180-day period. Clin Appl Thromb Hemost. 2006;12:389–96.

47. Lee AY, Kamphuisen PW, Meyer G, Bauersachs R, Janas MS, Jarner MF, et al. Tinzaparin vs warfarin for treatment of acute venous thromboembolism in patients with active cancer: A randomized clinical trial. JAMA. 2015;314:677–86.

48. Vedovati MC, Germini F, Agnelli G, Becattini C. Direct oral anticoagulants in patients with VTE and cancer: a systematic review and meta-analysis. Chest. 2015;147:475–83.

49. van Es N, Di Nisio M, Bleker SM, Segers A, Mercuri MF, Schwocho L, et al. Edoxaban for treatment of venous thromboembolism in patients with cancer. Rationale and design of the Hokusai VTE-cancer study. Thromb Haemost. 2015;114:1268–76.

50. Agnelli G, Buller HR, Cohen A, Curto M, Gallus AS, Johnson M, et al. Apixaban for extended treatment of venous thromboembolism. N Engl J Med. 2013;368:699–708.

51. Schulman S, Kearon C, Kakkar AK, Schellong S, Eriksson H, Baanstra D, et al. Extended use of dabigatran, warfarin, or placebo in venous thromboembolism. N Engl J Med. 2013;368:709–18.

52. Becattini C, Agnelli G, Schenone A, Eichinger S, Bucherini E, Silingardi M, et al. Aspirin for preventing the recurrence of venous thromboembolism. N Engl J Med. 2012;366:1959–67.

53. Brighton TA, Eikelboom JW, Mann K, Mister R, Gallus A, Ockelford P, et al. Low-dose aspirin for preventing recurrent venous thromboembolism. N Engl J Med. 2012;367:1979–87.

54. Simes J, Becattini C, Agnelli G, Eikelboom JW, Kirby AC, Mister R, et al. Aspirin for the prevention of recurrent venous thromboembolism: the INSPIRE collaboration. Circulation. 2014;130:1062–71.

55. Castellucci LA, Cameron C, Le Gal G, Rodger MA, Coyle D, Wells PS, et al. Efficacy and safety outcomes of oral anticoagulants and antiplatelet drugs in the secondary prevention of venous thromboembolism: systematic review and network meta-analysis. BMJ. 2013;347:f5133.

56. Wiener RS, Schwartz LM, Woloshin S. When a test is too good: how CT pulmonary angiograms find pulmonary emboli that do not need to be found. BMJ. 2013;347:f3368.

57. Carrier M, Righini M, Le Gal G. Symptomatic subsegmental pulmonary embolism: what is the next step? J Thromb Haemost. 2012;10:1486–90.

58. Stein PD, Goodman LR, Hull RD, Dalen JE, Matta F. Diagnosis and management of isolated subsegmental pulmonary embolism: review and assessment of the options. Clin Appl Thromb Hemost. 2012;18:20–6.

59. Musset D, Parent F, Meyer G, Maître S, Girard P, Leroyer C, et al. Diagnostic strategy for patients with suspected pulmonary embolism: a prospective multicentre outcome study. Lancet. 2002;360:1914–20.

60. Eyer BA, Goodman LR, Washington L. Clinicians' response to radiologists' reports of isolated subsegmental pulmonary embolism or inconclusive interpretation of pulmonary embolism using MDCT. AJR Am J Roentgenol. 2005;184:623–8.

61. Donato AA, Khoche S, Santora J, Wagner B. Clinical outcomes in patients with isolated subsegmental pulmonary emboli diagnosed by multidetector CT pulmonary angiography. Thromb Res. 2010;126:e266–70.

62. Pena E, Kimpton M, Dennie C, Peterson R, LE Gal G, Carrier M. Difference in interpretation of computed tomography pulmonary angiography diagnosis of subsegmental thrombosis in patients with suspected pulmonary embolism. J Thromb Haemost. 2012;10:496–8.

63. Mehta D, Barnett M, Zhou L, Woulfe T, Rolfe-Vyson V, Rowland V, et al. Management and outcomes of single subsegmental pulmonary embolus: a retrospective audit at North Shore Hospital. New Zealand Intern Med J. 2014;44:872–6.

64. Goy J, Lee J, Levine O, Chaudhry S, Crowther M. Sub-segmental pulmonary embolism in three academic teaching hospitals: a review of management and outcomes. J Thromb Haemost. 2015;13:214–8.

65. Ghazvinian R, Gottsäter A, Elf J. Is it safe to withhold long-term anticoagulation therapy in patients with small pulmonary emboli diagnosed by SPECT scintigraphy? Thromb J. 2016;14:12.

66. den Exter PL, van Es J, Klok FA, Kroft LJ, Kruip MJ, Kamphuisen PW, et al. Risk profile and clinical outcome of symptomatic subsegmental acute pulmonary embolism. Blood. 2013;122:1144–9.

67. White RH, Brunson A, Romano PS, Li Z, Wun T. Outcomes after vena cava filter use in non-cancer patients with acute venous thromboembolism: A population-based study. Circulation. 2016;133:2018–29.

68. Decousus H, Leizorovicz A, Parent F, Page Y, Tardy B, Girard P, et al. A clinical trial of vena caval filters in the prevention of pulmonary embolism in patients with proximal deep-vein thrombosis. Prévention du Risque d'Embolie Pulmonaire par Interruption Cave Study Group. N Engl J Med. 1998;338:409–15.

69. PREPIC Study Group. Eight-year follow-up of patients with permanent vena cava filters in the prevention of pulmonary embolism: the PREPIC (Prevention du Risque d'Embolie Pulmonaire par Interruption Cave) randomized study. Circulation. 2005;112:416–22.

70. Mismetti P, Laporte S, Pellerin O, Ennezat PV, Couturaud F, Elias A, et al. Effect of a retrievable inferior vena cava filter plus anticoagulation vs anticoagulation alone on risk of recurrent pulmonary embolism: a randomized clinical trial. JAMA. 2015;313:1627–35.

71. Streiff MB. Vena caval filters: a comprehensive review. Blood. 2000;95:3669–77.

72. Wu A, Helo N, Moon E, Tam M, Kapoor B, Wang W. Strategies for prevention of iatrogenic inferior vena cava filter entrapment and dislodgement during central venous catheter placement. J Vasc Surg. 2014;59:255–9.

14

Individualized prophylaxis for optimizing hemophilia care: can we apply this to both developed and developing nations?

Man-Chiu Poon[1,2,3,4]* and Adrienne Lee[1,4]

From The 9th Congress of the Asian-Pacific Society on Thrombosis and Hemostasis
Taipei, Taiwan.

Abstract

Prophylaxis is considered optimal care for hemophilia patients to prevent bleeding and to preserve joint function thereby improving quality of life (QoL). The evidence for prophylaxis is irrefutable and is the standard of care in developed nations. Prophylaxis can be further individualized to improve outcomes and cost effectiveness. Individualization is best accomplished taking into account the bleeding phenotype, physical activity/lifestyle, joint status, and pharmacokinetic handling of specific clotting factor concentrates, all of which vary among individuals. Patient acceptance should also be considered. Assessment tools (e.g. joint status imaging and function studies/ scores, QoL) for determining and monitoring risk factors and outcome, as well as population PK profiling have been developed to assist the individualization process. The determinants of optimal prophylaxis include (1) factor dose/ dosing frequency, hence, cost/affordability (2) bleeding triggers (physical activity/lifestyle, chronic arthropathy and synovitis) and (3) bleeding rates. Altering one determinant results in adjustment of the other two. Thus, the trough level to protect from spontaneous bleeding can be increased in patients who have greater bleeding risks; and prophylaxis to achieve zero joint bleeds is achievable through optimal individualization. Prophylaxis in economically constrained nations is limited by the ill-affordability of clotting factor concentrates. However, at least 5 studies on children and adults from Thailand, China and India have shown superiority of low dose (~5–10 IU kg^{-1} 2-3× per week) prophylaxis over episodic treatment in terms of bleed reduction, and quality of life, with improved physical activity, independent functioning, school attendance and community participation. In these nations, the prophylaxis goals should be for improved QoL rather than "zero bleeds" and perfect joints. Prophylaxis can still be individualized to affordability. Higher protective trough level can be achieved by using smaller doses given more frequently without an increase in consumption/cost. The bleeding trigger can also be down-regulated by avoiding unnecessary injury, and by engaging in judicious strengthening exercises appropriate to the joint status to improve balance and joint stabilization. Central to the success of prophylaxis are clinics with comprehensive care that provide the necessary professional expertise, support, and counseling, to educate patients, families, and other healthcare professionals, and to support research for improved hemophilia care.

Keywords: Hemophilia, Individualized prophylaxis, Personalized prophylaxis, Pharmacokinetics, Population pharmacokinetics, Low-dose prophylaxis, Terminal half-life

* Correspondence: mcpoon@ucalgary.ca
[1]Department of Medicine, Cumming School of Medicine, University of Calgary, Calgary, Alberta, Canada
[2]Department of Pediatrics, Cumming School of Medicine, University of Calgary, Calgary, Alberta, Canada
Full list of author information is available at the end of the article

Background

Individualized prophylaxis has become an important topic in how prophylaxis can be optimized based on various patient factors such as bleeding risk, pharmacokinetic (PK) profile, joint status and physical activity/lifestyle. With the understanding of interpatient heterogeneity influencing these factors, individualized prophylaxis should be the ideal strategy to optimize factor utilization while improving patient quality of life (QoL) and joint health. In developed nations where there are fewer constraints in terms of factor affordability, the ultimate goal of "zero bleeds" and possibly perfect joints is achievable with the right peak and trough levels adjusted for individual risk factors and PK handling. Assessment tools (e.g. MRI/ultrasound imaging for joint status, QoL tools, joint scores) for determining and monitoring risk factors and outcome, as well as population PK profiling have been developed to assist us in this individualization process. Although prophylaxis in general is expensive, and the proposed tools to assist with individualization are time consuming and resource intensive, the overall economic savings from improved QoL with almost no bleeding and bleed-related complications, should be more than enough to offset the costs of its implementation in resource adequate nations. The question is whether it is possible for the developing world to practice individualized prophylaxis when there are barely enough resources and affordable factor concentrate to ensure all bleeds are treated adequately or even treated at all. Approximately 75–80 % of the world's hemophilia population lives in developing nations and we are at risk of leaving this large proportion of patients behind and undertreated if we assume the goal for prophylaxis should always be "zero bleeds". Prophylaxis regimens that focus on using resource intensive measurement tools, and PK profiling models may not be attainable to all. However, this does not mean developing nations should not strive to achieve some form of prophylaxis in the interim. Simply the goals of prophylaxis need to be adjusted such that it is individualized for QoL rather than "zero bleeds", for independent function and gainful employment rather than pristine joints, and for trough levels that minimize bleed events rather than PK profiling to ensure a certain pre-defined trough level. For resource-limited countries, prophylaxis must be individualized to include affordability as a major determinant in order to optimize low-dose regimens that have demonstrated superiority compared to episodic treatment. This review aims to communicate the current concepts of individualized prophylaxis and how this might be adapted and applied in both developed and developing nations.

Review

The evolution of prophylaxis

Prophylaxis is considered optimal care for hemophilia patients to prevent bleeding and to preserve joint function [1]. The original idea being that keeping factor levels above 1 % converts severe hemophilia to a moderate severity phenotype where spontaneous joint bleeds and chronic arthropathy is less frequently observed. The Swedish have been practicing prophylaxis in young boys since the 1960's and demonstrated continuous prophylaxis started at an early age to prevent factor levels from falling below 1 %, preserved joint function, and allowed patients to lead normal lives [2]. The superiority of primary prophylaxis (for definition, see Table 1) compared to episodic treatment is no longer questioned based on pivotal randomized controlled studies [3, 4]. Studies of secondary and tertiary prophylaxis in adolescents and adults have also shown benefit in reducing annual bleeding rate (ABR), rate of joint deterioration, and number of days lost from school or work compared to episodic treatment [5–7] With this irrefutable evidence, prophylaxis (over episodic treatment) should be the standard of care to all severe hemophilia individuals.

However, practical issues related to the cost and burden of prophylaxis, together with the recognized heterogeneity in bleeding risk and PK handling of factor concentrates, have lead us to question what the ideal prophylaxis regimen for severe hemophilia should be. High-dose (Malmö) prophylaxis regimen is considered "gold standard" [2]. Unfortunately, the costs associated with such a regimen and patient acceptance of frequent infusions starting at a very young age has been prohibitive for its widespread implementation. Alternatively, intermediate-dose prophylaxis has been used by the Dutch since 1968 (Table 2) [8]. A long-term outcome study that compared the high-dose Malmö to the intermediate-dose Dutch prophylaxis showed comparable QoL (EQ-5D 0.84 vs 1.0), despite a small but significant reduction in median annual joint bleeding rate (AJBR, 1.3 vs. 0) and hemophilia joint health score (HJHS, 9 vs 4) [8]. However, annual factor consumption was 2150 IU kg^{-1} per year lower for the Dutch regimen resulting in a sizeable cost difference (US\$159,000 based on US\$1.10 per unit [8]) that argued against cost-

Table 1 Definitions of continuous prophylaxis (see reference [1])

	No. large joint bleeds*	Age to start (year)	Clinical arthropathy, osteochondral disease
Primary	≤1	≤3	absent
Secondary	≥2	any	absent
Tertiary	≥2	any	present

All refer to continuous prophylaxis intended for 52 weeks per year, and taken for at least 45 weeks of the year under consideration
*large joints = knees, ankles, elbows, hips, shoulders

Table 2 Primary prophylaxis regimens

	Dosing
High/full-dose (Malmö/Swedish) [2]	25–40 IU kg^{-1} 3 times a week or every other days starting at age 1–2 years, irrespective of bleeding history
Intermediate-dose (Dutch) [8]	15–25 IU kg^{-1} 2–3 times per week, usually started after ≥1 hemarthrosis
Escalating-dose (Canadian) [9]	50 IU kg^{-1} once a week, with dose increased to 30 IU kg^{-1} twice a week, then 25 IU kg^{-1} every other day, in response to bleeding frequency

effectiveness for quality-adjusted life years (QALY) for high-dose prophylaxis.

The Canadian Hemophilia Primary Prophylaxis Study (CHPS) looked at reduced-intensity escalating dose prophylaxis (Table 2) [9]. The impetus for this regimen followed observations that about 10–15 % of severe hemophilia patients have infrequent bleeding and hemarthroses, and little or no joint damage [10]. The CHPS study aimed to tailor the prophylaxis regimen to balance the burden of IV injections, need for central venous catheter (CVC) insertions, and the costs of factor concentrate, against the level of arthropathy and patient's QoL. In this study, patients were able to preserve reasonable joint function with a mean AJBR of 0.78. At 15 years follow up 9 % of subjects remained on step one (50 IU/ kg^{-1} once weekly prophylaxis) and 32 % on step two (30 IU kg^{-1} twice weekly) [9]). The mean annual factor consumption was 3228 IU kg^{-1} per year, less than the ~ 6000 IU kg^{-1} per year for full-dose alternate day regimen [11]. In addition only 30 % of subjects in CHPS required CVCs compared to 82 % from a survey of North American centres of children on full-dose prophylaxis [12]. A cost-utility analysis using Markov modelling taking into account costs of factor, medical resources, effectiveness and health-related QoL (HR-QoL) showed the QALY for full-dose and escalating dose (CHPS) prophylaxis were the same due to the trade-off in greater number of CVCs needed for full-dose and the higher number of bleeds with escalating dose prophylaxis. However, the incremental cost per QALY gained with full-dose was > CAD$1,000,000, suggesting escalating dose prophylaxis is the greater cost-saving strategy of the two regimens [13].

The shift in paradigm: individualized prophylaxis

CHPS was a pioneer in tailoring prophylaxis and was able to produce adequate preservation of joint status using less factor with some cost saving. However, CHPS takes into account only one aspect of bleeding risk, bleed frequency, and its applicability is limited to pediatric patients initiating primary prophylaxis. Individualizing prophylaxis that is applicable to all age groups should take into consideration additional factors that contribute to bleeding risk such as level of physical activity/lifestyle, existing joint arthropathy, chronic synovitis, and time spent below an acceptable trough level, as well as patient's acceptability, burden of frequent venipunctures and venous access issues especially in children, and ability to self-guided care. The intrinsic half-life of a factor concentrate and the variation in patient PK handling influences the strategies for individualizing prophylaxis. This has generated intense interest in measuring an individual's PK profile, particularly elimination half-life of factor concentrates for an individual patient. Full PK profiling requires measuring multiple time points following factor infusion to generate an accurate estimate of elimination half-life. To circumvent the inconvenience of multiple venipunctures, population PK models have been developed for various factor concentrates to predict individual PK parameters with only 2 or 3 time points. Understanding a patient's PK profile allows tailoring a prophylaxis regimen to a dose and interval that achieves a predetermined optimal trough level that will minimize bleeding and maximize cost effectiveness for that particular patient.

What target trough level should be used has been an issue of debate. It is widely accepted that keeping trough levels above 1 % should be a minimum as few joint bleeds occur above this level. However, there is emerging evidence to suggest that maybe 1 % is not sufficient and that targeting higher trough levels should be pursued to maintain the healthiest joints possible. Epidemiologic evaluation on a Dutch cohort at diagnosis demonstrates that a FVIII level at 1 % may still have upwards of 5 joint bleeds per year, while levels >10–12 % have essentially zero joint bleeds [14]. It has been argued that even one bleed into the healthy joint of a growing child is one too many [15]. Canine studies demonstrate that a single joint bleed produces enough inflammation to cause permanent damage to developing cartilage. It is possible that the same in a maturing human joint may have deleterious effects as the individual ages [16]. We currently have limited long term data on primary prophylaxis regimens with the most mature data coming from the Swedish versus Dutch prophylaxis study that supports the idea that higher troughs achieve the healthiest joints due to near zero AJBR [8]. Additionally the US joint outcome study showed MRI-detectable joint damage still occurred in individuals who had no clinically evident joint bleeding [4]. Presumably, this resulted from subclinical joint bleeds which theoretically may be averted by a prophylaxis regimen that maintained higher trough levels.

Determinants of individualized prophylaxis

In a recent review on optimizing prophylaxis [17], Oldenburg proposed 3 main determinants for prophylaxis (Fig. 1): (1) a target trough level dictated by dose and interval of prophylaxis based on patient PK parameters and the availability and cost of factor concentrate, (2) the bleeding triggers which includes degree of physical activity/lifestyle, presence and severity of joint arthropathy and chronic synovitis, and (3) the number of bleeds, specifically joint bleeds, that are deemed acceptable (Fig. 1). These 3 factors form a dynamic triangle for optimizing prophylaxis. When 1 determinant is changed, the other 2 will adjust. For example, in the setting of unlimited resources "zero bleeds" and normal or even intense physical activity is achievable by using high dose, frequent injections to target higher troughs (5–10 % or more). At the centre, patient acceptance and ability to

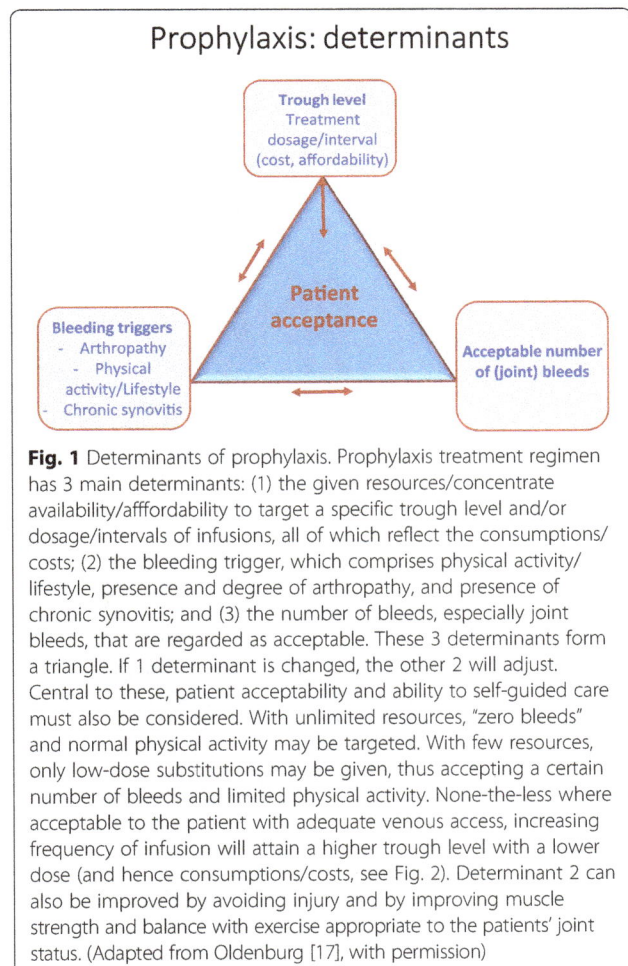

Fig. 1 Determinants of prophylaxis. Prophylaxis treatment regimen has 3 main determinants: (1) the given resources/concentrate availability/afffordability to target a specific trough level and/or dosage/intervals of infusions, all of which reflect the consumptions/ costs; (2) the bleeding trigger, which comprises physical activity/ lifestyle, presence and degree of arthropathy, and presence of chronic synovitis; and (3) the number of bleeds, especially joint bleeds, that are regarded as acceptable. These 3 determinants form a triangle. If 1 determinant is changed, the other 2 will adjust. Central to these, patient acceptability and ability to self-guided care must also be considered. With unlimited resources, "zero bleeds" and normal physical activity may be targeted. With few resources, only low-dose substitutions may be given, thus accepting a certain number of bleeds and limited physical activity. None-the-less where acceptable to the patient with adequate venous access, increasing frequency of infusion will attain a higher trough level with a lower dose (and hence consumptions/costs, see Fig. 2). Determinant 2 can also be improved by avoiding injury and by improving muscle strength and balance with exercise appropriate to the patients' joint status. (Adapted from Oldenburg [17], with permission)

self-guided care will play a role in how much weight can be placed on each corner of this triangle.

In the developed world where affordability of factor is not a major constraint, determinant (1), has a proportionally greater influence on the triangle since the trough level is the determinant we have the greatest control over. For determinant (2), bleeding triggers such as degree of arthropathy, presence of chronic synovitis, are inherent to the individual and cannot be easily changed. However, physical activity/lifestyle can be adapted to the degree of arthropathy, and the leeway to intensify physical activity is driven by trough level and number/intensity of peaks that determinant (1) can afford. Determinant (3), number of bleeds, is then a direct consequence of mostly how much determinant (1) can be changed. Therefore, in the developed world prophylaxis regimens should be adjusted to achieve the lowest number of bleeds possible. Given that the terminal half-life has the greatest impact on the trough, simply shortening the interval between infusions, even by 24 h, will cumulatively increase the trough level. Recent introduction of extended half-life products will provide patients with more options on frequency of infusion for a desired trough level.

Prophylaxis in resource limited nations: using low-dose and how it can still be individualized

The determinants of prophylaxis remain the same for developing nations, however; the freedom to adjust the determinants is impaired by lack of resources and affordable product. Thus, the majority of patients in developing countries continue to receive episodic treatment rather than prophylaxis. Full dose, and even intermediate dose prophylaxis is clearly not affordable/possible. Thus, adjusting trough levels to achieve a predefined target may become a moot point in the prophylaxis triangle. Without prophylaxis, these patients suffer tremendous disability, leaving them with crippling arthropathy, and unable to integrate fully to society. Many become wheelchair bound, unable to attend school or secure gainful employment.

It seems unacceptable to deny 75–80 % of the world's hemophilia population of prophylaxis when the benefits of this treatment are so clear. However, studies from Thailand, China and India are providing evidence that even low-dose prophylaxis can have major impact on number of bleeds, QoL, and functional participation in society. Four pediatric pilot studies, 3 from Thailand and China, and a small randomized study from India, used low-dose prophylaxis 8–10 IU kg^{-1} twice a week. Even though the numbers were small and the follow up ≤1 year, these studies demonstrate significant reductions in ABRs, AJBRs, fewer days absenteeism from school, and improved QoL despite only 37 % of children in the

Indian study had measured trough levels ≥1 % [18–21]. Factor consumption with prophylaxis was higher compared to on demand (1050 vs 675 IU kg^{-1} per year) in the Indian study [21] but is significantly lower when compared to full dose (~6000 IU kg^{-1} per year) [11] and escalating dose (~3228 IU kg^{-1} per year) [9] prophylaxis.

Only one study has looked at low-dose tertiary prophylaxis in adult patients who at baseline already have established severe arthropathy. This Chinese study used 5–10 IU kg^{-1} 2–3 times per week depending on what the patient can afford, and demonstrated a 77 % reduction in ABR and significant improvement in

functional independence scores (FISH) [22]. Although there was no measurable structural improvement (unchanged radiologic joint scores), some of the wheelchair-bound patients were able to walk on their own again, highlighting the significant impact low-dose prophylaxis made. Although solid evidence from large clinical trials on the benefits of low-dose prophylaxis is still lacking, it appears to be a feasible way to deliver prophylaxis treatment in resource-limited nations; at least until higher dose prophylaxis becomes economically possible.

As use of low-dose prophylaxis begins to gain support and is implemented in other resource-limited countries;

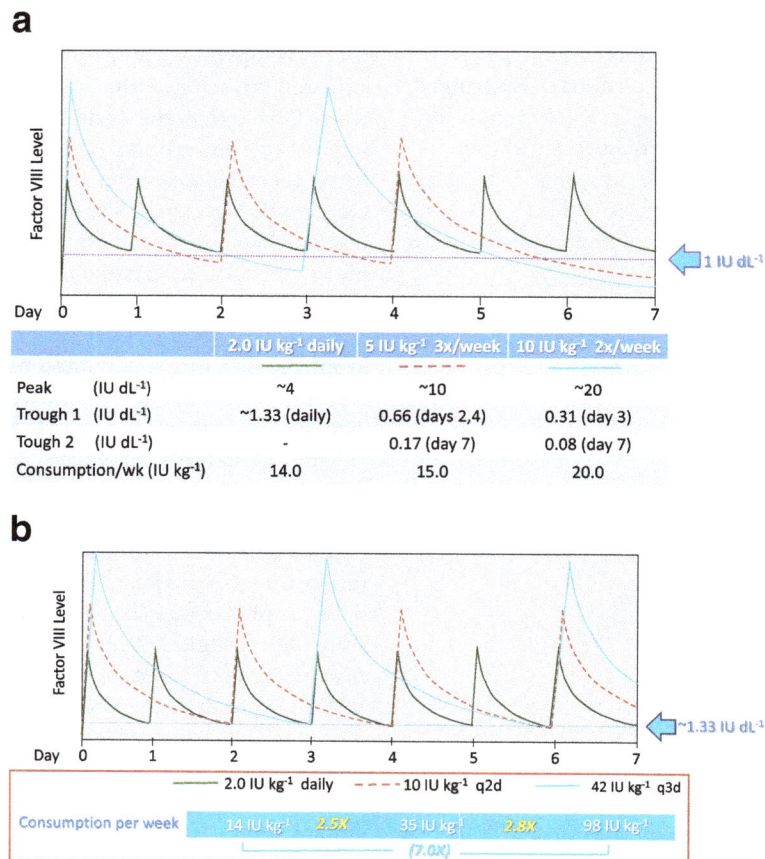

a

	2.0 IU kg^{-1} daily	5 IU kg^{-1} 3x/week	10 IU kg^{-1} 2x/week
Peak (IU dL^{-1})	~4	~10	~20
Trough 1 (IU dL^{-1})	~1.33 (daily)	0.66 (days 2,4)	0.31 (day 3)
Tough 2 (IU dL^{-1})	-	0.17 (day 7)	0.08 (day 7)
Consumption/wk (IU kg^{-1})	14.0	15.0	20.0

b

——— 2.0 IU kg^{-1} daily	– – – 10 IU kg^{-1} q2d	——— 42 IU kg^{-1} q3d
Consumption per week	14 IU kg^{-1} 2.5X 35 IU kg^{-1} 2.8X 98 IU kg^{-1}	
	(7.0X)	

Fig. 2 Low dose prophylaxis in economically constrained environment: Influence of FVIII infusion frequency on trough level and factor consumption. (Modeled based on an average FVIII recovery of 2 IU dL^{-1} per IU kg^{-1} infused and a T$_{1/2}$ of 12 h). **a** A dosage of 10 IU kg^{-1} two-times a week as well as 5 IU kg^{-1} three-times a week (weekly consumption 20 and 15 IU kg^{-1} per week respectively) each results in a trough level <1 IU dL^{-1} in 3–4 of the 7 days in the week (but with trough levels always higher with three-times a week than with two-times a week prophylaxis even at lower dose with lower consumption), whereas as little as 2 IU kg^{-1} daily (qd, weekly consumption 14 IU kg^{-1} per week) produces daily trough of ~1.33 IU dL^{-1}. [For three-times weekly prophylaxis, doubling the infusion dose from 5 to 10 IU kg^{-1} will double the day 2, 4 and 6 trough levels to ~1.33 IU dL^{-1}, but still leave trough level on day 7 at 0.66 IU dL^{-1} (i.e. <1 IU dL^{-1}, figure not shown)]. Prophylaxis at 10 IU kg^{-1} every-two-day (q2d) is shown in Fig. 2b. **b** In order for an every-three-day (q3d) regimen to produce a trough level similar to that obtained by every-two-day (q2d) infusion (e.g.1.33 IU/dL), the dosage per infusion has to be increased, whereas daily infusion requires a lower per infusion dosage. Compared to the q2d regimen, factor consumption is 2.8× more for the q3d regimen but 2.5× less for the qd regimen. These relative consumption multiples are the same for other target trough levels and other PK handling of clotting factors for a particular individual. (Figures not drawn to scale. Peak and trough levels will be different for different patients depending on their individual pharmacokinetic handling of the particular clotting factor, but the principles remain the same. Peak and trough levels tend to increase slightly with infusions but remain more or less constant after the first few infusions and steady state is achieved. Values for peak levels represent value range during steady state with each regimen)

we believe that the principles of individualization can still be used to optimize prophylaxis for any given patient within their fiscal limitations to maximize benefits. By determining how much factor a patient can afford over a given period of time, much more effective prophylaxis with higher trough levels can be achieved for that individual by giving smaller doses more frequently (Fig. 2). Figure 2a shows how increasing dose frequency can improve troughs without increasing consumption or costs. Assuming an average FVIII recovery of 2 IU dL^{-1} per IU kg^{-1} infused and a $T_{1/2}$ of 12 h, a dosage of 10 IU kg^{-1} two-times a week or 5 IU kg^{-1} three-times a week (weekly consumption 20 and 15 IU kg^{-1} per week respectively) each results in a trough level <1 IU dL^{-1} in 3–4 out of the 7 days per week, whereas as little as 2 IU kg^{-1} daily (qd, weekly consumption 14 IU kg^{-1} per week) produces daily troughs of ~1.33 IU dL^{-1}. This is an example of adjusting determinant (1) to individualize prophylaxis based on affordability in environments of resource constraint. This is particularly important for older children and adults with higher weight (hence, total dose) but have good veins for more frequent infusion. Conversely, to maintain any given trough level (e.g. 1.33 IU dL^{-1}), clotting factor consumption per week is decreased by ~2.5× when given daily, and increased by ~2.8× when given every 3rd day in comparison to "standard" every-other-day prophylaxis (Fig. 2b).

In order for prophylaxis to work in developing nations, there must be a clinic where by injections are given or patients are taught to self-inject (home care), and education for self-care and prophylaxis acceptance/adherence can be provided. Clinic support is also needed to educate patients on appropriate physical activity and life style adjustment, bleeding triggers that can be controlled. Hemophilia patients in developing nations often shy away from exercising because of the fear of bleeding. However, proper education on preventing avoidable injuries (including use of protective gear) and exercises that are appropriate to their joint status and degree of arthropathy requires professional help from trained-physiotherapists and physicians. Exercises to improve muscle strength and balance help stabilize joints and can avert joint bleeds in patients who are less protected on low dose prophylaxis. A dedicated hemophilia clinic with comprehensive care remains fundamental to prophylaxis irrespective of economic capacity, and should also be the priority in all developing nations.

Conclusion

Prophylaxis has significantly changed the lives of many hemophilia patients. Those living in developed nations have already benefited from prophylaxis, but room remains for improvement. Individualized prophylaxis by understanding bleeding triggers and PK profiles would allow us to target appropriate trough levels that can achieve "zero bleeds", provide the greatest chance of preserving joint health, and ultimately meet the specific goals for each patient. Although prophylaxis is expensive, this is not a reason for developing nations to remain complacent with inferior episodic treatment. Low and very-low dose prophylaxis and individualizing it to what is affordable for a given patient or nation, may bridge this gap created by global economic disparity. Greater efforts must be made in establishing comprehensive care and home care in developing nations in order for any type of prophylaxis to be successful. And finally maximizing the amount of time spent per week above target by using small but frequent doses of factor within one's fiscal constraints may individualize prophylaxis treatment for greater returns in functional independence and quality of life.

Acknowledgements

The authors thank Dr. Shannon Jackson (University of British Columbia, St. Paul's Hospital, Vancouver, Canada), Dr. John KM Wu (University of British Columbia, BC Children's Hospital, Vancouver, Canada) and Dr. Robert Card (University of Saskatchewan, Royal University Hospital, Saskatoon, Canada) for their helpful comments on the manuscript.

Authors' contributions

M-C Poon and A Lee contributed equally to the design, development, review and revision of the manuscript. They both approved the final submission version.

Competing interests

The authors declare that they have no competing interests.

Author details

[1]Department of Medicine, Cumming School of Medicine, University of Calgary, Calgary, Alberta, Canada. [2]Department of Pediatrics, Cumming School of Medicine, University of Calgary, Calgary, Alberta, Canada. [3]Department of Oncology, Cumming School of Medicine, University of Calgary, Calgary, Alberta, Canada. [4]Southern Alberta Rare Blood and Bleeding Disorders Comprehensive Care Program, Foothills Hospital, Alberta Health Services, Calgary, Alberta, Canada.

References

1. Srivastava A, Brewer AK, Mauser-Bunschoten EP, Key NS, Kitchen S, Llinas A, et al. Guidelines for the management of hemophilia. Haemophilia. 2013;19(1):e1–47.

2. Nilsson IM, Berntorp E, Lofqvist T, Petterssont H. Twenty-five years'
    experience of prophylactic treatment in severe haemophilia A and B.
    J Intern Med. 1992;232:25–32.

3. Gringeri A, Lundin B, Von Mackensen S, Mantovani L, Mannucci PM. A
    randomized clinical trial of prophylaxis in children with hemophilia A
    (the ESPRIT Study). J Thromb Haemost. 2011;9:700–10.

4. Manco-Johnson MJ, Abshire TC, Shapiro A, Riske B, Hacker MR, Kilcoyne R,
    et al. Prophylaxis versus episodic treatment to prevent joint disease in boys
    with severe hemophilia. N Engl J Med. 2007;357:535–44.

5. Manco-Johnson MJ, Kempton CL, Reding MT, Lissitchkov T, Goranov S, Gercheva
    L, et al. Randomized, controlled, parallel-group trial of routine prophylaxis vs.
    on-demand treatment with sucrose-formulated recombinant factor VIII in adults
    with severe hemophilia A. J Thromb Haemost. 2013;11:1119–27.

6. Aledort LM, Haschmeyer RH, Pettersson H. A longitudinal study of orthopaedic
    outcomes for severe fac tor-VIII-deficien t haemophiliacs. J Intern Med.
    1994;236:391–9.

7. Tagliaferri A, Feola G, Molinari AC, Santoro C, Rivolta GF, Cultrera DB, et al.
    Benefits of prophylaxis versus on-demand treatment in adolescents and
    adults with severe hemophilia A: the POTTER study. Thromb Haemost.
    2015;114:35–45.

8. Fischer K, Steen Carlsson K, Petrini P, Holmström M, Ljung R, van den Berg
    HM, et al. Intermediate-dose versus high-dose prophylaxis for severe
    hemophilia : comparing outcome and costs since the 1970s. Blood. 2013;
    122(7):1129–37.

9. Blanchette V, Israels S, Chan A, Rivard G, Cloutier S, Steele M, et al. Fifteen years
    of Canadian "tailored" prophylaxis: results from the Canadian Hemophilia
    Primary Prophylaxis Study (CHPS). Haemophilia. 2014;20 Suppl 3:94.

10. Molho P, Rolland N, Lebrun T, Dirat G, Courpied JP, Croughs T, et al.
    Epidemiological survey of the orthopaedic status of severe haemophilia A
    and B patients in France. Haemophilia. 2000;2:23–32.

11. Ljung R, Aronis-Vournas S, Krunik-Auberger K, van den Berg M, Chambost H,
    Claeyssens S, et al. Treatment of children with haemophilia in Europe : a
    survey of 20 centres in 16 countries. Haemophilia. 2000;6:619–24.

12. Blanchette VS, Mccready M, Achonu C, Abdolell M, Rivard G, Manco-
    Johnson MJ. A survey of factor prophylaxis in boys with haemophilia
    followed in North American haemophilia treatment centres. Haemophilia.
    2003;9 Suppl 1:19–26.

13. Risebrough N, Oh P, Blanchette V, Curtin J, Hitzler J, Feldman BM. Cost-utility
    analysis of Canadian tailored prophylaxis, primary prophylaxis and on-demand
    therapy in young children with severe haemophilia A. Haemophilia.
    2008;14:743–52.

14. den Uijl IEM, Fischer K, van der Bom JG, Grobbee DE, Rosendaal FR, Plug I.
    Analysis of low frequency bleeding data : the association of joint bleeds
    according to baseline FVIII activity levels. Haemophilia. 2011;17:41–4.

15. Gringeri A, Ewenstein B, Reininger A. The burden of bleeding in
    haemophilia : is one bleed too many ? Haemophilia. 2014;20:459–63.

16. Jansen NWD, Roosendaal G, Wenting MJG, Bijlsma JWJ, Theobald M,
    Hazewinkle HAW, et al. Very rapid clearance after a joint bleed in the canine
    knee cannot prevent adverse effects on cartilage and synovial tissue.
    Osteoarthr Cart. 2009;17:433–40.

17. Oldenburg J. Optimal treatment strategies for hemophilia : achievements and
    limitations of current prophylactic regimens. Blood. 2015;125(13):2038–45.

18. Chuansumrit A, Isarangkura P, Hathirat P. Prophylactic treatment for
    hemophilia A patients: a pilot study. Southeast Asian J Trop Med Public
    Health. 1995;26(2):243–6.

19. Wu R, Luke K-H, Poon M-C, Wu X, Zhang N, Zhao L, et al. Low dose
    secondary prophylaxis reduces joint bleeding in severe and moderate
    haemophilic children : a pilot study in China. Haemophilia. 2011;17:70–4.

20. Tang L, Wu R, Sun J, Zhang X, Feng X, Zhang X, et al. Short-term low-dose
    secondary prophylaxis for severe / moderate haemophilia A children is
    beneficial to reduce bleed and improve daily activity, but there are obstacle in
    its execution : a multi-centre pilot study in China. Haemophilia. 2013;19:27–34.

21. Verma SP, Dutta TK, Mahadevan S, Nalini P, Basu D, Biswal N, et al. A
    randomized study of very low-dose factor VIII prophylaxis in severe
    haemophilia – A success story from a resource limited country.
    Haemophilia. 2016;22:342–8.

22. Hua B, Lian X, Li K, Lee A, Poon M-C, Zhao Y. Low-dose tertiary prophylactic
    therapy reduces total number of bleeds and improves the ability to perform
    activities of daily living in adults with severe haemophilia A : a single-
    centre experience from Beijing. Blood Coagul Fibrinolysis. 2016;27:136–40.

15

Reduced platelet hyper-reactivity and platelet-leukocyte aggregation after periodontal therapy

Efthymios Arvanitidis, Sergio Bizzarro, Elena Alvarez Rodriguez, Bruno G. Loos and Elena A. Nicu[*]

Abstract

Background: Platelets from untreated periodontitis patients are hyper-reactive and form more platelet-leukocyte complexes compared to cells from individuals without periodontitis. It is not known whether the improvement of the periodontal condition achievable by therapy has beneficial effects on the platelet function. We aimed to assess the effects of periodontal therapy on platelet reactivity.

Methods: Patients with periodontitis ($n = 25$) but unaffected by any other medical condition or medication were included and donated blood before and after periodontal therapy. Reactivity to ADP or oral bacteria was assessed by flow cytometric analysis of membrane markers (binding of PAC-1, P-selectin, CD63) and platelet-leukocyte complex formation. Reactivity values were expressed as ratio between the stimulated and unstimulated sample. Plasma levels of soluble (s) P-selectin were determined by enzyme-linked immunosorbent assay (ELISA).

Results: Binding of PAC-1, the expression of P-selectin and CD63 in response to the oral bacterium *P. gingivalis* were lower at recall (1.4 ± 1.1, 1.5 ± 1.2, and 1.0 ± 0.1) than at baseline (2.7 ± 4.1, $P = 0.026$, 6.0 ± 12.5, $P = 0.045$, and 2.7 ± 6.7, $P = 0.042$, respectively). Formation of platelet-leukocyte complexes in response to *P. gingivalis* was also reduced at recall compared to baseline (1.2 ± 0.7 vs. 11.4 ± 50.5, $P = 0.045$). sP-selectin levels were significantly increased post-therapy.

Conclusions: In periodontitis patients, the improvement of the periodontal condition is paralleled by a reduction in platelet hyper-reactivity. We suggest that periodontal therapy, as an intervention for improved oral health, can facilitate the management of thrombotic risk, and on the long term can contribute to the prevention of cardiovascular events in patients at risk.

Keywords: Periodontal treatment, Periodontitis, Platelet reactivity, Platelet-monocyte complexes, Platelet-neutrophil Complexes

Background

Periodontitis is a chronic inflammatory disease of the teeth-supporting tissues characterized by progressive loss of attachment, deepening and ulceration of the barrier epithelium [1]. Under these circumstances, bacteremia with oral microorganisms is a common phenomenon during everyday activities, such as chewing and tooth brushing [2]. Oral bacterial species (among them *Porphyromonas gingivalis* and *Streptococcus sanguis*) have been identified in atherosclerotic plaques [3] and are involved in the pathogenesis of infective endocarditis [4]. Mechanisms of action include the capacity of oral bacteria to activate platelets [5, 6] and the formation of platelet-leukocyte complexes, containing activated platelets and leukocytes [7, 8].

Although periodontitis is a common condition (47% of U.S. dentate adults aged 30 years and older [9]) associated with chronic low-grade inflammatory state and atherosclerotic vascular disease [10], it is only sparsely investigated as a potential source of ongoing platelet

* Correspondence: e.nicu@acta.nl
Department of Periodontology, Academic Centre for Dentistry Amsterdam (ACTA), University of Amsterdam and VU University Amsterdam, Gustav Mahlerlaan 3004, Amsterdam 1081LA, The Netherlands

activation. A previous study from our group has shown that platelets are more activated in periodontitis patients [11]. Besides the more activated state, the platelets and their complexes with leukocytes are hyper-reactive in response to ADP and oral bacteria [12].

It is not known whether periodontal therapy could affect platelet hyper-reactivity thereby facilitating a better management of the cardiovascular risk. We hypothesized that circulating platelets and platelet-leukocyte complexes from peripheral blood of periodontitis patients become less reactive upon stimulation after the provision of non-surgical periodontal therapy. Therefore, the aim of this study was to investigate the effect of non-surgical periodontal therapy on platelet reactivity. To this end, we analyzed platelet membrane-bound activation markers expression and the formation of platelet-leukocyte complexes in response to ADP and oral bacteria (*Aggregatibacter actinomycetemcomitans* [*Aa*], *Porphyromonas gingivalis* [*Pg*], *Tannerella forsythia* [*Tf*], *Streptococcus sanguis* [*Ss*] and *Streptococcus mutans* [*Sm*]).

Methods
Chemicals and antibodies
All chemicals were purchased from Sigma Chemical (St Louis, MO, USA). The HEPES buffer solution consisted of 137 mM NaCl, 2.7 mM KCl, 1.0 mM MgCl$_2$, 5.6 mM glucose, 20 mM HEPES, 1 mg/mL bovine serum albumin, 3.3 mM NaH$_2$PO$_4$, pH 7.4. The lysing solution contained 155 mM NH$_4$Cl, 10 mM KHCO$_3$, 0.1 mM EDTA, pH 7.4 and was stored at 4 °C. The antibodies against surface markers were: CD4-PE, CD14-PE, CD45-APC, CD61-PerCP, CD62P-PE, CD62P-FITC, CD63-PE, CD66b-FITC, PAC-1 FITC, and their isotype control antibodies (all from BD Pharmingen, San Jose, CA, USA). CD61-APC was from Dako (Glostrup, Denmark).

Bacterial strains and culture conditions
For this experiment, *Aa*, *Pg*, *Tf*, *Ss* and *Sm* were grown as described in a previous study [12]. The bacterial suspensions were washed by centrifugation, reduced to an optical density of 1 at 600 nm in HEPES-buffer and stored in aliquots at −20 °C.

Patient selection and study protocol
The study population is part of a cohort of moderate-to-severe adult periodontitis patients participating in a clinical trial in the Department of Periodontology at the Academic Centre for Dentistry of Amsterdam (the Netherlands) [13]. Within a period of eighteen months (February 2012-September 2013), all consecutive patients fulfilling the inclusion criteria were included in this study. Patients were recruited if they fulfilled the following inclusion criteria: presence of chronic periodontitis, self-reported good general health and not being aware of any form of diabetes, cardiovascular disease, (auto) immune disease or any other systemic or metabolic disease, and not receiving any medication for hypertension, dyslipidemia of hyperglycemia. Further exclusion criteria were: regular use of medications that could influence platelet function (i.e. NSAIDs, acetylsalicylic acid, dipyridamole, thienopyridines), use of antibiotics in the past 6 months, periodontal treatment in the last 2 years, pregnancy or lactation, presence of implants or orthodontic appliances and presence of <20 natural teeth.

Participants were scheduled for two sessions of non-surgical periodontal therapy (average duration of 5 h) under local anesthesia conducted by two experienced staff oral hygienists. All subjects received a demonstration of basic oral hygiene principles with an electric toothbrush (Philips Sonicare®, Bothell, WA, USA) and were instructed to use interdental means of cleaning followed by rinsing with chlorhexidine 0.12% twice daily. The patients were recalled at six weeks for reinforcement of oral hygiene and localized rescaling of bleeding pockets. Patients were subsequently enrolled in a 3-monthly maintenance program. At baseline and recall (3 months after treatment) blood samples were taken into 0.32% citrate vacuum tubes (BD Vacutainer blood collection tube, Becton Dickinson, Oxford, UK). Citrated plasma was prepared by centrifugation (2000 g, 4 °C, 10 min). Aliquots were stored at −80 °C.

Platelet reactivity
At baseline and the 3 months-recall (twelve weeks after completion of active periodontal therapy), fasting blood samples for platelet assays were collected between 08:00–10:00 a.m. by venipuncture of the antecubital fossa (0.32% sodium citrate containing blood collection tubes). Blood was kept at room temperature and processed within 30 min of collection.

Aliquots of whole blood (10 μL) were diluted in 30 μL of HEPES-buffer (unstimulated control) or incubated with bacterial suspensions of Aa, Pg, Tf, Ss and Sm. Adenosine diphosphate (ADP, 10 μM) was used as a positive control [14]. The reaction vials contained APC-labeled anti-CD61, FITC-labeled PAC-1 plus PE-labeled anti-CD62P or APC-labeled anti-CD61 plus PE-labeled anti-CD63 (4 μg/mL, final concentration) [15]. To set fluorescence thresholds, 4 μg/mL PE-IgG$_1$ and 4 μg/mL FITC-IgM isotype control antibodies were used. The mixes were allowed to incubate for 30 min at room temperature in the dark. The samples were fixed by adding HEPES-buffer containing 0.3% paraformaldehyde (PFA, 2.5 mL). Whole blood flow cytometry was conducted on Accuri™ flow cytometer employing C6 software (Becton Dickinson, Michigan, USA). Forward (size) and side (granularity) scatter were set at logarithmic gain and the geometric mean fluorescent intensity (MFI) was recorded. Platelets were identified on basis of a characteristic forward and side scatter and specific binding of CD61. Within the platelet gate, fluorescence was employed to distinguish between PAC-1, CD62P or CD63 positive cells. Exposure of platelet activation markers was determined on 2500 platelets. The threshold for platelet activation was set at 1% of the appropriate isotype control-antibody.

Platelet-leukocyte complexes

For the platelet-leukocytes essays, fresh citrated blood (20 μL) was incubated with or without stimulants (see Platelet Reactivity), at room temperature in the dark. Leukocytes were identified using the 90°-light scatter and the expression of CD45 (Fig. 1a). Within each subpopulation gate (neutrophils, monocytes, lymphocytes), the expression of CD61 was determined (Fig.1b-g). The identity of neutrophils, monocytes, and lymphocytes was confirmed by the characteristic expression of CD66b, CD14 and CD4, respectively. The threshold for platelet-leukocyte binding was set at 1% using an isotype control antibody corresponding to the non-specific binding; above this threshold all leukocytes were considered to be CD61 positive reflecting the platelet-leukocyte complexes. After a 15 min incubation, 500 μL of cold (4 °C) lysing solution was added and each sample was placed on ice. Upon lysis, fixation was achieved with the addition of 0.3% PFA solution.

Soluble P-selectin determination

The concentration of circulating P-selectin in plasma was measured with a commercial enzyme-linked immunosorbent assay (sP-Selectin/CD62p ELISA kit, R&D Systems Inc., Minneapolis, MN, USA). The measurements were performed following the manufacturer's instructions. For sP-selectin determination, plasma samples were diluted 20 fold. The diluted plasma specimens were added together with an anti-sP-selectin antibody conjugated to peroxidase into a 96-well plate precoated with another anti-sP-selectin monoclonal antibody (MAb) and incubated for 1 h. Substrate was then added, and absorbance values were measured at 450 nm with a plate reader (Synergy HT, BioTek, Winooski, VT, USA). The concentration of each sample was determined by extrapolation from a standard curve estimated from a panel of sP-selectin standards of known concentrations and corrected for the dilution effect of the liquid anti-coagulant (citrate). Plasma levels of sP-selectin were expressed as ng/mL. The intra-assay and inter-assay co-efficients of variance were 5.2% and 8.7%, respectively.

Statistical analysis

Our sample size calculation was based on the observed mean ± SD of the fold increase in P-selectin (CD62p) expression on platelets after bacterial stimulation as reported by Nicu et al. [12]. We calculated that we needed to include 29 patients to be able to detect a reduction in

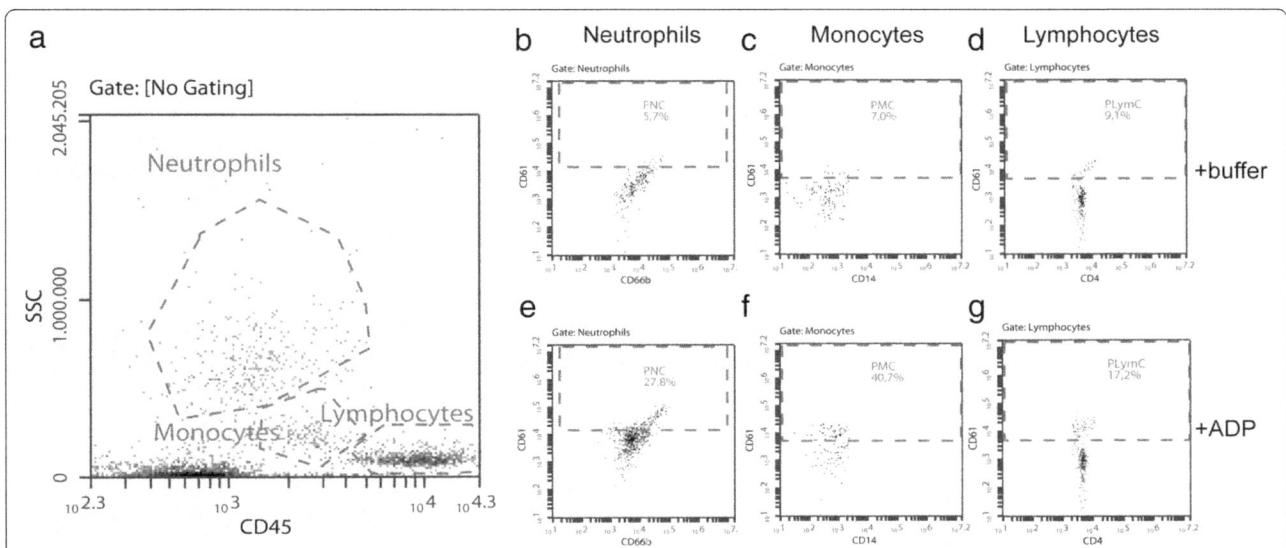

Fig. 1 Flow cytometric features of leukocytes, neutrophils, monocytes, and lymphocytes and their complexes with platelets. Panel **a** is showing all events. The Neutrophils gate is characterized by high side scatter and low CD45 expression, the Monocytes gate is characterized by intermediate side scatter and intermediate CD45 expression, and the Lymphocyte gate is characterized by low side scatter and high CD45 expression. All events within the Neutrophils gate in **a** were represented in a CD66b and CD61 plot. Events characterized by high expression of both CD66b and CD61 designate the platelet-neutrophil complexes (PNCs, dotted box in **b**. Similar strategy was employed for the monocytes (using CD14, the platelet-monocyte complexes, PMCs, are in the dotted box in **c** and lymphocytes (using CD4, the platelet-lymphocyte complexes, PLymCs, are in the dotted box in **d**. An example of an unstimulated sample (incubated in HEPES buffer) is shown in **b**, **c**, and **d**, whereas flow cytometric analysis of a stimulated sample (incubated in ADP) is shown in **e**, **f**, and **g**

platelet reactivity after periodontal therapy with a power of 85% (using a two-sided alpha level of 0.05).

Statistical analysis was performed using SPSS software (v.20.0; IBM, Chicago, Illinois, USA). GraphPad Prism (v. 6.0; GraphPad Software, San Diego, California, USA) was used for the graphic representation of all data. Normality of the data distribution was assessed by Kolmogorov-Smirnov test. When using parametric testing, the data sets showing a non-normal distribution were log-transformed before statistical analysis. The anthropometric, biochemical and clinical characteristics at baseline and recall were compared using the paired t-test.

Platelet reactivity was expressed as the ratio between the mean fluorescent intensity (MFI) of the indicated activation marker after stimulation and the MFI of the same marker in the absence of stimulation (cells in HEPES-buffer). The number of CD61-positive (equivalent to platelet-conjugated) leukocytes, neutrophils, monocytes and lymphocytes was recorded as a percentage of the total population of each respectively. Ratios were calculated [% platelet-bound cells after stimulation/% platelet-bound cells in HEPES-buffer] representing the change in number of complexes formed in response to stimulation with oral bacteria or ADP. A general linear model (repeated measures ANOVA using the Huyhn-Feldt correction followed by Bonferroni correction for multiple comparisons), was applied. In this model, comparisons between stimulated (ADP, Aa, Pg, Tf, Ss, Sm) and unstimulated samples (Hepes) were acquired (*within timepoint* comparisons, at baseline and recall). Secondly, *between timepoints* (baseline and recall) comparisons for each stimulus were assessed by applying the paired t-test. P-values < 0.05 were considered statistically significant.

The fold changes over time in PAC-1, CD62p, CD63, platelet-leukocyte, platelet-neutrophil or platelet-monocyte complexes, LDL levels, systolic blood pressure, waist circumference, number of periodontal pockets deeper than 6 mm were calculated by dividing the value of each parameter at recall by its value at baseline. The *fold changes over time* in PAC-1 (in response to ADP, Pg, Sm), CD62p (Pg), CD63 (Pg), platelet-leukocyte (Pg), platelet-neutrophil (Tf, Ss) or platelet-monocyte complexes (Ss) were entered as dependent variables, and the amount of smoking (pack-years), change in LDL levels, change in systolic blood pressure, change in waist circumference, change in number of periodontal pockets deeper than 6 mm as predictors. Multiple linear regression (Enter method) was used to model the relationship between the calculated platelet-related parameters and these predictors.

Results

Patient characteristics and effect of treatment
Within the study period thirty consecutive patients were included in this study; however, due to scheduling conflicts (regarding blood collection and processing), only 25 data sets were available as a complete set (baseline and recall at 12 weeks post-therapy). Demographic and dental characteristics of the participants are described in Table 1. The prevalence of chronic smokers (>10 years) within this group was high (56%). Interestingly, six patients successfully quitted smoking within the duration of the study. Two subjects were classified as obese (BMI > 30 kg/m^2, waist circumference > 124 cm), while hypercholesterolemia (total cholesterol > 6.2 mmol/L) was noted for three subjects. Using the biochemistry results (summarized in Table 1) we gave the patients a composite score of metabolic syndrome at baseline, according to the presence of central obesity (WC ≥102 cm in men or ≥88 cm in women) together with ≥2 of the following risk determinants: triglycerides ≥1.7 mmol/l, HDL <1.03 mmol/l in males or <1.29 mmol/l in females, blood pressure ≥130/85 mmHg, fasting glucose ≥5.6 mmol/l [16]. Based on this composite score, only 3 out of the 25 participants scored as having metabolic syndrome. LDL levels were lower at recall compared to baseline ($P = 0.03$). Further, seven patients received systemic antimicrobials (375 mg amoxicillin and 250 mg metronidazole, t.i.d, 7 days) as an adjunct to non-surgical periodontal therapy. The leukocyte and platelet counts were comparable before and after periodontal therapy ($P = 0.852$ and 0.570, respectively). As expected, the treatment resulted in significant improvement in all clinical periodontal variables ($P < 0.001$, Table 1). Four teeth were extracted in total, three of them in one individual.

Platelet reactivity
To determine the reactivity of circulating platelets, P-selectin and CD63 expression, and PAC-1 binding in response to stimulation was assessed (Fig. 2). Stimulation with ADP led to a significant many-fold increase in platelet activation over the unstimulated sample (Fig. 2a, b, c). Similarly, co-incubation of whole blood with oral bacteria induced a smaller but significant amount of platelet activation (overall $P < 0.001$ for the ***within timepoint*** analysis for all three markers). More specifically, Ss was the strongest inducer of platelet activation (post hoc $P < 0.05$ for all three markers). The PAC-1 binding was lower at recall than at baseline in response to stimulation with ADP (mean ratio MFI$_{recall}$ = 14.3 vs. mean ratio MFI$_{baseline}$ = 21.6, $P = 0.042$), Pg (mean ratio MFI$_{recall}$ = 1.4 vs. mean ratio MFI$_{baseline}$ = 2.7, $P = 0.026$) and Sm (mean ratio MFI$_{recall}$ = 2.9 vs. mean ratio MFI$_{baseline}$ = 3.9, $P = 0.017$, Fig. 2a). A non-significant reduction in PAC-1 binding was measured at recall in response to Aa and Ss. The P-selectin expression in response to Pg was lower at recall than baseline (mean ratio MFI$_{recall}$ = 1.6 vs. mean ratio MFI$_{baseline}$ = 6.0, $P = 0.045$, Fig. 2b). Similarly, CD63 expression after Pg stimulation was lower at

Table 1 Summary of the study population characteristics ($n = 25$) at baseline and recall (12 weeks post-therapy)

	Baseline	Recall	P-value
Age	44.7 ± 9.3	-	-
Gender (male/female)	11/14	-	-
Ethnicity (Caucasian/non-Caucasian)	21/4	-	-
Smoking (current/former/never)	14/5/6	8/11/6	-
Packyears	16.5 ± 13.8	-	-
BMI (kg/m^2)	25.0 ± 5.1	25.3 ± 5.2	NS
Waist circumference (cm)	95.6 ± 17.2	94.8 ± 16.9	NS
Blood pressure (mm Hg)			
Systolic	124.8 ± 19.4	127.2 ± 16.1	NS
Diastolic	76.1 ± 13.4	77.2 ± 11.9	NS
Total cholesterol (mmol/L)	5.2 ± 0.8	4.9 ± 0.9	NS
HDL (mmol/L)	1.5 ± 0.4	1.4 ± 0.5	NS
LDL (mmol/L)	3.2 ± 0.8	2.8 ± 0.7	$P = 0.03$
Triglycerides (mmol/L)	1.2 ± 1.0	1.4 ± 1.1	NS
C-reactive protein (mg/L)	2.1 ± 2.8	2.0 ± 3.9	NS
Fibrinogen (g/L)	2.9 ± 0.6	2.8 ± 0.6	NS
Leukocyte counts (× 10^9/L)	6.7 ± 2.0	6.6 ± 2.2	NS
Neutrophils	3.9 ± 1.6	3.8 ± 1.9	NS
Lymphocyte counts	2.0 ± 0.6	2.2 ± 1.1	NS
Platelet counts (× 10^3)	250.4 ± 66.1	246.6 ± 56.6	NS
Number of teeth	27.6 ± 2.6	27.4 ± 2.6	NS
#teeth with > 50% bone loss	4.4 ± 3.1	4.1 ± 3.1	NS
Sites with plaque (%)	74.6 ± 20.0	19.0 ± 13.0	$P < 0.001$
Sites with bleeding on probing	65.9 ± 15.0	18.7 ± 9.1	$P < 0.001$
Probing Pocket Depth (mm)	4.0 ± 0.6	2.9 ± 0.4	$P < 0.001$
Pockets ≥ 5 mm (%)	32.4 ± 14.5	11.7 ± 9.0	$P < 0.001$
Clinical Attachment Level (mm)	4.3 ± 0.9	3.6 ± 0.8	$P < 0.001$

Values are presented as means ± standard deviations or number of subjects
BMI (body mass index), *HDL* (high density lipoproteins), *LDL* (low density lipoproteins)

recall compared to baseline (mean ratio $MFI_{recall} = 1.0$ vs. mean ratio $MFI_{baseline} = 2.7$, $P = 0.042$, Fig. 2c).

Formation of platelet-leukocyte complexes

Incubation of fresh platelets with ADP or oral bacteria resulted in formation of platelet-leukocyte complexes (PLC) both at baseline and recall (overall $P < 0.001$ for the ***within timepoints*** analysis, Fig. 3). Specifically, formation of platelet-neutrophil (PNC) and platelet-monocyte complexes (PMC) was significantly induced by stimulation (Table 2). The strongest inducers of PLC, PNC or PMC were ADP, *Tf* and *Ss* (*post-hoc $P < 0.05$*). Formation of platelets-lymphocyte complexes (PLymC) appeared less influenced either by ADP or oral bacteria (Table 2, $P > 0.05$).

Less PLC formation could be observed at recall compared to baseline in response to *Pg* (mean ratio $\%PLC_{recall} = 1.2$ vs. mean ratio $\%PLC_{baseline} = 11.4$, $P = 0.045$, Fig. 3). Furthermore, less PNC were formed at recall compared to baseline in response to *Tf* ($P = 0.045$) and *Ss* ($P = 0.009$, Table 2). Similarly, less PMCs were formed at recall in response to *Tf* ($P = 0.065$), *Ss* ($P = 0.004$), and *Sm* ($P = 0.093$). PLymC formation was unaffected by time or bacterial stimulation ($P > 0.05$, Table 2).

The intrinsic platelet activation status at recall compared to baseline is presented in Additional file 1, in which raw data of the unstimulated condition (samples incubated in HEPES buffer) are summarized. None of the tested parameters were significantly different between baseline and recall. We noted a trend towards higher PAC-1 binding 3 months post-treatment ($P = 0.061$) and higher percentage of platelet-neutrophils complexes ($P = 0.077$), which however did not reach statistical significance.

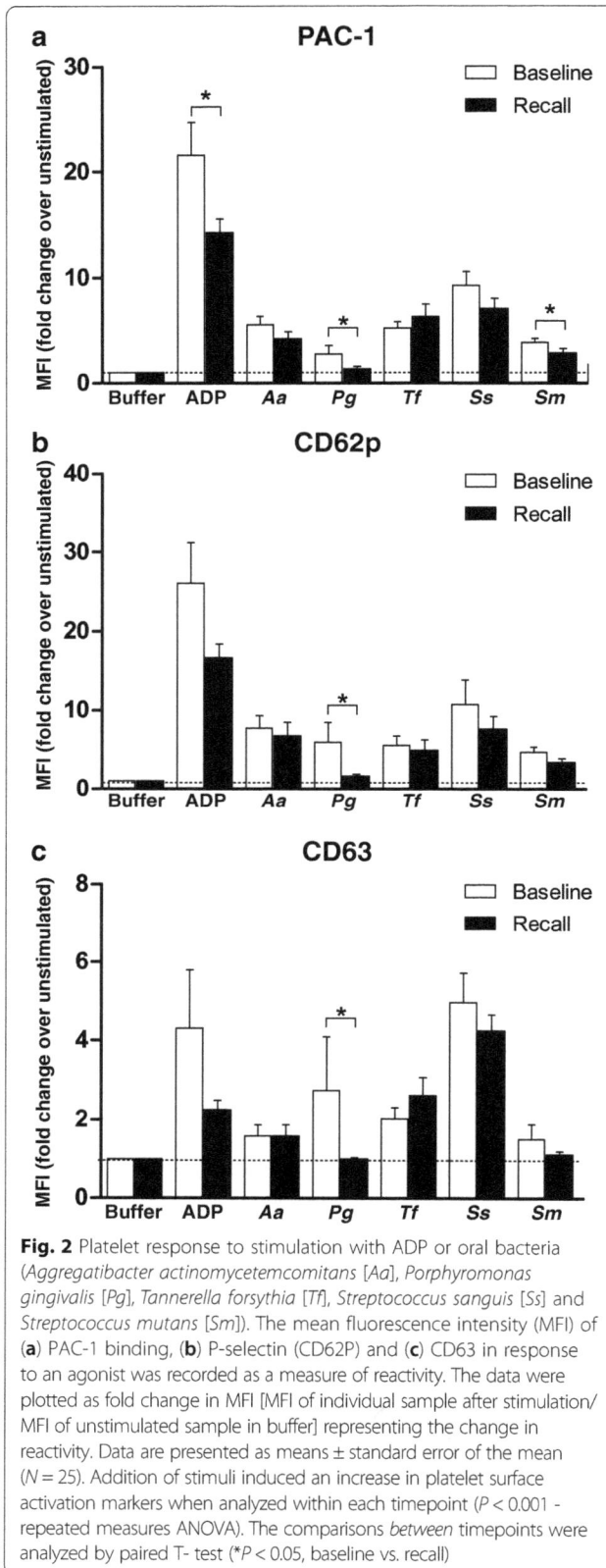

Fig. 2 Platelet response to stimulation with ADP or oral bacteria (*Aggregatibacter actinomycetemcomitans* [*Aa*], *Porphyromonas gingivalis* [*Pg*], *Tannerella forsythia* [*Tf*], *Streptococcus sanguis* [*Ss*] and *Streptococcus mutans* [*Sm*]). The mean fluorescence intensity (MFI) of (**a**) PAC-1 binding, (**b**) P-selectin (CD62P) and (**c**) CD63 in response to an agonist was recorded as a measure of reactivity. The data were plotted as fold change in MFI [MFI of individual sample after stimulation/ MFI of unstimulated sample in buffer] representing the change in reactivity. Data are presented as means ± standard error of the mean (*N* = 25). Addition of stimuli induced an increase in platelet surface activation markers when analyzed within each timepoint (*P* < 0.001 - repeated measures ANOVA). The comparisons *between* timepoints were analyzed by paired T- test (**P* < 0.05, baseline vs. recall)

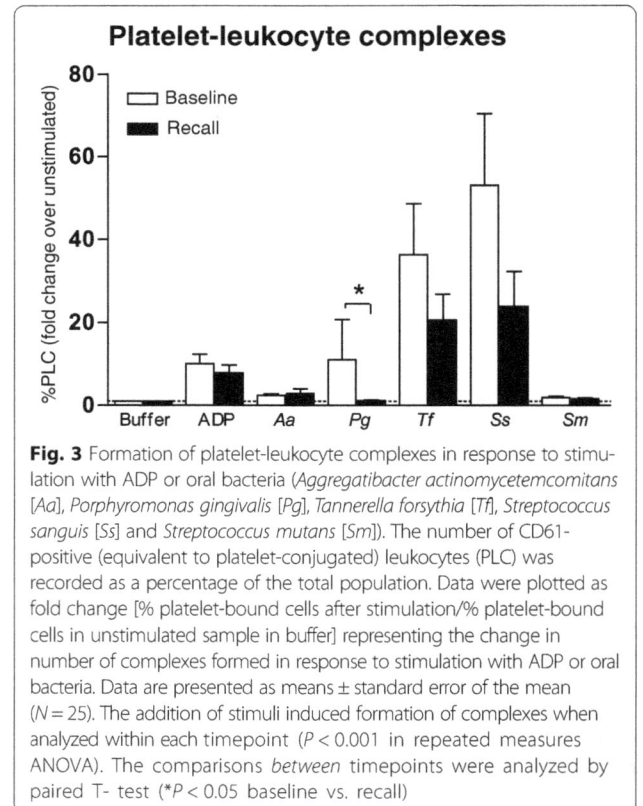

Fig. 3 Formation of platelet-leukocyte complexes in response to stimulation with ADP or oral bacteria (*Aggregatibacter actinomycetemcomitans* [*Aa*], *Porphyromonas gingivalis* [*Pg*], *Tannerella forsythia* [*Tf*], *Streptococcus sanguis* [*Ss*] and *Streptococcus mutans* [*Sm*]). The number of CD61-positive (equivalent to platelet-conjugated) leukocytes (PLC) was recorded as a percentage of the total population. Data were plotted as fold change [% platelet-bound cells after stimulation/% platelet-bound cells in unstimulated sample in buffer] representing the change in number of complexes formed in response to stimulation with ADP or oral bacteria. Data are presented as means ± standard error of the mean (*N* = 25). The addition of stimuli induced formation of complexes when analyzed within each timepoint (*P* < 0.001 in repeated measures ANOVA). The comparisons *between* timepoints were analyzed by paired T- test (**P* < 0.05 baseline vs. recall)

Soluble P-selectin concentration

At baseline, sP-selectin values ranged between 15.8 ng/mL and 72.8 ng/mL (mean ± standard deviation 40.5 ± 15.1 ng/ mL, Fig. 4). The plasma levels of sP-selectin at recall (range 21.1 - 123.8 ng/mL, mean ± SD: 56.4 ± 22.8 ng/mL) were significantly increased compared to baseline (*P* = 0.0008). The plasma concentration of sP-selectin was not correlated with the platelet expression of P-selectin (CD62p expression in unstimulated samples) at baseline (R = −0.37, *P* = 0.863) or recall (*R* = 0.006, *P* = 0.979).

Linear regression models

Linear regression analyses were run for all the platelet parameters showing a significant decrease post-treatment (PAC-1 binding in response to ADP, *Pg*, and *Sm*, CD62 response to *Pg*, CD63 response to *Pg*, PLC formation in response to *Pg*, PNC formation in response to *Tf*, PNC formation in response to *Ss*, PMC formation in response to *Ss*). The regression models included the following variables as predictors: smoking amounts, LDL (ratio recall/ baseline), waist circumference (ratio recall/baseline), systolic blood pressure (ratio recall/baseline) and the clinical response to periodontal treatment (ratio between the number of periodontal pockets deeper than 6 mm at recall/baseline). The results of these regression models are presented in Additional file 2. The final regression

Table 2 Summary of platelet-neutrophil, platelet-monocyte and platelet-lymphocyte complexes formation in response to stimulation

Platelet-neutrophil complexes (Fold change over unstimulated)				Platelet-monocyte complexes (Fold change over unstimulated)				Platelet-lymphocyte complexes (Fold change over unstimulated)		
	Baseline	Recall	P-value		Baseline	Recall	P-value		Baseline	Recall	P-value
+ADP	6.9 ± 7.9	8.6 ± 19.3	0.468	+ADP	13.0 ± 19.4	8.4 ± 16.8	0.339	+ADP	4.7 ± 8.1	7.1 ± 10.5	0.072
+Aa	2.1 ± 1.8	6.1 ± 17.5	0.766	+Aa	2.7 ± 2.5	1.9 ± 1.3	0.265	+Aa	7.7 ± 19.2	3.9 ± 8.2	0.483
+Pg	9.4 ± 40.1	2.4 ± 5.6	0.462	+Pg	2.1 ± 3.2	1.2 ± 1.0	0.100	+Pg	1.8 ± 2.1	2.0 ± 3.0	0.535
+Tf	32.9 ± 56.2	14.9 ± 30.5	**0.028**	+Tf	8.7 ± 8.3	7.7 ± 19.6	0.072	+Tf	11.5 ± 23.2	9.3 ± 12.1	0.431
+Ss	51.3 ± 93.4	15.4 ± 31.9	**0.003**	+Ss	13.2 ± 20.1	7.0 ± 25.1	**0.004**	+Ss	4.1 ± 10.6	3.9 ± 5.9	0.529
+Sm	1.4 ± 1.4	2.7 ± 7.8	0.906	+Sm	2.2 ± 2.0	1.2 ± 1.2	**0.046**	+Sm	1.4 ± 0.8	2.7 ± 3.8	0.087

Values are presented as means ± standard deviations. The platelet-neutrophil complexes, platelet-monocyte complexes, platelet-lymphocyte complexes were calculated as percentages platelet-positive neutrophils, monocytes or lymphocytes from the total number of neutrophils, monocytes or lymphocytes, respectively. The fold change over unstimulated values represent the ratios between the measured values after stimulation with ADP, Aa, Pg, Tf, Ss or Sm and in the absence of stimulation (cells in buffer). P-values were obtained by paired T-test and the significant values are given in bold
ADP (adenosine diphosphate), Aa (Aggregatibacter actinomycetemcomitans), Pg (Porphyromonas gingivalis), Tf (Tannerella forsythia), Ss (Streptococcus sanguis), Sm (Streptococcus mutans)

equation for the PAC-1 binding in response to ADP yielded R^2: 0.584, F = 3.083; P = 0.05. From this regression model it became apparent that the clinical response to periodontal treatment positively predicted the improvement in PAC-1 binding in response to ADP (B = 3.26, t = 2.76, P = 0.02) and Sm (B = 2.41, t = 2.29, P = 0.04). The positive relation between PAC-1 binding and response to treatment translates into: the reduction in the number of periodontal pockets deeper than 6 mm after treatment is positively correlated with the reduction in PAC-1 binding in response to ADP or Sm.

None of the other variables included in the models predicted the change in platelet parameters (P > 0.05).

Discussion

Many inflammatory states, e.g. systemic lupus erythematosus, pneumonia, or inflammatory bowel disease feature

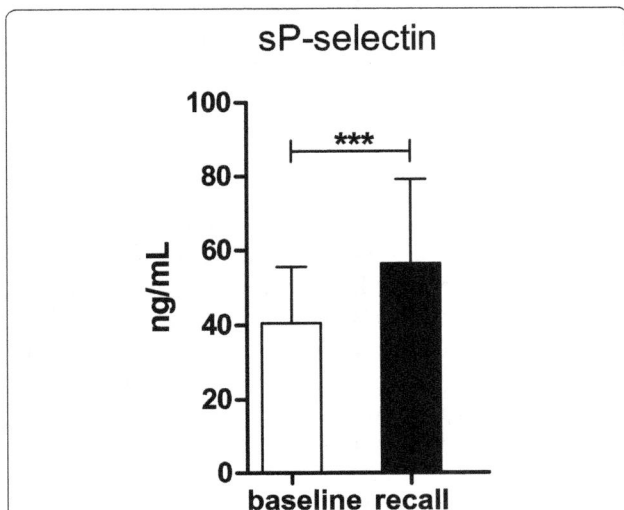

Fig. 4 Concentration of sP-selectin (N = 24) in citrate plasma at baseline (white bars) and recall (black bars). Data are presented as means ± standard deviation. P-value calculated by paired t- test (***P = 0.0008)

increased platelet reactivity, and potentially hypercoagulability with an increased risk for cardiovascular events [17–20]. Periodontitis is a condition characterized by low-grade inflammatory and infectious burden with systemic distribution of pro-inflammatory cytokines or bacterial products. We have previously documented hyper-reactivity of platelets in response to ADP and oral bacteria in untreated periodontitis patients as compared to matched controls [12]. In the current study we show that the improvement in the periodontal condition after non-surgical periodontal therapy is accompanied by a significant reduction in platelet reactivity, as reflected by lower PAC-1 binding, lower P-selectin expression and lower induction of platelet-leukocyte complexes in response to an agonist.

The circulation of leukocytes across the vascular endothelium is required for immune surveillance and for leukocyte recruitment at inflammatory sites. Platelet binding alters the adhesive and migratory phenotype of leukocytes, with platelet-monocyte and platelet-neutrophil complexes being more adhesive, thus resulting in enhanced transmigration through vascular endothelium [21]. Conversely, when the periodontal inflammatory lesions heal after periodontal therapy, the need for recruitment of inflammatory cells will decrease. This could explain our finding of reduced propensity to form platelet-leukocyte complexes after periodontal treatment. A positive side effect of this therapy could result in a reduced participation of platelets and leukocytes to the progression of atherothrombosis [22–24], potentially benefitting the patients at cardiovascular risk.

It has been reported in (systematic) reviews that successful treatment of periodontitis is accompanied by a decrease in systemic markers of inflammation such as CRP or leukocyte counts [25, 26]. In our study the CRP levels and leukocyte counts did not change after periodontal therapy. However, this finding must be interpreted in the context of the strict exclusion criteria we have applied. In this work, patients with any known co-morbidities were excluded. Although inclusion in the study was based on the self-reported health status, which might underestimate the prevalence of a medical condition when compared to diagnosis based on laboratory data [17], we have strong indications that the large majority of our participants were healthy, as only 3 out of 25 fulfilled the criteria for metabolic syndrome [16]. In the most recent meta-analysis of the effects of periodontal treatment on CRP levels, Teeuw and co-workers analyzed and presented separately the results from subjects with periodontitis, but otherwise healthy (without co-morbidities) and those from subjects with co-morbidities. From their meta-analysis it was concluded that it is the patients with co-morbidities that benefit the most from periodontal therapy, showing consistent reduction in CRP levels after treatment, whereas in the group without co-morbidities the change in CRP levels over time after periodontal treatment was not different than in the untreated control group [27]. An explanation for this finding might be the low baseline CRP values in most of the participants in our study (only 3 patients had CRP above the high risk AHA threshold of 3.0 mg/L). Ridker and co-workers reported a significant reduction in the risk for myocardial infarction after aspirin administration in the highest quartile of baseline CRP levels, but not in the lowest quartile [28]. The authors concluded that a certain inflammatory threshold might be necessary before anti-infective/inflammatory treatments can deliver measurable effects, and we suggest that this is the mechanism behind the non-significant change in inflammatory markers in our study population after periodontal treatment.

Interestingly, in the current study, the LDL levels were reduced after periodontal therapy. Our results are in line with previous reports of improved serum lipid levels post periodontal therapy in patients with periodontitis, but otherwise healthy, in the absence of any adjunctive lipid-lowering intervention (dietary advice or pharmacological cholesterol reduction medication) [29, 30]. Similar to the effects that periodontal therapy has on CRP levels, the lipid profiles show greater improvement in periodontitis patients with co-morbidities, e.g. hyperlipidemia, diabetes [31–33].

P-selectin is expressed on the cell surface of platelets and endothelial cells after activation [34], and mediates leukocyte adhesion to these activated cell types. We found a statistically significant, albeit modest, increase 3 months after periodontal therapy of sP-selectin levels. A similar trend post-treatment was observed by Marcaccini et al. [35]. Interestingly, also the unstimulated platelet activation values, representing intrinsic activity, showed a trend of slight increase (Additional file 1). It would be interesting to see in future studies

longer term results (more than 6 months) for these parameters. Activated platelets rapidly shed their membrane-bound P-selectin, which subsequently can be found as circulating sP-selectin [36], while platelets remain functional and responsive to stimulation. Possibly, this latter phenomenon explains why in periodontitis patients we found increased sP-selectin post-therapy, while their platelet reactivity was reduced. However, the increased sP-selectin post-therapy might be a marker of early endothelial function recovery. Previous observations have shown that in vivo, the adhesiveness of the endothelium is controlled by shedding of P-selectin [37]. Moreover, the shed soluble P-selectin is likely to inhibit additional leukocyte adhesion and may have a "calming" effect on the recruited neutrophils [38], which again may be part of the healing processes initiated post-therapy. Indeed, periodontal therapy has been shown to improve endothelial dysfunction [39], and our results provide insights into the cellular players involved.

Although slightly increased post-treatment, the sP-selectin levels in our periodontitis patients were lower than previously reported for both untreated periodontitis or healthy (periodontally unaffected) controls [11, 35]. We are cautious in interpreting these results, mainly because in the current study we measured sP-selectin in citrate plasma, and not in EDTA-plasma, like in the studies by Marcaccini et al. and Papapanagiotou et al. It has been shown that sP-selectin is lower in citrate than in EDTA [40], rendering comparisons between studies employing different anticoagulants highly hazardous.

The most widely used methods for the analysis of platelet function in vitro include global tests for whole blood such as the Platelet Function Analyzer 100 (PFA-100®), Plateletworks®, VerifyNow® or thromboelastography and specific tests such as the light transmission aggregometry (LTA), the flow cytometry-based tests or the ELISA-based tests [41]. Global tests are useful in monitoring the individual on-treatment platelet reactivity in clinical settings [42], however, they lack sensitivity and specificity due to interplay with multiple non-platelet related factors, e.g. plasma-derived adhesion and (anti)-coagulation factors, red blood cells and leukocytes [41]. LTA, on the other hand, enables the analysis of distinct activation mechanisms on isolated platelets (platelet-rich plasma or plasma-depleted platelet preparations) and represents the "gold standard" of platelet function analysis in vitro. However, LTA lacks the attributes needed for a point-of-care test: it requires sample preparation, is time consuming, operator-sensitive and has limited recommendation for monitoring anti-platelet therapy responses [41].

The methods employed in the current study, i.e. the flow cytometric evaluation of platelet surface markers and the determination of soluble P-selectin concentration in plasma by ELISA are both of a static nature. Ideally, platelet functions should be assessed under flow conditions, since some biologically relevant interactions such as that of GP1bα and VWF are relevant under shear stress. The hospital based analyzers such as the PFA-100® and Verify-Now® incorporate some aspect of shear stress, but are limited by the incomplete analysis of hemostasis they generate, the relative big volume of donor blood required and the low throughput [43]. Promising results have been obtained with microfluidic devices demonstrating the ability to obtain a large number of data points per single patient sample using small blood volumes and high throughput approach [44]. Although none of these flow-based assays were available for the current work, a future study should address the effect of periodontal therapy on platelet functions under flow conditions.

One limitation of the current study is the absence of an untreated (control) group. This would consist of periodontitis patients left untreated for the whole duration of the study. However, the inclusion of such a group is unethical, and would be met with strong opposition by the University Ethical Board. Furthermore, such a control group has been shown to be susceptible to a high dropout rate by patients who seek periodontal therapy elsewhere [45]. Nevertheless, on the basis of the current study it is not possible to establish whether the improvement in platelet reactivity is solely related to the professionally-applied periodontal therapy. It cannot be excluded that some patients have changed their lifestyle after receiving information about the negative effects of smoking, over-weight, lack of physical activity or unhealthy diet. The study protocol did not include the assessment of changes in physical activity or diet, which might have been of influence on the measured platelet functions. The LDL levels were lower post-treatment and, by the time of the recall (3 months post-periodontal therapy), six out of the 14 smokers in the current study had quitted smoking. As both LDL and smoking could influence platelet function [46–48], we sought of estimating their effect on the measured platelet parameters by regression analysis. When exploring the predictive value of smoking or the changes in LDL, systolic blood pressure, waist circumference for the measured platelet parameters, no significant effect of these variables was found. However, the study cohort is rather limited, so this conclusion might be underpowered.

In conclusion, our results support the notion of a longitudinal beneficial effect of periodontitis treatment on platelet function. Our results are a promising step towards an increased awareness of the medical community for periodontal therapy as a non-pharmacological intervention for improving platelet function, and given the high prevalence of periodontitis, could potentially benefit a large proportion of the adult population.

Conclusion

In conclusion, we suggest that periodontal therapy as an intervention for improved oral health is one of the emerging factors, in addition to lifestyle changes (nutrition, physical activity and psychological wellbeing) contributing to a reduction of the intrinsic platelet hyper-reactivity, which on the long term can have substantial benefits in preventing major cardiovascular events.

Acknowledgements
We are grateful to all clinical staff and participating patients who made this study possible. We thank S. van Leeuwen and B. Kuypers for their contribution to data analysis.

Funding
B.G. Loos and E.A. Nicu are supported in part by a grant from the University of Amsterdam for the focal point 'Oral infection and inflammation'. Part of the intervention study was supported by an unrestricted grant from Philips Oral Healthcare, Bothell, WA, USA.

Authors' contributions
EA performed experiments, analyzed and interpreted the data and wrote the first draft of the manuscript. SB and EAR selected patients and performed clinical measurements. BGL designed the study and revised the manuscript. EAN designed the study, performed experiments, analyzed and interpreted the data and wrote the manuscript. The final version of the manuscript has been read and approved for submission by all authors.

Competing interests
The authors declare that they have no competing interests.

References
1. Nanci A, Bosshardt DD. Structure of periodontal tissues in health and disease. Periodontol 2000. 2006;40:11–28.
2. Forner L, Larsen T, Kilian M, Holmstrup P. Incidence of bacteremia after chewing, tooth brushing and scaling in individuals with periodontal inflammation. J Clin Periodontol. 2006;33(6):401–7.
3. Chiu B. Multiple infections in carotid atherosclerotic plaques. Am Heart J. 1999;138(5 Pt 2):S534–6.
4. Von Reyn CF, Levy BS, Arbeit RD, Friedland G, Crumpacker CS. Infective endocarditis: An analysis based on strict case definitions. Ann Intern Med. 1981;94(4 pt 1):505–18.
5. Herzberg MC, Brintzenhofe KL, Clawson CC. Aggregation of human platelets and adhesion of streptococcus sanguis. Infect Immun. 1983;39(3):1457–69.
6. Yu KM, Inoue Y, Umeda M, Terasaki H, Chen ZY, Iwai T. The periodontal anaerobe porphyromonas gingivalis induced platelet activation and increased aggregation in whole blood by rat model. Thromb Res. 2011; 127(5):418–25.
7. Assinger A, Laky M, Schabbauer G, Hirschl AM, Buchberger E, Binder BR, et al. Efficient phagocytosis of periodontopathogens by neutrophils requires plasma factors, platelets and tlr2. J Thromb Haemost. 2011;9(4):799–809.
8. Borgeson E, Lonn J, Bergstrom I, Brodin VP, Ramstrom S, Nayeri F, et al. Lipoxin a(4) inhibits porphyromonas gingivalis-induced aggregation and reactive oxygen species production by modulating neutrophil-platelet interaction and cd11b expression. Infect Immun. 2011;79(4):1489–97.
9. Eke PI, Dye BA, Wei L, Thornton-Evans GO, Genco RJ. Cdc Periodontal Disease Surveillance workgroup: James Beck GDRP. Prevalence of periodontitis in adults in the united states: 2009 and 2010. J Dent Res. 2012; 91(10):914–20.

10. Lockhart PB, Bolger AF, Papapanou PN, Osinbowale O, Trevisan M, Levison ME, et al. Periodontal disease and atherosclerotic vascular disease: Does the evidence support an independent association?: A scientific statement from the american heart association. Circulation. 2012;125(20):2520–44.

11. Papapanagiotou D, Nicu EA, Bizzarro S, Gerdes VE, Meijers JC, Nieuwland R, et al. Periodontitis is associated with platelet activation. Atherosclerosis. 2009;202(2):605–11.

12. Nicu EA, Van der Velden U, Nieuwland R, Everts V, Loos BG. Elevated platelet and leukocyte response to oral bacteria in periodontitis. J Thromb Haemost. 2009;7(1):162–70.

13. Bizzarro S, Loos BG, Laine ML, Crielaard W, Zaura E. Subgingival microbiome in smokers and non-smokers in periodontitis: An exploratory study using traditional targeted techniques and a next-generation sequencing. J Clin Periodontol. 2013;40(5):483–92.

14. Shattil SJ, Cunningham M, Hoxie JA. Detection of activated platelets in whole blood using activation-dependent monoclonal antibodies and flow cytometry. Blood. 1987;70(1):307–15.

15. Metzelaar MJ, Sixma JJ, Nieuwenhuis HK. Detection of platelet activation using activation specific monoclonal antibodies. Blood Cells. 1990;16(1):85–93. discussion –6.

16. Grundy SM. Metabolic syndrome pandemic. Arterioscler Thromb Vasc Biol. 2008;28(4):629–36.

17. Akdogan A, Kilic L, Akman U, Dogan I, Karadag O, Bilgen SA, et al. Aspirin resistance in systemic lupus erythematosus. A pilot study. Lupus. 2013;22(8):835–8.

18. Cangemi R, Casciaro M, Rossi E, Calvieri C, Bucci T, Calabrese CM, et al. Platelet activation is associated with myocardial infarction in patients with pneumonia. J Am Coll Cardiol. 2014;64(18):1917–25.

19. Santos-Gallego CG, Badimon JJ. The sum of two evils: Pneumonia and myocardial infarction: Is platelet activation the missing link? J Am Coll Cardiol. 2014;64(18):1926–8.

20. Senchenkova E, Seifert H, Granger DN. Hypercoagulability and platelet abnormalities in inflammatory bowel disease. Semin Thromb Hemost. 2015;41(6):582–9.

21. Page C, Pitchford S. Neutrophil and platelet complexes and their relevance to neutrophil recruitment and activation. Int Immunopharmacol. 2013;17(4):1176–84.

22. Badrnya S, Schrottmaier WC, Kral JB, Yaiw KC, Volf I, Schabbauer G, et al. Platelets mediate oxidized low-density lipoprotein-induced monocyte extravasation and foam cell formation. Arterioscler Thromb Vasc Biol. 2014;34(3):571–80.

23. Santos-Gallego CG, Bayon J, Badimon JJ. Thrombi of different pathologies: Implications for diagnosis and treatment. Curr Treat Options Cardiovasc Med. 2010;12(3):274–91.

24. Santos-Gallego CG, Picatoste B, Badimon JJ. Pathophysiology of acute coronary syndrome. Curr Atheroscler Rep. 2014;16(4):401.

25. Loos BG. Systemic markers of inflammation in periodontitis. J Periodontol. 2005;76(11 Suppl):2106–15.

26. Paraskevas S, Huizinga JD, Loos BG. A systematic review and meta-analyses on c-reactive protein in relation to periodontitis. J Clin Periodontol. 2008;35(4):277–90.

27. Teeuw WJ, Slot DE, Susanto H, Gerdes VE, Abbas F, D'Aiuto F, et al. Treatment of periodontitis improves the atherosclerotic profile: A systematic review and meta-analysis. J Clin Periodontol. 2014;41(1):70–9.

28. Ridker PM, Cushman M, Stampfer MJ, Tracy RP, Hennekens CH. Inflammation, aspirin, and the risk of cardiovascular disease in apparently healthy men. N Engl J Med. 1997;336(14):973–9.

29. Pejcic A, Kesic L, Brkic Z, Pesic Z, Mirkovic D. Effect of periodontal treatment on lipoproteins levels in plasma in patients with periodontitis. South Med J. 2011;104(8):547–52.

30. D'Aiuto F, Parkar M, Nibali L, Suvan J, Lessem J, Tonetti MS. Periodontal infections cause changes in traditional and novel cardiovascular risk factors: Results from a randomized controlled clinical trial. Am Heart J. 2006;151(5):977 84.

31. Fu YW, Li XX, Xu HZ, Gong YQ, Yang Y. Effects of periodontal therapy on serum lipid profile and proinflammatory cytokines in patients with hyperlipidemia: A randomized controlled trial. Clin Oral Investig. 2016;20(6):1263–9.

32. Oz SG, Fentoglu O, Kilicarslan A, Guven GS, Tanrtover MD, Aykac Y, et al. Beneficial effects of periodontal treatment on metabolic control of hypercholesterolemia. South Med J. 2007;100(7):686–91.

33. Sun WL, Chen LL, Zhang SZ, Wu YM, Ren YZ, Qin GM. Inflammatory cytokines, adiponectin, insulin resistance and metabolic control after periodontal intervention in patients with type 2 diabetes and chronic periodontitis. Intern Med. 2011;50(15):1569–74.

34. McEver RP, Beckstead JH, Moore KL, Marshall-Carlson L, Bainton DF. Gmp-140, a platelet alpha-granule membrane protein, is also synthesized by vascular endothelial cells and is localized in weibel-palade bodies. J Clin Invest. 1989;84(1):92–9.

35. Marcaccini AM, Meschiari CA, Sorgi CA, Saraiva MC, de Souza AM, Faccioli LH, et al. Circulating interleukin-6 and high-sensitivity c-reactive protein decrease after periodontal therapy in otherwise healthy subjects. J Periodontol. 2009;80(4):594–602.

36. Michelson AD, Barnard MR, Hechtman HB, MacGregor H, Connolly RJ, Loscalzo J, et al. In vivo tracking of platelets: Circulating degranulated platelets rapidly lose surface p-selectin but continue to circulate and function. Proc Natl Acad Sci U S A. 1996;93(21):11877–82.

37. Hartwell DW, Mayadas TN, Berger G, Frenette PS, Rayburn H, Hynes RO, et al. Role of p-selectin cytoplasmic domain in granular targeting in vivo and in early inflammatory responses. J Cell Biol. 1998;143(4):1129–41.

38. Gamble JR, Skinner MP, Berndt MC, Vadas MA. Prevention of activated neutrophil adhesion to endothelium by soluble adhesion protein gmp140. Science. 1990;249(4967):414–7.

39. Orlandi M, Suvan J, Petrie A, Donos N, Masi S, Hingorani A, et al. Association between periodontal disease and its treatment, flow-mediated dilatation and carotid intima-media thickness: A systematic review and meta-analysis. Atherosclerosis. 2014;236(1):39–46.

40. Thom J, Gilmore G, Yi Q, Hankey GJ, Eikelboom JW. Measurement of soluble p-selectin and soluble cd40 ligand in serum and plasma. J Thromb Haemost. 2004;2(11):2067–9.

41. Jurk K. Analysis of platelet function and dysfunction. Hamostaseologie. 2015;35(1):60–72.

42. Gurbel PA, Becker RC, Mann KG, Steinhubl SR, Michelson AD. Platelet function monitoring in patients with coronary artery disease. J Am Coll Cardiol. 2007;50(19):1822–34.

43. Branchford BR, Ng CJ, Neeves KB, Di Paola J. Microfluidic technology as an emerging clinical tool to evaluate thrombosis and hemostasis. Thromb Res. 2015;136(1):13–9.

44. Conant CG, Nevill JT, Zhou Z, Dong J-F, Schwartz MA, Ionescu-Zanetti C. Using well-plate microfluidic devices to conduct shear-based thrombosis assays. J Assoc Lab Autom. 2011;16(2):148–52.

45. Couper DJ, Beck JD, Falkner KL, Graham SP, Grossi SG, Gunsolley JC, et al. The periodontitis and vascular events (pave) pilot study: Recruitment, retention, and community care controls. J Periodontol. 2008;79(1):80–9.

46. Barua RS, Ambrose JA. Mechanisms of coronary thrombosis in cigarette smoke exposure. Arterioscler Thromb Vasc Biol. 2013;33(7):1460–7.

47. Korporaal SJ, Akkerman JW. Platelet activation by low density lipoprotein and high density lipoprotein. Pathophysiol Haemost Thromb. 2006;35(3–4):270–80.

48. Relou IA, Hackeng CM, Akkerman JW, Malle E. Low-density lipoprotein and its effect on human blood platelets. Cell Mol Life Sci. 2003;60(5):961–71.

16

Preimplantation genetic diagnosis of hemophilia A

Ming Chen[1,2,3,4,5,6*†], Shun-Ping Chang[1,2†], Gwo-Chin Ma[1,2,7,8†], Wen-Hsian Lin[1,2], Hsin-Fu Chen[3], Shee-Uan Chen[3], Horng-Der Tsai[7], Feng-Po Tsai[9] and Ming-Ching Shen[10]

From The 9th Congress of the Asian-Pacific Society on Thrombosis and Hemostasis
Taipei, Taiwan.

Abstract

Preimplantation genetic diagnosis (PGD) is a powerful tool to tackle the transmission of monogenic inherited disorders in families carrying the diseases from generation to generation. It currently remains a challenging task, despite PGD having been developed over 25 years ago. The major difficulty is it does not have an easy and general formula for all mutations. Different gene locus needs individualized, customized design to make the diagnosis accurate enough to be applied on PGD, in which the quantity of DNA is scanty, whereas timely laboratory diagnosis is mandatory if fresh embryo transfer is desired occasionally. Indicators for outcome assessment of a successful PGD program include the successful diagnosis rate on blastomeres (Day 3 cleavage-stage embryo biopsy) or trophectoderm cells (Day 5/6 blastocyst biopsy), the implantation rate per embryo transferred, and the livebirth rate per oocyte retrieval cycle. Hemophilia A (HA) is an X-linked recessive bleeding disorder caused by various types of pathological defects in the factor VIII gene (*F8*). The mutation spectrum of the *F8* is complex, according to our previous report, including large segmental intra-gene inversions, large segmental deletions spanning a few exons, point mutations, and total deletion caused by chromosomal structural rearrangements. In this review, the molecular methodologies used to tackle different mutants of the *F8* in the PGD of HA are to be explained, and the experiences of successful use of amplification refractory mutation system-quantitative polymerase chain reaction (ARMS-qPCR) and linkage analysis for PGD of HA in our laboratory are also provided.

Keywords: PGD, ARMS-qPCR, Linkage analysis, STR marker, Polymorphism

Abbreviations: ADO, Allele dropout; ARMS-qPCR, Amplification refractory mutation system-quantitative polymerase chain reaction; FISH, Fluorescence in situ hybridization; HA, Hemophilia A; HGMD, Human gene mutation database; INV1, Intron 1 inversion; INV22, Intron 22 inversion; I-PCR, Inverse polymerase chain reaction; long-distance PCR, Long-distance polymerase chain reaction; MLPA, Multiplex ligation-dependent probe amplification; NGS, Next generation sequencing; PGD, Preimplantation genetic diagnosis; PGS, Preimplantation genetic screening; STR, Short tandem repeat; WGA, Whole genome amplification

* Correspondence: mingchenmd@gmail.com; mchen_cch@yahoo.com
†Equal contributors
[1]Department of Genomic Medicine and Center for Medical Genetics, Changhua Christian Hospital, Changhua, Taiwan
[2]Department of Genomic Science and Technology, Changhua Christian Hospital Healthcare System, Changhua, Taiwan
Full list of author information is available at the end of the article

Background

Preimplantation genetic diagnosis (PGD) had become a standard of care when dealing with stopping the transmission of the heritable disease from generation to generation since it was firstly introduced in 1990 [1, 2]. The gold standard of molecular technology used for PGD nowadays is the coamplification of the polymorphic microsatellite linkage markers [3, 4]. However, such techniques cannot avoid the possibility of recombination occurred within the segment which separated the linked polymorphic markers and the disease loci, and it is advised to combine more informative linkage markers to reduce the chance of misdiagnosis. On the other hand, direct mutation detection assay, either rapid PCR-based or the more time-consuming sequencing-based genotyping platforms, is prone to allele dropout (ADO), which may ensue a catastrophic false-negative misdiagnosis in PGD of autosomal dominant monogenic disorder [4, 5].

Hemophilia A (HA) (OMIM 306700), a bleeding disorder which causes long-term disability, is a X-linked recessive disorder and its causative gene is situated at Xq28, the factor VIII (*F8*) gene, is a serious threat for public health in Taiwan, and we had first published its mutation spectrum in the Taiwanese population in 2008 [6]. The mutation spectrum included rearrangements such as intron 1 inversions (INV1) and intron 22 inversions (INV22), large deletions spanning for consecutive exons, small deletions involving only a few base pairs, and point mutations [6]. The broad spectra of F8 mutations have also been reported in several other studies [7–9]. The genotyping itself for the *F8* is already a daunting task given its complicated existing mutations patterns, let alone the PGD. In spite of the challenges, we managed to tackle these difficulties in a few families who came to our hospital seeking for PGD. Meanwhile, a few similar efforts had been reported from other laboratories [10, 11], which indicates PGD for HA is feasible, at least in those families the mutation has been confirmed. Here we will give a concise review of PGD for HA, including the different molecular technologies used to tackle different mutation patterns, and also to cite a few of our experience with successful outcome, that is, to give birth to normal unaffected babies in families suffered from HA.

Review

Mutation spectrum of the F8 gene, genotyping strategies, and possible PGD approaches

Since the publication of the sequence of the *F8* in 1984, more than 2000 gene mutations causing HA have been described and these are catalogued in the Human Gene Mutation Database (HGMD; http://www.hgmd.cf.ac.uk/ac/index.php) and Factor VIII Variant Database (http://www.factorviii-db.org/). In 2008, we had first published the mutation spectrum in the Taiwanese population [6]. Of 31 unrelated HA patients (19 severe and 10 moderate/mild males, and 2 severe females), 12 (38.7 %) and 1 (3.2 %) severe males were genotyped with INV22 and INV1 respectively. The *F8* defects in the remaining 18 inversion-negative patients cover a wide spectrum, in which 17 different mutations were identified (10 missense and 3 nonsense mutations, and 2 small and 2 large deletions). Eleven of these mutations are novel and unique, confirming a high diversity of molecular defects in HA [6]. A systematic review for data from 30 studies on 5383 patients had been reported and showed 45 % of HA had INV22, 2 % INV1, 3 % large deletions, 16 % small deletions or insertions, and 28 % point mutations (15 % missense mutations, 10 % nonsense mutations, and 3 % splicing site mutations). In 4.6 % of patients, the mutation was unknown [12]. Overall, with the exceptions of recurrent INV22 and INV1, no mutation hot spots have been identified.

There are a number of different approaches for the genotyping of HA (Table 1). For reasons of rapid and smart screening, however, targeted mutation analysis for the recurrent INV22 and INV1 has become the first test assessed in patients (particularly in severely affected hemophiliacs). INV22 can be detected by Southern blotting or, more time- and labor-saving choice, by long-distance polymerase chain reaction (long-distance PCR) or inverse PCR (I-PCR) [13, 14]. INV1 is typically detected by multiplex PCR [15]. Other mutations responsible for HA are mostly point mutation and small deletion/insertion in the *F8* gene and their spectrum is quite complex. In these cases, mutation can be detected by PCR with a number of screening methods (e.g., single strand conformational polymorphism, conformation sensitive gel electrophoresis, amplification and mismatch detection, denaturing gradient gel electrophoresis) followed by direct DNA sequencing [16–21]. For female patients with only one mutation detected and also in those females suspected to be carriers but no mutation could be found, gene dosage assays such as multiplex ligation-dependent probe amplification (MLPA) should be applied to screen for the underlying exon deletions since deletions in single allele usually escape detection by the PCR-based analysis, due to the masking of the non-deleted allele. In Fig. 1, we exemplified the MLPA finding of a female HA patient who was karyotyped as 45,X [22]/46,X,idic(X)(q21) [8] mosaicism. Her aberrant X-chromosome (idic(X)(q21)) do not contain the Xq22q28 (and thus *F8* gene) and familiar follow-up studies demonstrate this anomaly is of *de novo*. PCR amplification for exon1-22 of the *F8* is failure in patient but is successful in her parents. Through the MLPA analyses, it is evidenced that the patient carries an exon 1–22 deletion in the allele on her "morphologically-normal" X-chromosome, which is inherited from her mother (Fig. 1).

Table 1 Genotype-phenotype relationship, genetic testing and preimplantation genetic diagnosis (PGD) in hemophilia A

Mutation type	Frequency of occurrence[a]	Clinical severity[b]	Test method	PGD method
Inversion • INV22 • INV1	47 % • 45 % • 2 %	Severe	• I-PCR (for INV22) • Long-distance PCR (for INV22) • Southern blotting (for INV22) • Multiplex PCR (for INV1)	• Linkage analysis
Point mutation • Missense • Nonsense • Splicing site	28 % • 15 % • 10 % • 3 %	Mild, Moderate, Severe • Mild, Moderate (majority) • Severe (majority) • Severe (majority)	Direct DNA sequencing	• ARMS-qPCR • Linkage analysis
Small deletion/insertion (<1 exon)	16 %	Severe (majority)	Direct DNA sequencing	• ARMS-qPCR • Linkage analysis
Large deletion (≥1 exon)	3 %	Severe (majority)	MLPA	• Linkage analysis
Others (e.g., Complex rearrangement)	NA	Severe (majority)	Depending on mutation entities	• Linkage analysis

MLPA multiplex ligation-dependent probe amplification, *I-PCR* inverse polymerase chain reaction, *ARMS* amplification refractory mutation system, *NA* not available
[a]See the review in Gouw et al., [12]
[b]HA patients are clinically divided into three different severities based on the residual FVIII coagulant activity (FVIII:C): severe (FVIII:C < 1 % of normal level), moderate (FVIII:C is 1–5 % of normal level) and mild (FVIII:C is 5–30 % of normal level)

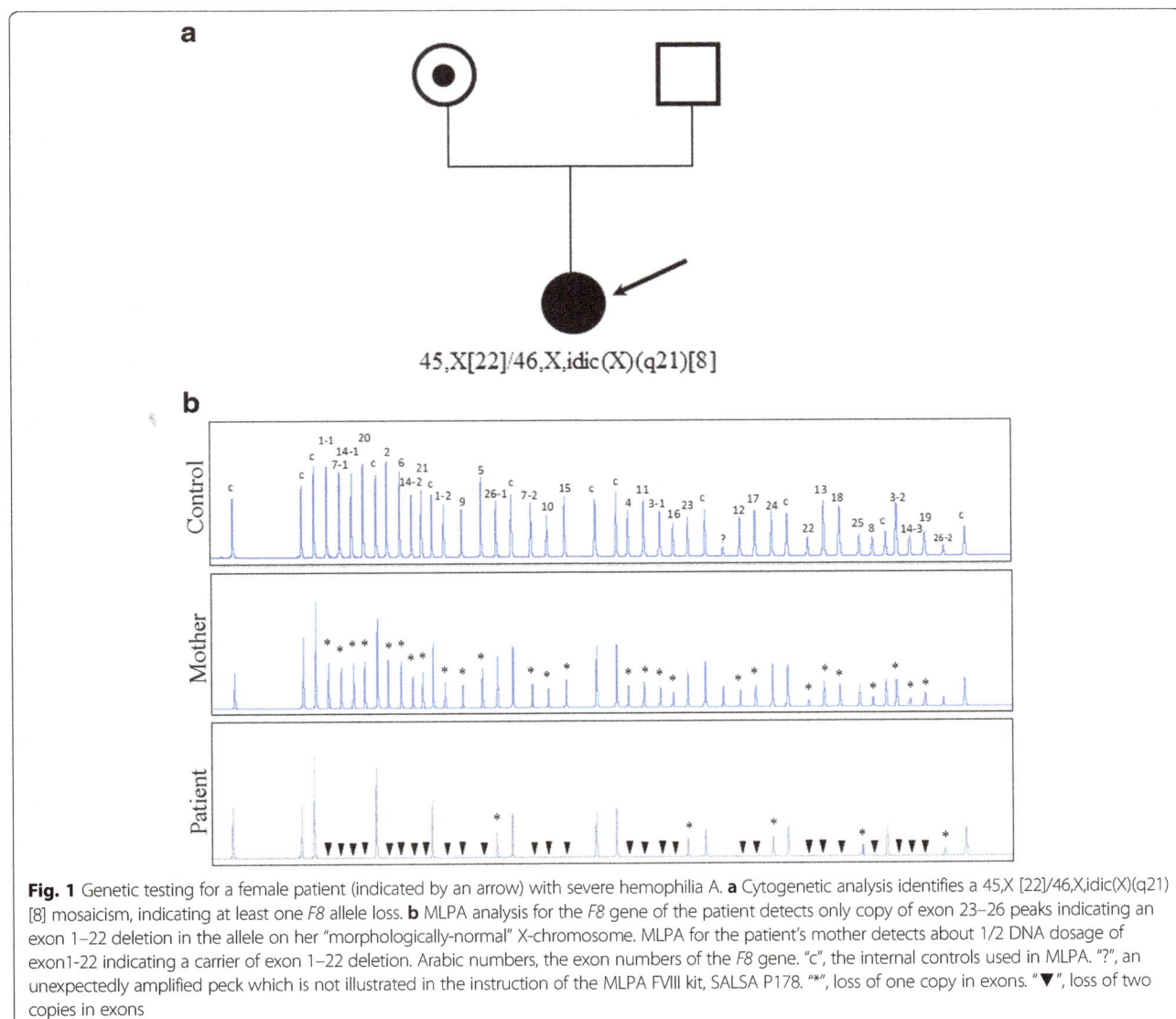

Fig. 1 Genetic testing for a female patient (indicated by an arrow) with severe hemophilia A. **a** Cytogenetic analysis identifies a 45,X [22]/46,X,idic(X)(q21) [8] mosaicism, indicating at least one *F8* allele loss. **b** MLPA analysis for the *F8* gene of the patient detects only copy of exon 23–26 peaks indicating an exon 1–22 deletion in the allele on her "morphologically-normal" X-chromosome. MLPA for the patient's mother detects about 1/2 DNA dosage of exon1-22 indicating a carrier of exon 1–22 deletion. Arabic numbers, the exon numbers of the *F8* gene. "c", the internal controls used in MLPA. "?", an unexpectedly amplified peck which is not illustrated in the instruction of the MLPA FVIII kit, SALSA P178. "*", loss of one copy in exons. "▼", loss of two copies in exons

Given the marked morbidity associated with severe HA, PGD has become a feasible option for couples at risk of having a child with HA since it reduces the risk of termination of affected pregnancies. Gender selection by fluorescence in situ hybridization (FISH) and transfer of only female embryos is a simple strategy for X-linked recessive disorders, such as HA, and has been adopted in many clinics [11]. However, in practice, gender selection is illegal in some countries (e.g., Taiwan) and methods allowing the correct and more definitive diagnosis of the HA status of every embryo are more desirable because the number of embryos available for transfer is increased. PGD involving whole genome amplification (WGA) step was broadly applied to mutation detection strategies, but the high rate of amplification bias renders WGA an imperfect option [22]. Recently, co-amplification of polymorphic microsatellite markers, linked with the targeted mutation, had been the gold-standard genotyping strategy for PGD [4, 23–26] (Table 1). A linkage approach using polymorphic markers located near the mutation allows monitoring the occurrence of allele dropout, a known problem associated with PCR amplification bias in PGD. Below, we describe our experience with two HA families seeking for PGD.

Experience of PGD of hemophilia A in our laboratory

Two Taiwanese couples were referred to our center for PGD of HA. Preliminary genetic testing of *F8* for two couples showed the two wives are both HA carriers: one has a splicing site mutation, c.1538-1G > A, and the other has a common INV22. For the family with c.1538-1G > A mutation, an in-house developed duplex-nested ARMS-qPCR was customized designed for PGD [4, 5]. The optimized PGD protocol was then performed to detect the disease-causing mutation in embryos acquired after ovarian stimulation. Seven single blastomeres biopsied from corresponding day-3 (8-cell cleavage-stage) embryos were collected and examined independently in a sterile PCR tube. Each blastomere cell was lysed with 125 µg/mL proteinase K at 50 °C for 60 min and inactivated at 99 °C for 4 min. Duplex-nested PCR was then used to amplify the intron 10–11 region of *F8* gene, which includes the targeted mutation. The two primer sets, designed based on the reverse strand's *F8* gene sequence, were OF: CTGAGGACCCATTACCCTGA and OR: CCTGCAACAGTGCTACATGC for the first PCR (amplicon size: 937 bp), and IF: CTTGCTCC CTTTCCTCACAG and IR: TGGGGAGGATCAGCTA-GAGA for the secondary PCR (amplicon size: 757 bp) (Fig. 2a). The first PCR was carried out in a 40 µL reaction, consisting of 1X PCR buffer, 1.25 mmol/L MgCl₂, 0.35 mmol/L dNTP, each 0.5 µmol/L of OF and OR primer, 1X GC-RICH solution, and 1U Faststart Taq

DNA polymerase (Roche Diagnostics GmbH, Mannheim, Germany). The cycling conditions were 95 °C, 5 min, followed by 25 cycles of 95 °C, 30 s, 55 °C, 30 s and 71 °C, 1 min, and a final extension at 71 °C, 2 min. The PCR products were directly subjected to the second round of PCR by adding 10 µL PCR supplement with a similar PCR mixture to that used in the first PCR, except for the primer set (IF and IR). Cycling conditions were similar to the first PCR, but the number of cycles in the second step was increased from 25 to 40. To ensure an accuracy of the PCR, amplified fragments were confirmed by direct sequencing. For ARMS-qPCR, two sequence-specific forward primers, modified with a mismatch at the penultimate nucleotide position of the mutation site to increase the specificity of the reaction, were designed: (MUF: TATGGTTTTGCTTGTGGGT GA for the mutant allele and WTF: TATGGTTTT GCTTGTGGGTGG for the wild-type allele). The two forward primers were respectively paired with the same reverse primer 3rdR: TGAGGAGAGGGCCAATGAGT (amplicon size:198 bp) (Fig. 2b). The ARMS-qPCR performed on the LightCycler 480 Real-Time PCR System (Roche, Mannheim, Germany) in a 20 µL reaction, consisted of 0.5 ng of the duplex-nested PCR product, 0.5 µmol/L of each primer, 1X SYBR Green PCR Master Mix (Finnzymes, Espoo, Finland). Cycling conditions were: 95 °C, 10 min, followed by 45 cycles at 95 °C, 10 s, 60 °C and 60 s. The exemplified results of ARMS-qPCR were shown in Fig. 2c. Of the seven blastomeres examined, two were reported as affected embryos with the homo- or hemizygous c.1538-1G > A mutation, one was known as a heterozygous carrier, and the remaining four were presented as same as wild-type pattern without the mutation. However, only one unaffected embryo kept good morphology and was transferred on day 5. After 39 weeks of uneventful gestation, one healthy baby girl was born successfully with a birth weight of 3040 g. Postnatal genotyping confirmed the girl to be an unaffected carrier and, interestingly, she was HLA-compatible with her older brother affected by HA (see family 1 in Fig. 3).

The INV22 of *F8* is one of the most frequent cause of severe HA, known as a result of homologous recombination between the int22h-1 region within the *F8* locus and either int22h-2 (Inv22 type II) or int22h-3 (Inv22 type I), which lie nearly 400 kb distal to *F8* [27]. The gene rearrangements tend to increase the difficulty of PGD experimental design performed in the affected families. In the second PGD family with *F8* INV22 mutation, the couple (2–1 and 2–2) has had a healthy boy and they would like to get more babies without HA. We performed 3 PGD cycles of HA during the period of Sep. 2014 to Dec. 2015 using short tandem repeat (STR) markers and capillary electrophoresis for direct linkage

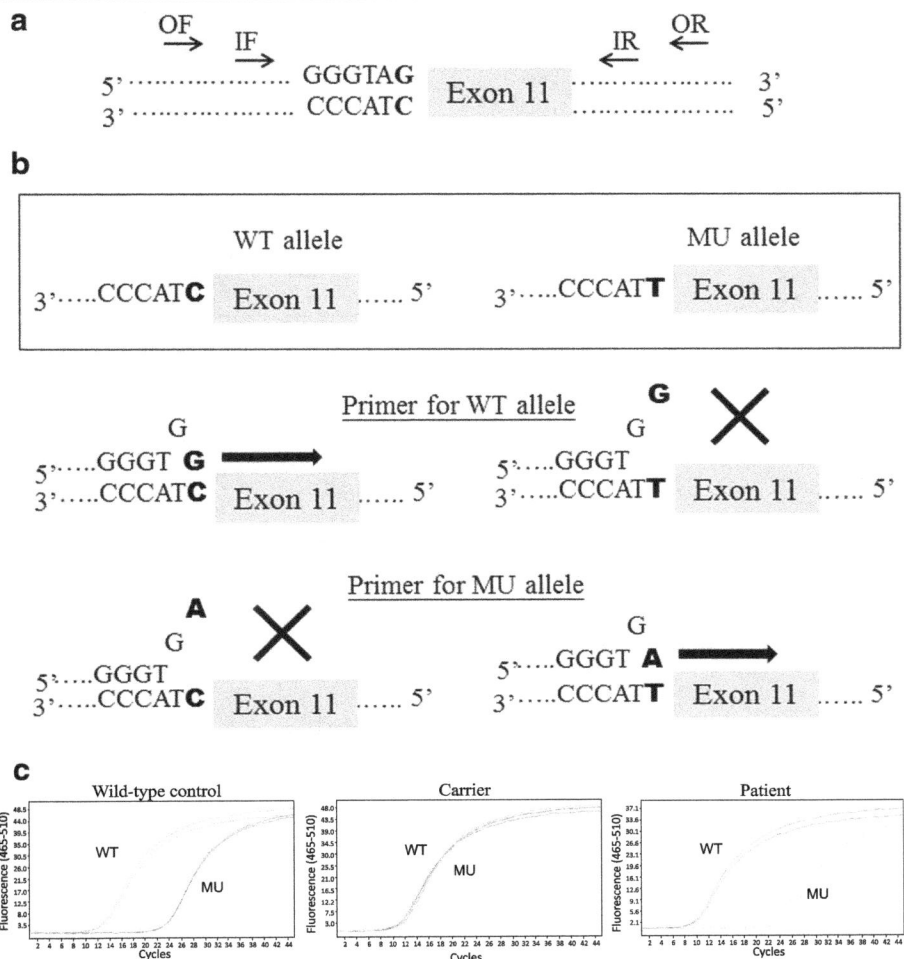

Fig. 2 Schematic diagram of a duplex-nested ARMS-qPCR for PGD of a splicing-site point mutation, located at the junction of intron 10 and exon 11 of *F8*, c.1538-1G > A (bold letter). **a** Primers for duplex-nested PCR were first designed to amplify the region covering the position of the mutation. OF and OR indicate the outer primer set, and IF and IR indicate inner primer set. **b** Primers specific for the amplification of the wild-type (WT) and mutant (MU) alleles, respectively, were subsequently used for ARMS-qPCR where the duplex-nested PCR amplicon was used as DNA template. **c** Representative ARMS-qPCR results for wild-type control (homozygous WT/WT or hemizygous WT), female carrier (heterozygous WT/MU), and affected male individual (hemizygous MU)

analysis. Five informative STR markers distributed within or near the flanking region of the *F8* were selected for PGD performing (see family 2 in Fig. 3). Among a total of 19 examined embryos, 5 wild types and 4 INV22 carriers were selected and transferred during the period. Unfortunately, pregnancy outcome did not occur as expected, possibly due to ad maternal age, embryo morphology, development and other abnormalities. Despite the fact that no pregnancy was achieved in the PGD experience so far, they are still willing to keep trying.

Discussion

The outcome indicators of PGD can be classified as successful diagnosis rate (the number of embryos which

diagnosis was made/the total number of embryos being biopsied), implantation rate (the number of embryos implanted/the total number of embryos being transferred), and the live-birth rate (the rate of liveborn pregnancy per transferred cycle or the rate of liveborn pregnancy per oocyte-retrieval). It is now still under debate whether frozen or fresh embryo transfer can achieve a better outcome against the other. However, it is vitally important that PGD laboratories developed a timely genotyping platform to cope with the need of fresh embryo transfer, especially when Day 5/6 blastocyst biopsy is undertaken. For rapid PGD of HA, the direct mutation detection, e.g., ARMS-qPCR, can greatly increase the reliability of mutation detection in embryos with small insertions/deletion and point mutations (see the exemplified

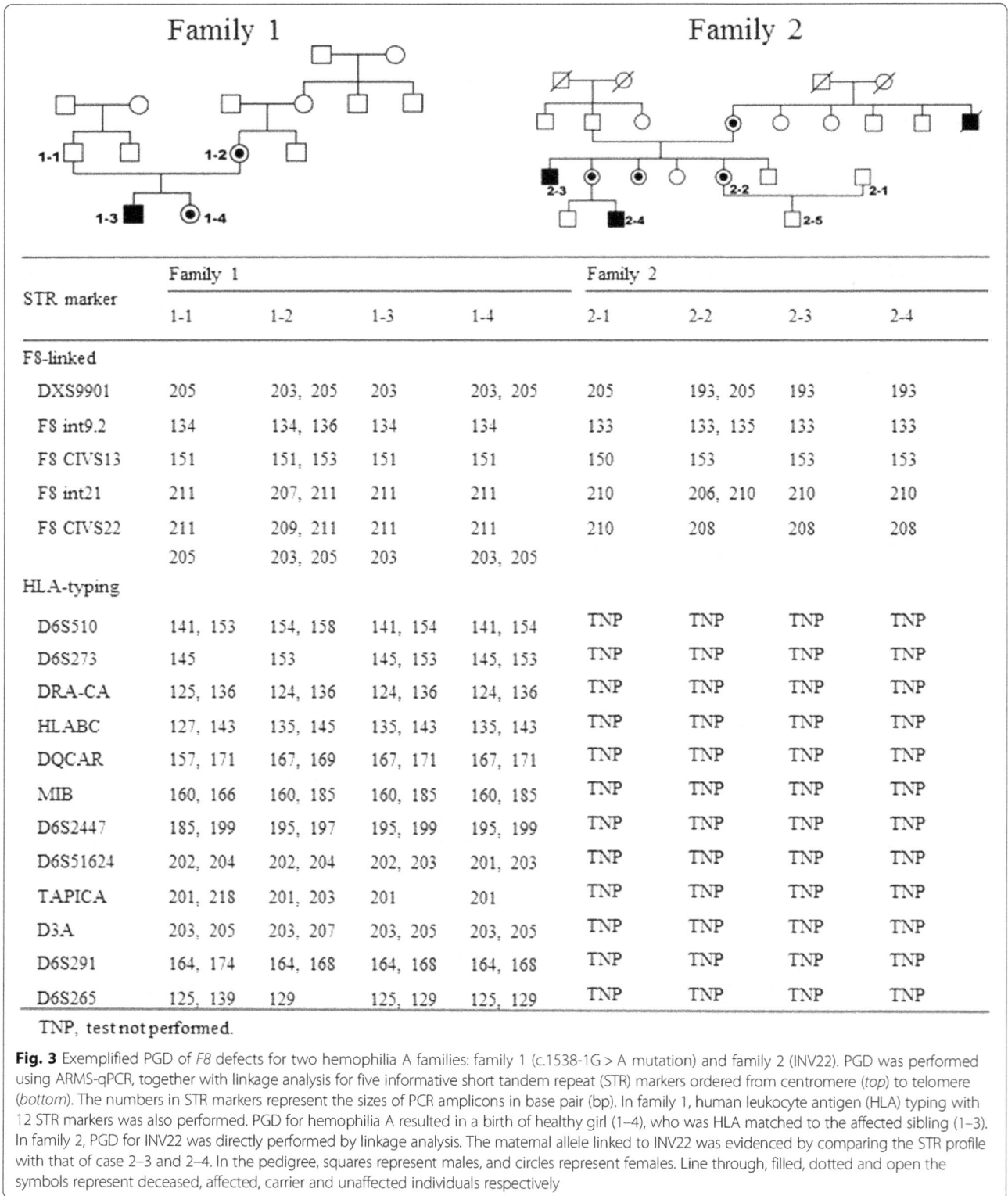

STR marker	Family 1				Family 2			
	1-1	1-2	1-3	1-4	2-1	2-2	2-3	2-4
F8-linked								
DXS9901	205	203, 205	203	203, 205	205	193, 205	193	193
F8 int9.2	134	134, 136	134	134	133	133, 135	133	133
F8 CIVS13	151	151, 153	151	151	150	153	153	153
F8 int21	211	207, 211	211	211	210	206, 210	210	210
F8 CIVS22	211	209, 211	211	211	210	208	208	208
	205	203, 205	203	203, 205				
HLA-typing								
D6S510	141, 153	154, 158	141, 154	141, 154	TNP	TNP	TNP	TNP
D6S273	145	153	145, 153	145, 153	TNP	TNP	TNP	TNP
DRA-CA	125, 136	124, 136	124, 136	124, 136	TNP	TNP	TNP	TNP
HLABC	127, 143	135, 145	135, 143	135, 143	TNP	TNP	TNP	TNP
DQCAR	157, 171	167, 169	167, 171	167, 171	TNP	TNP	TNP	TNP
MIB	160, 166	160, 185	160, 185	160, 185	TNP	TNP	TNP	TNP
D6S2447	185, 199	195, 197	195, 199	195, 199	TNP	TNP	TNP	TNP
D6S51624	202, 204	202, 204	202, 203	201, 203	TNP	TNP	TNP	TNP
TAPICA	201, 218	201, 203	201	201	TNP	TNP	TNP	TNP
D3A	203, 205	203, 207	203, 205	203, 205	TNP	TNP	TNP	TNP
D6S291	164, 174	164, 168	164, 168	164, 168	TNP	TNP	TNP	TNP
D6S265	125, 139	129	125, 129	125, 129	TNP	TNP	TNP	TNP

TNP, test not performed.

Fig. 3 Exemplified PGD of *F8* defects for two hemophilia A families: family 1 (c.1538-1G > A mutation) and family 2 (INV22). PGD was performed using ARMS-qPCR, together with linkage analysis for five informative short tandem repeat (STR) markers ordered from centromere (*top*) to telomere (*bottom*). The numbers in STR markers represent the sizes of PCR amplicons in base pair (bp). In family 1, human leukocyte antigen (HLA) typing with 12 STR markers was also performed. PGD for hemophilia A resulted in a birth of healthy girl (1–4), who was HLA matched to the affected sibling (1–3). In family 2, PGD for INV22 was directly performed by linkage analysis. The maternal allele linked to INV22 was evidenced by comparing the STR profile with that of case 2–3 and 2–4. In the pedigree, squares represent males, and circles represent females. Line through, filled, dotted and open the symbols represent deceased, affected, carrier and unaffected individuals respectively

couple 1). However, for large and complex *F8* defects, e.g., INV1 and INV22, PGD by direct genotyping is not easily feasible and indirect linkage analysis with informative markers may be considered (see the exemplified couple 2). Of noted, the chance of recombination between the markers and mutation can lead to small diagnostic error and some families may not be informative for any of the available markers.

Recently, it is noteworthy that because of the popularity of preimplantation genetic screening (PGS), there is a growing need of concurrent PGD/PGS. At the moment the strategies used in PGS, if we exclude the outdated FISH-based diagnostics [28], include array-based (either array comparative genomic hybridization or single nucleotide polymorphism chromosomal microarray) techniques [29–31], q-PCR based techniques [32, 33], and next generation sequencing (NGS)-based techniques [34, 35]. Some of the techniques had been reported to successfully being applied in PGD combined with PGS [36–39]. It is inevitable that in the near future, women will opt for select the unaffected embryos with certain heritable monogenic disorders, such as HA, as well as the euploid embryos which will reduce the chance of abortion due to aneuploidy in the later gestational period or improved the implantation rate as many researchers advocated [40]. However, it will be undisputable only after more convincing randomized trials to prove the efficacy of PGS, the combination of PGD and PGS should be offered to all women underwent PGD [41]. Those couple who opted for PGD combined with PGS should be counseled that double selection will inevitable reduce the number of embryos which are classified as "suitable" for transfer, thereby reducing all the outcome indicators of PGD, the most important live-birth rate is certainly included.

Conclusions

PGD of HA by direct mutation analysis or indirect linkage analysis has become a feasible option for couples at risk of having an affected child. However, given the broad spectra of the *F8* mutations, genetic counseling along with the technical aspects of the accuracy and limitations of tests should be provided for couples who request PGD.

Acknowledgements
This study was partially supported by grants from Changhua Christian Hospital to M. Chen and to M-C. Shen.

Authors' contributions
MC, SPC, GCM designed the study. MCS recruited the patients. MCS, HFC, SUC, HDT, FPT collected the clinical data. MC, SPC, GCM, WHL did the experiments and performed the analyses. MC, SPC, GCM wrote the paper. All authors read and approved the final manuscript.

Competing interests
The authors declare that they have no competing interests.

Author details
[1]Department of Genomic Medicine and Center for Medical Genetics, Changhua Christian Hospital, Changhua, Taiwan. [2]Department of Genomic Science and Technology, Changhua Christian Hospital Healthcare System, Changhua, Taiwan. [3]Department of Obstetrics and Gynecology, College of Medicine and Hospital, National Taiwan University, Taipei, Taiwan. [4]Department of Medical Genetics, National Taiwan University Hospital, Taipei, Taiwan. [5]Department of Life Science, Tunghai University, Taichung, Taiwan. [6]Department of Obstetrics and Gynecology, Changhua Christian Hospital, Changhua, Taiwan. [7]Institute of Biochemistry, Microbiology and Immunology, Chung Shan Medical University, Taichung, Taiwan. [8]Department of Medical Laboratory Science and Biotechnology, Central Taiwan University of Science and Technology, Taichung, Taiwan. [9]Po-Yuan Women's Clinic and IVF Center, Changhua, Taiwan. [10]Department of Internal Medicine, and Thrombosis and Hemostasis Center, Changhua Christian Hospital, Changhua, Taiwan.

References
1. Handyside A, Kontogianni EH, Hardy K, Winston RM. Pregnancies from biopsied human preimplantation embryos sexed by Y-specific DNA amplification. Nature. 1990;344:768–70.
2. Brezina PR, Brezina DS, Kearns WG. Preimplantation genetic testing. BMJ. 2012;345:e5908.
3. Harton GL, De Rycke M, Fiorentino F, Moutou C, SenGupta S, Traeger-Synodinos J, et al. European Society for Human Reproduction and Embryology (ESHRE) PGD Consortium: ESHRE PGD consortium best practice guidelines for amplification-based PGD. Human Reprod. 2011;26:33–40.
4. Chen HF, Chang SP, Wu SH, Lin WH, Lee YC, Ni YH, et al. Validating a rapid, real-time, PCR-based direct mutation detection assay for preimplantation genetic diagnosis. Gene. 2014;548:299–305.
5. Kuo SJ, Ma GC, Chang SP, Wu HH, Chen CP, Chang TM, et al. Preimplantation and prenatal genetic diagnosis of aromatic L-amino acid decarboxylase deficiency with an amplification-refractory mutation system-quantitative polymerase chain reaction. Taiwan J Obstet Gynecol. 2011;50:468–73.
6. Ma GC, Chang SP, Chen M, Kuo SJ, Chang CS, Shen MC. The mutation spectrum of the factor 8 (F8) defects in Taiwanese patients with severe hemophilia A. Haemophilia. 2008;14:787–95.
7. Bogdanova N, Markoff A, Pollmann H, Nowak-Göttl U, Eisert R, Wermes C, et al. Spectrum of molecular defects and mutation detection rate in patients with severe hemophilia A. Hum Mutat. 2005;26:249–54.
8. Guillet B, Lambert T, d'Oiron R, Proulle V, Plantier JL, Rafowicz A, Peynet J, et al. Detection of 95 novel mutations in coagulation factor VIII gene F8 responsible for hemophilia A: results from a single institution. Hum Mutat. 2006;27:676–85.
9. Bogdanova N, Markoff A, Eisert R, Wermes C, Pollmann H, Todorova A, et al. Spectrum of molecular defects and mutation detection rate in patients with mild and moderate hemophilia A. Hum Mutat. 2007;28:54–60.
10. Laurie AD, Hill AM, Harraway JR, Phillipson GT, Benny PS, Smith MP, et al. Preimplantation genetic diagnosis of hemophilia A using indirect linkage analysis and direct genotyping approaches. J Thrombo Haemost. 2010;8:783–9.
11. Fernández RM, Peciña A, Sánchez B, Lozano-Arana MD, García-Lozano JC, Pérez-Garrido R, et al. Experience of preimplantation genetic diagnosis for hemophilia at the University Hospital Virgen Del Rocio in Spain: Technical and clinical overview. Biomed Res Int. 2015;2015:406096.
12. Gouw SC, van den Berg HM, Oldenburg J, Astermark J, de Groot PG, Margaglione M, et al. F8 gene mutation type and inhibitor development in patients with severe hemophilia A: systematic review and meta-analysis. Blood. 2012;119:2922–34.
13. Liu Q, Nozari G, Sommer SS. Single-tube polymerase chain reaction for rapid diagnosis of the inversion hotspot of mutation in haemophilia A. Blood. 1998;92:1458–9.
14. Rossetti LC, Radic CP, Larripa IB, De Brasi CD. Genotyping the hemophilia inversion hotspot by use of inverse PCR. Clin Chem. 2005;51:1154–8.
15. Bagnall RD, Waseem N, Green PM, Giannelli F. Recurrent inversion breaking intron 1 of the factor VIII gene is a frequent cause of severe hemophilia A. Blood. 2002;99:168–74.

16. Tantawy AAG. Molecular genetics of hemophilia A: clinical perspectives. Egypt J Med Hum Genet. 2010;11:105–14.

17. Shetty S, Ghosh K, Mohanty D. Alternate strategies for carrier detection and antenatal diagnosis in haemophilias in developing countries. Indian J Hum Genet. 2003;9:5–9.

18. Mitchell M, Keeney S, Goodeve A. UK Haemophilia Centre Doctors' Organization Haemophilia Genetics Laboratory Network. The molecular analysis of haemophilia A: a guideline from the UK haemophilia centre doctors' organization haemophilia genetics laboratory network. Haemophilia. 2005;11:387–97.

19. Peyvandi F, Jayandharan G, Chandy M, Srivastava A, Nakaya SM, Johnson MJ, et al. Genetic diagnosis of haemophilia and other inherited bleeding disorders. Haemophilia. 2006;12 Suppl 3:82–9.

20. Castaldo G, D'Argenio V, Nardiello P, Zarrilli F, Sanna V, Rocino A, et al. Haemophilia A: molecular insights. Clin Chem Lab Med. 2007;45:450–61.

21. Goodeve A. Molecular genetic testing of hemophilia A. Semin Thromb Hemost. 2008;34:491–501.

22. Renwick PJ, Lewis CM, Abbs S, Ogilvie CM. Determination of the genetic status of cleavage-stage human embryos by microsatellite marker analysis following multiple displacement amplification. Prenat Diagn. 2007;27:206–15.

23. Laurie AD, Hill AM, Harraway JR, Fellowes AP, Phillipson GT, Benny PS, et al. Preimplantation genetic diagnosis for hemophilia A using indirect linkage analysis and direct genotyping approaches. J Thromb Haemost. 2010;8:783–9.

24. Chang LJ, Huang CC, Tsai YY, Hung CC, Fang MY, Lin YC, et al. Blastocyst biopsy and vitrification are effective for preimplantation genetic diagnosis of monogenic diseases. Hum Reprod. 2013;28:1435–44.

25. De Rycke M, Georgiou I, Sermon K, Lissens W, Henderix P, Joris H, et al. PGD for autosomal dominant polycystic kidney disease type 1. Mol Hum Reprod. 2005;11:65–71.

26. Korzebor A, Derakhshandeh-Peykar P, Meshkani M, Hoseini A, Rafati M, Purhoseini M, et al. Heterozygosity assessment of five STR loci located at 5q13 region for preimplantation genetic diagnosis ofspinal muscular atrophy. Mol Biol Rep. 2013;40:67–72.

27. Naylor JA, Buck D, Green P, Williamson H, Bentley D, Gianneill F. Investigation of the factor VIII intron 22 repeated region (int22h) and the associated inversion junctions. Hum Mol Genet. 1995;4:1217–24.

28. Mastenbroek S, Twisk M, van der Veen F, Repping S. Preimplantation genetic screening: a systematic review and meta-analysis of RCTs. Hum Reprod Update. 2011;17:454–66.

29. Schoolcraft WB, Treff NR, Stevens JM, Ferry K, Katz-Jaffe M, Scott Jr RT. Live birth outcome with trophectoderm biopsy, blastocyst vitrification, and single-nucleotide polymorphism microarray-based comprehensive chromosome screening in infertile patients. Fertil Steril. 2011;96:638–40.

30. Treff NR, Levy B, Su J, Taylor D, Scott Jr RT. Development and validation of an accurate quantitative real-time polymerase chain reaction- based assay for human blastocyst comprehensive chromosomal aneuploidy screening. Fertil Steril. 2012;97:819–24.

31. Rubio C, Rodrigo L, Mir P, Mateu E, Peinado V, Milán M, et al. Use of array comparative genomic hybridization (array-CGH) for embryo assessment: clinical results. Fertil Steril. 2013;99:1044–8.

32. Treff NR, Tao X, Ferry KM, Su J, Taylor D, Scott Jr RT. Development and validation of an accurate quantitative real-time polymerase chain reaction-based assay for human blastocyst comprehensive chromosomal aneuploidy screening. Fertil Steril. 2012;97:819–24.

33. Yang YS, Chang SP, Chen HF, Ma GC, Lin WH, Lin CF, et al. Preimplantation genetic screening of blastocysts by multiplex qPCR followed by fresh embryo transfer: validation and verification. Mol Cytogenet. 2015;8:49.

34. Wells D, Kaur K, Grifo J, Glassner M, Taylor JC, Fragouli E, et al. Clinical utilisation of a rapid low-pass whole genome sequencing technique for the diagnosis of aneuploidy in human embryos prior to implantation. J Med Genet. 2014;51:553–62.

35. Ma GC, Chen HF, Yang YS, Lin WH, Tsai FP, Lin CF, et al. A pilot proof-of-principle study to compare fresh and vitrified cycle preimplantation genetic screening by chromosome microarray and next generation sequencing. Mol Cytogenet. 2016;9:25.

36. Giménez C, Sarasa J, Arjona C, Vilamajó E, Martínez-Pasarell O, Wheeler K, et al. Karyomapping allows preimplantation genetic diagnosis of a de-novo deletion undetectable using conventional PGD technology. Reprod Biomed Online. 2015;31:770–5.

37. Zimmerman RS, Jalas C, Tao X, Fedick AM, Kim JG, Northrop LE, et al. Development and validation of concurrent preimplantation genetic diagnosis for single gene disorders and comprehensive chromosomal aneuploidy screening without whole genome amplification. Fertil Steril. 2016;105:286–94.

38. Gui B, Yang P, Yao Z, Li Y, Liu D, Liu N, et al. A new next-generation sequencing-based assay for concurrent preimplantation genetic diagnosis of Charcot-Marie-Tooth disease yype 1A and aneuploidy screening. J Genet Genomics. 2016;43:155–9.

39. Goldman KN, Nazem T, Berkeley A, Palter S, Grifo JA. Preimplantation genetic diagnosis (PGD) for monogenic disorders: the value of concurrent aneuploidy screening. J Genet Couns. 2016. [Epub ahead of print]

40. Forman EJ, Hong KH, Franasiak JM, Scott Jr RT. Obstetrical and neonatal outcomes from the BEST Trial: single embryo transfer with aneuploidy screening improves outcomes after in vitro fertilization without compromising delivery rates. Am J Obstet Gynecol. 2014;210:157.e1-6.

41. Yang Z, Lin J, Zhang J, Fong WI, Li P, Zhao R, et al. Randomized comparison of next-generation sequencing and array comparative genomic hybridization forpreimplantation genetic screening: a pilot study. BMC Med Genomics. 2015;8:30.

17

Reduced cardiac function and risk of venous thromboembolism in Asian countries

Ruiqi Zhu[†], Yu Hu[*] and Liang Tang[†]

Abstract

Patients with reduced cardiac function are thought to have a higher risk of venous thromboembolism (VTE). Additionally, they are vulnerable to complications of pulmonary embolism (PE) as well as right heart failure (HF), which in return is supposed to increase the rate of mortality. Studies focusing on VTE in heart failure patients were rare in Asian countries before the 21st century. Nowadays, more and more data are becoming available in this field in Asia. It is already known that heart failure can increase the risk of VTE, but so far a consensus on this issue has not been reached for many years, not only in Asian countries but all over the world. This condition may be due to the detailed pathological advancement in Virchow's triad and some other theories. In clinical practice, VTE, especially PE is difficult to diagnose in patients with heart failure because of overlapping symptoms (e.g. cough and chest pain) and the elevation of laboratory markers (e.g. probrain natriuretic peptide (NT-proBNP) and D-dimer in both heart failure and VTE patients). Management of VTE in heart failure patients is also controversial because heart failure patients always have complications, such as renal failure and hepatic failure, which increase the risk of bleeding. In this study, we analyzed data from China, Japan, Korea, Singapore and India mainly to get a better understanding of the research progress in VTE in patients with heart failure. The aim of this review is to discuss the risk, incidence, advancement of diagnosis, management and prevention of VTE in patients with heart failure in Asian countries.

Background

Venous thromboembolism (VTE) is considered to be a common global health problem. It includes two major clinical manifestations, namely deep vein thrombosis (DVT) and pulmonary embolism (PE), the latter is commonly generated from DVT, but it is associated with higher mortality. The incidence of VTE was considered to be rare in the Asians population in early publications [1, 2]. It is estimated that the incidence is only about 21–29 cases per 100,000 individuals per year in Asians and Pacific Islanders compared to that of African Americans (138–141 cases per 100,000 individuals per year) and Caucasians (80–117 cases per 100,000 per year) [3, 4]. However, along with the increase in the proportion of elderly people in Asia and the development of diagnostic technology, as well as a better understanding of VTE by Asian clinicians, a huge number of VTE patients have been recognized and the incidence of VTE still shows a rising trend in Asians [5].

Reduced heart function with symptoms of congested lungs, fluid and water retention, rapid or irregular heartbeats as a result of congestive heart failure has recently been determined to be an independent risk factor for VTE in Asians in a SMART study [6]. Additionally, according to a meta-analysis, hospitalized patients with heart failure had an RR of 1.49 (1.16–1.92) for VTE in Asians [7].

Management of patients diagnosed with heart failure and VTE is difficult. Once this kind of patients develop symptoms of heart failure (e.g. dyspnea, cardiogenic shock, elevated jugular venous pressure), symptoms of heart failure may overshadow that of VTE and impede its diagnosis [8]. Moreover, PE increases pulmonary vascular resistance and right ventricular afterload through several mechanisms, including physical obstruction and hypoxemia, which in return deteriorate heart function. In addition, heart failure patients often have severe

* Correspondence: dr_huyu@126.com
†Equal contributors
Department of Hematology, Wuhan Union Hospital of Huazhong University of Science and Technology, Wuhan 430030, China

complications and multiple risk factors that amplify the risk of VTE which make the treatment complicated (e.g., heart failure patients with renal or liver dysfunction have a higher risk of bleeding during or after fibrinolysis) [9]. A study shows that PE with heart failure have a higher overall mortality rate compared to those without heart failure (17% vs 10%) [10] and PE has also been considered as an independent predictor of death in patients with heart failure [10, 11].

Risk factor and incidence

In Asian patients with heart failure, the incidence of VTE is considered to be lower than that of Western patients. However, some studies have shown that the incidences are neck and neck. It is reported that the incidence of VTE in decompensated heart failure patients ranges from 4 to 26% in Western countries [12], the incidence of PE with congestive heart failure at autopsy ranges from 28 to 48% [13, 14]. A research in Japan reported that the incidence of DVT in heart failure patients was 11.2%, and the incidence is highest in patients classified as NYHA IV (NYHA II: 4.4%, NYHA III: 4.8%, NYHA IV: 25.5%, $P < 0.01$) [15]. One study in Thailand suggested that chronic pulmonary diseases and chronic heart failure were the two most common VTE risk factors in Caucasians, but this study revealed that the highest incidence of VTE was in rheumatologic diseases and the incidence of VTE in congestive heart failure was only 0.5% [16]. This result may due to the study design. The study excluded patients in coronary care units because coronary care unit patients are usually given anticoagulants for cardiac indications, thus the number of heart failure patients in this research is relatively low, the group is too small to get accurate information.

Whether symptomatic reduced heart function is a risk factor for VTE has been a controversial topic for many years, RR for venous thrombosis in patients with heart failure varies from high risk (96.–32.4) [17, 18] to mild risk (1.7–2.6) [19, 20], and even no increase in risk (0.7–0.8) [21, 22]. Data from Asian countries is rare. Nevertheless, it has also shown that Asians have similar non-genetic risk factors as Caucasians, which include severe medical diseases such as heart failure. A prospective, international, multicenter, observational study of a cohort of consecutive Asian patients indicates that congestive heart failure is a risk factor for venous thromboembolic events, whose odds ratio is within the range of Western patients [6]. Some recent studies found that reduced cardiac function is an independent risk factor for VTE in Asians as well as in Caucasians [6, 23–25].

VTE risk is also correlated with the severity of heart failure, as defined by the N-terminal prohormone of brain natriuretic peptide (NT-proBNP) study, which is a multicenter one that was also carried out in China. In this study, the NT-proBNP is suggested to be useful to identify high short-term (Day 10) risk and elevated D-dimer may be useful in recognizing high midterm (Day 35) risk [26]. Elevated NT-proBNP concentration is supposed to be an independent predictor of recurrent VTE in a Chinese study [27], but the result is not consistent with data from the Acute Decompensated Heart Failure National Registry, which indicate that the BNP levels in patients aged ≥65 years is not associated with an increased risk of thromboembolism [28].

Pathophysiology

Virchow's triad, which originated more than 150 years ago, proposes that endothelial damage and dysfunction, abnormal blood stasis, and a hypercoagulable state are the three main elements for thromboembolism (Fig. 1).

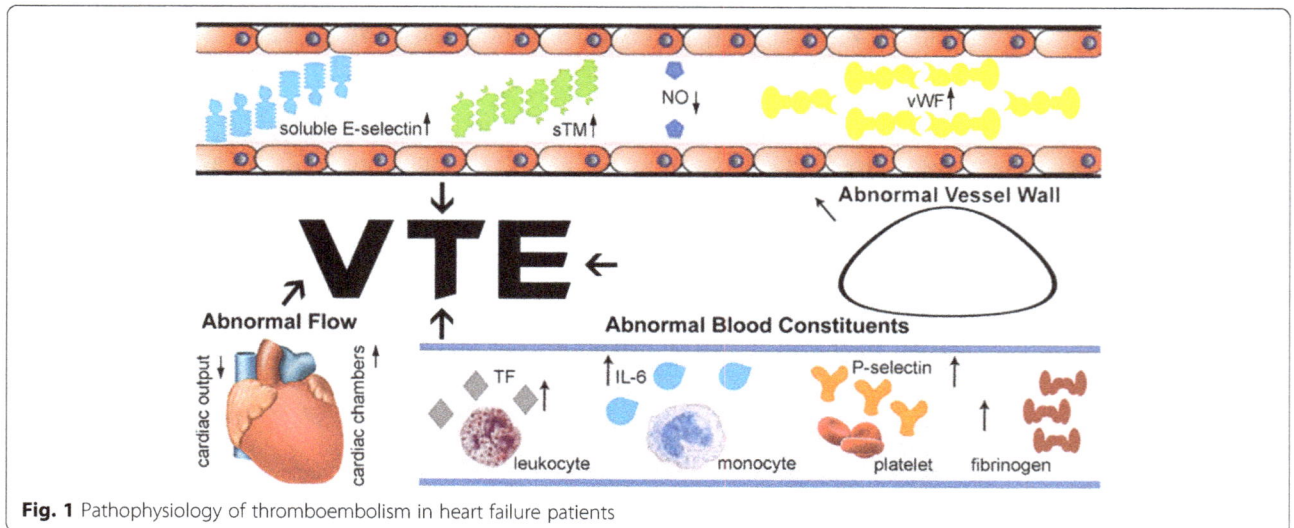

Fig. 1 Pathophysiology of thromboembolism in heart failure patients

Endothelial damage and dysfunction occurs at the start of endothelial and vascular remodeling, and it is also the start of heart failure in most cases, as most of the heart failure cases are caused by coronary heart disease and hypertension [29], both of them begin with endothelial damage. Endothelial cells stand between the blood vessels and tissues, sense and respond to local hydrodynamics and circulating chemical agents. First, their damage arise as a result of many risk factors for atherosclerosis (e.g. cholesterol, low-density lipoprotein) [30]. Then, endothelial damage is accompanied by pro- and anti-coagulant dysfunction, which puts patients in a pro-thrombotic state. Not only plasma markers of endothelial dysfunction increase in heart failure patients, but also inflammatory cytokines (e.g. interleukin-1) generated by damaged endothelial cell [31].

In addition, heart failure contributes to abnormalities of homeostasis through low cardiac output, the dysfunctional cardiac chambers creates areas of blood stasis, then the abnormalities of homeostasis accelerate the activation of the coagulation system and fibrin formation [31], which makes heart failure patients more vulnerable to VTE.

In addition, increased plasma viscosity, platelet activation, thrombin formation [32] and high levels of circulating coagulant factors and thrombin agents (e.g. fibrinogen, D-dimer) [33] and decreased soluble thrombomodulin [34] in patients with heart failure may lead to a hypercoagulable state and contribute to thrombogenesis.

Although Virchow's triad explains why heart failure patients are, to some extent, prone to VTE, the exact pathophysiology mechanisms of VTE and heart failure remain to be discovered. Some primary mechanisms include: 1) Impairment of the protein C pathway, specifically, the endothelial protein C receptor (EPCR) is down regulated through inflammatory cytokines elevated in patients with heart failure, which impairs the protein C pathway-mediated anticoagulation [35]. 2) Enhancement of procoagulant reactions resulting in hypercoagulability. 3) Activated receptor (PAR) activation. 4) Neuro-hormonal activation 5) Stasis after low cardiac output [36] and 6) Endothelial dysfunction due to hypoperfusion and systemic inflammation [37]. Tumor necrosis factor and Interleukin-6 are elevated in heart failure patients [38], the former is associated with the activation of coagulation system and the latter has been shown to be associated with procoagulant tissue factor in heart failure patients [39].

Reduced heart failure patients have increased risk of VTE. In addition, immobilization, infections, central venous catheters and leads from implantable cardiac defibrillators and pacemakers are related to VTE and are common among heart failure patients [9]. Also heart failure and VTE patients both tend to be older [40]. Moreover, in return, acute PE deteriorates the right ventricular (RV) function, which makes the condition complicated and leads to high mortality rates in heart failure patients with VTE.

Diagnosis of PE in heart failure patients

Reduced cardiac function with PE is likely to go undiagnosed. Indeed, it is often misdiagnosed as worsening heart failure because of the overlapping symptoms and signs and the lack of specific laboratory markers, like dyspnea and D-dimer. Dyspnea occurs both in heart failure and PE patients. The D-dimer laboratory marker is used to help diagnose PE, but it is also elevated in heart failure patients.

Routine imaging examination such as X-ray, electrocardiogram and ultrasonic cardiogram also have specificity problems for the diagnosis of PE. Contrast-enhanced chest computerized tomography (CT) is accurate in the diagnosis of PE.

Diagnosis programs of PE in Asian and Western countries do not show significant difference.

China follows the ESC guidelines on the diagnosis and management of acute PE [41] and the diagnosis program follows three steps: 1) PE possibility assessment 2) Risk stratification 3) Proper examination for diagnosis.

The PE assessment systems used in China are the Wells and Geneva score systems, while the simplified PE severity index (sPESI) is adopted for risk stratification.

However, if patients with heart failure are suspected of suffering from PE after the assessment, they are recommended to undergo contrast-enhanced CT immediately, if they do not have contraindications such as renal failure. The reasons are the followings:

1) In risk stratification strategy, patients who suffer persistent hypotension or shock (systolic pressure under 90 mmHg or drop 40 mmHg) are considered to be high risk and recommended to undergo ultrasonic cardiogram. Ultrasonic cardiogram is used to detect RV overload, however, heart patients can develop RV dysfunction, which makes this examination less useful.
2) For patients who do not suffer persistent hypotension or shock, the D-dimer test or Chest contrast CT is recommended. However, patients with heart failure also have elevated D-dimer levels, which makes it difficult to diagnose PE in heart failure patients.

In brief, a heart failure patient is recommended to take contrast-enhanced chest CT if he/she is highly suspected to have PE.

A previous study in China has shown that in PE patients, heart failure is the third most commonly misdiagnosed disease by clinicians, with a proportion of 8.5%. Additionally, between 2002 and 2006, the number of misdiagnosis of this diseases is four times that between 1984 and 2000, which indicates that the specificity of the various kinds of examinations is not adequate for the diagnosis of PE [42].

The development of molecular biological techniques offers new approaches to help in the diagnosis of this disease. For example, microRNA-134 is reported to be a potential plasma biomarker for the diagnosis of acute PE in Chinese patients [43], but whether it can distinguish PE from heart failure remains to be determined.

In Japan, if a suspected patient has circulatory collapse or cardiopulmonary arrest, or if clinical findings suggest severe risk of PE, the patient is first recommended to receive percutaneous cardiopulmonary support and then undergo contrast CT, pulmonary angiography and transesophageal echocardiography to diagnose PE. If this patient does not have circulatory collapse and clinical findings suggest mild or moderate risk of PE, the D-dimer test is recommended for this patient. If the D-dimer level is high, then the patient should undergo examinations as in the circulatory collapse group [44]. Different conditions of venous thromboembolism in HF patients in Japan and Western Countries are shown in Table 1.

Management of PE in China and Japan

Management of PE in reduced cardiac function patients depends on the hemodynamics, right ventricle function and complications in these patients. Conditions are complicated in heart failure patients with severe clinical issues (e.g. renal failure) due to the increased risk of bleeding.

Thus, risk stratifications are also applied in heart failure patients. Various clinical probability scores, calculated according to combinations of known PE risk factors, are used in the management approaches. Heart failure is considered to be the moderate risk level in Asian countries [45, 46], as well as in Western countries.

An agreement has been reached in Asian countries that reduced cardiac function patients who are suffering circulatory collapse should be given hemodynamic and respiratory support immediately. Specifically, percutaneous cardiopulmonary support should be performed according to the Japanese VTE and PE guidelines [44].

Volume loading, limited to 250 to 500 mL, is prescribed in Western countries for systemic arterial hypotensive heart failure patients with PE, without evidence of increased right-sided filling pressures. In China, patients with low cardiac index and normal blood pressure patients are recommended to receive 500 mL of fluid bolus, and this therapy helps to increase cardiac output [9]. However, the Japan VTE guidelines do not suggest volume loading and excessive loading in the right ventricle decreases left cardiac output [44]. Oxygen therapy and drugs, such as dopamine and dobutamine, are also important for the treatment of heart failure patients in all guidelines.

Anticoagulation therapy and thrombolytic therapy are used in PE patients with heart failure without contradictions in China. But in Japan, anticoagulation therapy is for normotensive patients without right heart dysfunction and thrombolytic therapy is the choice for patients with persistent shock and hypotension. In the past, unfractionated heparin was used as anticoagulation agent in Asian countries, just following ESC and ACCP

Table 1 Different conditions of venous thromboembolism in HF patients in Japan and Western Countries

Items	Japan	Western Countries
Incidence of VTE with HF	11.20%	4%–26%
Risk level of VTE in HF	Moderate	Moderate
Diagnosis		
Steps when suspected PE with shock or hypotension	Percutaneous Cardiopulmonary Support	CT angiography
	Angiography, Echocardiography	Echocardiography
	Treatment or other examine	Treatment or other examine
	43.50%	50.20%
Steps when suspected PE without shock or hypotension	Screening: D-dimer, Echocardiography, X-ray etc.	PE Clinical probability evaluation
	Angiography or MRA or CT angiography	D-dimer
	Treatment or other examine	CT angiography when D-dimer positive
		Treatment or other examine
Prophylaxis rate for prevention	43.50%	50.20%

guidelines. However, in 2014, ESC started to strongly recommend non-vitamin K-dependent new oral anticoagulants (NOAC) as an alternative to combined parenteral anticoagulation with a VKA. NOACs have been proven to be not inferior to conditional anticoagulants in efficacy outcome and primary safety outcome and can be used to treat VTE in Western countries. In recent worldwide Hokusai-VTE clinical trial, edoxaban, the oral factor Xa inhibitor, which is a kind of NOACs, administered once daily after initial treatment with heparin was shown noninferior to high-quality standard therapy and could decreased bleeding events significantly [47]. And in patients with right ventricular dysfunction with elevated NT-proBNP levels, a reduction in recurrences was observed in edoxaban group compared with that in warfarin group [47]. When paying attention to Hokusai-VTE trial of East Asia area, Asian patients might get extra benefit from edoxaban compared with warfarin than non-East Asian patients [48]. The major concern was that warfarin may be associated with a higher rate of bleeding in Asians and its efficacy in curing thrombosis was sometimes questioned [49, 50]. Warfarin is difficult to control and is more sensitive in Asians. Edoxaban should be considered an effective and safer alternative to warfarin in East Asian venous thromboembolism patients possessing heart failure at the same time who require anticoagulant treatment. However, data are still limited in Asia, and NOAC treatment is only used in a few medical centers in countries such as China.

Thrombolytic therapy is necessary for reduced heart failure patients because it promptly improves pulmonary circulation [44]. Japan uses monteplase as the only drug officially approved to treat acute PE, whereas in China, the drugs used include alteplase, reteplase and urokinase.

Other treatments for PE do not show significant differences between China and Japan, or between Asian and Western countries. Significant differences in management between areas are shown in Table 2.

Prevention

Many VTE guidelines in Asian countries are based on ESC and ACCP guidelines, these guidelines are regarded as 'gold standard' in diagnosis, management and prevention of VTE. In 2004, the recommendation grade for the use of anticoagulant prophylaxis in heart failure patients with VTE was Grade 1C+ in the ACCP guidelines, until recently pathophysiological evidence of retrospective data showed that antithrombotic substances can improve outcomes in patients with heart failure. The recommendation grade shifted to Grade 1A. Low-molecular-weight heparin (LMWH), unfractionated heparin (UFH) or fondaparinux (Grade 1A) are recommended in the VTE prophylaxis plan. If anticoagulant prophylaxis is contraindicated, then GCS or IPC should be used.

Although mechanical prophylaxis devices, such as intermittent pneumatic compression devices (IPC), have been shown to be effective in preventing VTE [51, 52], and they are recommended in acutely ill medical patients who have a high bleeding risk in the ACCP guidelines with Grade 1A [53], these devices should be carefully prescribed in cardiac failure patients with VTE, because cardiac function may be worsened by leg compression [5].

Data from some Asian countries also suggest that thromboprophylaxis should be applied in patients with heart failure to prevent VTE events, but the national guidelines for preventing VTE in heart failure patients have not been established in all Asian countries. Recently, consensus has been reached in some Asian countries, including China, Korea, India, etc. [54, 55]. Additionally, VTE prophylaxis rates are high in Asian countries, such as Korea and Japan, but they are still low compared to the higher use of prophylaxis worldwide

Table 2 Management shows significant differences between areas

Management	Western countries	China	Japan
Volume loading	250–500 ml	500 ml	None
Anticoagulation therapy	Recommended in PE patients with HF	Recommended in PE patients with HF	For normotensive PE patients without right heart dysfunction
Thrombolytic therapy	Considered for PE patients with HF without contradictions	Recommended in PE patients with HF without contradictions	For PE patients with persistent shock and hypotension
Anticoagulation drugs	NOACs combined parenteral anticoagulation	Unfractionated heparin only except in few medical centers	Unfractionated heparin only except in few medical centers
Thrombolytic drugs	Tenecteplase	Monteplase	Alteplase, reteplase, urokinase

(50.2%) [56]. The rate in heart/respiratory failure prescribing VTE prophylaxis is estimated to be 46.9% in Korea [55] and 43.5% of heart failure patients received anticoagulant therapy according to a research in Japan [15]. The prophylaxis rates are extremely low in developing countries such as India, although the accurate prophylaxis rate has not been obtained in heart failure patients in this country. In fact, it has been reported that only 19.1% of medical patients received the ACCP recommended thromboprophalaxis [25].

Despite the guidelines recommendation that heart failure patients should receive prophylaxis, a study whose authors including a team in China suggests that only severe heart failure patients whose NT-proBNP concentration is ≥ 1906 pg/ml should receive prophylaxis; less severe heart failure patients do not show a significant difference in VTE incidence compared with patients who do not have heart failure [26]. This study also indicated that rivaroxaban (Clotting Factor X inhibitor) may reduce the risk of VTE in patients with severe heart failure, but enoxaparin (LMWH, 40 mg/d) does not show similar trend [26]. Nevertheless, enoxaparin is widely used in preventing VTE in medically ill patients and several studies provide evidence for the use of enoxaparin. Meanwhile, a study has shown that, in medically ill patients, an extended course of thromboprophylaxis with apixaban is not superior to a shorter course with enoxaparin and the former is significantly associated with more major bleeding events [57]. Another study published in the New England Journal of Medicine in 1999 suggested that enoxaparin is useful to reduce the risk of VTE [58]. Additionally, in the EXCLAIM trial, it was revealed that extended prophylaxis with enoxaparin reduced the rate of VTE in medically ill patients (including congestive heart failure patients) from 4.0 to 0.5%, but increased the rate of major bleeding from 0.3 to 0.8% [59].

In the 2014 Korean guidelines for the prevention of VTE, patients are recommended to be assessed for VTE risk and bleeding risk (Grade 1A, a strong recommendation with high-quality evidence) and prophylaxis is based on risk stratification [60]. Congestive heart failure is considered to be in the moderate risk group for VTE, and may not increase the risk for bleeding according to a study in France [26, 60]. Patients with congestive heart failure only are recommended pharmacological prophylaxis or mechanical prophylaxis, and the recommendation level is Grade 2C (a weak recommendation with low- or very-low-quality evidence). If a patient is admitted to an intensive care unit with multiple risk factors (including heart failure) for VTE, the patient should be routinely assessed and prescribed pharmacological prophylaxis or mechanical prophylaxis (Grade 2A, a weak recommendation with high-quality evidence).

Pharmacological prophylaxis mainly comprises LMWH, 0.2–1 mg/kg, subcutaneously daily and low-dose of unfractionated heparin (LDUH), 5000U subcutaneously every 8–12 hours [55]. The recommendation levels in Asian countries are different from the ACCP guidelines, more evidence remain to be discovered in Asian countries.

Conclusion

In this article, we make a review on the topic of reduced cardiac function and risk of VTE, especially PE in Asian countries in aspects of risk factor, incidence, pathophysiology, diagnosis, management and prevention. Despite genetic risk factors for Eastern and Western countries are different, non-genetic risk factors are similar all over the world. Reduced cardiac function is considered an intermediate risk factor for VTE and should be given attention in Department of Cardiology and Intensive Care Unit. Besides, diagnosis in PE patients with cardiac failure is also intractable because of overlapping of symptoms and signs of these two diseases. Contrast-enhanced chest computerized tomography is necessary when a patient is suspected. Management shows large disparity in different countries. Prevention of PE in Asian countries are mainly based on ESC guideline and developed rapidly in recent years although prophylaxis rate are still lower than western countries. VTE incidence is considered lower than western countries in the past, however emerging evidence suggests the incidence may be nearly the same. Companying with high incidence and mortality in cardiovascular diseases in nowadays Asia, the topic of heart failure and venous thromboembolism should be issued. More studies should be done and a guideline appropriate for Asians is needed.

Abbreviations
CT: Computerized tomography; DVT: Deep vein thrombosis; ERCP: Endothelial Protein C Receptor; HF: Heart failure; IPC: Intermittent pneumatic compression devices; LDUH: Low-dose of unfractionated heparin; LMWH: Low-molecular-weight heparin; NOAC: Non-vitamin K-dependent new Oral Anticoagulants; NT pro-BNP: Pro-brain Natriuretic Peptide; PAR: Activated receptor; PE: Pulmonary embolism; RV: Right ventricular; sPESI: Simplified PE severity index; UHF: Unfractionated heparin; VTE: Venous thromboembolism

Acknowledgements
Not applicable.

Funding
No funding evolved.

Authors' contributions
RZ searching for and reading studies about the topic in depth and draft this manuscript, LT participate in its design and coordination. YH conceived of

the study, and participated in its design and coordination and helped to draft the manuscript. All authors read and approved the final manuscript.

Competing interests
The authors declare that they have no competing interests.

References
1. Hwang WS. The rarity of pulmonary thromboembolism in asians. Singapore Med J. 1968;9(4):276–9.
2. Kishimoto M, et al. Prevalence of venous thromboembolism at a teaching hospital in Okinawa, Japan. Thromb Haemost. 2005;93(5):876–9.
3. Stein PD, et al. Pulmonary thromboembolism in Asians/Pacific Islanders in the United States: analysis of data from the National Hospital Discharge Survey and the United States Bureau of the Census. Am J Med. 2004;116(7):435–42.
4. White RH, et al. Effect of ethnicity and gender on the incidence of venous thromboembolism in a diverse population in California in 1996. Thromb Haemost. 2005;93(2):298–305.
5. Liew NC, et al. Asian venous thromboembolism guidelines: prevention of venous thromboembolism. Int Angiol. 2012;31(6):501–16.
6. Leizorovicz A, et al. Epidemiology of venous thromboembolism in Asian patients undergoing major orthopedic surgery without thromboprophylaxis. The SMART study. J Thromb Haemost. 2005;3(1):28–34.
7. Tang L, et al. Heart failure and risk of venous thromboembolism: a systematic review and meta-analysis. Lancet Haematol. 2016;3(1):e30–44.
8. Piazza G, Seddighzadeh A, Goldhaber SZ. Heart failure in patients with deep vein thrombosis. Am J Cardiol. 2008;101(7):1056–9.
9. Piazza G, Goldhaber SZ. Pulmonary embolism in heart failure. Circulation. 2008;118(15):1598–601.
10. Monreal M, et al. Pulmonary embolism in patients with chronic obstructive pulmonary disease or congestive heart failure. Am J Med. 2006;119(10):851–8.
11. Darze ES, et al. Acute pulmonary embolism is an independent predictor of adverse events in severe decompensated heart failure patients. Chest. 2007;131(6):1838–43.
12. Alikhan R, Spyropoulos AC. Epidemiology of venous thromboembolism in cardiorespiratory and infectious disease. Am J Med. 2008;121(11):935–42.
13. Goldhaber SZ, et al. Risk factors for pulmonary embolism. The Framingham study. Am J Med. 1983;74(6):1023–8.
14. Greenstein J. Thrombosis and pulmonary embolism. S Afr Med J. 1945;19:377–80.
15. Ota S, et al. Incidence and clinical predictors of deep vein thrombosis in patients hospitalized with heart failure in Japan. Circ J. 2009;73(8):1513–7.
16. Aniwan S, Rojnuckarin P. High incidence of symptomatic venous thromboembolism in Thai hospitalized medical patients without thromboprophylaxis. Blood Coagul Fibrinolysis. 2010;21(4):334–8.
17. Heit JA, et al. Risk factors for deep vein thrombosis and pulmonary embolism: a population-based case–control study. Arch Intern Med. 2000;160(6):809–15.
18. Sorensen HT, et al. Heart disease may be a risk factor for pulmonary embolism without peripheral deep venous thrombosis. Circulation. 2011;124(13):1435–41.
19. Howell MD, Geraci JM, Knowlton AA. Congestive heart failure and outpatient risk of venous thromboembolism: a retrospective, case–control study. J Clin Epidemiol. 2001;54(8):810–6.
20. Ocak G, et al. Risk of venous thrombosis in patients with major illnesses: results from the MEGA study. J Thromb Haemost. 2013;11(1):116–23.
21. Sellier E, et al. Risk factors for deep vein thrombosis in older patients: a multicenter study with systematic compression ultrasonography in postacute care facilities in France. J Am Geriatr Soc. 2008;56(2):224–30.
22. Zakai NA, Wright J, Cushman M. Risk factors for venous thrombosis in medical inpatients: validation of a thrombosis risk score. J Thromb Haemost. 2004;2(12):2156–61.
23. Matsuo H, et al. Frequency of deep vein thrombosis among hospitalized non-surgical Japanese patients with congestive heart failure. J Cardiol. 2014;64(6):430–4.
24. Lee CH, et al. Universal pharmacological thromboprophylaxis for total knee arthroplasty may not be necessary in low-risk populations: a nationwide study in Taiwan. J Thromb Haemost. 2012;10(1):56–63.
25. Pinjala R. Venous thromboembolism risk & prophylaxis in the acute hospital care setting (ENDORSE), a multinational cross-sectional study: results from the Indian subset data. Indian J Med Res. 2012;136(1):60–7.
26. Mebazaa A, et al. Predicting the risk of venous thromboembolism in patients hospitalized with heart failure. Circulation. 2014;130(5):410–8.
27. Wang Y, et al. Association of elevated NTproBNP with recurrent thromboembolic events after acute pulmonary embolism. Thromb Res. 2012;129(6):688–92.
28. Kociol RD, et al. B-type natriuretic peptide level and postdischarge thrombotic events in older patients hospitalized with heart failure: insights from the Acute Decompensated Heart Failure National Registry. Am Heart J. 2012;163(6):994–1001.
29. McMurray JJ, Pfeffer MA. Heart failure. Lancet. 2005;365(9474):1877–89.
30. Heusch G, et al. Cardiovascular remodelling in coronary artery disease and heart failure. Lancet. 2014;383(9932):1933–43.
31. Shantsila E, Lip GY. The risk of thromboembolism in heart failure: does it merit anticoagulation therapy? Am J Cardiol. 2011;107(4):558–60.
32. O'Connor CM, Gurbel PA, Serebruany VL. Usefulness of soluble and surface-bound P-selectin in detecting heightened platelet activity in patients with congestive heart failure. Am J Cardiol. 1999;83(9):1345–9.
33. Yamamoto K, et al. The coagulation system is activated in idiopathic cardiomyopathy. J Am Coll Cardiol. 1995;25(7):1634–40.
34. Kapur NK, et al. Hemodynamic modulation of endocardial thromboresistance. Circulation. 2007;115(1):67–75.
35. Loubele ST, et al. Activated protein C protects against myocardial ischemia/reperfusion injury via inhibition of apoptosis and inflammation. Arterioscler Thromb Vasc Biol. 2009;29(7):1087–92.
36. Zannad F, et al. Is thrombosis a contributor to heart failure pathophysiology? Possible mechanisms, therapeutic opportunities, and clinical investigation challenges. Int J Cardiol. 2013;167(5):1772–82.
37. Chen D, et al. Cytokines and acute heart failure. Crit Care Med. 2008;36(1 Suppl):S9–16.
38. van der Poll T, et al. Activation of coagulation after administration of tumor necrosis factor to normal subjects. N Engl J Med. 1990;322(23):1622–7.
39. Chin BS, et al. Interleukin-6, tissue factor and von Willebrand factor in acute decompensated heart failure: relationship to treatment and prognosis. Blood Coagul Fibrinolysis. 2003;14(6):515–21.
40. Piazza G, Seddighzadeh A, Goldhaber SZ. Deep-vein thrombosis in the elderly. Clin Appl Thromb Hemost. 2008;14(4):393–8.
41. Konstantinides SV. 2014 ESC Guidelines on the diagnosis and management of acute pulmonary embolism. Eur Heart J. 2014;35(45):3145–6.
42. Jia WB, Zhang CX, Xu ZM. [Pulmonary embolism misdiagnosis in China: a literature review (2001 to 2004)]. Zhonghua Xin Xue Guan Bing Za Zhi. 2006;34(3):277–80.
43. Xiao J, et al. MicroRNA-134 as a potential plasma biomarker for the diagnosis of acute pulmonary embolism. J Transl Med. 2011;9:159.
44. JCS Joint Working Group. et al. Guidelines for the diagnosis, treatment and prevention of pulmonary thromboembolism and deep vein thrombosis (JCS 2009). Circ J. 2011;75(5):1258–81.
45. Yorozu T. Prevention of venous thromboembolism and anticoagulant therapy. Masui. 2014;63(3):278–86.
46. Cohen A, et al. Treating pulmonary embolism in Pacific Asia with direct oral anticoagulants. Thromb Res. 2015;136(2):196–207.
47. Buller HR, et al. Edoxaban versus warfarin for the treatment of symptomatic venous thromboembolism. N Engl J Med. 2013;369(15):1406–15.
48. Nakamura M, et al. Efficacy and safety of edoxaban for treatment of venous thromboembolism: a subanalysis of East Asian patients in the Hokusai-VTE trial. J Thromb Haemost. 2015;13(9):1606–14.
49. Shen AY, et al. Racial/ethnic differences in the risk of intracranial hemorrhage among patients with atrial fibrillation. J Am Coll Cardiol. 2007;50(4):309–15.
50. Chiang CE, Wang KL, Lip GY. Stroke prevention in atrial fibrillation: an Asian perspective. Thromb Haemost. 2014;111(5):789–97.
51. Kakkos SK, et al. The efficacy of a new portable sequential compression device (SCD Express) in preventing venous stasis. J Vasc Surg. 2005;42(2):296–303.
52. Urbankova J, et al. Intermittent pneumatic compression and deep vein thrombosis prevention. A meta-analysis in postoperative patients. Thromb Haemost. 2005;94(6):1181–5.
53. Geerts WH, et al. Prevention of venous thromboembolism: American college of chest physicians evidence-based clinical practice guidelines (8th edition). Chest. 2008;133(6 Suppl):381s–453s.

54. Ramakrishnan N. Thrombolysis is not warranted in submassive pulmonary embolism: a systematic review and meta-analysis. Crit Care Resusc. 2007; 9(4):357–63.

55. Lee J, et al. Prevention of venous thromboembolism in medical intensive care unit: a multicenter observational study in Korea. J Korean Med Sci. 2014;29(11):1572–6.

56. Cohen AT, et al. Venous thromboembolism risk and prophylaxis in the acute hospital care setting (ENDORSE study): a multinational cross-sectional study. Lancet. 2008;371(9610):387–94.

57. Goldhaber SZ, et al. Apixaban versus enoxaparin for thromboprophylaxis in medically ill patients. N Engl J Med. 2011;365(23):2167–77.

58. Samama MM, et al. A comparison of enoxaparin with placebo for the prevention of venous thromboembolism in acutely ill medical patients. Prophylaxis in Medical Patients with Enoxaparin Study Group. N Engl J Med. 1999;341(11):793–800.

59. Hull RD, et al. Extended-duration venous thromboembolism prophylaxis in acutely ill medical patients with recently reduced mobility: a randomized trial. Ann Intern Med. 2010;153(1):8–18.

60. Bang SM, Jang MJ. Prevention of venous thromboembolism, 2nd edition: Korean Society of Thrombosis and Hemostasis Evidence-based Clinical Practice Guidelines. J Korean Med Sci. 2014;29(2):164–71.

18

Recombinant human soluble thrombomodulin improves mortality in patients with sepsis especially for severe coagulopathy: a retrospective study

Takahiro Kato[1][*] and Katsuhiko Matsuura[2]

Abstract

Background: Disseminated intravascular coagulation (DIC) is associated with high mortality in patients with sepsis. Several studies reporting that recombinant human soluble thrombomodulin (rhTM) reduced mortality in sepsis patients. This retrospective cohort study aimed to evaluate the efficacy of rhTM for patients with mild coagulopathy compared with those with severe coagulopathy.

Methods: We evaluated about 90-day mortality and SOFA score. SOFA score was also evaluated for the following components: respiratory, cardiovascular, hepatic, renal and coagulation.

Results: All 69 patients were diagnosed with sepsis, fulfilled Japanese Association for Acute Medicine criteria for DIC, and were treated with rhTM. Patients were assigned to either the mild coagulopathy group (did not fulfill the International Society on Thrombosis and Haemostasis overt DIC criteria) or the severe coagulopathy group (fulfilled overt DIC criteria). The 90-day mortality was significant lower in severe coagulopathy group than mild coagulopathy group ($P = 0.029$). Although the SOFA scores did not decrease in the mild coagulopathy group, SOFA scores decreased significantly in the severe coagulopathy group. Furthermore the respiratory component of the SOFA score significant decreased in severe coagulopathy group compared with mild coagulopathy group.

Conclusions: rhTM administration may reduce mortality by improving organ dysfunction especially for respiratory in septic patients with severe coagulopathy.

Keywords: Thrombomodulin, Sepsis, Disseminated intravascular coagulation, Severe coagulopathy

Background

Sepsis and septic shock remain the most common cause of death in critically ill patients [1], and new therapeutic approaches are urgently needed. Ideal management of sepsis and septic shock remains controversial. Current evidence suggests that compliance with the Surviving Sepsis Campaign (SSC) guidelines is associated with decreased mortality [2–4]. Furthermore, it has been reported recently that early lactate clearance has a lower mortality risk than early goal-directed therapy [5].

Disseminated intravascular coagulation (DIC) is associated with high mortality in patients with sepsis [6]. Excessive coagulation activation, inhibition of fibrinolysis, and consumption of coagulation inhibitors lead to a hypercoagulable state, resulting in fibrin deposition in microvessels and inflammatory reactions [7]. Current management of DIC is primarily focused on treating any associated underlying medical condition, although use of supplemental clotting factors or platelets, or anticoagulant therapy may occasionally be required [8]. In particular, therapeutic intervention directly against coagulation

* Correspondence: takkato1@aichi-med-u.ac.jp
[1]Departments of Pharmacy, Aichi Medical University, 1 -1 Yazakokarimata, Nagakute, Aichi 480-1195, Japan
Full list of author information is available at the end of the article

and inflammation for DIC associated with sepsis is effective [9, 10], and it is generally accepted that early, aggressive treatment of the underlying disease is important. The revised Japanese Association for Acute Medicine (JAAM) criteria allows diagnosis of DIC in the earlier phase of disease than the overt DIC criteria published by the International Society on Thrombosis and Haemostasis (ISTH) [11].

Recombinant human soluble thrombomodulin (rhTM) is the only agent for the treatment of DIC [12]. rhTM was approved in 2008 and has been used clinically for DIC treatment in Japan. Several animal studies have demonstrated a reduction in mortality with the administration of rhTM in sepsis models [13]. Moreover, rhTM prevents endotoxin-induced lung injury in rats by leukocyte activation [14]. Multicenter retrospective study and meta-analysis have shown that rhTM improves mortality in sepsis patients [15, 16]. Yamakawa et al. shown that rhTM improves coagulopathy and decreases SOFA score compared with control group in patients with sepsis [17].

We hypothesized that mortality would be improved after treatment with rhTM in septic patients especially for mild coagulopathy. Therefore, the purpose of this study was to evaluate the efficacy of rhTM for patients with mild coagulopathy compared with those with severe coagulopathy.

Methods

Patients and study design

This was a retrospective cohort study. All patients were admitted to Aichi Medical University Hospital intensive care unit (ICU) between May 2008 and and December 2014. Although the criteria for ICU admission were not standardized, all patients included in this study were diagnosed with sepsis what is according to SEPSIS-3 [18] and DIC diagnosed by JAAM criteria (Score ≥ 4) [11] (Table 1), and were treated with rhTM. rhTM doses were 0.06 mg/kg/day (or 0.02 mg/kg/day for patients who required renal replacement therapy for acute kidney injury [AKI]); rhTM was administered for 30 min once daily. All patients were principally treated according to the SSC guidelines [19]. The exclusion criteria were: acute pancreatitis, burns, treatment with danaparoid sodium at the start of treatment, treatment with cyclosporine or tacrolimus until sepsis diagnosis, age ≤ 15 years, and those not diagnosed with DIC due to a lack of laboratory data. A flow diagram of patient inclusion is shown in Fig. 1. The study protocol was reviewed and approved by an institutional review board. Informed consent was not required because blood samples were taken as part of the routine patient care for clinical laboratory testing, but the highest standard of privacy policy was applied.

Data collection

Relevant clinical background, medication history, and laboratory data of all patients were collected at appropriate times during the treatment for sepsis. We collected the patients' demographic and laboratory test data, including age, sex, clinical outcome (mortality at 90 days), shock (hypotension not reversed with fluid resuscitation) , presence of AKI as defined by the AKI network [20], acute physiologic and chronic health evaluation II

Table 1 JAAM criteria [11] and ISTH overt DIC criteria [22]

	JAAM		ISTH		
Score	1	3	1	2	3
SIRS	≥3 items				
Platelet Count (10^3/mL)	≥80 and < 120, or > 30% decrease within 24 h	< 80 or 50% decrease within 24 h	< 100	< 50	
FDP (μg/mL)	≥10 and < 25	≥25		≥10 and < 25 (Moderate increase)	≥25 (Strong increase)
PT Ratio	≥1.2				
Prolonged prothrombin time (sec)			3<, < 6	6<	
Fibrinogen level (g/L)			< 1.0		
Diagnosis	4 points or more		5 points or more		

These score was assessed using d-dimer if FDP was not measured. The cut off value of d-dimer level were "moderate increase; 5.4–13.2 μg/mL, strong increase; ≥13.2 μg/mL"

JAAM: The revised Japanese Association for Acute Medicine
ISTH: The International Society on Thrombosis and Haemostasis
SIRS: systemic inflammatory response syndrome
Criteria for SIRS (systemic inflammatory response syndrome)
• Temperature: > 38 °C or < 36 °C
• Heart rate: > 90 beats/min
• Respiratory rate: > 20 breath /min or PaCO2 < 32 Torr (< 4.3 kPa)
• White cell blood counts: > 12,000/mm3, < 4,000cells/mm3, or 10% immature (band) forms

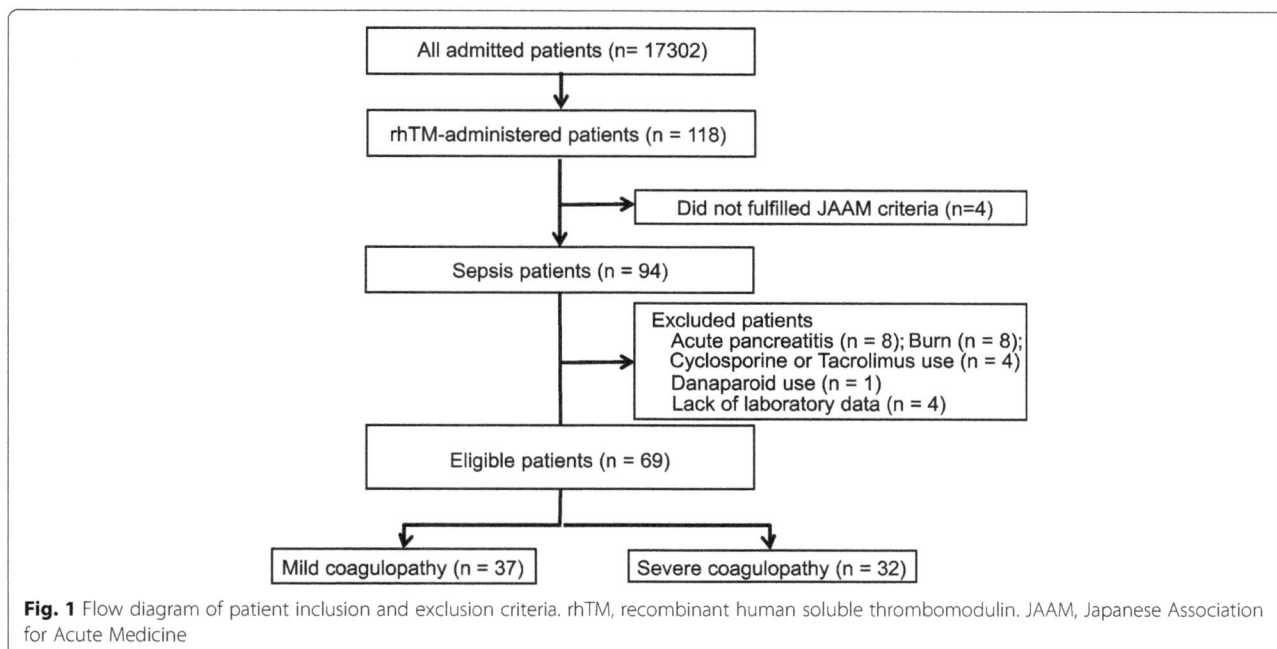

Fig. 1 Flow diagram of patient inclusion and exclusion criteria. rhTM, recombinant human soluble thrombomodulin. JAAM, Japanese Association for Acute Medicine

(APACHE II) score, sequential organ failure assessment (SOFA) score (Table 2) [21], presence of DIC as defined by the ISTH overt DIC criteria [22], mechanical ventilation, renal replacement therapy, vasopressor use, presence of cancer, prothrombin time (PT) ratio, antithrombin III (AT III) activity, D-dimer level, platelet count, fibrinogen level and lactate level. The SOFA score was recorded on days 1, 3, 5, 7 and 28 after administration of rhTM.

Evaluation of clinical response

Patients were assigned to either the severe coagulopathy group or the mild coagulopathy group. Severe coagulopathy was defined as diagnosed DIC by not only JAAM criteria (Score ≥ 4) but also ISTH overt DIC criteria (Score ≥ 5). Mild coagulopathy was defined as fulfilled the JAAM criteria only (Table 1).

We evaluated about 90-day mortality and SOFA score at day 1, 3, 5, 7 and 28. An animal study has been reported that rhTM prevents endotoxin-induced lung injury [14]. Therefore SOFA score was also evaluated for the following components: respiratory, cardiovascular, hepatic, renal and coagulation. Moreover, changes over time in coagulation test results (D-dimer level, PT ratio and fibrinogen level) were assessed from day 1 to day 7. PT and fibrinogen were measured by electric impedance methods (PT: Thrombocheck PT; Sysmex CO., LTD., fibrinogen: Coagpia®Fbg; Sekisui medical CO., LTD.). FDP and D-dimer were measured by latex nephelometric immunoassay (Nanopia®P-FDP; Sekisui medical CO., LTD., LIAS AUTO® D-Dimer NEO; Sysmex CO., LTD.). AT III activity was measured by synthetic substrate method (Testzym®S AT III; Sekisui medical CO., LTD.).

Table 2 SOFA score [21]

SOFA score	1	2	3	4
Respiratory PaO2/FiO2, mmHg	< 400	< 300	< 200 (With respiratory support)	< 100 (With respiratory support)
Coagulation Platelets × 103/µl	< 150	< 100	< 50	< 20
Hepatic Bilirubin, mg/dl	1.2–1.9	2.0–5.9	6.0–11.9	> 12.0
Cardiovascular (Adrenergic agents dose is in µg/kg/min)	MAP < 70 mmHg	Dopamine ≤5 or dobutamine (any dose)	Dopamine > 5 or epinephrine ≤0.1 or norepinephrine ≤0.1	Dopamine > 15 or epinephrine > 0.1 or norepinephrine > 0.1
Central nervous system	13–14	10–12	5–9	< 6
Renal Creatinine, mg/dl or Urine output	1.2–1.9	2.0–3.4	3.5–4.9 Or < 500 ml/day	> 5.0 Or 200 ml/day

Statistical analysis

Data were expressed as group mean ± standard deviation, or percentages. Continuous variables were compared between groups using the Student's t-test. Noncontinuous variables were compared between groups using the Mann–Whitney U test. Categorical variables were analyzed using the chi-squared test or Fisher's exact test. Log-rank analysis was used to evaluate 90-day mortality. Multivariate Cox regression analysis was used to assess the covariates that were associated with time to mortality. SOFA scores, Platelet count, D-dimer level, PT ratio and fibrinogen level between groups over time were analyzed by repeated measures analysis of variance and post hoc Dunnett's test. Independent predictive variables with a P value of less than 0.05 were considered statistically significant. Statistical analyses were performed using JMP for Windows version 5.0.1 software (SAS Institute, Inc., U.S.).

Results

Baseline characteristics

Although 94 patients were diagnosed with sepsis and treated with rhTM during the study period, only 69 patients met the requirements of our study (Fig. 1). Thirty-seven patients were in the mild coagulopathy group and 32 patients were in the severe coagulopathy group. The characteristics of the study population are shown in Table 3. FDP levels were not measured in most of patients. ISTH overt DIC score, JAAM DIC score, D-dimer level and Platelet count were significant difference between mild coagulopathy group and severe coagulopathy group. These score was assessed using d-dimer if FDP was not measured. The cut off value of d-dimer level were "moderate increase; 5.4-13.2 µg/mL, strong increase; ≥13.2 µg/mL".

Influence of treatment for mild or severe coagulopathy on mortality

The Kaplan–Meier plot of survival function during the 90-day study period is given for both the mild coagulopathy group and the severe coagulopathy group in Fig. 2. There was trend toward lower 90-day mortality in the severe coagulopathy group than mild coagulopathy group (P = 0.029). We performed a Cox regression analysis to assessed four possible confounders related to

Table 3 Characteristics of patients

	Mild coagulopathy (n = 37)	Severe coagulopathy (n = 32)	P value
Male, n (%)	25 (67.6)	23 (71.9)	0.796
Age (years)	69 [38–94]	72.5 [33–91]	0.110
Shock, n (%)	14 (42.4)	13 (40.6)	1.000
AKI, n (%)	15 (42.9)	18 (56.3)	0.332
APACHE II score	26.6 ± 8.1	29.8 ± 10.8	0.229
SOFA score	6.2 ± 3.5	7.5 ± 2.5	0.114
ISTH overt DIC score	3.4 ± 0.7	5.3 ± 0.6	< 0.001
Mechanical ventilation, n (%)	31 (88.6)	30 (93.8)	0.675
Renal replacement therapy, n (%)	25 (71.4)	22 (68.8)	1.000
Vasopressor use, n (%)	24 (68.6)	24 (75.0)	0.598
Lactate (mmol/L)	32.0 ± 22.8	38.3 ± 21.5	0.289
Time for normalize lactate level (h)	94.8 ± 142.6	88.3 ± 87.0	0.854
Cancer, n (%)	6 (16.7)	5 (15.6)	1.000
rhTM dose (mg/kg)	0.041 ± 0.018	0.048 ± 0.023	0.218
Duration of rhTM administration (days)	5.4 ± 1.8	6.3 ± 3.5	0.181
Coagulation tests			
Prothrombin time ratio	1.34 ± 0.28	1.42 ± 0.26	0.212
Antithrombin III activity (%)	57.7 ± 20.6	54.5 ± 21.8	0.581
D-dimer (10^3 ng/ml)	14.0 ± 15.4	40.0 ± 65.0	< 0.001
Platelet count (10^3/µl)	10.0 ± 10.1	5.3 ± 3.2	0.004
Fibrinogen (mg/dl)	420.3 ± 216.7	410.0 ± 117.7	0.813

Collected data are when rhTM administration start

Data are presented as mean ± standard deviation unless otherwise stated. DIC: disseminated intravascular coagulation, *AKI*: acute kidney injury, *APACHE II*: acute physiologic and chronic health evaluation, *SOFA*: sequential organ failure assessment, *ISTH*: International Society on Thrombosis and Haemostasis, rhTM: recombinant human soluble thrombomodulin

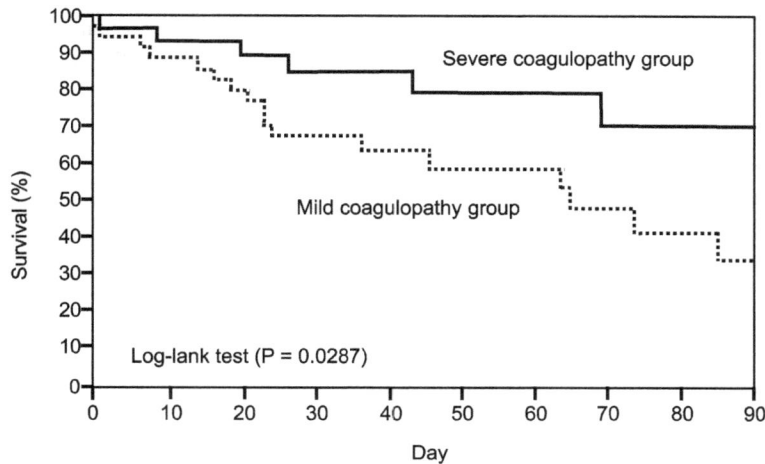

Fig. 2 Kaplan–Meier plot of survival at 90 daysThe solid line represents patients in the severe coagulopathy group, and the dotted line represents patients in the mild coagulopathy group. The mortality rate was significantly different between the two groups.

outcome: age, APACHE II score, SOFA score (day1) and severe coagulopathy. Consequently, severe coagulopathy influenced lower mortality ($p = 0.015$). (Table 4).

Sequential organ failure assessment score

Although the SOFA score did not decrease in the mild coagulopathy group, it decreased significantly in the severe coagulopathy group at day7 and 28 ($P = 0.001$). There was trend toward lower SOFA scores in severe coagulopathy group than mild coagulopathy group on day 28 ($p = 0.08$) (Fig. 3). The respiratory component of the SOFA score significant decreased in severe coagulopathy group ($p = 0.029$) (Table 5).

Coagulation tests

Prothrombin time ratio and D-dimer were improved in the severe coagulopathy group significantly compared with baseline. Although D-dimer level was higher in the severe coagulopathy group than mild coagulopathy group at day 1, D-dimer was not different between two groups.

Platelet count improved in both groups (not significant). Platelet count, Prothrombin time ratio, D-dimer and fibrinogen levels were not significantly different at day 7 between the groups. (Fig. 4).

Table 4 Cox regression analysis

	Risk ratio	95% CI	P value
Age	0.985	0.950–1.024	0.422
APACHE II score	0.996	0.934–1.060	0.909
SOFA score (day 1)	1.171	0.985–1.411	0.074
Severe coagulopathy	0.554	0.314–0.897	0.015

CI: confidence intervals, *SOFA*: sequential organ failure assessment, *APACHE*: acute physiologic and chronic health evaluation

Discussion

Although several trials have shown that rhTM reduced mortality in septic patients with DIC [13, 14, 17], the timing of treatment initiation was unclear. The present study represents the first attempt to evaluate efficacy of rhTM in septic patients with different degree of coagulopathy. This study suggested that treatment with rhTM in septic patients with severe coagulopathy improves mortality compared with those without severe coagulopathy.

The present study included 69 patients with sepsis. There was no difference in baseline characteristics except coagulation tests between severe coagulopathy group and mild coagulopathy group. Platelet count was significantly lower and D-dimer level was significantly higher in the severe coagulopathy group than mild coagulopathy group. The sensitivity of a low fibrinogen level for the diagnosis of DIC according to ISTH criteria was 28% and hypofibrinogenemia has been detected in only severe cases of DIC [8]. Fibrinogen levels were normal in most of patients in the present study. Therefore, fibrinogen levels showed no significant differences between the two groups. PT ratio was improved significantly in the severe coagulopathy group at day 7. There was significant reduction of SOFA score in severe coagulopathy group within 7 days compared with baseline. Furthermore, at day 7 and 28, the score was trends in lower of the severe coagulopathy group, as compared with mild coagulopathy group. On the other hand, there was no significant reduction of SOFA score in the mild coagulopathy group compared with baseline.

Severe coagulopathy is associated with high mortality in patients with sepsis. Patients with severe coagulopathy had higher mortality than those with mild coagulopathy [6, 23]. The phase II study shown that rhTM trend

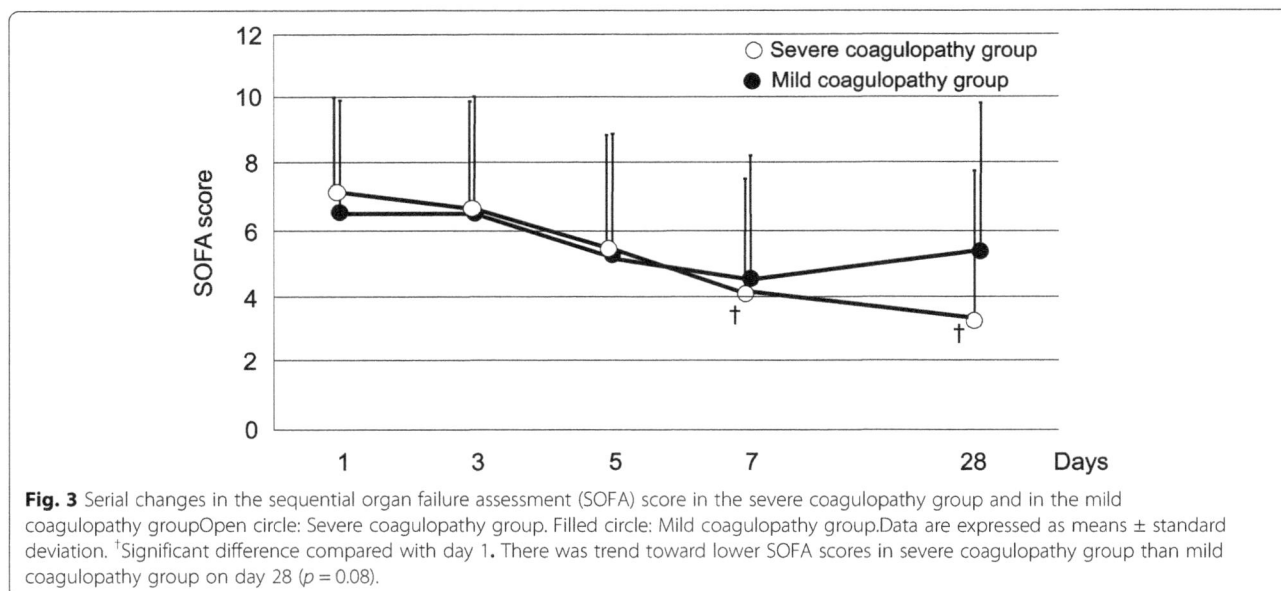

Fig. 3 Serial changes in the sequential organ failure assessment (SOFA) score in the severe coagulopathy group and in the mild coagulopathy groupOpen circle: Severe coagulopathy group. Filled circle: Mild coagulopathy group.Data are expressed as means ± standard deviation. †Significant difference compared with day 1. There was trend toward lower SOFA scores in severe coagulopathy group than mild coagulopathy group on day 28 (p = 0.08).

toward to improve mortality compared with placebo in patients with sepsis [24]. The majority of patients included in the study were not severe coagulopathy state (ISTH DIC score < 5). It was considered in the study that rhTM may be more beneficial for subjects with greater coagulation abnormality. Multicenter retrospective study has shown that rhTM improved mortality significantly [16]. Yoshimura et al. reported that rhTM improves mortality in high risk septic patients (APACHEII 24–29). On the other hand, rhTM did not improve mortality in moderate risk of septic patients (APACHE II score < 24) [25]. Moreover ISTH score was significantly higher in high risk and very high risk of septic patients compared with moderate risk of septic patients. In addition, the patients included in this study were high risk of septic patients (APACHE II score; 27.1 ± 8.1 and 29.4 ± 11.0).

Generally, it is difficult to determine the survival benefit of a particular lifesaving therapy in a set of patients with a low risk of mortality. This may be one of the reasons why thTM administration does not reduce the mortality risk in patients who are not at high risk in the first place. On the other hand, these results are congruent with recent pathophysiological findings concerning

the innate immune response. Under certain circumstances, thrombosis is considered to play a major physiological role, which is specifically named immunothrombosis, in immune defense [26]. However, aberrant of uncontrolled activation of immunothrombosis is likely to constitute a key event in the development of thrombotic disorders [27]. In patients in the mild coagulopathy state, rhTM could have inhibited host-defensive thrombosis, which suppress to capture and ensnare pathogens circulating in the blood, and therefore failed to improve mortality. In contrast, immunothrombosis could have been aberrantly activated and proved detrimental to the host in patients in the severe coagulopathy state, which may have improved mortality. SOFA score was trends in lower of the severe coagulopathy group, as compared with mild coagulopathy group. It is considered that rhTM may improve organ dysfunction by improving severe coagulopathy. Furthermore, respiratory component of the SOFA score was significant reduction in the severe coagulopathy group than mild coagulopathy group in the present study.

Several studies have shown that rhTM improves coagulopathy in disseminated intravascular coagulation [28, 29].

Yamakawa et al. showed that rhTM improves coagulopathy, mortality and SOFA score compared with control group [17]. It was discussed in the study that suppressing the hypercoagulative state by rhTM administration may potentially prevent the progression to multiple organ failure. rhTM has the effect of directly combining with thrombin. Thrombin – rhTM complex activates protein C. Therefore the anticoagulative effect of rhTM depends on the amount of thrombin available. The subgroup analysis of PROWESS trial has shown that activated protein C improves respiratory dysfunction in patients with sepsis [30]. Moreover, Ogawa et al.,

Table 5 The components of the SOFA score at day 7

	Mild coagulopathy (n = 37)	Severe coagulopathy (n = 32)	P value
Respiratory	0.93 ± 0.18	0.44 ± 0.18	0.029
Cardiovascular	0.83 ± 0.25	1.08 ± 0.27	0.438
Hepatic	1.50 ± 0.29	1.43 ± 0.30	0.843
Renal	1.12 ± 0.25	0.78 ± 0.26	0.673
Coagulation	1.54 ± 0.19	1.23 ± 0.20	0.253

Data are presented as mean ± standard error unless otherwise stated

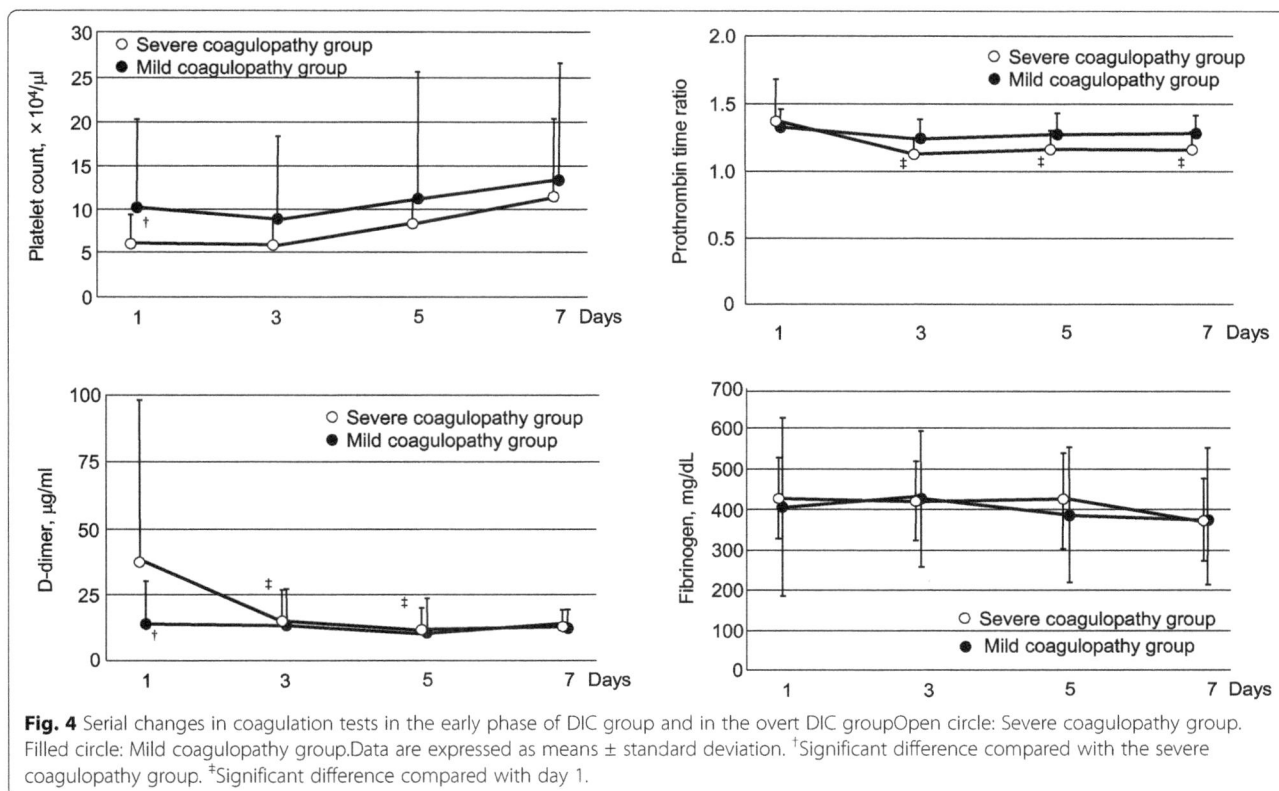

Fig. 4 Serial changes in coagulation tests in the early phase of DIC group and in the overt DIC groupOpen circle: Severe coagulopathy group. Filled circle: Mild coagulopathy group.Data are expressed as means ± standard deviation. [†]Significant difference compared with the severe coagulopathy group. [‡]Significant difference compared with day 1.

reported the respiratory component of the SOFA score reduced significantly in patients with DIC who treated by rhTM compared with placebo [31]. The results of this study indicate that respiratory component of the SOFA score was more reduced in the severe coagulopathy group than the mild coagulopathy group. rhTM was considered to improve respiratory dysfunction by more activating protein C in severe coagulopathy state than mild coagulopathy state. Therefore, administrating rhTM might more improve not only coagulopathy but also respiratory dysfunction in patients with severe coagulopathy compared with those without rhTM. We considered that there might be relation among SOFA score and mortality, SOFA score was not selected as covariate for mortality in current study. We considered reason of above was because of small sample size.

We acknowledge several limitations of our observational study design. First, this study was retrospective small scale trial. Second, this study is not a randomized placebo controlled trial. Multiple unmeasured variables might account for the outcome differences observed in this study. Third, this study was carried out in a single institution. Further multicenter, prospective randomized trials are needed to thoroughly evaluate the effects of rhTM on the treatment of septic patients with coagulopathy.

Conclusion

In conclusion, we found that rhTM administration may reduce mortality by improving organ dysfunction especially for respiratory in septic patients with severe coagulopathy. The present study represents the first attempt to evaluate efficacy of rhTM in septic patients with different degree of coagulopathy. Further clinical investigations are necessary to evaluate the effect of rhTM in several degree of coagulopathy.

Abbreviations
AKI: Acute kidney injury; APACHE II: Acute Physiologic and Chronic Health Evaluation II; AT III: Antithrombin III; DIC: Disseminated intravascular coagulation; ICU: Intensive care unit; ISTH: Subcommittee of the International Society on Thrombosis and Haemostasis; JAAM: Japanese Association for Acute Medicine; PT: Prothrombin time; rhTM: Recombinant human soluble thrombomodulin; SOFA: Sequential Organ Failure Assessment; SSC: Surviving sepsis campaign

Authors' contributions
TK and KM contributed to the study conception and design, collected and assembled the study data, contributed to the writing and revising of the manuscript, and provided final approval of the manuscript. TK performed the statistical analysis. All authors read and approved the final manuscript.

Competing interests
The authors declare that they have no competing interests.

Author details
[1]Departments of Pharmacy, Aichi Medical University, 1 -1 Yazakokarimata, Nagakute, Aichi 480-1195, Japan. [2]Laboratory of Clinical Pharmacodynamics, Aichi Gakuin University School of Pharmacy, Nagakute, Japan.

References

1. Martin GS, Mannino DM, Eaton S, Moss M. The epidemiology of sepsis in the United States from 1979 through 2000. N Engl J Med. 2003;348:1546–54.
2. Levy MM, Dellinger RP, Townsend SR, Linde-Zwirble WT, Marshall JC, Bion J, et al. The surviving Sepsis campaign: results of an international guideline-based performance improvement program targeting severe sepsis. Intensive Care Med. 2010;36:222–31.
3. Miller RR 3rd, Dong L, Nelson NC, Brown SM, Kuttler KG, Probst DR, et al. Multicenter implementation of a severe sepsis and septic shock treatment bundle. Am J Respir Crit Care Med. 2013;188:77–82.
4. Ferrer R, Artigas A, Levy MM, Blanco J, González-Díaz G, Garnacho-Montero J, et al. Improvement in process of care and outcome after a multicenter severe sepsis educational program in Spain. JAMA. 2008;299:2294–303.
5. Zhang L, Zhu G, Han L, Fu P. Early goal-directed therapy in the management of severe sepsis or septic shock in adults: a meta-analysis of randomized controlled trials. BMC Med. 2015;13:71.
6. Bakhtiari K, Meijers JC, de Jonge E, Levi M. Prospective validation of the International Society of Thrombosis and Haemostasis scoring system for disseminated intravascular coagulation. Crit Care Med. 2004;32:2416–21.
7. Zeerleder S, Hack CE, Wuillemin WA. Disseminated intravascular coagulation in sepsis. Chest. 2005;128:2864–75.
8. Levi M, Toh CH, Thachil J, Watson HG. Guidelines for the diagnosis and management of disseminated intravascular coagulation. Br J Haematol. 2009;145:24–33.
9. Wada H, Wakita Y, Nakase T, Shimura M, Hiyoyama K, Nagaya S, et al. Outcome of disseminated intravascular coagulation in relation to the score when treatment was begun. Mie DIC Study Group Thromb Haemost. 1995;74:848–52.
10. Dhainaut JF, Yan SB, Joyce DE, Pettilä V, Basson B, Brandt JT, et al. Treatment effects of drotrecogin alfa (activated) in patients with severe sepsis with or without overt disseminated intravascular coagulation. J Thromb Haemost. 2004;2:1924–33.
11. Gando S, Iba T, Eguchi Y, Ohtomo Y, Okamoto K, Koseki K, Mayumi T, Murata A, Ikeda T, Ishikura H, Ueyama M, Ogura H, Kushimoto S, Saitoh D, Endo S. Shimazaki S; a multicenter, prospective validation of disseminated intravascular coagulation diagnostic criteria for critically ill patients: comparing current criteria. Crit Care Med. 2006;34:625–31.
12. Saito H, Maruyama I, Shimazaki S, Yamamoto Y, Aikawa N, Ohno R, et al. Efficacy and safety of recombinant human soluble thrombomodulin (ART-123) in disseminated intravascular coagulation: results of a phase III, randomized, double-blind clinical trial. J Thromb Haemost. 2007;5:31–41.
13. Iba T, Nakarai E, Takayama T, Nakajima K, Sasaoka T, Ohno Y. Combination effect of antithrombin and recombinant human soluble thrombomodulin in a lipopolysaccharide induced rat sepsis model. Crit Care. 2009;13:R203.
14. Uchiba M, Okajima K, Murakami K, Johno M, Okabe H, Takatsuki K. Recombinant thrombomodulin prevents endotoxin-induced lung injury in rats by inhibiting leukocyte activation. Am J Phys. 1996;271:L470–5.
15. Yamakawa K, Aihara M, Ogura H, Yuhara H, Hamasaki T, Shimazu T. Recombinant human soluble thrombomodulin in severe sepsis: a systematic review and meta-analysis. J Thromb Haemost. 2015;13:508–19.
16. Hayakawa M, Yamakawa K, Saito S, Uchino S, Kudo D, Iizuka Y, et al. Recombinant human soluble thrombomodulin and mortality in sepsis-induced disseminated intravascular coagulation. A multicentre retrospective study. Thromb Haemost. 2016;115:1157–66.
17. Yamakawa K, Fujimi S, Mohri T, Matsuda H, Nakamori Y, Hirose T, et al. Treatment effects of recombinant human soluble

thrombomodulin in patients with severe sepsis: a historical control study. Crit Care. 2011;15:R123.
18. Seymour CW, Liu VX, Iwashyna TJ, Brunkhorst FM, Rea TD, Scherag A, et al. Assessment of clinical criteria for Sepsis: for the third international consensus definitions for Sepsis and septic shock (Sepsis-3). JAMA. 2016;315:762–74.
19. Dellinger RP, Levy MM, Rhodes A, Annane D, Gerlach H, Opal SM, et al. Surviving Sepsis campaign: international guidelines for Management of Severe Sepsis and Septic Shock, 2012. Intensive Care Med. 2013;39:165–228.
20. Mehta RL, Kellum JA, Shah SV, Molitoris BA, Ronco C, Warnock DG, et al. Acute kidney injury network: report of an initiative to improve outcomes in acute kidney injury. Crit Care. 2007;11:R31.
21. Vincent JL, Moreno R, Takala J, Willatts S, De Mendonça A, Bruining H, et al. The SOFA (Sepsis-related organ failure assessment) score to describe organ dysfunction/failure. On behalf of the working group on Sepsis-related problems of the European Society of Intensive Care Medicine. Intensive Care Med. 1996;22:707–10.
22. Taylor FB Jr, Toh CH, Hoots WK, Wada H, Levi M. Towards definition, clinical and laboratory criteria, and a scoring system for disseminated intravascular coagulation. Thromb Haemost. 2001;86:1327–30.
23. Gando S, Iba T, Eguchi Y, Ohtomo Y, Okamoto K, Koseki K, et al. A multicenter, prospective validation of disseminated intravascular coagulation diagnostic criteria for critically ill patients: comparing current criteria. Crit Care Med. 2006;34:625–31.
24. Vincent JL, Ramesh MK, Ernest D, LaRosa SP, Pachl J, Aikawa N, et al. A randomized, double-blind, placebo-controlled, phase 2b study to evaluate the safety and efficacy of recombinant human soluble thrombomodulin, ART-123, in patients with sepsis and suspected disseminated intravascular coagulation. Crit Care Med. 2013;41:2069–79.
25. Yoshimura J, Yamakawa K, Ogura H, Umemura Y, Takahashi H, Morikawa M, et al. Benefit profile of recombinant human soluble thrombomodulin in sepsis-induced disseminated intravascular coagulation: a multicenter propensity score analysis. Crit Care. 2015;19:78.
26. Engelmann B, Massberg S. Thrombosis as an intravascular effector of innate immunity. Nat Rev Immunol. 2013;13:34–45.
27. Esmon CT. The interactions between inflammation and coagulation. Br J Haematol. 2005;131:417–30.
28. Yasuda N, Goto K, Ohchi Y, Abe T, Koga H, Kitano T, et al. The efficacy and safety of antithrombin and recombinant human thrombomodulin combination therapy in patients with severe sepsis and disseminated intravascular coagulation. J Crit Care. 2016;36:29–34.
29. Hashimoto D, Chikamoto A, Miyanari N, Ohara C, Kuramoto M, Horino K, et al. Recombinant soluble thrombomodulin for postoperative disseminated intravascular coagulation. J Surg Res. 2015;197:405–11.
30. Vincent JL, Angus DC, Artigas A, Kalil A, Basson BR, Jamal HH, et al. Effects of drotrecogin alfa (activated) on organ dysfunction in the PROWESS trial. Crit Care Med. 2003;31:834–40.
31. Ogawa Y, Yamakawa K, Ogura H, Kiguchi T, Mohri T, Nakamori Y, et al. Recombinant human soluble thrombomodulin improves mortality and respiratory dysfunction in patients with severe sepsis. J Trauma. 2012;72:1150–7.

19

The diagnosis and treatment of venous thromboembolism in Asian patients

Kang-Ling Wang[1,2], Eng Soo Yap[3,4], Shinya Goto[5], Shu Zhang[6], Chung-Wah Siu[7] and Chern-En Chiang[1,2]*

Abstract: Although the incidence of venous thromboembolism (VTE) in Asian populations is lower than in Western countries, the overall burden of VTE in Asia has been considerably underestimated. Factors that may explain the lower prevalence of VTE in Asian populations relative to Western populations include the limited availability of epidemiological data in Asia, ethnic differences in the genetic predisposition to VTE, underdiagnoses, low awareness toward thrombotic disease, and possibly less symptomatic VTE in Asian patients. The clinical assessment, diagnostic testing, and therapeutic considerations for VTE are, in general, the same in Asian populations as they are in Western populations. The management of VTE is based upon balancing the treatment benefits against the risk of bleeding. This is an especially important consideration for Asian populations because of increased risk of intracranial hemorrhage with vitamin K antagonists. Non-vitamin K antagonist oral anticoagulants have shown advantages over current treatment modalities with respect to bleeding outcomes in major phase 3 clinical trials, including in Asian populations. Although anticoagulant therapy has been shown to reduce the risk of postoperative VTE in Western populations, VTE prophylaxis is not administered routinely in Asian countries. Despite advances in the management of VTE, data in Asian populations on the incidence, prevalence, recurrence, risk factors, and management of bleeding complications are limited and there is need for increased awareness. To that end, this review summarizes the available data on the epidemiology, risk stratification, diagnosis, and treatment considerations in the management of VTE in Asia.

Keywords: Venous thromboembolism, Asia, Epidemiology, Risk factors, Treatment

Background

Venous thromboembolism (VTE), which includes deep vein thrombosis (DVT) and pulmonary embolism (PE), is a significant healthcare burden that remains under-recognized [1–3]. Even with anticoagulant therapy, the mortality rate and the risk of recurrence are high in the early phase of VTE [4–6], and it has serious long-term complications, including chronic pulmonary hypertension and post-thrombotic syndrome, both of which require substantial healthcare resources for their management and are associated with considerable morbidity [7, 8].

VTE is a common cause of preventable mortality for both medical and surgical patients. In addition to early mortality related to PE, VTE associated with hospitalization is a leading cause of lost disability-adjusted life years across low-, middle-, and high-income countries. Although anticoagulant therapy has been shown to reduce the risk of postoperative

VTE in Western populations, VTE prophylaxis is not administered routinely in Asian countries [9–11].

The disease burden associated with VTE is high, as the incidence of VTE in Western countries is approximately 100 cases per 100,000 patient-years [12]. The incidence of VTE has risen in Asia over recent years but remains lower than in Western countries [13, 14]. In this review, we summarize the epidemiology, risk stratification, diagnosis, and treatment considerations in the management of VTE in Asia.

Epidemiology

Although Asian populations are subject to the same major acquired risk factors for VTE as Western populations, studies conducted in Asia have consistently reported lower rates of VTE in Asian populations than in Caucasians (Table 1) [3, 13, 15–20]. These data are comparable to those obtained from Asian patients in Western countries [21, 22]. There are several possibilities that may explain the lower rate of VTE in Asian populations relative to Western populations. Firstly, the estimates may be lower than the true numbers because

* Correspondence: cechiang@vghtpe.gov.tw
[1]General Clinical Research Center, Taipei Veterans General Hospital, No. 201, Sec. 2, Shipai Rd., 11217 Taipei, Taiwan
[2]School of Medicine, National Yang-Ming University, Taipei, Taiwan
Full list of author information is available at the end of the article

Table 1 Estimated incidence of VTE from studies in Western and Asian populations [3, 13, 15–20]

Incidence[a]	Western countries			Asian countries				
	UK	Norway	US (age-adjusted)	Taiwan[b]	Hong Kong	Japan[c]	Korea[c] (age-adjusted)	Singapore[d]
VTE	75	143	117	16	17	NR	14	57
DVT	40	93	48	NR	NR	12	5	NR
PE	34	50	69	NR	NR	6	7	15

[a]First incidence per 100,000 person-years unless indicated otherwise
[b]Crude incidence
[c]Overall incidence
[d]Overall incidence (Chinese, Indian, Malay)
DVT deep vein thrombosis, *NR* not reported, *PE* pulmonary embolism, *VTE* venous thromboembolism

of the limited availability of epidemiological data in Asia and the asymptomatic nature of VTE. Secondly, historically, the difference in incidence rates reflects underdiagnosis in Asian patients as a result of low awareness toward thrombotic disease and/or manifestations, low clinical suspicion due to the perceived low incidence rate, and limited access to healthcare resources [23–25]. In addition, low autopsy rates—mainly because of cultural and religious practices—may partially account for the perceived low incidence rate of VTE in Asia [25]. Autopsies reveal high rates of asymptomatic thrombosis [2], and autopsy studies indicate that the incidence of PE in Asian countries is comparable with that in Western countries [2, 26, 27]. Finally, the low rates of VTE in Asian populations may be attributed to the low prevalence of risk factors, such as obesity and mutations, in prothrombin or factor V Leiden genes [28–31]. Accordingly, these data suggest that the rate of VTE in Asia may be underestimated, particularly because the thrombi tend not to advance to symptomatic thrombosis in Asian patients [32].

Risk factors

Heritable risk factors arise from genetic abnormalities in the components of the coagulation pathway that lead to hereditary thrombophilia, including mutations in factor V and prothrombin; and deficiencies of protein S, protein C, and antithrombin [28]. While factor V Leiden and prothrombin G20210A polymorphisms are exclusive to Caucasians, the prevalence of protein S, protein C, and

antithrombin deficiencies in Asian populations are higher than those found in Caucasians (Table 2) [30, 33–38].

Although the major inherited risk factors for VTE are different between Asian and Western populations, the major acquired risk factors in Asians are similar to those of the Western populations [39]. Risk factors, such as surgery, trauma, prolonged bed rest, immobility, and pregnancy, are transient and reversible, while risk factors, such as malignancy and paralysis due to nerve damages, are irreversible. The most common acquired risk factor for VTE in Asians is malignancy; 16% to 40% of VTE cases are cancer-associated [40–42]. Other common acquired risk factors for VTE in Asians include surgery, immobility, obesity, advanced age, and the use of oral contraceptives [39, 43].

VTE is a serious complication after high-risk surgeries even when preventive measures are taken. The rates for symptomatic DVT and PE with low-molecular-weight heparin (LMWH) after orthopedic surgery are 0.8% and 0.35%, respectively [10]. Since Asian patients have a perceived lower risk for symptomatic VTE following surgery than in Western populations, regular prophylaxis in Asian patients at high risk for VTE is not always administered [44]. However, in studies involving Asian patients undergoing major surgery, the incidence of postoperative DVT was noted to be similar to that reported in Western populations [39, 45–50]. The Assessment of the Incidence of Deep Vein Thrombosis in Asia (AIDA) study, which was conducted in 19 centers across Asia (China, Indonesia, Korea, Malaysia, the Philippines, Taiwan, and Thailand) in patients

Table 2 Ethnic differences in the distribution of inherited thrombophilias

	Healthy subjects		Patients with VTE	
	Western [123]	Asian [33, 39]	Western [123]	Asian [39]
Factor V Leiden mutation	4.8%	0%–0.2%	18.8%	0%
Prothrombin G20210A mutation	2.7%	0%–0.2%	7.1%	0%
Protein S deficiency	0.03%–0.13%	0.06%–6.4%	2.3%	10.7%–17.8%
Protein C deficiency	0.2%–0.4%	0.3%–4.0%	3.7%	8.9%–10.7%
Antithrombin deficiency	0.02%	0%–6.4%	1.9%	4.7%–8.1%

VTE venous thromboembolism

undergoing total hip or knee arthroplasty or hip fracture surgery and did not receive thromboprophylaxis, assessed the rate of DVT of the lower limbs using bilateral venography; DVT was diagnosed in 41% of patients (121/295) [51]. A meta-analysis of 22 studies done in Asian patients undergoing orthopedic procedures showed that Asian patients have similar overall DVT rates detected by venography, but a lower rate of symptomatic and proximal DVT than Western populations [52]. The Epidemiologic International Day for the Evaluation of Patients at Risk for Venous Thromboembolism in the Acute Hospital Care Setting EN-DORSE) study was a multinational cross-sectional survey designed to assess the prevalence of VTE in accordance with the 2004 American College of Chest Physicians (ACCP) guidelines in the acute hospital care setting. In Asian countries (India, Thailand, Pakistan, and Bangladesh), the proportion of surgical patients at risk for VTE ranged from 44% to 62%, which was similar to the proportion reported for all countries studied (overall: 64%; range: 44%–80%) [9]. These findings suggest that surgical patients at risk for VTE in Asian countries should receive appropriate VTE prophylaxis.

Diagnosis considerations

In general, the clinical assessment and diagnostic testing for VTE are the same in Asian populations as they are in non-Asian populations. DVT usually originates in the deep veins of the calf and can extend into the popliteal and femoral veins [53]. DVT at the calf is generally asymptomatic, but it may produce symptoms once it extends proximally and obstructs venous outflow [53, 54]. Symptomatic DVT is suspected primarily on the basis of unilateral leg pain, swelling, and/or redness [55]. Once extended proximally, venous thrombi may give rise to fatal PE [54]. Common symptoms of PE include palpitation, dyspnea, chest pain, cough, and/or syncope [56, 57].

Careful clinical examinations of signs, symptoms, and risk factors associated with suspected VTE, and distinguishing it from other medical conditions, are important for accurate diagnosis of the disease. Clinical assessment, plasma D-dimer measurement, and imaging tests are recommended and validated for the diagnosis of DVT and PE. The most commonly proposed systematic diagnostic management techniques for VTE are illustrated in Fig. 1.

Clinical assessment

The Wells scoring system is the most widely used pretest probability scoring system stratifying patients with suspected DVT or PE [58, 59]. The clinical features used for DVT stratification are (1) active cancer; (2) immobilization of the lower extremities; (3) bed rest for more than 3 days or major surgery within 12 weeks; (4) tenderness along the distribution of the deep venous system; (5) swollen leg; (6) affected calf swelling by more than 3 cm as being compared with the asymptomatic leg; (7) pitting edema; (8) collateral superficial (nonvaricose) veins; and (9) alternative diagnoses as likely as DVT [60]. The clinical features used for PE stratification are (1) signs and symptoms of DVT; (2) heart rate higher than 100 beats/min; (3) immobilization for ≥3 consecutive days or surgery in the previous 4 weeks; (4) previous objectively diagnosed DVT or PE; (5) hemoptysis; (6) active cancer; (7) and PE as likely as, or more likely than, an alternative diagnosis [61]. Although the reliability of the Wells scoring system has been established in Western populations, among Asian countries it has only been validated for DVT in Japan and Singapore with relatively small number of patients [62–64]. Based on the results of 2 Japanese studies, the combination of Wells scoring system and D-dimer testing was effective in excluding DVT and reducing the need for venous duplex scanning. In a study conducted in Singapore, the combination of Wells scoring system and D-dimer testing was effective in reducing unnecessary ultrasound scans for excluding DVT in patients with suspected DVT presenting to the emergency department. Despite these promising results from Asian patients, confirmatory studies with a larger number of patients will help establish the effectiveness of the Wells scoring system in Asia.

Diagnostic tests

D-dimer, a degradation product of cross-linked fibrin, is typically elevated in VTE, but also in conditions such as infection, malignancy, pregnancy, surgery, trauma, and stroke [65]. The value of D-dimer testing, due to its moderate specificity, lies in its ability as a negative predictor in patients with suspected DVT or PE when used in combination with clinical pretest probability in both Asian and Western populations [60, 66–70], simplifying the diagnostic process (illustrated in Fig. 1). Although D-dimer testing alone was not accurate enough to detect DVT after total knee arthroplasty in Asian patients [70], it was useful in excluding DVT in hospitalized Japanese patients with acute medical diseases. Among 42 hospitalized patients with acute medical diseases in which plasma D-dimer was measured, the sensitivity and negative predictive value of D-dimer reached 100%, while the positive predictive value (31.6%) and specificity (13.3%) were low [68].

Commercially available D-dimer assays include latex agglutination, whole blood agglutination, and enzyme-linked immunosorbent assays [71]. The Taiwan Society of Cardiology guidelines recommend using D-dimer enzyme-linked immunofluorescence, enzyme-linked

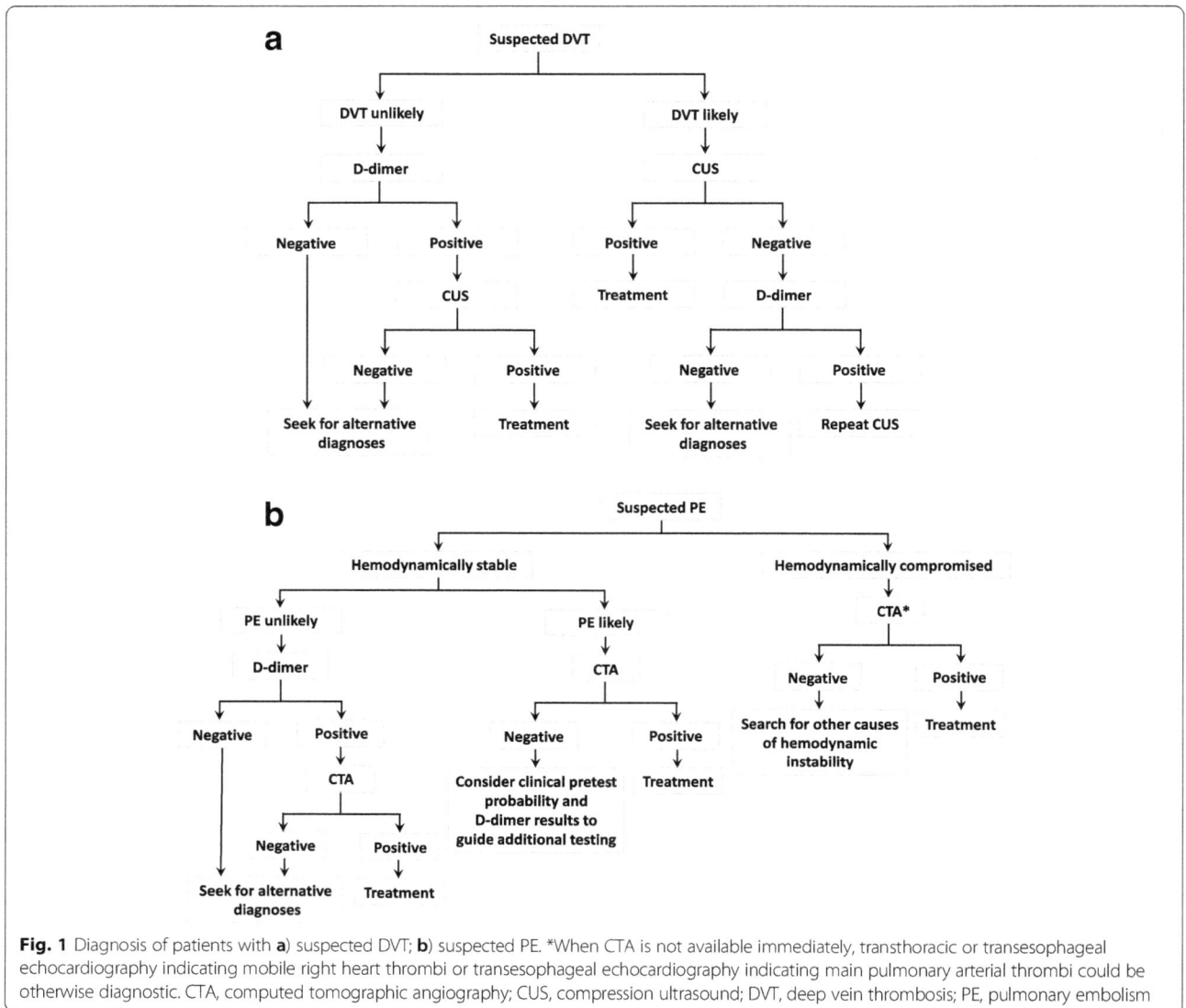

Fig. 1 Diagnosis of patients with **a**) suspected DVT; **b**) suspected PE. *When CTA is not available immediately, transthoracic or transesophageal echocardiography indicating mobile right heart thrombi or transesophageal echocardiography indicating main pulmonary arterial thrombi could be otherwise diagnostic. CTA, computed tomographic angiography; CUS, compression ultrasound; DVT, deep vein thrombosis; PE, pulmonary embolism

immunosorbent, and latex quantitative assays over whole blood, latex semiquantitative, and latex qualitative assays due to their higher sensitivity. Furthermore, since the specificity of D-dimer assay seems to decrease with age, age-adjusted cutoffs (age × 10 µg/L above 50 years) are suggested to improve the specificity of D-dimer testing [72]. Due to the difficulty in standardization of the different available assays, the D-dimer assays used in the diagnostic processes should be of equivalent sensitivity and specificity to ones used in clinical trials in order to be able to compare results obtained with different methods.

In both Asian and Western populations, compression ultrasound (CUS) and multidetector computed tomographic angiography (CTA) have become the methods of choice for effectively imaging the vasculature with high sensitivity and specificity in patients with suspected DVT and PE, respectively [73, 74]. The sensitivity and specificity

of CUS for DVT (proximal and distal) is 90.3% and 97.8%, respectively. The sensitivity and specificity of CTA for PE is 83.0% and 96.0%, respectively [75, 76].

Risk stratification

Selection of patients who are at low or high risk of VTE is crucial when considering prevention options for VTE. The development of VTE in patients is affected by the aforementioned risk factors, such as age, previous history of VTE, cancer, and surgery. Although orthopedic surgeries, such as total hip or knee arthroplasty and hip fracture surgery, are classified as high risk for VTE in Asia, VTE risk stratification is not routine and there is a strong need for a hospital VTE management protocol for VTE risk assessment [77].

The Pulmonary Embolism Severity Index (PESI) and its simplified version (sPESI) are the most extensively used prediction scores for the risk stratification in patients diagnosed with PE in order to guide therapeutic decision making [78, 79]. PE patients with a sPESI score of 0 have a 30-day all-cause mortality rate of 1%, whereas PE patients with a sPESI score of 1 or more have a 30-day all-cause mortality rate of 9% to 11% [79]. PE patients with a sPESI score of 0 are considered to be low risk and may be considered for outpatient treatment [57]. However, patients estimated to be high risk may benefit from inpatient management and/or higher levels of care (ie, intensive care setting). The Hestia criteria are also widely used for selecting patients with PE, including those with right ventricular (RV) dysfunction, for outpatient treatment [80, 81].

The bleeding risk assessment tools may be useful for distinguishing which patients are at low or high risk of bleeding and for identifying patients who might benefit from extended anticoagulation [82–86]. A risk score based on VTE patients included in the RIETE registry identified VTE patients at low, intermediate, or high risk of major bleeding during the first 3 months of therapy. This score was based on 6 variables documented at entry—recent major bleeding, anemia, cancer, abnormal creatinine levels, age > 75 years, and PE diagnosis at baseline [84]. Similarly, the VTE-BLEED score was based on 6 variables—active cancer, male with uncontrolled arterial hypertension, anemia, history of bleeding, age ≥ 60 years, and renal dysfunction—and accurately predicted major bleeding events in VTE patients on anticoagulation [86, 87]. The predictive value of these bleeding risk scores is uncertain in Asian populations and needs to be validated with careful examination of independent risk factors in Asians.

VTE prevention and treatment guidelines in Asia
The effectiveness of postoperative thromboprophylaxis in Western countries is well recognized [10, 11]. Recent studies conducted in Asia reported that postoperative thromboprophylaxis reduces VTE risk without significantly increasing the risk of bleeding [88]. For the prevention of VTE in patients undergoing high-risk surgeries, thromboprophylaxis with anticoagulants and/or mechanical prophylaxis are typically recommended based on patients' risk of bleeding [11, 14]. The Asian Venous Thrombosis Forum—composed of experts from China, Hong Kong, Malaysia, the Philippines, Singapore, Taiwan, Thailand, India, Indonesia, Korea, Australia, and Europe—recommends using mechanical prophylaxis for patients with increased risk of bleeding, and mechanical prophylaxis in combination with pharmacological prophylaxis for patients with high risk of VTE [77]. Korean Society of Thrombosis and Hemostasis guidelines also recommend using mechanical prophylaxis for patients with increased risk of bleeding and pharmacological

prophylaxis, including LMWH, fondaparinux, dabigatran, apixaban, rivaroxaban, low-dose unfractionated heparin, vitamin K antagonist (VKA; ie, warfarin), or aspirin, for patients undergoing major orthopedic surgery of the lower limbs, such as total hip or knee arthroplasty [89]. According to the latest update, the Asia-Pacific Thrombosis Advisory Board suggests routine use of postoperative thromboprophylaxis for VTE after major orthopedic surgery. They further suggest that the use of non-vitamin K antagonist oral anticoagulants (NOACs) may simplify patient management in Asia primarily due to no regular coagulation monitoring requirement because of their predictable pharmacokinetic (PK) and pharmacodynamic (PD) properties, and demonstrating no interactions with nonsteroidal anti-inflammatory drugs [88]. The Asian Venous Thrombosis Forum recommends LMWH (ie, enoxaparin), fondaparinux, NOACs, VKA, or aspirin with intermittent pneumatic compression for thromboprophylaxis in patients undergoing total hip or knee arthroplasty or hip fracture surgery [77]. Enoxaparin and fondaparinux are the standard therapy for the prevention of VTE in Japanese patients undergoing abdominal surgery or orthopedic surgery of the lower limbs [14]. However, results of a small sized randomized controlled trial conducted in Japan suggested that dabigatran reduces incidence of VTE in patients undergoing total knee arthroplasty with a safety profile comparable to placebo [90]. Furthermore, results from small sized phase 3 trials (STARS [Studying Thrombosis After Replacement Surgery]) indicated that edoxaban is superior to enoxaparin in preventing VTE in Japanese patients undergoing total hip and knee arthroplasty, and has similar safety and efficacy as enoxaparin in hip fracture surgery [91–93]. The results of these clinical trials led to the approval of edoxaban for venous thromboprophylaxis in patients undergoing major orthopedic surgery in Japan [94]. In a postmarketing surveillance study done to monitor the adverse drug reactions of edoxaban during the first 6 months after its commercial launch in Japan, edoxaban's safety data were consistent with its known safety profile [95].

The goal of the VTE treatment is to prevent thrombus extension and recurrence through pharmacological or mechanical interventions [96]. Japanese and Taiwanese guidelines were issued by the Japanese Circulation Society (JCS) in 2011 and by the Taiwan Society of Cardiology in 2016 [14, 72]. The ACCP VTE treatment guidelines and European Society of Cardiology PE guidelines are also widely used in Asia [57, 97]. According to the latest update, treatment with NOACs is suggested over VKA therapy. The suggested duration of treatment for symptomatic DVT (distal or proximal) or PE is at least 3 months, and patients should be evaluated for the risk-benefit ratio to determine the need for extended therapy (no scheduled stop date) (Fig. 2) [96]. However, the JCS guidelines recommend using intravenous unfrac-tionated heparin (UFH) overlapped with, and followed by, VKA for a minimum of 3 months, and the recom-mended target international normalized ratio (INR) range is 1.5 – 2.5. This target INR range is lower than the range recommended in Western countries (ie, 2.0–3.0) perhaps because of increased bleeding tendency in Japanese patients [14, 43]. Although use of LMWH was adopted in the US and Europe to overcome the limitations of UFH for the treatment of VTE, LMWH has yet to be approved for this indication in Japan due to limited clinical evidence from Japanese patients [98]. The Taiwanese guidelines recommend using either intra-venous UFH or LMWH overlapped with, and followed by, VKA with a maintenance target INR of 2.0 to 3.0 [72].

NOACs have been approved for the treatment of VTE in many countries in Asia; however, only a few countries provide reimbursements to patients. Dabigatran has been approved in Korea, Singapore, the Philippines, China, Thailand, and Taiwan; rivaroxaban and apixaban have been approved in Korea, Singapore, Japan, China, Thailand, and Taiwan; and edoxaban has been approved in Japan, South Korea, Hong Kong, Thailand, and Taiwan at the time of this review [94, 99, 100].

Anticoagulants for the treatment of VTE
Parenteral anticoagulants
Treatment of DVT and PE has traditionally been initial parenteral anticoagulation overlapping with, or followed by, longer-term VKAs [96]. While the UFH therapy has been proven effective in anticoagulation, it has limita-tions that include the requirement for activated partial thromboplastin time monitoring and the risk of heparin-induced thrombocytopenia and osteoporosis. On the contrary, LMWH and fondaparinux have predictable PK and PD properties and are associated with a lower risk of nonhemorrhagic side effects [101]. On average, Asian

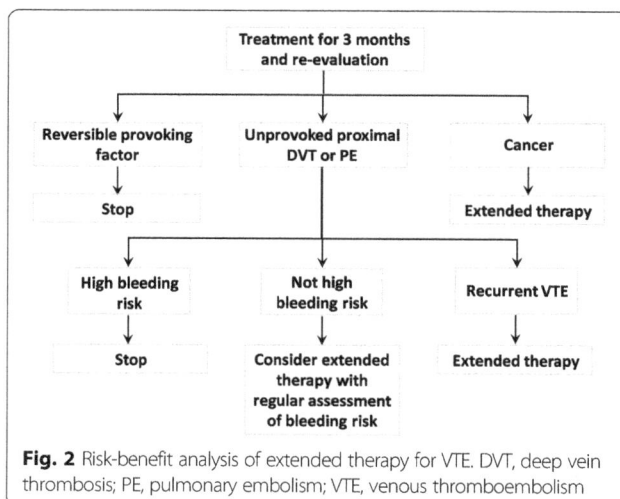

Fig. 2 Risk-benefit analysis of extended therapy for VTE. DVT, deep vein thrombosis; PE, pulmonary embolism; VTE, venous thromboembolism

patients have lower body mass index than non-Asian populations [102]. Weight-based dose adjustments without routine monitoring are required for parenteral anticoagulants [101, 103]; however, the need for paren-teral administration limits their use for outpatient treatment [104]. Regular monitoring of LMWH therapy is recommended only for patients who have an increased risk of bleeding, such as patients with extremely low or high body weight, renal insufficiency (creatinine clear-ance <30 mL/min), and advanced age [105–107].

Vitamin K antagonists
VKAs have been the most widely used anticoagulants for the treatment of VTE, but they have several limitations in terms of patient acceptance, including a slow onset and offset of action and a narrow thera-peutic window that requires individualized dosing based on INR with the need for regular monitoring [108]. In addition, Asian patients are at an increased risk for bleeding when treated with VKAs. As shown in a post hoc analysis of RE-LY (Randomized Evaluation of Long-term Anticoagulation Therapy), ROCKET AF (Rivaroxaban Once Daily Oral Direct Factor Xa Inhibition Compared with Vitamin K Antagonism for Prevention of Stroke and Embolism Trial in Atrial Fibrillation), and ARISTOTLE (Apixa-ban for Reduction in Stroke and Other Thrombo-embolic Events in Atrial Fibrillation) trials, VKA use in Asian patients with atrial fibrillation (AF) is associ-ated with a higher risk of bleeding when compared with non-Asian patients [109]. There is limited information on risk of bleeding with VKAs in Asian patients with VTE. However, according to the available reports from the Hokusai-VTE trial, Asian patients with VTE randomized to VKAs had higher rates of overall and major or clinically relevant nonmajor (CRNM) bleeding than non-Asian patients randomized to VKAs [110]. In a subgroup analysis that examined the results of the Chinese patients included in the EINSTEIN-DVT (Oral Direct Factor Xa Inhibitor Rivaroxaban in Patients with Acute Symptomatic Deep Vein Thrombosis) and EINSTEIN-PE (Oral Direct Factor Xa Inhibitor Rivaroxaban in Patients with Acute Symptomatic Pulmonary Embol-ism) trials, 9.2% (20/218) of patients receiving VKA therapy experienced a major or CRNM bleeding event [111]. In the AMPLIFY-J (Apixaban for the Initial Management of Pulmonary Embolism and Deep Vein Thrombosis as First-Line Therapy-Japan) trial, 28.2% (11/39) of Japanese patients receiving VKA therapy experienced a major or CRNM bleeding event [112]. On the basis of these data, alternatives to VKAs for the treatment of VTE may be of particular import-ance for Asian populations.

Non-vitamin K antagonist oral anticoagulants

The rapid onset of action, minimal drug and food interactions, predictable PKs, no regular monitoring requirement, and lower risk of bleeding make NOACs an attractive alternative to VKAs [108]. These attributes also make NOACs more applicable for outpatient treatment. The NOACs include the direct thrombin inhibitor dabigatran and the direct factor Xa inhibitors rivaroxaban, apixaban, and edoxaban [113]. Table 3 shows a summary of the efficacy and safety outcomes of clinical trials with NOACs for the treatment of VTE, including in Asian patients.

In both RE-COVER (Efficacy and Safety of Dabigatran Compared to Warfarin for 6 Month Treatment of Acute Symptomatic Venous Thromboembolism) and RE-COVER II trials, patients were randomized to receive dabigatran (150 mg twice daily) or warfarin for 6 months after initial parenteral anticoagulation therapy. Both studies indicated that dabigatran is as efficacious as warfarin, with respect to recurrent VTE, and has a lower risk of CRNM bleeding. Although only 2.6% (65/2539) of patients with acute VTE enrolled in the RE-COVER trial were Asian, 20.9% (537/2568) of patients in the RE-COVER II trial were Asian [114, 115].

Both EINSTEIN-DVT and EINSTEIN-PE trials compared rivaroxaban (15 mg twice daily for 3 weeks, followed by 20 mg once daily) with subcutaneous enoxaparin followed by VKA therapy for 3, 6, or 12 months. In both trials, rivaroxaban was as efficacious as the conventional therapy with respect to recurrent VTE, with a similar safety

profile with respect to major or CRNM bleeding [116, 117]. A subgroup analysis examined the results of the Chinese patients included in the EINSTEIN-DVT and EINSTEIN-PE trials. The relative efficacy and safety of rivaroxaban compared with the conventional therapy in Chinese patients were consistent with that of the overall population [111]. However, the incidence of major or CRNM bleeding for rivaroxaban was lower in Chinese patients compared with the overall population (5.9% vs 9.4%) [111, 118].

J-EINSTEIN DVT and PE trial compared rivaroxaban (10 or 15 mg twice daily for 3 weeks, followed by 15 mg once daily) with UFH/warfarin for 3, 6, or 12 months in Japanese patients. The relative efficacy of rivaroxaban compared with UFH/warfarin in Japanese patients was consistent with that of the overall population of EINSTEIN-DVT and EINSTEIN-PE. Major bleeding did not occur during the study, and CRNM bleeding occurred in 7.8% (6/77) of patients in the rivaroxaban group and 5.3% (1/19) of patients in the UFH/warfarin group [73]. These results suggest the safety of rivaroxaban for the treatment of VTE in Asian patients.

In the AMPLIFY trial, patients with acute VTE were randomly assigned to apixaban (10 mg twice daily for 7 days, followed by 5 mg twice daily) or subcutaneous enoxaparin followed by warfarin for 6 months. Overall, apixaban was found to be noninferior to the conventional therapy, with respect to recurrent VTE, and had a significant lower risk of major or CRNM bleeding [119]. AMPLIFY-J, which was designed based on the AMPLIFY study, compared apixaban with UFH/warfarin for

Table 3 Efficacy and safety outcomes of clinical trials with NOACs for the treatment of VTE

All Patients				Asian Patients			
Trial	N	VTE recurrence[a]	Major or CRNM bleeding[a]	Trial	N	VTE recurrence[a]	Major or CRNM bleeding[a]
Dabigatran				**Dabigatran**			
RE-COVER [114]	2539	1.10 (0.65–1.84)	0.63 (0.47–0.84)	RE-COVER RE-COVER II Asian subanalysis[b]	557	2.55 (0.66–9.90)	0.63 (0.33–1.19)
RE-COVER II [115]	2568	1.08 (0.64–1.80)	0.62 (0.45–0.84)				
Rivaroxaban				**Rivaroxaban**			
EINSTEIN-DVT [116]	3449	0.68 (0.44–1.04)	0.97 (0.76–1.22)	EINSTEIN-DVT and PE Asian subanalysis [111]	439	1.04 (0.36–3.0)	0.63 (0.31–1.26)
EINSTEIN-PE [117]	4832	1.12 (0.75–1.68)	0.90 (0.76–1.07)	J-EINSTEIN DVT and PE [73]	100	3.9% (−3.4 to 23.8)[c]	Rivaroxaban 7.8% UFH/warfarin 5.3%[d]
Apixaban				**Apixaban**			
AMPLIFY [119]	5395	0.84 (0.60–1.18)	0.44 (0.36–0.55)	AMPLIFY-J [112]	80	Apixaban 0/40 UFH/warfarin 1/40[e]	Apixaban 7.5% UFH/warfarin 28.2%[f]
Edoxaban				**Edoxaban**			
Hokusai-VTE [120]	8240	0.89 (0.70–1.13)	0.81 (0.71–0.94)	Hokusai-VTE Asian subanalysis [110]	1109	0.64 (0.34–1.19)	0.56 (0.40–0.78)

[a]Values are hazard ratio (95% confidence interval) unless otherwise indicated
[b]Data on file
[c]Absolute risk difference (95% confidence interval)
[d]Percentage of patients with CRNM bleeding
[e]Number of patients
[f]Percentage of patients
CRNM clinically relevant nonmajor, DVT deep vein thrombosis, NOAC non-vitamin K antagonist oral anticoagulant, PE pulmonary embolism, UFH unfractionated heparin, VTE venous thromboembolism

24 weeks in Japanese patients with acute VTE. Recurrent VTE did not occur in patients receiving apixaban, but occurred in 1 patient receiving UFH/warfarin. Apixaban had a lower risk of major or CRNM bleeding compared with UFH/warfarin, suggesting the safety of apixaban for the treatment of VTE in Japanese patients [112].

Hokusai-VTE trial compared edoxaban (60 mg [reduced to 30 mg in patients with a creatinine clearance 30–50 mL/min or a body weight ≤ 60 kg or in patients receiving potent P-glycoprotein inhibitors concomitantly] once daily) with warfarin for 3 to 12 months after initial heparin therapy. Edoxaban was as efficacious as warfarin, with respect to recurrent VTE, and had a significantly lower risk of major or CRNM bleeding [120]. In a subgroup of PE patients with evident RV dysfunction (N-terminal probrain natriuretic peptide level of ≥500 pg/mL), edoxaban, compared with warfarin, was associated with a lower rate of recurrent VTE. A subgroup analysis evaluated the results of the East Asian patients included in the Hokusai-VTE trial. The relative efficacy of edoxaban compared with warfarin in East Asian patients was consistent with that of the overall population; however, edoxaban had a better safety profile with respect to major or CRNM bleeding than warfarin in East Asian patients, as compared to that of the overall population, confirming the safety of edoxaban for the treatment of VTE in Asia [110]. Hokusai-VTE is the only VTE trial where a NOAC was dose-adjusted by weight or creatinine clearance. Since Asians are known to have lower body mass index than non-Asian populations, future phase 2/3 and PK/PD studies, specifically in Asian patients, will afford new treatment algorithms and dosing regimens by increasing the understanding of specific characteristics of VTE in Asia.

Taken together, based on the results of these pivotal clinical trials, NOACs provide a strong alternative to conventional therapy with similar efficacy and superior safety profiles in the treatment of VTE [121]. Importantly, the results of the analyses that evaluated NOACs in Asian patients and Asian subgroup analyses—specifically EINSTEIN-DVT, EINSTEIN-PE, and Hokusai-VTE—suggest that NOACs present a possible safety advantage for the treatment of VTE in Asian populations. However, the lack of clinical trials assessing the efficacy and safety of NOACs for the treatment and prevention of VTE specifically in Asian populations makes it difficult to change the standard of care in Asian countries.

Conclusions

The overall burden of VTE in Asia has been considerably underestimated. Despite advances in the management of VTE globally, more data on epidemiology in the form of first incidence, prevalence, recurrence and risk factors, management of bleeding complications, as well as increased awareness in Asian populations, are necessary. Although regional standard of care may vary based upon physicians' preference or clinical experience, increased collaborative studies among the Asian countries and participation in international trials may lead to different treatment algorithms and dosing regimens by providing more data on the epidemiology, pharmacology, and bleeding complications of the disease in Asian patients which may differ significantly from Western populations. The ongoing international registry of acute VTE, which includes a substantial number of patients from both Asian and Western countries, will provide important insights for understanding specific characteristics of VTE in Asia [122]. VTE requires considerable healthcare resources for its management due to its chronic nature, high recurrence rate, and associated long-term complications. Decisions for VTE management are based upon balancing the treatment benefits against the risk of bleeding from the treatment. This is an especially important consideration for Asian populations because of increased bleeding tendency of Asians, intracranial hemorrhage in particular. Given this risk, timely and accurate diagnosis of the disease and ruling it out safely when absent are crucial. NOACs have shown advantages over existing options with respect to bleeding outcomes in major clinical trials, which renders them a safe and preferable strategy for VTE treatment.

Abbreviations

ACCP: American College of Chest Physicians; AF: Atrial fibrillation; AIDA: Assessment of the Incidence of Deep Vein Thrombosis in Asia; AMPLIFY: Apixaban for the Initial Management of Pulmonary Embolism and Deep Vein Thrombosis as First-Line Therapy; ARISTOTLE: Apixaban for Reduction in Stroke and Other Thromboembolic Events in Atrial Fibrillation; CRNM: Clinically relevant nonmajor; CTA: Computed tomographic angiography; CUS: Compression ultrasound; DVT: Deep vein thrombosis; EINSTEIN-DVT: Oral Direct Factor Xa Inhibitor Rivaroxaban in Patients with Acute Symptomatic Deep Vein Thrombosis; EINSTEIN-PE: Oral Direct Factor Xa Inhibitor Rivaroxaban in Patients with Acute Symptomatic Pulmonary Embolism; ENDORSE: Epidemiologic International Day for the Evaluation of Patients at Risk for Venous Thromboembolism in the Acute Hospital Care Setting; INR: International normalized ratio; JCS: Japanese Circulation Society; LMWH: Low-molecular-weight heparin; NOAC: Non-vitamin K antagonist oral anticoagulant; PD: Pharmacodynamic; PESI: Pulmonary Embolism Severity Index; PK: Pharmacokinetic; RE-COVER: Efficacy and Safety of Dabigatran Compared to Warfarin for 6 Month Treatment of Acute Symptomatic Venous Thromboembolism; RE-LY: Randomized Evaluation of Long-term Anticoagulation Therapy; ROCKET AF: Rivaroxaban Once Daily Oral Direct Factor Xa Inhibition Compared with Vitamin K Antagonism for Prevention of Stroke and Embolism Trial in Atrial Fibrillation; RV: Right ventricular; SPESI: Simplified Pulmonary Embolism Severity Index; STARS: Studying Thrombosis After Replacement Surgery; UFH: Unfractionated heparin; VKA: Vitamin K antagonist; VTE: Venous thromboembolism

Acknowledgments
Medical writing and editorial support were provided by Senem Kurtoglu, PhD, of AlphaBioCom, LLC (King of Prussia, PA).

Funding
Medical writing and editorial support were funded by Daiichi-Sankyo, Inc. (Basking Ridge, NJ).

Authors' contributions

All authors made substantial intellectual contributions to the conception and design of this manuscript. All authors were involved in drafting the manuscript and revising it critically for important intellectual content, and all gave consent for the publication of the manuscript. All authors read and approved the final manuscript.

Competing interests

Kang-Ling Wang has received honoraria from AstraZeneca, Bayer, Boehringer Ingelheim, and Daiichi-Sankyo. Eng Soo Yap has received honoraria from Bayer and Leo Pharma. Chern-En Chiang has been on the speaker bureau for AstraZeneca, Bayer, Boehringer Ingelheim, Chugai, Daiichi-Sankyo, GSK, MSD, Novartis, Pfizer, Roche, Sanofi, Servier, Tanabe, Takeda, and TTY. The other authors report no conflict of interest.

Author details

[1]General Clinical Research Center, Taipei Veterans General Hospital, No. 201, Sec. 2, Shipai Rd., 11217 Taipei, Taiwan. [2]School of Medicine, National Yang-Ming University, Taipei, Taiwan. [3]Department of Haematology-Oncology, National University Cancer Institute, Singapore, Singapore. [4]Department of Laboratory Medicine, National University Hospital, Singapore, Singapore. [5]Department of Medicine, Tokai University School of Medicine, Kanagawa, Japan. [6]Arrhythmia Center, National Center for Cardiovascular Diseases and Beijing Fuwai Hospital, Chinese Academy of Medical Sciences and Pekin Union Medical College, Beijing, China. [7]Cardiology Division, Department of Medicine, Li Ka Shing Faculty of Medicine, The University of Hong Kong, Hong Kong SAR, China.

References

1. Vaitkus PT, Leizorovicz A, Cohen AT, Turpie AG, Olsson CG, Goldhaber SZ, Group PMTS. Mortality rates and risk factors for asymptomatic deep vein thrombosis in medical patients. Thromb Haemost. 2005;93:76–9.
2. Sandler DA, Martin JF. Autopsy proven pulmonary embolism in hospital patients: are we detecting enough deep vein thrombosis? J R Soc Med. 1989;82:203–5.
3. Sakuma M, Nakamura M, Yamada N, Ota S, Shirato K, Nakano T, Ito M, Kobayashi T. Venous thromboembolism: deep vein thrombosis with pulmonary embolism, deep vein thrombosis alone, and pulmonary embolism alone. Circ J. 2009;73:305–9.
4. Goldhaber SZ, Visani L, De Rosa M. Acute pulmonary embolism: clinical outcomes in the international cooperative pulmonary embolism registry (ICOPER). Lancet. 1999;353:1386–9.
5. Nijkeuter M, Sohne M, Tick LW, Kamphuisen PW, Kramer MH, Laterveer L, van Houten AA, Kruip MJ, Leebeek FW, Buller HR, et al. The natural course of hemodynamically stable pulmonary embolism: clinical outcome and risk factors in a large prospective cohort study. Chest. 2007;131:517–23.
6. Heit JA, Lahr BD, Petterson TM, Bailey KR, Ashrani AA, Melton LJ 3rd. Heparin and warfarin anticoagulation intensity as predictors of recurrence after deep vein thrombosis or pulmonary embolism: a population-based cohort study. Blood. 2011;118:4992–9.
7. Pengo V, Lensing AW, Prins MH, Marchiori A, Davidson BL, Tiozzo F, Albanese P, Biasiolo A, Pegoraro C, Iliceto S, et al. Incidence of chronic thromboembolic pulmonary hypertension after pulmonary embolism. N Engl J Med. 2004;350:2257–64.
8. Cohen AT, Agnelli G, Anderson FA, Arcelus JI, Bergqvist D, Brecht JG, Greer IA, Heit JA, Hutchinson JL, Kakkar AK, et al. Venous thromboembolism (VTE) in Europe. The number of VTE events and associated morbidity and mortality. Thromb Haemost. 2007;98:756–64.
9. Cohen AT, Tapson VF, Bergmann JF, Goldhaber SZ, Kakkar AK, Deslandes B, Huang W, Zayaruzny M, Emery L, Anderson FA Jr,

Investigators E. Venous thromboembolism risk and prophylaxis in the acute hospital care setting (ENDORSE study): a multinational cross-sectional study. Lancet. 2008;371:387–94.
10. Falck-Ytter Y, Francis CW, Johanson NA, Curley C, Dahl OE, Schulman S, Ortel TL, Pauker SG, Colwell CW Jr, American College of Chest P. Prevention of VTE in orthopedic surgery patients: antithrombotic therapy and prevention of thrombosis, 9th ed: American College of Chest Physicians Evidence-Based Clinical Practice Guidelines. Chest. 2012;141:e278S–325S.
11. Gould MK, Garcia DA, Wren SM, Karanicolas PJ, Arcelus JI, Heit JA, Samama CM, American College of Chest P. Prevention of VTE in nonorthopedic surgical patients: antithrombotic therapy and prevention of thrombosis, 9th ed: American College of Chest Physicians Evidence-Based Clinical Practice Guidelines. Chest. 2012;141:e227S–77S.
12. White RH. The epidemiology of venous thromboembolism. Circulation. 2003;107:I4–8.
13. Jang MJ, Bang SM, Oh D. Incidence of venous thromboembolism in Korea: from the Health Insurance Review and Assessment Service database. J Thromb Haemost. 2011;9:85–91.
14. JCS. Guidelines for the diagnosis, treatment and prevention of pulmonary thromboembolism and deep vein thrombosis (JCS 2009). Circ J. 2011;75:1258–81.
15. Huerta C, Johansson S, Wallander MA, Garcia Rodriguez LA. Risk factors and short-term mortality of venous thromboembolism diagnosed in the primary care setting in the United Kingdom. Arch Intern Med. 2007;167:935–43.
16. Naess IA, Christiansen SC, Romundstad P, Cannegieter SC, Rosendaal FR, Hammerstrom J. Incidence and mortality of venous thrombosis: a population-based study. J Thromb Haemost. 2007;5:692–9.
17. Silverstein MD, Heit JA, Mohr DN, Petterson TM, O'Fallon WM, Melton LJ 3rd. Trends in the incidence of deep vein thrombosis and pulmonary embolism: a 25-year population-based study. Arch Intern Med. 1998;158:585–93.
18. Lee CH, Lin LJ, Cheng CL, Kao Yang YH, Chen JY, Tsai LM. Incidence and cumulative recurrence rates of venous thromboembolism in the Taiwanese population. J Thromb Haemost. 2010;8:1515–23.
19. Liu HS, Kho BC, Chan JC, Cheung FM, Lau KY, Choi FP, Wu WC, Yau TK. Venous thromboembolism in the Chinese population–experience in a regional hospital in Hong Kong. Hong Kong Med J. 2002;8:400–5.
20. Molina JA, Jiang ZG, Heng BH, Ong BK. Venous thromboembolism at the National Healthcare Group, Singapore. Ann Acad Med Singap. 2009;38:470–8.
21. Liao S, Woulfe T, Hyder S, Merriman E, Simpson D, Chunilal S. Incidence of venous thromboembolism in different ethnic groups: a regional direct comparison study. J Thromb Haemost. 2014;12:214–9.
22. White RH, Zhou H, Murin S, Harvey D. Effect of ethnicity and gender on the incidence of venous thromboembolism in a diverse population in California in 1996. Thromb Haemost. 2005;93:298–305.
23. Zakai NA, McClure LA. Racial differences in venous thromboembolism. J Thromb Haemost. 2011;9:1877–82.
24. Wendelboe AM, McCumber M, Hylek EM, Buller H, Weitz JI, Raskob G, Day ISCfWT. Global public awareness of venous thromboembolism. J Thromb Haemost. 2015;13:1365–71.
25. Lee LH. Clinical update on deep vein thrombosis in Singapore. Ann Acad Med Singap. 2002;31:248–52.
26. Kakkar N, Vasishta RK. Pulmonary embolism in medical patients: an autopsy-based study. Clin Appl Thromb Hemost. 2008;14:159–67.
27. Dickens P, Knight BH, Ip P, Fung WS. Fatal pulmonary embolism: a comparative study of autopsy incidence in Hong Kong and Cardiff, Wales. Forensic Sci Int. 1997;90:171–4.
28. Margaglione M, Grandone E. Population genetics of venous thromboembolism. A narrative review. Thromb Haemost. 2011;105:221–31.
29. Barnes PM, Adams PF, Powell-Griner E: Health characteristics of the Asian adult population: United States, 2004–2006. Adv Data 2008:1–22.
30. Jun ZJ, Ping T, Lei Y, Li L, Ming SY, Jing W. Prevalence of factor V Leiden and prothrombin G20210A mutations in Chinese patients with deep venous thrombosis and pulmonary embolism. Clin Lab Haematol. 2006;28:111–6.

31. Ageno W, Becattini C, Brighton T, Selby R, Kamphuisen PW. Cardiovascular risk factors and venous thromboembolism: a meta-analysis. Circulation. 2008;117:93–102.

32. Lee WS, Kim KI, Lee HJ, Kyung HS, Seo SS. The incidence of pulmonary embolism and deep vein thrombosis after knee arthroplasty in Asians remains low: a meta-analysis. Clin Orthop Relat Res. 2013;471:1523–32.

33. Shen MC, Lin JS, Tsay W. Protein C and protein S deficiencies are the most important risk factors associated with thrombosis in Chinese venous thrombophilic patients in Taiwan. Thromb Res. 2000;99:447–52.

34. Suehisa E, Nomura T, Kawasaki T, Kanakura Y. Frequency of natural coagulation inhibitor (antithrombin III, protein C and protein S) deficiencies in Japanese patients with spontaneous deep vein thrombosis. Blood Coagul Fibrinolysis. 2001;12:95–9.

35. Akkawat B, Rojnuckarin P. Protein S deficiency is common in a healthy Thai population. J Med Assoc Thail. 2005;88(Suppl 4):S249–54.

36. Rees DC, Cox M, Clegg JB. World distribution of factor V Leiden. Lancet. 1995;346:1133–4.

37. Rosendaal FR, Doggen CJ, Zivelin A, Arruda VR, Aiach M, Siscovick DS, Hillarp A, Watzke HH, Bernardi F, Cumming AM, et al. Geographic distribution of the 20210 G to a prothrombin variant. Thromb Haemost. 1998;79:706–8.

38. Ho CH, Chau WK, Hsu HC, Gau JP, Yu TJ. Causes of venous thrombosis in fifty Chinese patients. Am J Hematol. 2000;63:74–8.

39. Angchaisuksiri P. Venous thromboembolism in Asia–an unrecognised and under-treated problem? Thromb Haemost. 2011;106:585–90.

40. Peng YY, Jeng JS, Shen MC, Tsay W, Wang BS, Lin WH, Chang YC, Yip PK. Aetiologies and prognosis of Chinese patients with deep vein thrombosis of the lower extremities. QJM. 1998;91:681–6.

41. Lee HC, Liao WB, Bullard MJ, Hsu TS. Deep venous thrombosis in Taiwan. Jpn Heart J. 1996;37:891–6.

42. Mutirangura P, Rüengsethakit C, Wongwanit C. Epidemiologic analysis of proximal deep vein thrombosis in Thai patients: malignancy, the predominant etiologic factor. Int J Angiol. 2004;13:81–3.

43. Nakamura M, Miyata T, Ozeki Y, Takayama M, Komori K, Yamada N, Origasa H, Satokawa H, Maeda H, Tanabe N, et al. Current venous thromboembolism management and outcomes in Japan. Circ J. 2014;78:708–17.

44. Chung LH, Chen WM, Chen CF, Chen TH, Liu CL. Deep vein thrombosis after total knee arthroplasty in asian patients without prophylactic anticoagulation. Orthopedics. 2011;34:15.

45. Wang CJ, Wang JW, Chen LM, Chen HS, Yang BY, Cheng SM. Deep vein thrombosis after total knee arthroplasty. J Formos Med Assoc. 2000;99:848–53.

46. Dhillon KS, Askander A, Doraismay S. Postoperative deep-vein thrombosis in Asian patients is not a rarity: a prospective study of 88 patients with no prophylaxis. J Bone Joint Surg Br. 1996;78:427–30.

47. Kadono Y, Yasunaga H, Horiguchi H, Hashimoto H, Matsuda S, Tanaka S, Nakamura K. Statistics for orthopedic surgery 2006-2007: data from the Japanese diagnosis procedure combination database. J Orthop Sci. 2010;15:162–70.

48. Fujita Y, Nakatsuka H, Namba Y, Mitani S, Yoshitake N, Sugimoto E, Hazama K. The incidence of pulmonary embolism and deep vein thrombosis and their predictive risk factors after lower extremity arthroplasty: a retrospective analysis based on diagnosis using multidetector CT. J Anesth. 2015;29:235–41.

49. Liew NC, Moissinac K, Gul Y. Postoperative venous thromboembolism in Asia: a critical appraisal of its incidence. Asian J Surg. 2003;26:154–8.

50. Wu PK, Chen CF, Chung LH, Liu CL, Chen WM. Population-based epidemiology of postoperative venous thromboembolism in Taiwanese patients receiving hip or knee arthroplasty without pharmacological thromboprophylaxis. Thromb Res. 2014;133:719–24.

51. Piovella F, Wang CJ, Lu H, Lee K, Lee LH, Lee WC, Turpie AG, Gallus AS, Planes A, Passera R, et al. Deep-vein thrombosis rates after major orthopedic surgery in Asia. An epidemiological study based on postoperative screening with centrally adjudicated bilateral venography. J Thromb Haemost. 2005;3:2664–70.

52. Kanchanabat B, Stapanavatr W, Meknavin S, Soorapanth C, Sumanasrethakul C, Kanchanasuttirak P. Systematic review and meta-analysis on the rate of postoperative venous thromboembolism in orthopaedic surgery in Asian patients without thromboprophylaxis. Br J Surg. 2011;98:1356–64.

53. Kakkar VV, Howe CT, Flanc C, Clarke MB. Natural history of postoperative deep-vein thrombosis. Lancet. 1969;2:230–2.

54. Hirsh J, Hoak J. Management of deep vein thrombosis and pulmonary embolism. A statement for healthcare professionals. Council on thrombosis (in consultation with the council on cardiovascular radiology), American Heart Association. Circulation. 1996;93:2212–45.

55. Wells P, Anderson D. The diagnosis and treatment of venous thromboembolism. Hematology Am Soc Hematol Educ Program. 2013;2013:457–63.

56. Prandoni P, Lensing AW, Prins MH, Ciammaichella M, Perlati M, Mumoli N, Bucherini E, Visona A, Bova C, Imberti D, et al. Prevalence of pulmonary embolism among patients hospitalized for syncope. N Engl J Med. 2016;375:1524–31.

57. Konstantinides SV, Torbicki A, Agnelli G, Danchin N, Fitzmaurice D, Galie N, Gibbs JS, Huisman MV, Humbert M, Kucher N, et al. 2014 ESC guidelines on the diagnosis and management of acute pulmonary embolism. Eur Heart J. 2014;35:3033–69. 3069a-3069k

58. Wells PS, Hirsh J, Anderson DR, Lensing AW, Foster G, Kearon C, Weitz J, D'Ovidio R, Cogo A, Prandoni P. Accuracy of clinical assessment of deep-vein thrombosis. Lancet. 1995;345:1326–30.

59. Wells PS, Ginsberg JS, Anderson DR, Kearon C, Gent M, Turpie AG, Bormanis J, Weitz J, Chamberlain M, Bowie D, et al. Use of a clinical model for safe management of patients with suspected pulmonary embolism. Ann Intern Med. 1998;129:997–1005.

60. Wells PS, Anderson DR, Rodger M, Forgie M, Kearon C, Dreyer J, Kovacs G, Mitchell M, Lewandowski B, Kovacs MJ. Evaluation of D-dimer in the diagnosis of suspected deep-vein thrombosis. N Engl J Med. 2003;349:1227–35.

61. Wells PS, Anderson DR, Rodger M, Stiell I, Dreyer JF, Barnes D, Forgie M, Kovacs G, Ward J, Kovacs MJ. Excluding pulmonary embolism at the bedside without diagnostic imaging: management of patients with suspected pulmonary embolism presenting to the emergency department by using a simple clinical model and d-dimer. Ann Intern Med. 2001;135:98–107.

62. H'Ng MW, Loh SS, Earnest A, Wansaicheong GK. Effectiveness of an algorithm in reducing the number of unnecessary ultrasound scans for deep vein thrombosis: an evaluation report. Singap Med J. 2012;53:595–8.

63. Yamaki T, Nozaki M, Sakurai H, Takeuchi M, Soejima K, Kono T. Uses of different D-dimer levels can reduce the need for venous duplex scanning to rule out deep vein thrombosis in patients with symptomatic pulmonary embolism. J Vasc Surg. 2007;46:526–32.

64. Yamaki T, Nozaki M, Sakurai H, Kikuchi Y, Soejima K, Kono T, Hamahata A, Kim K. Combined use of pretest clinical probability score and latex agglutination D-dimer testing for excluding acute deep vein thrombosis. J Vasc Surg. 2009;50:1099–105.

65. Righini M, Perrier A, De Moerloose P, Bounameaux H. D-Dimer for venous thromboembolism diagnosis: 20 years later. J Thromb Haemost. 2008;6:1059–71.

66. van Belle A, Buller HR, Huisman MV, Huisman PM, Kaasjager K, Kamphuisen PW, Kramer MH, Kruip MJ, Kwakkel-van Erp JM, Leebeek FW, et al. Effectiveness of managing suspected pulmonary embolism using an algorithm combining clinical probability, D-dimer testing, and computed tomography. JAMA. 2006;295:172–9.

67. Wells PS, Anderson DR, Bormanis J, Guy F, Mitchell M, Gray L, Clement C, Robinson KS, Lewandowski B. Value of assessment of pretest probability of deep-vein thrombosis in clinical management. Lancet. 1997;350:1795–8.

68. Matsuo H, Nakajima Y, Ogawa T, Mo M, Tazaki J, Doi T, Yamada N, Suzuki T, Nakajima H: Evaluation of D-dimer in screening deep vein thrombosis in hospitalized Japanese patients with acute medical diseases/episodes. Ann Vasc Dis 2016, 2016 July. [Epub ahead of print].

69. Park R, Seo YI, Yoon SG, Choi TY, Shin JW, Uh ST, Kim YK. Utility of D-dimer assay for diagnosing pulmonary embolism: single institute study. Korean J Lab Med. 2008;28:419–24.

70. Chen CJ, Wang CJ, Huang CC. The value of D-dimer in the detection of early deep-vein thrombosis after total knee arthroplasty in Asian patients: a cohort study. Thromb J. 2008;6:5.

71. Prisco D, Grifoni E. The role of D-dimer testing in patients with suspected venous thromboembolism. Semin Thromb Hemost. 2009;35:50–9.

72. Wang KL, Chu PH, Lee CH, Pai PY, Lin PY, Shyu KG, Chang WT, Chiu KM, Huang CL, Lee CY, et al. Management of Venous Thromboembolisms: part I. The consensus for deep vein thrombosis. Acta Cardiol Sin. 2016;32:1–22.

73. Yamada N, Hirayama A, Maeda H, Sakagami S, Shikata H, Prins MH, Lensing AW, Kato M, Onuma J, Miyamoto Y, et al. Oral rivaroxaban for Japanese patients with symptomatic venous thromboembolism - the J-EINSTEIN DVT and PE program. Thromb J. 2015;13:2.

74. Anderson DR, Kahn SR, Rodger MA, Kovacs MJ, Morris T, Hirsch A, Lang E, Stiell I, Kovacs G, Dreyer J, et al. Computed tomographic pulmonary angiography vs ventilation-perfusion lung scanning in patients with suspected pulmonary embolism: a randomized controlled trial. JAMA. 2007;298:2743–53.

75. Goodacre S, Sampson F, Thomas S, van Beek E, Sutton A. Systematic review and meta-analysis of the diagnostic accuracy of ultrasonography for deep vein thrombosis. BMC Med Imaging. 2005;5:6.

76. Stein PD, Fowler SE, Goodman LR, Gottschalk A, Hales CA, Hull RD, Leeper KV Jr, Popovich J Jr, Quinn DA, Sos TA, et al. Multidetector computed tomography for acute pulmonary embolism. N Engl J Med. 2006;354:2317–27.

77. Liew NC, Chang YH, Choi G, Chu PH, Gao X, Gibbs H, Ho CO, Ibrahim H, Kim TK, Kritpracha B, et al. Asian venous thromboembolism guidelines: prevention of venous thromboembolism. Int Angiol. 2012;31:501–16.

78. Aujesky D, Obrosky DS, Stone RA, Auble TE, Perrier A, Cornuz J, Roy PM, Fine MJ. Derivation and validation of a prognostic model for pulmonary embolism. Am J Respir Crit Care Med. 2005;172:1041–6.

79. Jimenez D, Aujesky D, Moores L, Gomez V, Lobo JL, Uresandi F, Otero R, Monreal M, Muriel A, Yusen RD, Investigators R. Simplification of the pulmonary embolism severity index for prognostication in patients with acute symptomatic pulmonary embolism. Arch Intern Med. 2010;170:1383–9.

80. Zondag W, den Exter PL, Crobach MJ, Dolsma A, Donker ML, Eijsvogel M, Faber LM, Hofstee HM, Kaasjager KA, Kruip MJ, et al. Comparison of two methods for selection of out of hospital treatment in patients with acute pulmonary embolism. Thromb Haemost. 2013;109:47–52.

81. Zondag W, Vingerhoets LM, Durian MF, Dolsma A, Faber LM, Hiddinga BI, Hofstee HM, Hoogerbrugge AD, Hovens MM, Labots G, et al. Hestia criteria can safely select patients with pulmonary embolism for outpatient treatment irrespective of right ventricular function. J Thromb Haemost. 2013;11:686–92.

82. Landefeld CS, Goldman L. Major bleeding in outpatients treated with warfarin: incidence and prediction by factors known at the start of outpatient therapy. Am J Med. 1989;87:144–52.

83. Kuijer PM, Hutten BA, Prins MH, Buller HR. Prediction of the risk of bleeding during anticoagulant treatment for venous thromboembolism. Arch Intern Med. 1999;159:457–60.

84. Ruiz-Gimenez N, Suarez C, Gonzalez R, Nieto JA, Todoli JA, Samperiz AL, Monreal M. Predictive variables for major bleeding events in patients presenting with documented acute venous thromboembolism. Findings from the RIETE registry. Thromb Haemost. 2008;100:26–31.

85. Kearon C, Ginsberg JS, Kovacs MJ, Anderson DR, Wells P, Julian JA, MacKinnon B, Weitz JI, Crowther MA, Dolan S, et al. Comparison of low-intensity warfarin therapy with conventional-intensity warfarin therapy for long-term prevention of recurrent venous thromboembolism. N Engl J Med. 2003;349:631–9.

86. Klok FA, Hosel V, Clemens A, Yollo WD, Tilke C, Schulman S, Lankeit M, Konstantinides SV. Prediction of bleeding events in patients with venous thromboembolism on stable anticoagulation treatment. Eur Respir J. 2016;48:1369–76.

87. Klok FA, Barco S, Konstantinides SV. External validation of the VTE-BLEED score for predicting major bleeding in stable anticoagulated patients with venous thromboembolism. Thromb Haemost. 2017;117:1164–70.

88. Cohen AT. Asia-Pacific thrombosis advisory B: Asia-Pacific thrombosis advisory board consensus paper on prevention of venous thromboembolism after major orthopaedic surgery. Thromb Haemost. 2010;104:919–30.

89. Bang SM, Jang MJ, Kim KH, Yhim HY, Kim YK, Nam SH, Hwang HG, Bae SH, Kim SH, Mun YC, et al. Prevention of venous thromboembolism, 2nd edition: Korean Society of Thrombosis and Hemostasis Evidence-Based Clinical Practice Guidelines. J Korean Med Sci. 2014;29:164–71.

90. Fuji T, Fujita S, Ujihira T, Sato T. Dabigatran etexilate prevents venous thromboembolism after total knee arthroplasty in Japanese patients with a safety profile comparable to placebo. J Arthroplast. 2010;25:1267–74.

91. Fuji T, Fujita S, Kawai Y, Nakamura M, Kimura T, Fukuzawa M, Abe K, Tachibana S. Efficacy and safety of edoxaban versus enoxaparin for the prevention of venous thromboembolism following total hip arthroplasty: STARS J-V. Thromb J. 2015;13:27.

92. Fuji T, Fujita S, Kawai Y, Nakamura M, Kimura T, Kiuchi Y, Abe K, Tachibana S. Safety and efficacy of edoxaban in patients undergoing hip fracture surgery. Thromb Res. 2014;133:1016–22.

93. Fuji T, Wang CJ, Fujita S, Kawai Y, Nakamura M, Kimura T, Ibusuki K, Ushida H, Abe K, Tachibana S. Safety and efficacy of edoxaban, an oral factor Xa inhibitor, versus enoxaparin for thromboprophylaxis after total knee arthroplasty: the STARS E-3 trial. Thromb Res. 2014;134:1198–204.

94. Lee YJ. Use of novel oral anticoagulants for the treatment of venous thromboembolism and its considerations in Asian patients. Ther Clin Risk Manag. 2014;10:841–50.

95. Kuroda Y, Hirayama C, Hotoda H, Nishikawa Y, Nishiwaki A. Postmarketing safety experience with edoxaban in Japan for thromboprophylaxis following major orthopedic surgery. Vasc Health Risk Manag. 2013;9:593–8.

96. Kearon C, Akl EA, Ornelas J, Blaivas A, Jimenez D, Bounameaux H, Huisman M, King CS, Morris TA, Sood N, et al. Antithrombotic therapy for VTE disease: CHEST guideline and expert panel report. Chest. 2016;149:315–52.

97. Cohen A, Chiu KM, Park K, Jeyaindran S, Tambunan KL, Ward C, Wong R, Yoon SS. Managing venous thromboembolism in Asia: winds of change in the era of new oral anticoagulants. Thromb Res. 2012;130:291–301.

98. Nakamura M, Yamada N, Ito M. Current management of venous thromboembolism in Japan: current epidemiology and advances in anticoagulant therapy. J Cardiol. 2015;66:451–9.

99. Wong WH, Yip CY, Sum CL, Tan CW, Lee LH, Yap ES, Kuperan P, Ting WC, Ng HJ. A practical guide to ordering and interpreting coagulation tests for patients on direct oral anticoagulants in Singapore. Ann Acad Med Singap. 2016;45:98–105.

100. Pradaxa® (dabigatran etexilate) now approved in more than 100 countries for stroke prevention in atrial fibrillation. Available at: https://www.boehringer-ingelheim.com/press-release/pradaxa-dabigatran-etexilate-now-approved-more-100-countries-stroke-prevention-atrial, March 6, 2014. Accessed October 19, 2017.

101. Garcia DA, Baglin TP, Weitz JI, Samama MM, American College of Chest P. Parenteral anticoagulants: antithrombotic therapy and prevention of thrombosis, 9th ed: American college of chest physicians evidence-based clinical practice guidelines. Chest. 2012;141:e24S–43S.

102. Consultation WHOE. Appropriate body-mass index for Asian populations and its implications for policy and intervention strategies. Lancet. 2004;363:157–63.

103. Kearon C, Ginsberg JS, Julian JA, Douketis J, Solymoss S, Ockelford P, Jackson S, Turpie AG, MacKinnon B, Hirsh J, et al. Comparison of fixed-dose weight-adjusted unfractionated heparin and low-molecular-weight heparin for acute treatment of venous thromboembolism. JAMA. 2006;296:935–42.

104. Haas S. New oral Xa and IIa inhibitors: updates on clinical trial results. J Thromb Thrombolysis. 2008;25:52–60.

105. Samama MM, Poller L. Contemporary laboratory monitoring of low molecular weight heparins. Clin Lab Med. 1995;15:119–23.

106. Abbate R, Gori AM, Farsi A, Attanasio M, Pepe G. Monitoring of low-molecular-weight heparins in cardiovascular disease. Am J Cardiol. 1998;82:33L–6L.

107. Nieuwenhuis HK, Albada J, Banga JD, Sixma JJ. Identification of risk factors for bleeding during treatment of acute venous thromboembolism with heparin or low molecular weight heparin. Blood. 1991;78:2337–43.

108. Bauer KA. Pros and cons of new oral anticoagulants. Hematology Am Soc Hematol Educ Program. 2013;2013:464–70.

109. Chiang CE, Wang KL, Lip GY. Stroke prevention in atrial fibrillation: an Asian perspective. Thromb Haemost. 2014;111:789–97.

110. Nakamura M, Wang YQ, Wang C, Oh D, Yin WH, Kimura T, Miyazaki K, Abe K, Mercuri M, Lee LH, et al. Efficacy and safety of edoxaban for treatment of venous thromboembolism: a subanalysis of east Asian patients in the Hokusai-VTE trial. J Thromb Haemost. 2015;13:1606–14.

111. Wang Y, Wang C, Chen Z, Zhang J, Liu Z, Jin B, Ying K, Liu C, Shao Y, Jing Z, et al. Rivaroxaban for the treatment of symptomatic deep-vein thrombosis and pulmonary embolism in Chinese patients: a subgroup analysis of the EINSTEIN DVT and PE studies. Thromb J. 2013;11:25.

112. Nakamura M, Nishikawa M, Komuro I, Kitajima I, Uetsuka Y, Yamagami T, Minamiguchi H, Yoshimatsu R, Tanabe K, Matsuoka N, et al. Apixaban for the treatment of Japanese subjects with acute venous Thromboembolism (AMPLIFY-J study). Circ J. 2015;79:1230–6.

113. Ahrens I, Lip GY, Peter K. New oral anticoagulant drugs in cardiovascular disease. Thromb Haemost. 2010;104:49–60.

114. Schulman S, Kearon C, Kakkar AK, Mismetti P, Schellong S, Eriksson H, Baanstra D, Schnee J, Goldhaber SZ, Group R-CS. Dabigatran versus warfarin in the treatment of acute venous thromboembolism. N Engl J Med. 2009;361:2342–52.

115. Schulman S, Kakkar AK, Goldhaber SZ, Schellong S, Eriksson H, Mismetti P, Christiansen AV, Friedman J, Le Maulf F, Peter N, et al. Treatment of acute venous thromboembolism with dabigatran or warfarin and pooled analysis. Circulation. 2014;129:764–72.

116. Bauersachs R, Berkowitz SD, Brenner B, Buller HR, Decousus H, Gallus AS, Lensing AW, Misselwitz F, Prins MH, Raskob GE, et al. Oral rivaroxaban for symptomatic venous thromboembolism. N Engl J Med. 2010;363:2499–510.

117. Buller HR, Prins MH, Lensin AW, Decousus H, Jacobson BF, Minar E, Chlumsky J, Verhamme P, Wells P, Agnelli G, et al. Oral rivaroxaban for the treatment of symptomatic pulmonary embolism. N Engl J Med. 2012;366:1287–97.

118. Prins MH, Lensing AW, Bauersachs R, van Bellen B, Bounameaux H, Brighton TA, Cohen AT, Davidson BL, Decousus H, Raskob GE, et al. Oral rivaroxaban versus standard therapy for the treatment of symptomatic venous thromboembolism: a pooled analysis of the EINSTEIN-DVT and PE randomized studies. Thromb J. 2013;11:21.

119. Agnelli G, Buller HR, Cohen A, Curto M, Gallus AS, Johnson M, Masiukiewicz U, Pak R, Thompson J, Raskob GE, et al. Oral apixaban for the treatment of acute venous thromboembolism. N Engl J Med. 2013;369:799–808.

120. Buller HR, Decousus H, Grosso MA, Mercuri M, Middeldorp S, Prins MH, Raskob GE, Schellong SM, Schwocho L, Segers A, et al. Edoxaban versus warfarin for the treatment of symptomatic venous thromboembolism. N Engl J Med. 2013;369:1406–15.

121. van Es N, Coppens M, Schulman S, Middeldorp S, Buller HR. Direct oral anticoagulants compared with vitamin K antagonists for acute venous thromboembolism: evidence from phase 3 trials. Blood. 2014;124:1968–75.

122. Weitz JI, Haas S, Ageno W, Angchaisuksiri P, Bounameaux H, Nielsen JD, Goldhaber SZ, Goto S, Kayani G, Mantovani L, et al. Global anticoagulant registry in the field - venous Thromboembolism (GARFIELD-VTE). Rationale and design. *Thromb Haemost*. 2016;116:1172–9.

123. Seligsohn U, Lubetsky A. Genetic susceptibility to venous thrombosis. N Engl J Med. 2001;344:1222–31.

20

Differential impact of diabetes mellitus on antiplatelet effects of prasugrel and clopidogrel

Satoshi Niijima[1], Tsukasa Ohmori[2]* and Kazuomi Kario[1]

Abstract

Background: Although prasugrel exerts stronger antiplatelet effects compared with clopidogrel, the factors affecting platelet reactivity under prasugrel have not been fully determined. This study aimed to find the novel mechanistic differences between two thienopyridines and identify the factor that influence platelet reactivity to each drug.

Methods: Forty patients with stable angina who underwent elective percutaneous coronary intervention were randomly assigned to receive either prasugrel (20 mg) or clopidogrel (300 mg) as a loading dose. Platelet function (light transmission, laser light scattering, and vasodilator-stimulated phosphoprotein phosphorylation) and plasma active metabolite levels were measured after the loading dose.

Results: Prasugrel consistently inhibited adenosine diphosphate receptor $P2Y_{12}$ signalling to abolish amplification of platelet aggregation. Prasugrel abolished even small platelet aggregates composed of less than 100 platelets. On the other hand, clopidogrel inhibited large aggregates but increased small and medium platelet aggregates. Diabetes was the only independent variable for determining antiplatelet effects and active metabolite concentration of prasugrel, but not clopidogrel. Sleep-disordered breathing was significantly correlated with platelet reactivity in patients who had clopidogrel.

Conclusions: Prasugrel efficiently abolishes residual $P2Y_{12}$ signalling that causes small platelet aggregates, but these small aggregates are not inhibited by clopidogrel. Considering the differential effect of diabetes on antiplatelet effects between these two drugs, the pharmacokinetics of prasugrel, other than cytochrome P450 metabolism, might be affected by diabetes.

Keywords: Thienopyridines, $P2Y_{12}$, Vasodilator-stimulated phosphoprotein phosphorylation

Background

Dual antiplatelet therapy with aspirin and thienopyridine is a common therapy in patients who are undergoing percutaneous coronary intervention (PCI) to protect stent thrombosis [1, 2]. Clopidogrel is broadly used to inhibit the adenosine diphosphate (ADP) receptor $P2Y_{12}$, but it shows a delayed onset of action and a great inter-individual variability of drug efficacy [3, 4]. Absorbed clopidogrel is converted to an active metabolite through two oxidation steps by hepatic cytochrome P450 (CYP)

[5]. High on-treatment platelet reactivity under clopidogrel therapy because of genetic polymorphisms in *CYP2C19* and drug-interactions increases the risk of cardiovascular events after PCI [3, 4]. These limitations of clopidogrel have led to the development of alternative $P2Y_{12}$ inhibitors with a rapid onset of action and consistent antiplatelet activity.

Prasugrel is a new-generation thienopyridine that shows more potent inhibition of $P2Y_{12}$ with rapid onset of action, and significantly reduces ischaemic events after PCI compared with clopidogrel [6, 7]. Prasugrel is effectively converted to an active metabolite by esterases followed by a single oxidation step [8]. The peak plasma concentration of prasugrel is reached at 30 min after

* Correspondence: tohmori@jichi.ac.jp
[2]Department of Biochemistry, Jichi Medical University School of Medicine, 3311-1 Yakushiji, Shimotsuke, Tochigi 329-0498, Japan
Full list of author information is available at the end of the article

dosing in stable PCI patients, and is not affected by *CYP2C19* polymorphisms, body mass index, diabetes, smoking, and renal impairment [9]. Prasugrel treatment consistently results in fewer poor responders compared with clopidogrel, while inadequate platelet inhibition has also been reported. Platelet reactivity under prasugrel treatment is an independent risk factor for adverse events or bleeding after PCI [10, 11]. However, the factors that affect platelet reactivity under prasugrel treatment have not been fully determined. In this study, we prospectively compared the pharmacodynamics and platelet reactivity of clopidogrel and prasugrel in a randomized trial.

Methods

Patient population and study design

This study was a prospective, randomized, open-label, parallel-group, single-centre study that was conducted in Japan between November 2014 and April 2016 (UMIN000017624). The protocol was approved by the Institutional Review Board of Jichi Medical University on 14 October 2014. From the day on, we started to recruit patients, and total 10 patients were included before completion of clinical trial registration. Patients who were scheduled to undergo PCI with suspected angina pectoris were enrolled. Eligible subjects for the study met all of the following inclusion criteria: (1) typical ischaemic symptoms with coronary risk factors or a positive study for coronary computed tomography (CT), myocardial perfusion scintigraphy, or a treadmill exercise test; (2) on treatment with low-dose aspirin (100 mg/day) for at least 7 days; and (3) older than 20 years of age. Exclusion criteria were any of the following: (1) use of any antiplatelet agents other than aspirin, or oral anticoagulant agents within 7 days before admission; (2) body weight of 50 kg or less; (3) a history of active bleeding; (4) any active malignancy or collagen disease; (4) a platelet count of $<100,000/mm^3$ or $>400,000/mm^3$; (5) participation in other clinical trials;

(6) creatinine levels >2.5 mg/dl; and (7) liver disease (bilirubin levels >2 mg/dl). Hypertension was defined as a systemic blood pressure of 140 mmHg or higher or taking any antihypertensive drug. Dyslipidaemia was defined as serum low-density lipoprotein cholesterol levels of 140 mg/dl or higher or taking statins. Diabetes was diagnosed by taking oral hypoglycaemic agents or insulin, or glycosylated haemoglobin (HbA1c) was 6.5% or greater.

Patients who met all of the criteria listed above were randomized at admission to treatment of either an oral loading dose (LD) of prasugrel 20 mg followed by a 3.75-mg/day maintenance dose or an oral LD of clopidogrel 300 mg followed by a 75-mg/day maintenance dose for 14 days (Fig. 1). The randomization ratio was 1:1 between two treatment arms and assignment was determined with a computer-based table of randomization system by a secretary who was unaware of the study protocol. The same dose of aspirin was continued during the study. Primary outcomes of the study were to compare responses of platelets to the treatment with prasugrel and clopidogrel. Further, this study aimed to identify the factor that influence platelet reactivity to each drug. Here, we analyzed on the responses to LD. Platelet function analyses were performed at five time points (baseline, and 0.5, 3, 6, and 20 h) after the LD (Fig. 1). The concentrations of active metabolites were measured at 0.5 and 3 h after the LD (Fig. 1). Blood was collected before meal mainly. Blood at 3 h after dosing was only collected after meal.

Platelet function assays and measurement of active metabolites

Blood for platelet function analysis was collected from the antecubital vein using a 21-guage needle into a syringe containing 1/10 sodium citrate at pre-defined time points. Platelet functions were assessed by light transmission and light scattering intensity using a PA-200C platelet aggregation analyser (Kowa Co., Ltd., Tokyo, Japan) [12, 13]. This equipment is particularly sensitive for detecting the size of small platelet aggregates and

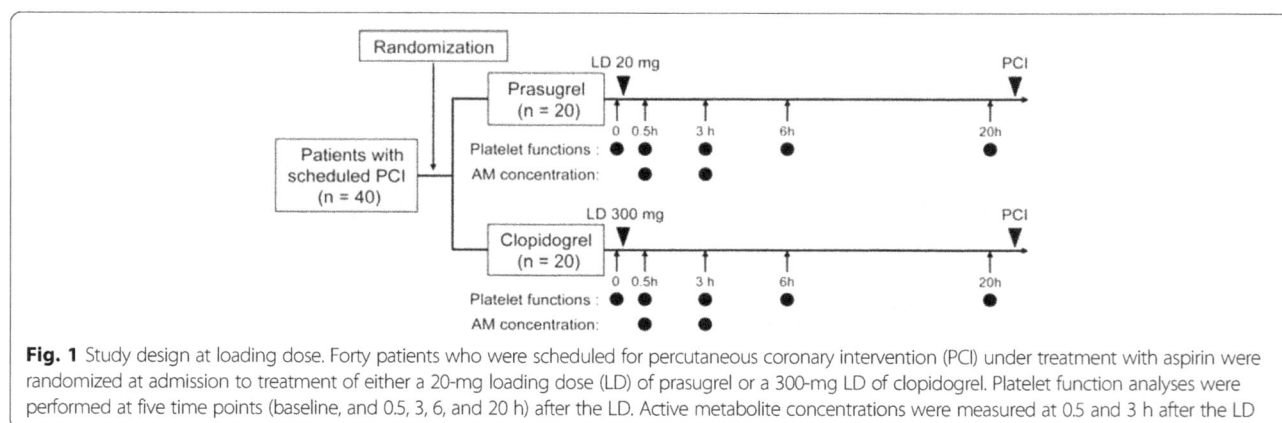

Fig. 1 Study design at loading dose. Forty patients who were scheduled for percutaneous coronary intervention (PCI) under treatment with aspirin were randomized at admission to treatment of either a 20-mg loading dose (LD) of prasugrel or a 300-mg LD of clopidogrel. Platelet function analyses were performed at five time points (baseline, and 0.5, 3, 6, and 20 h) after the LD. Active metabolite concentrations were measured at 0.5 and 3 h after the LD

can classify platelet aggregates according to size into small, medium, or large aggregates [14]. Platelet aggregation was induced by 5 and 20 µM ADP. Inhibition of platelet aggregation induced by ADP was expressed as absolute reduction of maximal platelet aggregation (baseline response – post-administration response). Phosphorylation of vasodilator-stimulated phosphoprotein (VASP) was measured according to the manufacturer's recommendation (PLT VASP/P2Y12; Biocytex Inc., Marseille, France), and quantified by flow cytometry (FACSAria II; BD Biosciences, San Jose, CA) and expressed as the platelet reactivity index (PRI).

To measure active metabolites of thienopyridines, blood was collected in a tube containing EDTA at 0.5 and 3 h after the loading dose, and 0.5 mol/L 3′-methoxyphenacyl bromide was immediately added to stabilize the active metabolite. The concentrations of active metabolites of prasugrel (R-138727) and clopidogrel (R-130964) were measured using liquid chromatography with tandem mass spectrometry at LSI Medience Co., Ltd. (Tokyo, Japan).

Statistical analysis

A sample size of 17 patients in each arm was required to provide at least 80% power to detect a 20% difference in the VASP-PRI at 3 h after the LD with a standard deviation of 20% at a two-tailed significance level of 0.05. Previous reports that compared the pharmacodynamics of clopidogrel with those of prasugrel reached the conclusion that 17 to 24 patients were required in each arm [15, 16].

Statistical analyses were performed using SPSS version 23.0 software (SPSS Inc., Chicago, IL). Normality was first assessed using the Kolmogorov–Smirnov test. Normally distributed variables were compared by the Student's t test, while non-normally distributed variables were compared by the Mann–Whitney U test. Categorical variables are expressed as frequency, and were compared using the chi-square test or Fisher's exact test. Differences in the time course of platelet reactivity (VASP-PRI, change in maximum light transmission, area under the curve of light intensity) between groups were determined by repeated measures ANOVA. All significance tests were two-tailed and $P < 0.05$ was considered statistically significant.

Results

VASP phosphorylation and platelet aggregation

Forty patients were randomly assigned to either prasugrel ($n = 20$) or clopidogrel ($n = 20$) (Fig. 1). Baseline characteristics are shown in Table 1. Fig. 2 shows the results of platelet $P2Y_{12}$ inhibition as assessed by the VASP-PRI and platelet aggregation, which was measured by light transmission after the LD. Baseline VASP-PRI

Table 1 Baseline Characteristics of the Study Population

Variable	Prasugrel ($n = 20$)	Clopidogrel ($n = 20$)	p-Value
Age, yrs	61.1 ± 11.0	66.1 ± 11.2	0.16
Male, n (%)	17 (85)	13 (65)	0.14
Body mass index, kg/m²	27.4 ± 3.6	26.3 ± 4.3	0.37
Current Smoker, n (%)	7 (35)	4 (20)	0.24
Hypertension, n (%)	13 (65)	17 (85)	0.14
Dyslipidemia, n (%)	15 (75)	11 (55)	0.19
Diabetes, n (%)	8 (40)	7 (35)	0.74
SDB (ODI 3%), n (%)	6 (30)	6 (30)	1.00
Previous MI, n (%)	0 (0)	0 (0)	1.0
Previous AP, n (%)	2 (10)	1 (5)	0.55
Previous PCI, n (%)	2 (10)	1 (5)	0.55
Previous CABG, n (%)	0 (0)	0 (0)	1.0
Previous stroke, n (%)	1 (5)	1 (5)	1.0
PAD, n (%)	0 (0)	0 (0)	1.0
Family History of CAD, n (%)	8 (40)	6 (30)	0.51
LVEF, %	69.9 ± 6.3	69.4 ± 6.2	0.74
eGFR, ml/min/1.73m²	65.8 ± 18.5	68.2 ± 17.2	0.68
Platelet counts, ×10³/µL	21.0 ± 5.9	20.0 ± 4.2	0.54
Medications			
Aspirin, n (%)	20 (100)	20 (100)	1.00
PPI, n (%)	15 (75)	11 (55)	0.19
OAD, n (%)	8 (40)	4 (20)	0.17
Insulin therapy, n (%)	0 (0)	1 (5)	0.31
Statins, n (%)	15 (75)	11 (55)	0.19
Nitrates, n (%)	6 (30)	3 (15)	0.26
CCB, n (%)	9 (45)	10 (50)	0.75
ACEIs/ ARBs, n (%)	11 (55)	11 (55)	1.00
Beta blockers, n (%)	15 (75)	12 (60)	0.31

Values are mean ± SD or n (%)
ACEIs Angiotensin converting enzyme inhibitors, AP Angina pectoris, ARBs Angiotensin receptor blockers, CABG Coronary artery bypass surgery, CAD Coronary artery disease, CCB Calcium channel blockers, LVEF Left ventricular ejection fraction, MI Myocardial infarction, OAD Oral antidiabetic drug, PCI Percutaneous coronary intervention, PPI Proton pump inhibitor, SDB Sleep-disordered breathing

and maximal platelet aggregation induced by ADP were similar in the prasugrel and clopidogrel groups (VASP-PRI: 84.0 ± 6.4 vs. 82.1 ± 4.4, $P = 0.24$; % of light transmission [ADP 20 µM]: 65.0 ± 11.2 vs. 67.5 ± 9.4, $P = 0.58$). Patients who were treated with prasugrel showed significant inhibition of platelet aggregation and the VASP-PRI at 3 h after administration (Fig. 2). The difference between the two drugs was consistent thereafter.

To examine the timing of $P2Y_{12}$ inhibition by active metabolites, we compared the correlation of the VASP-PRI with active metabolite concentrations. Active metabolite concentrations that were measured at 30 min were

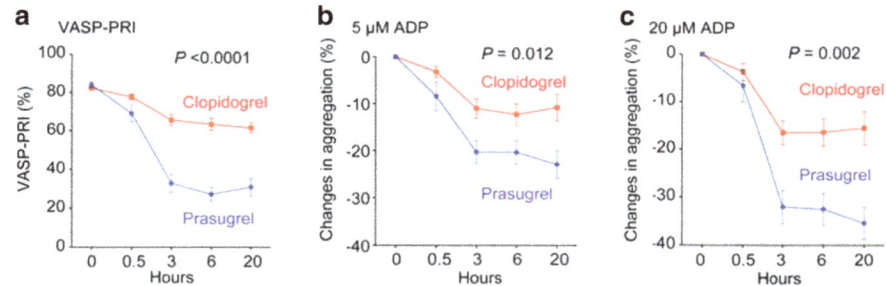

Fig. 2 Comparison of platelet function after the loading dose (LD) between clopidogrel and prasugrel. **a** The vasodilator-stimulated phosphoprotein-platelet reactivity index (VASP-PRI) was measured at the indicated time points after the LD. **b, c** Platelets in platelet-rich plasma obtained at the indicated time points were stimulated with 5 µM adenosine diphosphate (ADP) (**b**) or 20 µM ADP (**c**). The absolute change in maximal platelet aggregation as assessed by light transmission (baseline – an indicated point) was calculated. Blue lines and red lines represent the prasugrel LD (20 mg) and clopidogrel LD (300 mg), respectively. Values are means ± SEM. Differences in the time course between groups were determined by repeated measures ANOVA

highly correlated with the VASP-PRI in prasugrel-treated patients (Fig. 3a). A similar high association was also found between the VASP-PRI and platelet aggregation (Fig. 3b). However, these associations appeared to be weak and delayed in clopidogrel-treated patients (Fig. 3).

We next compared the profiles of platelet aggregates by the laser light scattering method. When platelets were stimulated with a low concentration of ADP (5 µM), formation of large aggregates was similarly inhibited in prasugrel and clopidogrel treatment (Fig. 4c). Formation of small aggregates was abolished only by prasugrel treatment (Fig. 4a). Inhibition of $P2Y_{12}$ signalling by clopidogrel appeared to be incomplete because clopidogrel treatment failed to inhibit platelet aggregate formation that was induced by higher concentrations of ADP (20 µM; Fig. 4d–f). Clopidogrel treatment increased formation of medium and small platelet aggregates after platelet stimulation (Fig. 4d, e).

Differences in determinants of drug efficacy after the LD
To determine the factors that are associated with the inter-individual variability of drug efficacy in both drugs, we analysed the correlation of the VASP-PRI with patients' characteristics and laboratory data after the LD. The presence of diabetes mellitus and active metabolite concentrations were consistently correlated with the VASP-PRI in prasugrel treatment (Table 2). Diabetes was only independent variable to associate with VASP-PRI in the multiple regression analysis adjusted for age, gender, body mass index, dyslipidemia, hypertension, sleep disordered breathing, platelet counts and PPI use (VASP-PRI 3 h; $R^2 = 0.93$, $P < 0.001$, 6 h; $R^2 = 0.92$, $P = 0.001$, 20 h; $R^2 = 0.86$, $P = 0.006$). Although diabetes did not affect VASP-PRI in clopidogrel-treated patients, sleep-disordered breathing assessed by the oxygen desaturation index showed a positive correlation. A positive association between the VASP-PRI and active metabolite

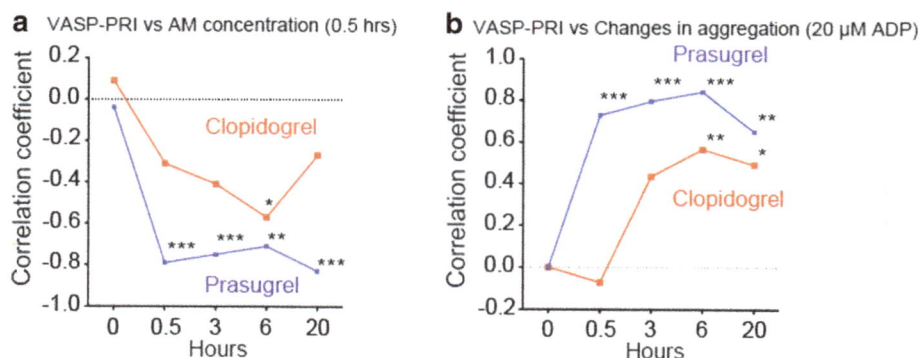

Fig. 3 Changes in the correlation coefficient between variables. **a** Changes in Spearman's correlation coefficient according to the time course between the vasodilator-stimulated phosphoprotein-platelet reactivity index (VASP-PRI) and active metabolite concentrations (AM) measured at 30 min after the LD. **b** Changes in Spearman's correlation coefficient according to the time course between the VASP-PRI and maximal platelet aggregation induced by 20 µM adenosine diphosphate (ADP). Blue lines and red lines represent the LD of prasugrel (20 mg) and that of clopidogrel (300 mg), respectively. *$P < 0.05$; **$P < 0.01$; ***$P < 0.001$

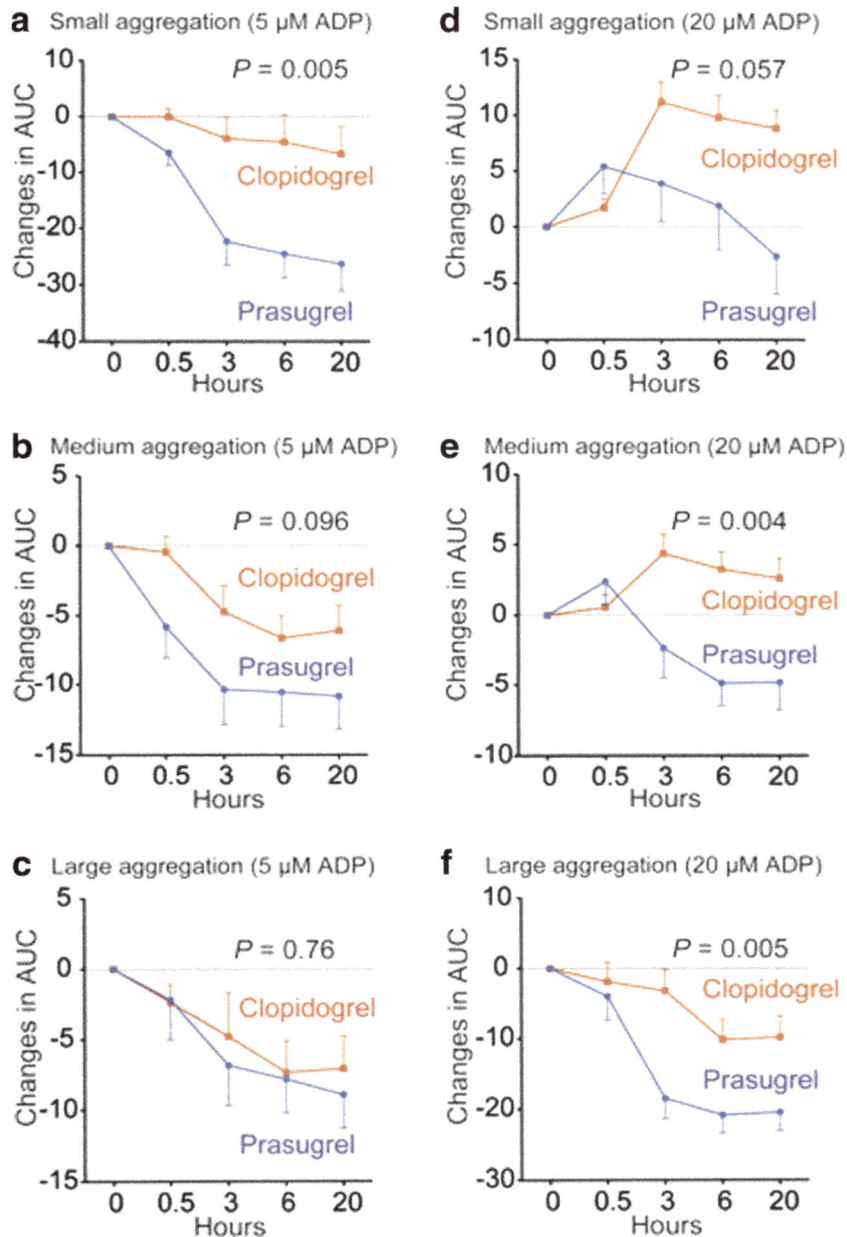

Fig. 4 Platelet aggregation as assessed by the laser light scattering method after the loading dose (LD). Platelets in platelet-rich plasma obtained at the indicated time points after the LD were stimulated with 5 μM adenosine diphosphate (ADP) (**a–c**) or 20 μM ADP (**d–f**). Small (**a, d**), medium (**b, e**), and large (**c, f**) platelet aggregate formation was measured by the laser light scattering method. This formation is expressed as changes in the area under curve (AUC) of each platelet aggregate number during 5 min (x 10^6 V/min). Blue lines and red lines represent the LD of prasugrel (20 mg) and that of clopidogrel (300 mg), respectively. Values are means ± SEM. Differences in the time course between groups were determined by repeated measures ANOVA

concentrations was observed only at 6 h after administration in the case of clopidogrel (Table 2).

To determine the importance of diabetes on drug metabolism and inhibition of platelet aggregation, we compared active metabolite concentrations, the VASP-PRI, and inhibition of platelet aggregation induced by 20 μM ADP in patients with diabetes and those without

diabetes. Eight patients in the prasugrel treatment group and seven in the clopidogrel treatment group were previously diagnosed with diabetes. Patients with diabetes had significantly lower levels of active metabolites with prasugrel treatment but not with clopidogrel treatment (Fig. 5a). Reflecting the lower levels of active metabolites, inhibition of the VASP-PRI and platelet aggregation

Table 2 Correlation of various factors with VASP-PRI

Variable	Prasugrel					Clopidogrel				
	R									
	pre	0.5 h	3 h	6 h	20 h	pre	0.5 h	3 h	6 h	20 h
Age, yrs	−0.28	−0.16	−0.33	−0.31	−0.27	0.14	−0.32	−0.18	−0.30	−0.13
Male	−0.29	−0.24	−0.13	−0.04	0.03	0.12	0.28	0.16	0.40	0.28
Body weight, kg	0.01	0.22	0.23	0.29	0.41	0.13	0.27	0.22	0.32	0.16
Body mass index, kg/m^2	−0.02	0.23	0.25	0.27	0.38	0.26	0.19	0.13	0.26	0.08
Body surface area, m^2	−0.06	0.16	0.21	0.28	0.39	0.14	0.40	0.21	0.37	0.17
Current Smoker	−0.02	0.32	0.14	0.26	0.20	0.13	0.31	0.33	0.41	0.41
Alcohol	0.06	−0.06	−0.14	0.10	0.0	0.02	0.36	0.22	0.38	0.1
Hypertension	0.38	0.20	0.28	0.38	0.30	0.46*	0.30	0.16	0.01	0.09
Dyslipidemia	0.02	0.44	0.22	0.50*	0.37	−0.17	−0.23	−0.12	−0.05	−0.11
Diabetes	0.14	0.62**	0.70***	0.64**	0.68***	−0.20	−0.17	−0.08	−0.12	−0.23
eGFR, ml/min/1.73m^2	0.14	0.30	0.39	0.57*	0.44	−0.02	0.19	0.34	0.32	0.37
Platelet counts, ×10^3/μL	0.43	0.24	0.52*	0.53*	0.39	−0.08	−0.16	−0.10	−0.20	−0.29
Proton pump inhibitor	−0.17	0.14	0.07	0.21	0.35	0.06	0.25	0.17	0.27	0.24
Concentration (0.5 h)	−0.04	−0.79***	−0.75***	−0.71**	−0.83***	0.09	−0.31	−0.41	−0.57*	−0.27
ODI3%	0.15	−0.16	0.18	0.05	0.03	0.12	0.50*	0.48*	0.49*	0.44*

Analysis was performed using the spearman's correlation coefficient. *$P < 0.05$; **$P < 0.01$; ***$P < 0.001$. ODI = oxygen desaturation index

in diabetes was attenuated in prasugrel treatment (Fig. 5b, c). In patients without diabetes, the VASP-PRI was already reduced 30 min after the prasugrel LD (non-diabetes vs. diabetes: 61.1% ± 5.5% vs. 82.7% ± 3.0%, $P = 0.009$). These differences were not observed in clopidogrel treatment. This finding suggests that diabetes has the potential to specifically interfere with pharmacokinetics of prasugrel after a LD.

Discussion

Application of the new generation of P2Y$_{12}$ inhibitor has improved clinical outcomes after PCI in several randomized, clinical trials [7, 17, 18] . The drug efficacy of thienopyridines affects not only the prognosis but also bleeding complications. Therefore, factors that affect the efficacy of thienopyridine to adequately inhibit P2Y$_{12}$ signalling should be identified in each individual. In the current study, we found reduced levels of active metabolites in diabetes after a LD of prasugrel but not clopidogrel. Further, incomplete inhibition of P2Y$_{12}$ by clopidogrel resulted in an increase in medium and small platelet aggregate formation, which could be overcome by prasugrel.

The most important finding in our study is the differential effect of diabetes on the efficacy between prasugrel and clopidogrel. Increase in active metabolites of prasugrel might be inhibited by the presence of diabetes, resulting in high on-treatment platelet reactivity. Numerous studies have suggested that patients with diabetes have increased platelet reactivity and a reduced

platelet response to clopidogrel [19, 20]. However, our study suggests a differential effect of diabetes on antiplatelet effects of thienopyridines. This phenomenon is probably due to variance in determining active metabolite concertation. Most absorbed clopidogrel is hydrolysed by esterase, and only 15% is transformed into the active metabolite by two CYP oxidation steps [5]. Therefore, the *CYP2C19* loss of function polymorphism has a strong effect to determine active metabolite concentration of clopidogrel. On the other hand, absorbed prasugrel is completely converted by esterase to an intermediate metabolite and then is easily oxidized independently of the *CYP2C19* polymorphism. This suggests that the absorbent process in the intestine may predominantly affect active metabolite concentration. Gastroenteropathy manifesting in delayed gastric emptying and constipation causes significant morbidity in patients with diabetes [21]. Gastrointestinal neuromuscular dysfunction in diabetes may reduce absorption of prasugrel after ingestion. Recently, a study reported that crushed prasugrel administration resulted in faster drug absorption and more prompt and potent antiplatelet effects [22]. Such a strategy may overcome the delayed absorption of prasugrel in diabetes.

We also found differences in the platelet aggregation process under treatment with thienopyridines ex vivo. Treatment with clopidogrel inhibited large platelet aggregation but increased small and medium platelet aggregation by stimulation with high ADP concentrations. Platelet aggregation consists of two phases as follows.

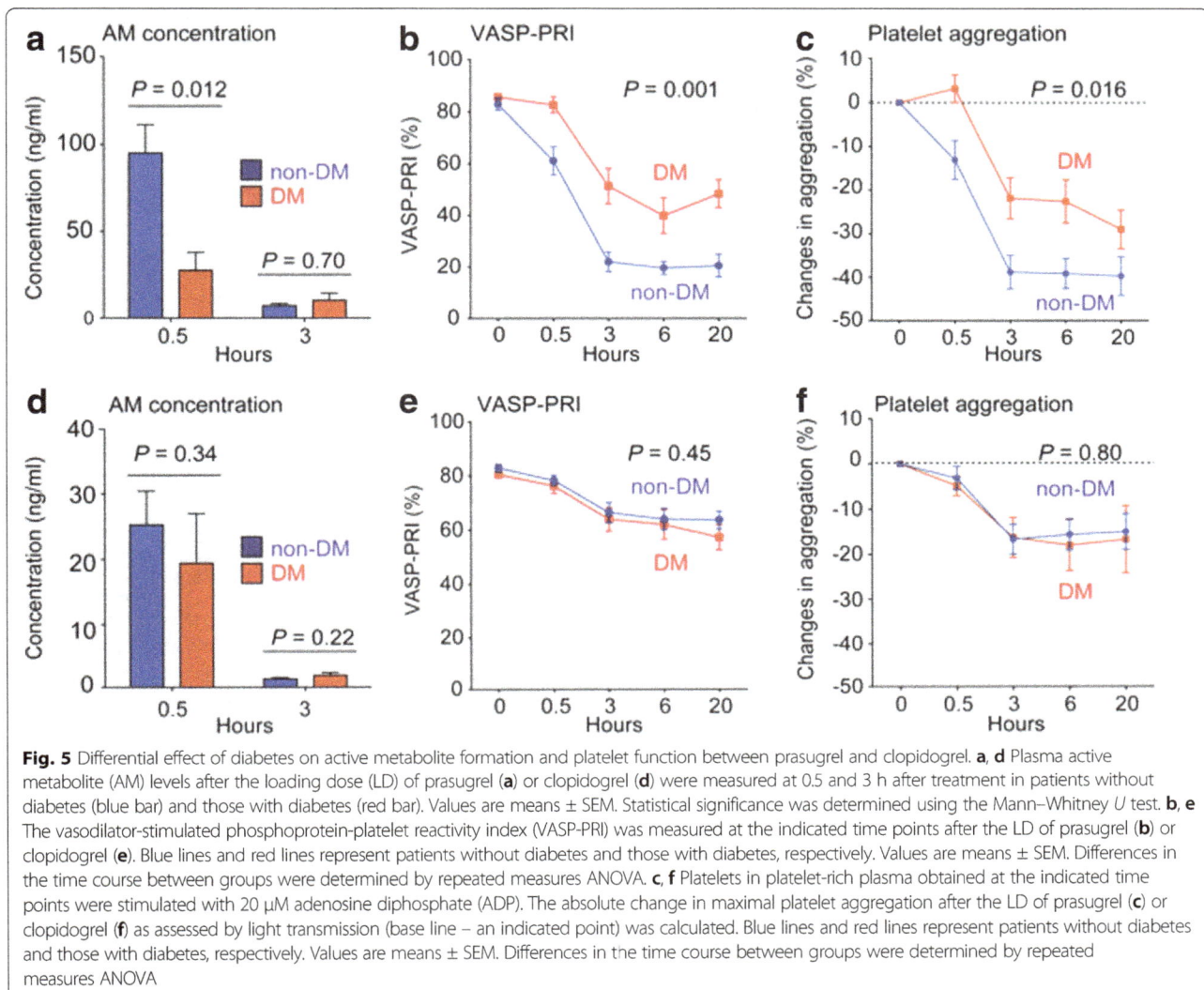

Fig. 5 Differential effect of diabetes on active metabolite formation and platelet function between prasugrel and clopidogrel. **a, d** Plasma active metabolite (AM) levels after the loading dose (LD) of prasugrel (**a**) or clopidogrel (**d**) were measured at 0.5 and 3 h after treatment in patients without diabetes (blue bar) and those with diabetes (red bar). Values are means ± SEM. Statistical significance was determined using the Mann–Whitney *U* test. **b, e** The vasodilator-stimulated phosphoprotein-platelet reactivity index (VASP-PRI) was measured at the indicated time points after the LD of prasugrel (**b**) or clopidogrel (**e**). Blue lines and red lines represent patients without diabetes and those with diabetes, respectively. Values are means ± SEM. Differences in the time course between groups were determined by repeated measures ANOVA. **c, f** Platelets in platelet-rich plasma obtained at the indicated time points were stimulated with 20 µM adenosine diphosphate (ADP). The absolute change in maximal platelet aggregation after the LD of prasugrel (**c**) or clopidogrel (**f**) as assessed by light transmission (base line – an indicated point) was calculated. Blue lines and red lines represent patients without diabetes and those with diabetes, respectively. Values are means ± SEM. Differences in the time course between groups were determined by repeated measures ANOVA

Formation of small-sized aggregates is followed by the phase of large aggregate formation with a concomitant decrease in the number of small aggregates [23]. $P2Y_{12}$ signalling is important for maintenance of GPIIb/IIIa (integrin $\alpha IIb\beta 3$) activation, which causes stable platelet aggregation to interact with fibrinogen [24]. This suggests that incomplete inhibition of $P2Y_{12}$ results in an increase in small and medium aggregates, despite inhibition of large aggregates. One reason why prasugrel reduces coronary events, including stent thrombosis, compared with clopidogrel, may be that this drug effectively abolishes formation of small aggregates. However, the increase in bleeding complications by strong inhibition of $P2Y_{12}$ should be considered. Because patients with $P2Y_{12}$ mutations demonstrate severe bleeding diathesis [25, 26], complete inhibition of $P2Y_{12}$ signalling by thienopyridines causes a tendency for severe bleeding. To identify the optimal range of $P2Y_{12}$ inhibition, evaluation of the ratio among small, medium, and large

platelet aggregate formation after ADP stimulation might become an index of adequate $P2Y_{12}$ inhibition in thienopyridine-treated patients.

We demonstrated the effect of diabetes on prasugrel metabolism, while previous reports showed inconsistent results for the role of diabetes [9, 27]. One possible explanation of this discrepancy between studies is the introduction of a lower LD in Japanese patients. This relative reduction in dose may lead to malabsorption of drugs in diabetes. There are several reasons to administrate low-dose prasugrel in Japan as follows: 1) bleeding complications, including cerebral haemorrhage, are more frequent in Japanese [28]; 2) the inhibitory effect on platelet aggregation is more potent [29]; and 3) a previous study was conducted at a lower dose and effectively inhibited platelet aggregation [16]. Further, we could not find any association of the efficacy of clopidogrel with diabetes, although a number of reports have described its relationship [20, 30]. The high ratio of poor and intermediate metabolizers of clopidogrel in Japanese might have reduced the importance of diabetes in our study. We found that the presence of sleep-disordered breathing was significantly correlated with the VASP-PRI in patients who had clopidogrel treatment. Because of the poor correlation among drug concentrations, the VASP-PRI, and platelet aggregation in patients who have clopidogrel, the cAMP signalling pathway, other than $P2Y_{12}$, may be modified by the presence of sleep-disordered breathing.

Study limitations

This study has some limitations. First, we applied a low LD of prasugrel (20 mg) compared with that in Western countries (60 mg). Our study included a relatively small number of patients, and did not include patients with acute coronary syndrome. Therefore, our findings may not be generalizable to the condition where prasugrel is indicated in Western countries. Additionally, we could not conclude that a higher LD could overcome defects in drug metabolism in diabetes. Finally, we could not assess bleeding and thrombotic events associated with antiplatelet therapy.

Conclusions

This study shows the differential effect of diabetes on antiplatelet activity between clopidogrel and prasugrel. We speculated that absorbed process of prasugrel, but not CYP metabolism, affected active metabolite concentration of prasugrel in diabetes. Further, prasugrel efficiently abolishes residual $P2Y_{12}$ signalling that leads to small platelet aggregation, but these small aggregates are not inhibited by clopidogrel. To efficiently apply dual antiplatelet therapy with potent $P2Y_{12}$ blockers, including prasugrel and ticagrelor, further studies are required to understand their optical range for inhibiting $P2Y_{12}$ signalling.

Abbreviations
ADP: Adenosine diphosphate; AM: Active metabolites; CT: Computed tomography; CYP: Cytochrome P450; LD: Loading dose; PCI: Percutaneous coronary intervention; PRI: Platelet reactivity index; VASP: Vasodilator stimulated phosphoprotein

Acknowledgements
The authors are grateful for the hard work of the Coronary Care Unit staff for recruitment and management of patients. We also thank Masanori Ito and Rumiko Ochiai (Jichi Medical University) for their technical assistance.

Funding
This work was supported by Daiichi Sankyo Co., Ltd. (Tokyo, Japan).

Author's contributions
All authors contributed sufficiently to the project. S.N. designed the protocol, recruited the patients, performed the experiments, analysed the data, and drafted the manuscript. T.O. designed the protocol, analysed data, and wrote the manuscript. K.K. designed the protocol, analysed the data, and revised the manuscript. All authors participated in subsequent revisions of the manuscript. We also declare that all of the authors have read and approved the final version of the manuscript.

Competing interests
T.O. has received research funding from Bayer AG. K.K. has received honoraria from Takeda Pharmaceutical Company Limited., Daiichi Sankyo Co., Ltd., and Omron Healthcare Co., Ltd., as well as research grants from Teijin Pharma Limited, Omron Healthcare Co., Ltd., Fukuda Denshi, Bayer Yakuhin Ltd., A&D Co., Ltd., Daiichi Sankyo Co., Ltd., Mochida Pharmaceutical Co., Ltd., EA Pharma, Otsuka Pharmaceutical Co., Ltd., Boehringer Ingelheim Japan Inc., Mitsubishi Tanabe Pharma Corporation, and Medtronic Japan Co., Ltd. The authors declare that they have no competing interests.

Author details
[1]Division of Cardiovascular Medicine, Department of Medicine, Jichi Medical University School of Medicine, 3311-1 Yakushiji, Shimotsuke, Tochigi 329-0498, Japan. [2]Department of Biochemistry, Jichi Medical University School of Medicine, 3311-1 Yakushiji, Shimotsuke, Tochigi 329-0498, Japan.

References
1. Yusuf S, Zhao F, Mehta SR, Chrolavicius S, Tognoni G, Fox KK. Effects of clopidogrel in addition to aspirin in patients with acute coronary syndromes without ST-segment elevation. N Engl J Med. 2001;345:494–502.
2. Steinhubl SR, Berger PB, Mann JT 3rd, Fry ET, DeLago A, Wilmer C, Topol EJ. Early and sustained dual oral antiplatelet therapy following percutaneous coronary intervention: a randomized controlled trial. JAMA. 2002;288:2411–20.
3. Holmes MV, Perel P, Shah T, Hingorani AD, Casas JP. CYP2C19 genotype, clopidogrel metabolism, platelet function, and cardiovascular events: a systematic review and meta-analysis. JAMA. 2011;306:2704–14.
4. Mega JL, Close SL, Wiviott SD, Shen L, Hockett RD, Brandt JT, Walker JR, Antman EM, Macias W, Braunwald E, Sabatine MS. Cytochrome p-450 polymorphisms and response to clopidogrel. N Engl J Med. 2009;360:354–62.
5. Kazui M, Nishiya Y, Ishizuka T, Hagihara K, Farid NA, Okazaki O, Ikeda T, Kurihara A. Identification of the human cytochrome P450 enzymes involved in the two oxidative steps in the bioactivation of clopidogrel to its pharmacologically active metabolite. Drug Metab Dispos. 2010;38:92–9.
6. Wallentin L, Varenhorst C, James S, Erlinge D, Braun OO, Jakubowski JA, Sugidachi A, Winters KJ, Siegbahn A. Prasugrel achieves greater and faster P2Y12receptor-mediated platelet inhibition than clopidogrel due to more efficient generation of its active metabolite in aspirin-treated patients with coronary artery disease. Eur Heart J. 2008;29:21–30.
7. Wiviott SD, Braunwald E, McCabe CH, Montalescot G, Ruzyllo W, Gottlieb S, Neumann FJ, Ardissino D, De Servi S, Murphy SA, et al. Prasugrel versus clopidogrel in patients with acute coronary syndromes. N Engl J Med. 2007; 357:2001–15.
8. Rehmel JL, Eckstein JA, Farid NA, Heim JB, Kasper SC, Kurihara A, Wrighton SA, Ring BJ. Interactions of two major metabolites of prasugrel, a thienopyridine antiplatelet agent, with the cytochromes P450. Drug Metab Dispos. 2006;34:600–7.
9. Wrishko RE, Ernest CS 2nd, Small DS, Li YG, Weerakkody GJ, Riesmeyer JR, Macias WL, Rohatagi S, Salazar DE, Antman EM, et al. Population pharmacokinetic analyses to evaluate the influence of intrinsic and extrinsic factors on exposure of prasugrel active metabolite in TRITON-TIMI 38. J Clin Pharmacol. 2009;49:984–98.
10. Sato T, Namba Y, Kashihara Y, Tanaka M, Fuke S, Yumoto A, Saito H. Clinical significance of platelet reactivity during prasugrel therapy in patients with acute myocardial infarction. J Cardiol. 2017;70:35–40.
11. Bonello L, Mancini J, Pansieri M, Maillard L, Rossi P, Collet F, Jouve B, Wittenberg O, Laine M, Michelet P, et al. Relationship between post-treatment platelet reactivity and ischemic and bleeding events at 1-year follow-up in patients receiving prasugrel. J Thromb Haemost. 2012;10:1999–2005.
12. Ohmori T, Yatomi Y, Nonaka T, Kobayashi Y, Madoiwa S, Mimuro J, Ozaki Y, Sakata Y. Aspirin resistance detected with aggregometry cannot be explained by cyclooxygenase activity: involvement of other signaling pathway(s) in cardiovascular events of aspirin-treated patients. J Thromb Haemost. 2006;4:1271–8.

13. Yano Y, Ohmori T, Hoshide S, Madoiwa S, Yamamoto K, Katsuki T, Mitsuhashi T, Mimuro J, Shimada K, Kario K, Sakata Y. Determinants of thrombin generation, fibrinolytic activity, and endothelial dysfunction in patients on dual antiplatelet therapy: involvement of factors other than platelet aggregability in Virchow's triad. Eur Heart J. 2008;29:1729–38.

14. Ozaki Y, Satoh K, Yatomi Y, Yamamoto T, Shirasawa Y, Kume S. Detection of platelet aggregates with a particle counting method using light scattering. Anal Biochem. 1994;218:284–94.

15. Angiolillo DJ, Badimon JJ, Saucedo JF, Frelinger AL, Michelson AD, Jakubowski JA, Zhu B, Ojeh CK, Baker BA, Effron MB. A pharmacodynamic comparison of prasugrel vs. high-dose clopidogrel in patients with type 2 diabetes mellitus and coronary artery disease: results of the optimizing anti-platelet therapy in diabetes MellitUS (OPTIMUS)-3 trial. Eur Heart J. 2011;32:838–46.

16. Yokoi H, Kimura T, Isshiki T, Ogawa H, Ikeda Y. Pharmacodynamic assessment of a novel P2Y12 receptor antagonist in Japanese patients with coronary artery disease undergoing elective percutaneous coronary intervention. Thromb Res. 2012;129:623–8.

17. James S, Angiolillo DJ, Cornel JH, Erlinge D, Husted S, Kontny F, Maya J, Nicolau JC, Spinar J, Storey RF, et al. Ticagrelor vs. clopidogrel in patients with acute coronary syndromes and diabetes: a substudy from the PLATelet inhibition and patient outcomes (PLATO) trial. Eur Heart J. 2010;31:3006–16.

18. Saito S, Isshiki T, Kimura T, Ogawa H, Yokoi H, Nanto S, Takayama M, Kitagawa K, Nishikawa M, Miyazaki S, Nakamura M. Efficacy and safety of adjusted-dose prasugrel compared with clopidogrel in Japanese patients with acute coronary syndrome: the PRASFIT-ACS study. Circ J. 2014;78:1684–92.

19. Angiolillo DJ, Shoemaker SB, Desai B, Yuan H, Charlton RK, Bernardo E, Zenni MM, Guzman LA, Bass TA, Costa MA. Randomized comparison of a high clopidogrel maintenance dose in patients with diabetes mellitus and coronary artery disease: results of the optimizing antiplatelet therapy in diabetes mellitus (OPTIMUS) study. Circulation. 2007;115:708–16.

20. Angiolillo DJ, Jakubowski JA, Ferreiro JL, Tello-Montoliu A, Rollini F, Franchi F, Ueno M, Darlington A, Desai B, Moser BA, et al. Impaired responsiveness to the platelet P2Y12 receptor antagonist clopidogrel in patients with type 2 diabetes and coronary artery disease. J Am Coll Cardiol. 2014;64:1005–14.

21. Ordog T, Hayashi Y, Gibbons SJ. Cellular pathogenesis of diabetic gastroenteropathy. Minerva Gastroenterol Dietol. 2009;55:315–43.

22. Rollini F, Franchi F, Hu J, Kureti M, Aggarwal N, Durairaj A, Park Y, Seawell M, Cox-Alomar P, Zenni MM, et al. Crushed Prasugrel tablets in patients with STEMI undergoing primary percutaneous coronary intervention: the CRUSH study. J Am Coll Cardiol. 2016;67:1994–2004.

23. Satoh K, Ozaki Y, Qi R, Yang L, Asazuma N, Yatomi Y, Kume S. Factors that affect the size of platelet aggregates in epinephrine-induced activation: a study using the particle counting method based upon light scattering. Thromb Res. 1996;81:515–23.

24. Kamae T, Shiraga M, Kashiwagi H, Kato H, Tadokoro S, Kurata Y, Tomiyama Y, Kanakura Y. Critical role of ADP interaction with P2Y12 receptor in the maintenance of alpha(IIb)beta3 activation: association with Rap1B activation. J Thromb Haemost. 2006;4:1379–87.

25. Lecchi A, Razzari C, Paoletta S, Dupuis A, Nakamura L, Ohlmann P, Gachet C, Jacobson KA, Zieger B, Cattaneo M. Identification of a new dysfunctional platelet P2Y12 receptor variant associated with bleeding diathesis. Blood. 2015;125:1006–13.

26. Lecchi A, Femia EA, Paoletta S, Dupuis A, Ohlmann P, Gachet C, Jacobson KA, Machura K, Podda GM, Zieger B, Cattaneo M. Inherited dysfunctional platelet P2Y12 receptor mutations associated with bleeding disorders. Hamostaseologie. 2016;36:279–83.

27. Erlinge D, Varenhorst C, Braun OO, James S, Winters KJ, Jakubowski JA, Brandt JT, Sugidachi A, Siegbahn A, Wallentin L. Patients with poor responsiveness to thienopyridine treatment or with diabetes have lower levels of circulating active metabolite, but their platelets respond normally to active metabolite added ex vivo. J Am Coll Cardiol. 2008;52:1968–77.

28. Mak KH, Bhatt DL, Shao M, Hankey GJ, Easton JD, Fox KA, Topol EJ. Ethnic variation in adverse cardiovascular outcomes and bleeding complications in the Clopidogrel for high Atherothrombotic risk and ischemic stabilization, management, and avoidance (CHARISMA) study. Am Heart J. 2009;157:658–65.

29. Small DS, Kothare P, Yuen E, Lachno DR, Li YG, Winters KJ, Farid NA, Ni L, Jakubowski JA, Salazar DE, et al. The pharmacokinetics and pharmacodynamics of prasugrel in healthy Chinese, Japanese, and Korean subjects compared with healthy Caucasian subjects. Eur J Clin Pharmacol. 2010;66:127–35.

30. Sweeny JM, Angiolillo DJ, Franchi F, Rollini F, Waksman R, Raveendran G, Dangas G, Khan ND, Carlson GF, Zhao Y, et al. Impact of diabetes mellitus on the Pharmacodynamic effects of Ticagrelor versus Clopidogrel in troponin-negative acute coronary syndrome patients undergoing ad hoc percutaneous coronary intervention. J Am Heart Assoc. 2017;6

21

Thromboembolic events in cancer patients on active treatment with cisplatin-based chemotherapy: another look!

Hikmat Abdel-Razeq[1]*[iD], Asem Mansour[2], Hazem Abdulelah[1], Anas Al-Shwayat[1], Mohammad Makoseh[1], Mohammad Ibrahim[1], Mahmoud Abunasser[1], Dalia Rimawi[3], Abeer Al-Rabaiah[4], Rozan Alfar[1], Alaa' Abufara[1], Alaa Ibrahim[2], Anas Bawaliz[1] and Yousef Ismael[5]

Abstract

Background: The risk of thromboembolic events is higher among cancer patients, especially in patients undergoing chemotherapy. Cisplatin-based regimens claim to be associated with a very high thromboembolic rate. In this study, we report on our own experience with thrombosis among patients on active cisplatin-based chemotherapy.

Methods: Medical records and hospital databases were searched for all the patients treated with any cisplatin-based regimen for any kind of cancer. Thrombosis was considered cisplatin-related if diagnosed any time after the first dose and up to 4 weeks after the last. The Khorana risk assessment model was performed in all cases.

Results: A total of 1677 patients (65.5% males, median age: 50 years) treated with cisplatin-based regimens were identified. Head and neck (22.9%), lung (22.2%), lymphoma and gastric (11.4% each) were the most common primary tumors. Thromboembolic events were reported in 110 (6.6%); the highest was in patients with gastric cancer (20.9%) and the lowest in patients with head and neck cancers (2.3%) and lymphoma (1.6%). Thrombosis included deep vein thrombosis (DVT) in 69 (62.7%), pulmonary embolism (PE) in 18 (16.9%) and arterial thrombosis in 17 (15.6%). A majority (51.1%) of the patients had stage IV disease and only 16% had stage I or II.

In a multivariate analysis, significantly higher rates of thrombosis were associated with gastric as the primary tumor, advanced-stage disease, female sex but not age, and the Khorana risk score or type of cisplatin regimen. While the presence of CVC was significantly associated with the risk of thrombosis ($p < 0.0001$) in the univariate analysis, and such significance was lost in the multivariate analysis (odds ratio, 1.098; 95%CI, 0.603–1.999, $p = 0.7599$).

Conclusions: Thromboembolic events in cancer patients on active cisplatin-based chemotherapy were commonly encountered. Gastric cancer, regardless of other clinical variables, was associated with the highest risk.

Keywords: Cisplatin, Chemotherapy, Thrombosis, Cancer

Background

Venous thromboembolism (VTE) and, to a lesser extent, arterial thrombosis are common complications encountered in patients with cancer during the course of their treatment and follow-up [1, 2].

Much of this high risk is attributed to the cancer itself or its therapy. However, patient-related factors such as age,

performance status, body mass index and underlying co-morbidities are also important factors [3, 4].

Thromboembolic events are one of the leading causes of death in patients with cancer [5]. Many studies show that the survival of cancer patients with thrombosis is significantly lower than those without [6–8].

Cisplatin is an old chemotherapeutic drug that was licensed in 1978 and is now listed on the World Health Organization's list of essential medicines. It is widely used, alone or in combination, to treat a number of cancers, including testicular, ovarian, cervical, bladder, head and neck, lung, esophageal and gastric cancers [9, 10].

* Correspondence: habdelrazeq@khcc.jo
[1]Department of Internal Medicine, King Hussein Cancer Center, 202 Queen Rania Al-Abdulla St., P.O. Box 1269, Amman 11941, Jordan
Full list of author information is available at the end of the article

Cisplatin is well known for its vascular and thrombotic complications, including both venous and arterial thrombosis [11–13]. In one study, researchers at Memorial Sloan-Kettering Cancer Center (MSKCC) and Michigan State University reported a thrombosis rate of 18.1% among 932 patients treated with cisplatin-based regimens for various kinds of cancers. All had their thromboembolic events while on active cisplatin therapy or within 4 weeks of the last dose. Deep vein thrombosis (DVT) and/or pulmonary embolism (PE) accounted for almost 90% of the events [14]. More recently, a higher risk of VTE [crude relative risk of 2.8 (95% CI, 1.4–4.2)] was also reported in a group of 200 patients with various malignancies undergoing treatment with cisplatin-based chemotherapy compared to 200 others who received non-cisplatin-based chemotherapy [15]. A meta-analysis that involved 8216 patients treated with different chemotherapy regimens for various advanced solid tumors from 38 randomized controlled trials was recently reported. Patients receiving cisplatin-based chemotherapy had a significantly increased risk of VTEs (RR, 1.67; 95% CI, 1.25 to 2.23; $P = 0.01$) [16].

Given the variation in the reported thromboembolic rates among such patients, this study highlights the observed thrombosis rate in real daily clinical practice. Factors that help predict the occurrence of thrombosis were also studied. Following this analysis, it was hypothesized that particular group(s) of patients with specific clinical features and particular primary tumors treated with cisplatin-based regimen could be identified as high risk for VTE to justify prophylaxis, even in the ambulatory setting. The results of this study could help design clinical trials addressing preventive measures for a subgroup of patients with the highest risk.

Methods

Medical records and the hospital database were searched for patients treated with any cisplatin-based regimen for any kind of cancer. All adult patients (≥ 18 years old) that were treated between January 2007 and December 2015 and had at least 4 weeks of follow-up after their last cisplatin dose were included.

The patients' medical records and imaging reports were searched for a diagnosis of venous or arterial thrombosis. To avoid any missing events, we also searched the pharmacy database for any anticoagulant therapy for all the patients who received cisplatin-based chemotherapy during this period.

The presence of central venous catheter (CVC) and other thrombotic risk factors used to calculate the Khorana risk score were collected, and such risk factors included hemoglobin level, platelet and WBC counts, primary cancer site, disease stage, and body mass index (BMI) [17]. Patients were then grouped into three risk

categories, including high, intermediate and low risk, as shown in Table 1. Thrombosis was considered cisplatin-related if it was diagnosed any time after the first dose and up to 4 weeks after the last. All DVT was diagnosed by Doppler ultrasound, while all the PE were diagnosed by CT angiogram. This study was approved by our institutional review board.

Statistical analysis

The primary objective of this study was to determine the overall incidence and characteristics of thrombosis in adult patients receiving cisplatin-based chemotherapy with or without radiation therapy. The secondary objectives were to analyze the importance of the patients' tumor and treatment characteristics in predicting the occurrence of thrombosis.

The association between such variables and the development of thromboembolic events during the defined treatment period was evaluated using the X^2 test for categorical variables and the Wilcoxon rank sum test for continuous variables. The variables found to be significant ($p < 0.05$) by the univariate analysis were subsequently entered into a multivariate logistic regression model. Following this analysis, it was hypothesized that particular group(s) of patients with specific clinical features and particular primary tumors treated with cisplatin-based regimen could be identified as high risk for VTE to justify prophylaxis, even in the ambulatory setting.

Results

During the study period, 1677 patients received at least one cycle of cisplatin-based regimen and were included in this study. The median age was 50 years (range: 18–83 years), and 1099 (65.5%) were male. The most common primary tumors encountered were head and neck (22.9%), lung (22.2%), lymphoma (11.4%), gastric (11.4%), and testicular (8.4%). A majority of the patients had advanced-

Table 1 Khorana Risk Assessment Model

Patient characteristic	Risk Score
1. Site of cancer	
• Very high risk (stomach, pancreas)	2
• High risk (Lung, Lymphoma, Gynecologic, bladder, testicular)	1
2. Prechemotherapy platelet count 350×10^9/L or more	1
3. Hemoglobin level less than 100 g/L or use of red cell growth factors	1
4. Prechemotherapy leukocyte count more than 11×10^9 /L	1
5. BMI: 35 kg/m² or more	1

Three Risk Groups:
• Low Risk 0
• Intermediate Risk 1–2
• High Risk ≥3

stage disease at the time of chemotherapy administration, and 858 (51.2%) patients were stage IV and 487 (29.0%) patients had stage III disease. Chemotherapy was delivered through a central venous catheter (CVC) in 303 (18.1%) patients as shown in Table 2. None of the patients had any form of thromboprophylaxis while in ambulatory settings.

Thromboembolic events were reported in 110 (6.6%) patients; 96 (5.7%) were venous thrombosis in the form of DVT and/or PE, and 14 (0.83%) had arterial thrombosis. The thrombosis rate was highest among patients with gastric cancer; it was reported in 40 (20.9%) of 191 patients compared to 70 (4.7%) of 1486 patients with other tumor types, $p < 0.0001$. The thromboembolic rates were particularly low among the patients with lymphoma (1.6%), head and neck (2.3%) and testicular cancers (2.8%).

The thrombosis rate was also studied in relation to the Khorana risk score. Patients with a high-risk score had higher rates of thromboembolic events, which were reported in 33 (13.1%) of 252 such patients compared to 77 (5.4%) of all the other patients with an intermediate or low-risk score, $p < 0.0001$, as shown in Table 3.

We also studied the effect of a combination chemotherapy regimen on the incidence of thrombosis. This rate was highest (30.0%) among a small group of 30 patients treated with ECF (epirubicin, cisplatin and fluorouracil (5-FU)); all of these patients had gastric cancer. The rate of thrombosis was 12.7% in the 245 treated with cisplatin, docetaxel and 5-FU, was only 2.1% among the 145 patients treated with cisplatin and etoposide and was 4.3% among the 116 patients treated with the BEP

Table 2 Patients Characteristics ($n = 1677$)

Characteristic	No. of Patients	Percentage
Age (Years)		
Median	50	
Range	18–83	
Sex		
Male	1099	65.5
Females	578	34.5
Primary Tumor		
Head and Neck	384	22.9
Lung	373	22.2
Gastric	191	11.4
Lymphoma	191	11.4
Cervical	121	7.2
Testicular	104	6.2
Bladder	77	4.6
Sarcoma	45	2.7
Esophageal	33	2.0
Others	158	9.4
Khorana Risk Score		
Low	350	20.9
Intermediate	1075	64.1
High	252	15.0
Central Venous Catheter		
Present	303	18.1%
Absent	1374	81.9%
Disease Stage		
I	56	3.3
II	213	12.7
III	487	29.0
IV	857	51.1
Unstageable/Unknown	64	3.8

Table 3 Thromboembolic events for the whole group

	Whole Group (1677)		Patients with thrombosis (110)		
	Number	%	Number	%	p-value
Sex					
Male	1099	65.5	58	5.3	0.003
Female	578	34.5	52	9.0	
Age (Years)					
Missed	1				0.6445
≤ 60	1276	76.1	81	6.3	
> 60	400	23.9	28	7.0	
Primary Tumor					
Head and Neck	384	22.9	9	2.3	<0.0001
Lung	373	22.2	25	6.7	
Gastric	191	11.4	40	20.9	
Lymphoma	191	11.4	3	1.6	
Testicular	104	6.2	4	3.8	
Cervical	121	7.2	7	5.8	
Bladder	77	4.6	3	3.9	
Sarcoma	45	2.7	3	6.7	
Esophageal	33	2.0	6	18.2	
Others	158	9.4	10	6.3	
Khorana Risk Score					
Low risk	350	20.9	16	4.6	<0.0001
Intermediate risk	1075	64.1	61	5.7	
High risk	252	15.0	33	13.1	
Disease Stage					
I	56	3.3	3	5.4	0.0038
II	213	12.7	8	3.8	
III	487	29	20	4.1	
IV	857	51.1	76	8.9	
Unstageable/Unknown	64	3.8	3	4.7	

(bleomycin, etoposide and cisplatin) regimen or cisplatin and radiation therapy. Table 4 shows the chemotherapy regimens and corresponding thromboembolic events.

To further address the effect of the chosen combination chemotherapy regimen in relation to a particular disease, we studied the three most commonly utilized regimens, including Cisplatin-Radiation (299 patients), Cisplatin-Docetaxel-5FU (245 patients) and Cisplatin-Docetaxel (193 patients). While none of the 95 patients with head and neck cancers treated with (Cisplatin-Docetaxel-5FU) had any thromboembolic events, 28 (20.6%) of the 136 patients with gastric cancer and 3 (42.9%) of the 7 patients with esophageal cancers treated with the same regimen had thrombosis, $p < 0.0001$. Further details are shown in Table 5.

We further analyzed the 191 gastric patients and studied the rate of thrombosis in relation to many other variables, including the chosen combination chemotherapy, the disease stage, the Khorana risk score and age. None of those clinical variables had a significant impact on the rates of thromboembolic events, as shown in Table 6.

To further address the association of the baseline and treatment variables with the development of thrombosis, a univariate analysis was conducted. Sex, the Khorana risk score, the presence of central venous catheter (CVC), and the primary tumor site and stage were all associated with a significantly higher rate of thrombosis as shown in Table 7.

The significant variables in the univariate analysis were subsequently entered into a multivariate logistic regression model. In the multivariate analysis, only sex (odds ratio,

1.732; 95% CI, 1.152–2.605, $p = 0.0083$), gastric cancer as the primary site (odds ratio, 3.377; 95% CI, 1.759–6.483, $p = 0.0003$) and disease stage (odds ratio, 1.665; 95% CI, 1.054–2.63, $p = 0.0289$) were significantly associated with thromboembolic events as shown in Table 8. In addition,

Table 5 Thromboembolic events according to Cisplatin-based chemotherapy regimen

Chemotherapy Regimen	Patients		Thromboembolic Events		p-value
	(n)	(%)	(n)	(%)	
Cisplatin-Docetaxel-5FU					
Head and Neck	95	38.8	0	0	<0.0001
Gastric	136	55.5	28	20.6	
Esophageal	7	2.9	3	42.9	
Others	7	2.9	0	0	
Total	245		31	12.7	
Cisplatin-XRT					
Cervical	101	33.8	7	6.9	0.2166
Head and Neck	184	61.5	5	2.7	
Others	14	4.7	1	7.1	
Total	299		13	4.3	
Cisplatin-Docetaxel					
Lung	181	93.3	12	6.6	0.9999
Others	13	6.7	1	7.7	
Total	194		13	6.7	

5FU 5-Flurouracil, *XRT* Radiation therapy

Table 4 Thromboembolic events according to chemotherapy regimen

Chemotherapy Regimen	Number of Patients	Thromboembolic Events	
		(n)	%
Cisplatin-XRT	299	13	4.3
Cisplatin-Docetaxel-5FU	245	31	12.7
Cisplatin-Docetaxel	194	13	6.7
DHAP	180	3	1.7
Cisplatin-Etoposide	145	3	2.1
Cisplatin-5FU	120	9	7.5
BEP	116	5	4.3
Cisplatin-Gemcitabine	95	9	9.5
Cisplatin-Doxorubicin	42	3	7.1
Cisplatin-Etoposide-XRT	38	4	10.5
ECF	30	9	30.0
Cisplatin-Pemetrexed	19	3	15.8
Others	154	5	3.2

5-FU 5-Flurouracil, *DHAP* Dexamethasone, High-dose
Ara-C and Cisplatin; *BEP* Bleomycin, Etoposide and Cisplatin, *ECF* Epirubicin, Cisplatin and 5-Flurouracil, *XRT* Radiation therapy

Table 6 Thromboembolic events in patients with Gastric cancer

Clinical Variables	Number of Patients	Thromboembolic Events		p-Value
		(n)	(%)	
Chemotherapy Regimen				
ECF	26	8	30.8	0.5982
Cisplatin-Docetaxel-5FU	137	28	20.4	
Cisplatin-5FU	20	4	20	
Others	8	0	0	
Disease Stage				
Early Stage	35	11	31.4	0.0916
Metastatic	156	29	18.5	
Khorana Risk Score				
Low[a]	1	1		0.5331
Intermediate	101	19	18.8	
High	89	20	22.5	
Age (years)				
Missed	1			0.8647
< 50	90	18	18.5	
≥ 50	100	21	23.5	

ECF Epirubicin, Cisplatin and 5-Flurouracil, *5-FU* 5-Flurouracil
[a] Only one patient and had thrombosis

Table 7 Univariate Analysis for thromboembolic events

Factors		Number of Patients	Thromboembolic Events 110 (6.6%)	P-value
Age	≤ 60	1276 (76.1%)	81 (6.3%)	0.6445
	> 60	401 (23.9%)	29 (7.2%)	
Gender	Female	578 (34.5%)	52 (9.0%)	0.003
	Male	1099 (65.5%)	58 (5.3%)	
Khorana risk	High	252 (15.0%)	33 (13.1%)	<0.0001
	Others	1423 (85.0%)	77 (5.4%)	
Central venous catheter	No	1374 (81.9%)	70 (5.1%)	<0.0001
	Yes	303 (18.1%)	40 (13.2%)	
Primary Tumor	Gastric	191 (11.4%)	40 (20.9%)	<0.0001
	Other	1486 (88.6%)	70 (4.7%)	
Stage	IV	857 (51.1%)	76 (8.9%)	<0.0001
	Early stage	756 (45.1%)	31 (4.1%)	

the presence of CVC was significantly associated with risk of thrombosis ($p < 0.0001$) in the univariate analysis, and this significance was lost in the multivariate analysis (odds ratio, 1.098; 95%CI, 0.603–1.999, $p = 0.7599$).

Discussion

The association of cisplatin with thrombosis is well-known. However, its pathogenesis remains unclear. Endothelial cell damage, as revealed by the increased plasma levels of the Von Willebrand factor during chemotherapy, is believed to be a major contributing factor [18]. Platelet activation and the up-regulation of prothrombotic factors are also implicated in cisplatin-associated thrombosis [19–21].

Table 8 Multivariate Analysis for thromboembolic events

Factor	Odds Ratio	95% Confidence Limits	P-value
Primary Tumor (Gastric vs. Others)	3.377	1.759–6.483	0.0003
Gender (Female vs. Male)	1.732	1.152–2.605	0.0083
Khorana risk group (High vs. Others)	1.387	0.842–2.285	0.1992
Central Venous Catheter (Presence vs. Absence)	1.098	0.603–1.999	0.7599
Stage (IV vs. Early stage)	1.665	1.054–2.63	0.0289

In addition to venous thrombosis, arterial thrombosis is also well-described. In one study, 25 cases of myocardial infarction (MI) and cerebrovascular accidents (CVA) were reported among a group of young patients treated with cisplatin-based regimens for testicular cancer. None of these patients had known risk factors and none had atherosclerotic features [22].

Given the high recurrence rates [23], poor quality of life, and worse overall survival associated with thrombosis in cancer patients [6–8, 24], antithrombotic prophylaxis is widely practiced. Much of the emphasis is given to patients admitted for medical illnesses or surgical procedures. Such practice was endorsed by many international clinical practice guidelines, including the American Society of Clinical Oncology (ASCO) and the National Comprehensive Cancer Network (NCCN) [25, 26].

However, many recent studies addressing thrombosis in cancer patients show that a significant portion of these patients had thrombosis while in an ambulatory setting and were never admitted at the time or just prior to their thrombotic events [27]. Many factors contributed to these findings, and routine oncology practice has recently shifted away from the inpatient setting to the ambulatory one. Additionally, we tend to offer chemotherapy to much older and sicker patients. Routine thrombotic prophylaxis for such ambulatory cancer patients is not endorsed by any of the published guidelines.

Several efforts have been made to address the issue of prophylaxis among ambulatory cancer patients on active chemotherapy. Khorana, et al. suggested a risk assessment model that assigns these patients into three risk levels, including high, intermediate, and low [17]. Despite its simplicity and the availability of the data needed to calculate the risk of VTE, this model failed to gain popularity in clinical practice, and several studies show that it can be only applied to a small portion of such ambulatory patients [28]. Additionally, although the Khorana score, detailed in Table 1, considered gastric cancer as a high-risk type (score of 2), it did not consider the type of chemotherapy offered as a risk category.

Enrolling high-risk patients in clinical trials to test the value of thromboembolic prophylaxis in a wide range of cancer patients was another promising approach. However, due to a higher risk of bleeding and despite the associated benefit in lowering the thrombosis rate, this approach also failed to show a significant overall clinical benefit [29, 30].

A third approach was offering VTE prophylaxis to a particular high-risk group of patients with a specific diagnosis, such as advanced pancreatic cancer, undergoing active chemotherapy. The benefit of this approach was also offset by the high rate of bleeding [31, 32]. Another approach, similar to the one under discussion in this study, is to link a specific kind of chemotherapy and thrombosis risk. Cisplatin, as discussed earlier, is a good example.

Our thrombosis rate was lower than the 18% reported by the MSKCC group [14]. Many factors could have contributed to this lower rate, including a lower risk-patient population enrolled and different diagnostic methods. However, clinically important observations were noted and deserve discussion. In our study, we identified a specific subgroup of cancer patients treated with cisplatin-based chemotherapy with a real high risk for thrombosis. Patients with gastric cancer had a significantly higher rate of thrombosis, which was 20.9% compared to 4.7% among other patients receiving a similar cisplatin-based chemotherapy regimen. This high rate of thrombosis among patients with gastric cancer was high regardless of their age, stage, Khorana risk score, or the combination chemotherapy regimen used as shown in Table 6.

Given this relatively high rate, we proposed here that such patients could be selected into a randomized clinical trial to test the value of thrombotic prophylaxis among them, and most of them were usually treated with chemotherapy in the ambulatory setting without prophylaxis.

Thromboembolic prophylaxis in particular disease entities undergoing specific combinations of chemotherapy is routinely practiced in diseases, such as multiple myeloma (MM). We now have strong evidence and clear guidelines to offer antithrombotic prophylaxis when these patients are treated with immune modulators (thalidomide and lenalidomide) when combined with dexamethasone [25, 26].

We hope that future clinical research will lead to clear guidelines recommending antithrombotic prophylaxis in high-risk cancer patients, such as those with gastric cancer treated with a cisplatin-based regimen, even when done in ambulatory settings similar to what we routinely do with MM patients.

Conclusions

Thromboembolic events among cancer patients on active cisplatin-based chemotherapy are relatively common. The highest thrombosis rates were encountered in patients with gastric cancer regardless of other clinical variables. Prospective randomized trials are needed to study the value of VTE prophylaxis in such high-risk patients.

Abbreviations

5-FU: Fluorouracil; ASCO: American Society of Clinical Oncology; BEP: Bleomycin, Etoposide and Cisplatin; BMI: Body mass index; CVA: Cerebrovascular accidents; CVC: Central venous catheter; DHAP: Dexamethasone, High-dose Ara-C and Cisplatin; DVT: Deep vein thrombosis; ECF: Epirubicin, Cisplatin and Fluorouracil; MI: Myocardial infarction; MM: Multiple myeloma; NCCN: National Comprehensive Cancer Network; PE: Pulmonary embolism; VTE: Venous thromboembolism; XRT: Radiation therapy

Acknowledgements
The authors would like to thank Mrs. Alice Haddadin, Haifa Al-Ahmad and Laila Alqatu for the help in preparing this manuscript.

Funding
None.

Authors' contributions
HA: Designed and coordinated the study, performed the data analysis and drafted and wrote the final version of the manuscript. AM: Helped in the study design, data analysis and writing the final draft. HA, AS, MM, MI, MA, AR, RA, AA, AI, AB, YI: Data collection, analysis and interpretation. DR: Performed the statistical analysis. All the authors read and approved the final manuscript.

Competing interests
The authors declare that they have no competing interests.

Author details
[1]Department of Internal Medicine, King Hussein Cancer Center, 202 Queen Rania Al-Abdulla St., P.O. Box 1269, Amman 11941, Jordan. [2]Radiology, King Hussein Cancer Center, Amman, Jordan. [3]Scientific and Reseaerch Office, King Hussein Cancer Center, Amman, Jordan. [4]Pharmacy, King Hussein Cancer Center, Amman, Jordan. [5]Radiation Oncology, King Hussein Cancer Center, Amman, Jordan.

References
1. Timp JF, Braekkan SK, Versteeg HH, Cannegieter SC. Epidemiology of cancer-associated venous thrombosis. Blood. 2013;122(10):1712–23.
2. Khorana AA, Francis CW, Culakova E, Kuderer NM, Lyman GH. Frequency, risk factors, and trends for venous thromboembolism among hospitalized cancer patients. Cancer. 2007;110(10):2339–46.
3. Falanga A, Marchetti M, Vignoli A. Coagulation and cancer: biological and clinical aspects. J Thromb Haemost. 2013;11(2):223–33.
4. Khorana AA. Risk assessment and prophylaxis for VTE in cancer patients. J Natl Compr Cancer Netw. 2011;9(7):789–97.
5. Khorana AA, Francis CW, Culakova E, Kuderer NM, Lyman GH. Thromboembolism is a leading cause of death in cancer patients receiving outpatient chemotherapy. J Thromb Haemost. 2007;5:632–4.
6. Agnelli G, Verso M, Mandala M, Gallus S, Cimminiello C, Apolone G, et al. A prospective study on survival in cancer patients with and without venous thromboembolism. Intern Emerg Med. 2014;9(5):559–67.
7. Sørensen HT, Mellemkjaer L, Olsen JH, Baron JA. Prognosis of cancers associated with venous thromboembolism. N Engl J Med. 2000;343(25):1846–50.
8. Mandalà M, Reni M, Cascinu S, Barni S, Floriani I, Cereda S, et al. Venous thromboembolism predicts poor prognosis in irresectable pancreatic cancer patients. Ann Oncol. 2007;18(10):1660–5.
9. Fischer J, Ganellin CR. Analogue-based drug discovery. John Wiley & Sons. 2006. p. 513. ISBN 9783527607495.
10. WHO Model List of Essential Medicines (19th List). Available at: http://www.who.int/medicines/publications/essentialmedicines/EML2015_8-May-15.pdf. Accessed 01 May 2017.
11. Anders JC, Grigsby PW, Singh AK. Cisplatin chemotherapy (without erythropoietin) and risk of life-threatening thromboembolic events in carcinoma of the uterine cervix: the tip of the iceberg? A review of the literature. Radiat Oncol. 2006;1:14.
12. Czaykowski PM, Moore MJ, Tannock IF. High risk of vascular events in patients with urothelial transitional cell carcinoma treated with cisplatin based chemotherapy. J Urol. 1998;160:2021–4.

13. Weijl NI, Rutten MF, Zwinderman AH, Keizer HJ, Nooy MA, Rosendaal FR, et al. Thromboembolic events during chemotherapy for germ cell cancer: a cohort study and review of the literature. J Clin Oncol. 2000;18:2169–78.

14. Moore RA, Adel N, Riedel E, Bhutani M, Feldman DR, Tabbara NE, et al. High incidence of thromboembolic events in patients treated with cisplatin-based chemotherapy: a large retrospective analysis. J Clin Oncol. 2011;29: 3466–73.

15. Zahir MN, Shaikh Q, Shabbir-Moosajee M, Jabbar AA. Incidence of venous Thromboembolism in cancer patients treated with Cisplatin based chemotherapy - a cohort study. BMC Cancer. 2017;17(1):57.

16. Seng S, Liu Z, Chiu SK, Proverbs-Singh T, Sonpavde G, Choueiri TK, et al. Risk of venous Thromboembolism in patients with cancer treated with Cisplatin: a systematic review and meta-analysis. J Clin Oncol. 2012;30:4416–26.

17. Khorana AA, Kuderer NM, Culakova E, Lyman GH, Francis CW. Development and validation of a predictive model for chemotherapy-associated thrombosis. Blood. 2008;111:4902–7.

18. Nuver J, Smit AJ, van der Meer J, van den Berg MP, van der Graaf WT, Meinardi MT, et al. Acute chemotherapy-induced cardiovascular changes in patients with testicular cancer. J Clin Oncol. 2005;23:9130–7.

19. Jafri M, Protheroe A. Cisplatin-associated thrombosis. Anti-Cancer Drugs. 2008;19:927–9.

20. Lechner D, Kollars M, Gleiss A, Kyrle PA, Weltermann A. Chemotherapy-induced thrombin generation via procoagulant endothelial microparticles is independent of tissue factor activity. J Thromb Haemost. 2007;5:24452452.

21. Fotopoulou C, duBois A, Karavas AN, Trappe R, Aminossadati B, Schmalfeldt B, Pfisterer J, et al. Incidence of venous thromboembolism in patients with ovarian cancer undergoing platinum/paclitaxel containing first-line chemotherapy: an exploratory analysis by the Arbeitsgemeinschaft Gynaekologische Onkologie ovarian cancer study group. J Clin Oncol. 2008; 26:2683–9.

22. Dieckmann KP, Gerl A, Witt J, Hartmann JT, German Testicular Cancer Study Group. Myocardial infarction and other major vascular events during chemotherapy for testicular cancer. Ann Oncol. 2010;21(8):1607–11.

23. Cohen AT, Katholing A, Rietbrock S, Bamber L, Martinez C. Epidemiology of first and recurrent venous thromboembolism in patients with active cancer. A population-based cohort study. Thromb Haemost. 2017;117:57–65.

24. Khorana AA, Francis CW, Culakova E, Fisher RI, Kuderer NM, Lyman GH. Thromboembolism in hospitalized neutropenic cancer patients. J Clin Oncol. 2006;24:484–90.

25. Lyman GH, Bohlke K, Khorana AA, Kuderer NM, Lee AY, Arcelus JI, et al. Venous thromboembolism prophylaxis and treatment in patients with cancer: American Society of Clinical Oncology clinical practice guideline update 2014. J Clin Oncol. 2015;33(6):654–6.

26. NCCN guidelines (Cancer-associated venous thromboembolic disease). Available at: https://www.nccn.org/professionals/physician_gls/pdf/vte.pdf. Accessed on 02 April 2017.

27. Abdel-Razeq H, Albadainah F, Hijjawi S, Mansour A, Treish I. Venous Thromboembolism (VTE) in hospitalized cancer patients: prophylaxis failure or failure to Prophylax. J Thromb Thrombolysis. 2011;3:107–12.

28. Abdel-Razeq H, Mansour A, Saadeh SS, Abu-Nasser M, Makoseh M, Salam M, et al. The application of current proposed venous Thromboembolism risk assessment model for ambulatory patients with cancer. Clin Appl Thromb Hemost. 2017:1076029617692880. https://doi.org/10.1177/ 1076029617692880.

29. Barni S, Labianca R, Agnelli G, Bonizzoni E, Verso M, Mandalà M, et al. Chemotherapy-associated thromboembolic risk in cancer outpatients and effect of nadroparin thromboprophylaxis: results of a retrospective analysis of the PROTECHT study. J Transl Med. 2011;9:179.

30. Agnelli G, George DJ, Kakkar AK, Fisher W, Lassen MR, Mismetti P, et al. Semuloparin for thromboprophylaxis in patients receiving chemotherapy for cancer. N Engl J Med. 2012;366:601–9.

31. Maraveyas A, Waters J, Roy R, Fyfe D, Propper D, Lofts F, et al. Gemcitabine versus gemcitabine plus dalteparin thromboprophylaxis in pancreatic cancer. Eur J Cancer. 2012;48:1283–92.

32. Pelzer U, Opitz B, Deutschinoff G, Stauch M, Reitzig PC, Hahnfeld S, et al. Efficacy of prophylactic low-molecular weight heparin for ambulatory patients with advanced pancreatic cancer: outcomes from the CONKO-004 trial. J Clin Oncol. 2015;33:2028–34.

22

Awareness of venous thromboembolism and thromboprophylaxis among hospitalized patients

Hind Almodaimegh[1,2]* ⓘ, Lama Alfehaid[1], Nada Alsuhebany[1], Rami Bustami[1], Shmylan Alharbi[1,2], Abdulmalik Alkatheri[1,2] and Abdulkareem Albekairy[1,2]

Abstract

Background: Patient awareness of venous thromboembolism (VTE) and thromboprophylaxis is essential for their safety. In this study, we evaluated patients' awareness of VTE and their perceptions of thromboprophylaxis.

Methods: We administered a cross-sectional survey to patients hospitalized at the King Abdulaziz Medical City, Riyadh, Saudi Arabia.

Results: Of 190 patients approached, 174 completed the survey, constituting a response rate of 95%. Most participants (72%) were receiving thromboprophylaxis. However, only 32 and 15% reported knowledge of deep vein thrombosis (DVT) and pulmonary embolism (PE), respectively. Fifty-five percent of participants with knowledge of DVT identified swelling of the leg as a symptom. Risk factors for blood clot development were correctly identified by about half of participants, although most agreed that blood clots can cause death (77%). The level of awareness of DVT or PE did not significantly differ by respondents' demographics. However, awareness of DVT or PE was significantly higher among those with a personal or family history of VTE. Participants had positive perceptions of thromboprophylaxis and were satisfied with treatment (> 69%), but perceived its adverse effects less favorably and reported lower satisfaction with the information provided about DVT and PE (46%).

Conclusion: This study demonstrates the lack of awareness of VTE, DVT, and PE among hospitalized patients. More attention must be paid to patient education to ensure safe and high-quality patient care.

Keywords: Venous thromboembolism, Deep vein thrombosis, Pulmonary embolism, Patient awareness, Patient safety

Key points

This paper shows that there is a lack of awareness about thromboembolism among hospitalized patients that emphasizes the need for improved education in at-risk patients.

Background

Venous thromboembolism (VTE) is the inappropriate formation of a blood clot in a vein. It can affect hospitalized

and non-hospitalized patients, and is associated with considerable mortality, morbidity, and costs [1, 2]. VTE is preventable, but the condition is also unpredictable, with few warning signs. Studies have shown that about 60–70% of cases of deep vein thrombosis (DVT) are clinically undiagnosed and only detected during autopsy. Similarly, at least 70% of cases of fatal pulmonary embolism (PE) detected post-mortem are neither suspected nor diagnosed before death [3]. The incidence of VTE rises during hospitalization as a result of increases in predisposing factors; reportedly, approximately 78% of hospitalized patients have more than one risk factor for VTE, and around 20% of patients have at least three risk factors [4]. The standard approach for the prevention of VTE is

* Correspondence: modaimeghh@ksau-hs.edu.sa
[1]King Abdullah International Medical Research Center/King Saud Bin Abdulaziz University for Health Sciences, College of Pharmacy, Ministry of National Guard Health Affairs, PO BOX 22490, Riyadh 11426, Saudi Arabia
[2]Pharmaceutical Care Department, King Abdulaziz Medical City, King Abdullah International Medical Research Center/King Saud Bin Abdulaziz University for Health Sciences, PO BOX 22490, Riyadh 11426, Saudi Arabia

pharmacologic thromboprophylaxis with unfractionated heparin or low-molecular weight heparin [5].

National Institute for Health and Care Excellence guidelines state that all patients should receive verbal and written information on the risks and consequences of VTE and the potential adverse effects of thromboprophylaxis and risk-reduction strategies prior to starting thromboprophylactic treatment [6]. Increased patient awareness of VTE and thromboprophylaxis may promote patient safety by facilitating active participation in recommended activities such as early ambulation and calf-pumping exercises. Reportedly, patient refusal is the most common reason for missed doses of thromboprophylactic treatment [7]. Therefore, patient education prior to the start of treatment may improve adherence, especially when patients understand the purpose of their medication. In addition, it has been shown that education on the potential adverse effects of thromboprophylactic treatment is not necessarily associated with its refusal by patients [8]. Rather, it may increase patient recognition of serious adverse effects and promote fast reporting. Moreover, knowledge of the signs and symptoms of VTE helps patients to assess and report them during hospital admission and after discharge to obtain timely medical help, especially in those at high risk of VTE recurrence.

Although, a number of general reports have focused on the importance of preventing VTE [9–11], few studies have assessed patients' awareness of VTE and their satisfaction with thromboprophylactic treatment, particularly in Arabic-speaking countries. Therefore, in this cross-sectional study, we evaluated patients' awareness of VTE, perceptions of thromboprophylaxis, and satisfaction with the information provided on VTE and thromboprophylactic treatment.

Methods

Study design

In this cross-sectional study, we distributed a survey to adult patients hospitalized in medical wards at the King Abdulaziz Medical City (KAMC), Riyadh, Saudi Arabia, between December 2015 and March 2016. The KAMC is a 1200-bed tertiary care academic hospital accredited by the Joint Commission International. Patients were selected by convenience sampling, and were included in the study if they had received thromboprophylaxis (5000 units of heparin subcutaneously (SC) q8–12 h, 7500 units of heparin SC q12 h, or 30–40 mg of enoxaparin SC once daily). Patients were excluded if they were critically ill, admitted to the emergency department, receiving ambulatory care, or cognitively impaired. The average number of adult patients receiving thromboprophylaxis during the study period was 350. With a confidence level of 95%, margin of error of 5%, and response distribution of 50%, the minimum recommended sample size for this study was 184 according to the software Sample Size Calculator (Raosoft, Inc., Seattle, WA, USA). Patients were approached on the third day of admission to allow adequate exposure to any kind of education on VTE or thromboprophylaxis. Eligible patients were provided with a description of the study and its objectives, and were then asked to participate. Those who agreed to participate were interviewed by one of the researchers to ensure that all survey items were clear and comprehensive.

Survey instrument

The survey was developed by combining two previously validated surveys [12, 13], and the questions were selected based on the study objectives. The survey was translated into Arabic and validated in a pilot study involving 43 Arabic-speaking participants. Analysis was also performed to assess the reliability of the combined survey.

The survey consisted of 18 closed-ended questions intended to discern:

1. demographic information including age, sex, level of education, and reason for admission;
2. personal or family history of VTE and thromboprophylaxis;
3. awareness of DVT and PE, including their underlying causes, risk factors, symptoms, and prevention;
4. perceptions of pharmacologic thromboprophylaxis and information received on VTE; and
5. satisfaction with thromboprophylactic treatment and related information received.

Responses to some of the survey items measuring awareness, perception, and satisfaction used a five-point Likert scale ranging from *strongly disagree* to *strongly agree*.

The content validity of the translated combined version of the survey was established by two expert individuals who examined the appropriateness of the content after making necessary modifications to items to ensure that they were sufficiently comprehensive and accurately assessed awareness of VTE and perceptions of thromboprophylaxis. In addition, the reliability of the survey was examined using Cronbach's alpha (α), a measure of internal consistency that indicates how closely related the set of items are as a group.

The completed questionnaires were collected and safely stored in the principal investigator's office. Data were saved into an appropriately designed Excel® spreadsheet (Microsoft Corp., Redmond, WA, USA).

Data were processed in accordance with the best practices for raw data management to identify any inaccuracies or omissions prior to statistical analysis. To accomplish this task, all interval variables were checked and summarized in terms of minimum and maximum values. These values were checked and compared against the possible minimum and maximum values of each variable, and variables with implausible values were flagged. A similar process was applied to categoric variables to identify any potential anomalies using a general frequency analysis.

Statistical analysis

Descriptive statistics including the number and percentage of respondents by demographic characteristics and personal and family history of DVT and PE were calculated. Percentage awareness of correct and incorrect signs and symptoms of DVT and PE were computed. Percentage positive perception and satisfaction (indicated by a response of *agree/strongly agree*) were also calculated. Awareness of DVT and PE were compared by a number of characteristics including age, sex, level of education, and personal and family history of VTE using the chi-squared test. Statistical significance was set at $p < 0.05$. All statistical analyses were performed using SPSS (Release 21.0.0.0; IBM Corp., Armonk, NY, USA).

Results

Out of 190 patients have been screened, 174 participants completed the questionnaire, constituting a response rate of 95%. Descriptive statistics for the respondents are displayed in Table 1. Fifty-six percent of respondents were aged over 50 years, and 52% were male. Most respondents had an educational level of high school or lower (77%). Sixty-three percent of respondents were admitted for medical treatment. Only 14 and 12% of respondents had personal or family histories of VTE, respectively. Most respondents (72%) were aware that they were receiving pharmacologic/non-pharmacologic thromboprophylaxis at the time of questionnaire completion, whereas only 31% reported a history of thromboprophylactic treatment.

As shown in Table 2, only 32 and 15% of participants reported knowledge of DVT and PE, respectively. Of the respondents aware of DVT, 55% (30/55) identified swelling of the leg as a symptom. Other correct symptoms, including pain/tenderness in the leg, noticeable changes in the color of the leg, and noticeable changes in the temperature of the leg, were selected by 49% (27/55), 29% (16/55), and 18% (10/55), respectively. Incorrect signs and symptoms of DVT, including leg paralysis, itching of the leg, and others, were selected by 36, 20, and 15% of respondents, respectively. Relatively higher accuracy levels were observed in response to questions

Table 1 Profile of participants ($N = 174$)

Factor	Number	Percent
Age Category (years)		
18–30	32	18.4%
31–50	45	25.9%
51–70	66	37.9%
71+	31	17.8%
Gender		
Male	90	51.7%
Female	84	48.3%
Education Level		
Uneducated	65	37.4%
Less than high school	42	24.1%
High school	27	15.5%
University	32	18.4%
Higher education	8	4.6%
Reason for Admission		
Surgical	60	34.5%
Medical treatment	110	63.2%
Oncology (nonsurgical)	3	1.7%
Palliative care	1	0.6%
Personal History of VTE		
Yes	25	14.4%
No	143	82.2%
Unknown	6	3.4%
Family History of VTE		
Yes	21	12.1%
No	141	81.0%
Unknown	12	6.9%
Currently Receiving Pharmacological/non-Pharmacological Thromboprophylaxis		
Yes	126	72.4%
No	36	20.7%
Unknown	12	6.9%
History of Receiving Pharmacological/non-Pharmacological Thromboprophylaxis		
Yes	54	31.0%
No	111	63.8%
Unknown	9	5.2%

reflecting patient awareness of the signs and symptoms of PE, where correct answers including chest pain, shortness of breath, lightheadedness, and coughing up blood were selected by 69% (18/26), 69% (18/26), 23% (6/26), and 23% (6/26) of respondents, respectively.

Sixty-eight percent of respondents correctly identified "not moving for a long time" as a risk factor for developing a blood clot. However, other risk factors including

Table 2 Awareness of VTE

Item	Options	No. of responses	Percent
Which of the following cause DVT?	Blood clot in vein[b]	82	47.1%
	Lack of oxygen in vein	5	2.9%
	A tumor in vein	7	4.0%
	None of the above	4	2.3%
	Not sure	76	43.7%
Know what a blood clot in your leg is or DVT?	Yes	55	31.6%
	No	119	68.4%
Which of following are signs/symptoms of DVT?[a, c]			
	Swelling of leg[b]	30	54.5%
	Itching of leg	11	20.0%
	Pain/tenderness in leg[b]	27	49.0%
	Noticeable changes in color of leg[b]	16	29.0%
	The leg feels warm[b]	10	18.1%
	Leg paralysis	20	36.3%
	Other	8	14.5%
	Not sure	2	3.6%
Know what a blood clot in your lung or PE?	Yes	26	14.9%
	No	148	85.1%
Which of following are signs/symptoms of PE?[a, d]			
	Shortness of breath[b]	18	69.2%
	Slow, shallow breathing	5	19.2%
	Chest pain (may be worse with deep breath)[b]	18	69.2%
	Rapid heart rate	7	26.9%
	Lightheadedness/passing out[b]	6	23.0%
	Pain radiating down arm	5	19.2%
	You cough up blood[b]	6	23.0%
	You have frequent headaches	4	15.4%
	Other	3	11.4%
	None of the above	1	3.8%
Which of the following might increase your risk of developing a blood clot?[a]			
	A hospital stay[b]	49	28.2%
	Surgery[b]	67	38.5%
	Cancer[b]	47	27.0%
	Not moving a long time[b]	119	68.4%
	Pregnancy/giving birth[b]	40	23.0%
	Using estrogen-based meds[b]	14	8.0%
	Family history of blood clots[b]	59	33.9%
	Older age (65+)[b]	72	41.4%
	Too much exercise	6	3.4%
	High blood cholesterol[b]	92	52.9%
	Donating blood	8	4.6%
	High blood pressure[b]	83	47.7%
	Other	24	14.1%

Table 2 Awareness of VTE *(Continued)*

	None of the above	2	1.1%
	Not sure	41	23.6%
Which of following help prevent a blood clot?[a, e]	Walking/stretching legs[b]	76	92.7%
	Drinking plenty of fluids	37	45.1%
	Eating lots of fiber	41	50.0%
	Bed rest	11	13.4%
	Washing/bathing regularly	27	32.9%
	Don't know	11	13.4%
	Other	9	5.2%

$N = 174$
[a]More than one response allowed
[b]Indicates correct response
[c]$N = 52$
[d]$N = 26$
[e]$N = 82$

hypocholesteremia and hypertension were correctly identified by about half of the respondents. Fewer respondents correctly selected other risk factors such as advanced age (41%), family history of blood clots (34%), and pregnancy/childbirth (23%). Most respondents were aware of the benefits of walking or stretching the legs for the prevention of blood clots (93%). However, a relatively high percentage of activities like drinking fluids (45%), eating lots of fiber (50%), and washing/bathing regularly (33%) were incorrectly identified as measures that may prevent blood clots.

The results for patient awareness as measured using a Likert scale (Fig. 1) showed that most respondents agreed that blood clots can cause death (77%), whereas just over half of them were aware that blood clots can develop at any age (56%), and are considered a medical emergency (57%). Only 42% of respondents thought that most blood clots can be prevented, and only 37% knew that they can travel to the lungs.

Figure 2 shows that respondents generally had a positive perception of thromboprophylaxis: about 70% reported that they considered the treatment beneficial and safe and were in favor of receiving it. However, less than half reported that the adverse effects of the treatment were tolerable. Most respondents were satisfied with the time they received the treatment (78%), but only 56 and 46% were satisfied with the information they received about the treatment and about DVT/PE, respectively.

The results of analyses of respondents' awareness of DVT or PE by age, sex, level of education, and personal and family history of VTE are shown in Table 3. The percentage of respondents reporting awareness of DVT or PE was significantly higher among those with a personal or family history of VTE: 68% versus 32%, $p = 0.001$, and 57% versus 35%, $p = 0.046$, respectively. Awareness of DVT was not associated with any of the other factors listed in the table.

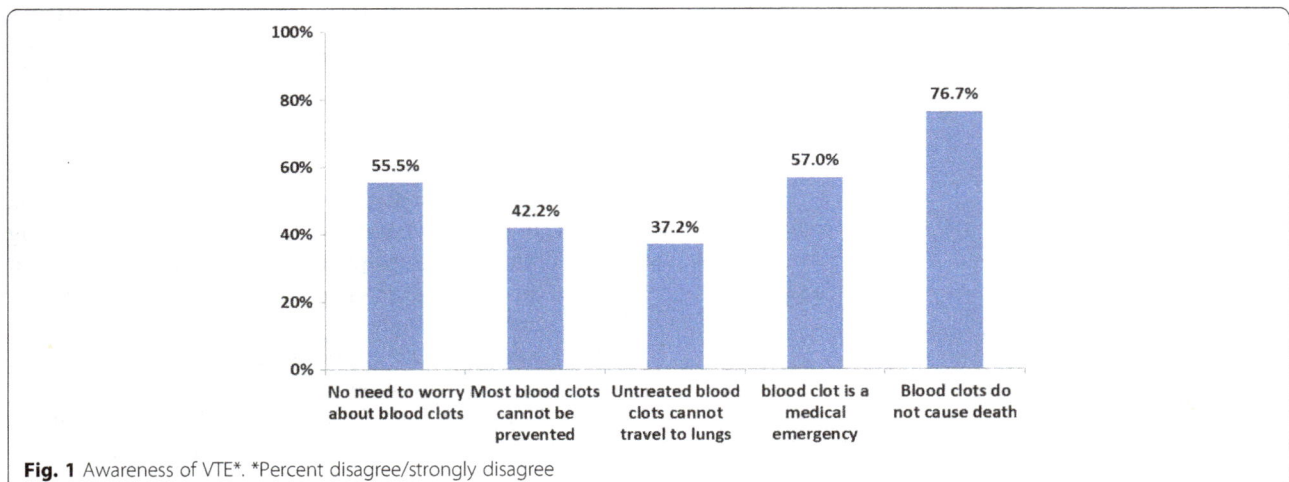

Fig. 1 Awareness of VTE*. *Percent disagree/strongly disagree

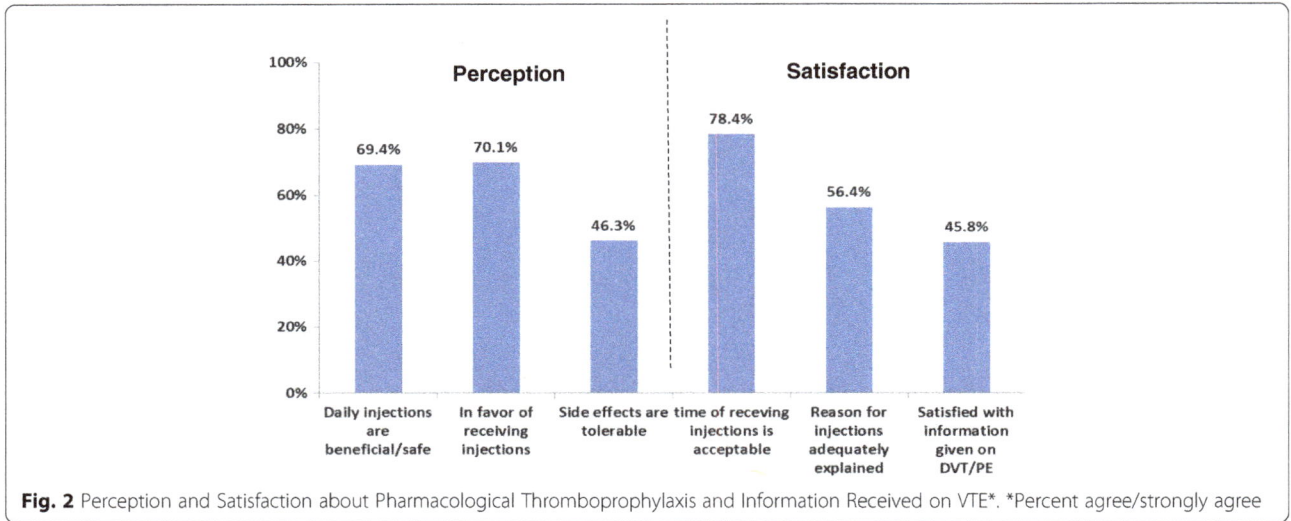

Fig. 2 Perception and Satisfaction about Pharmacological Thromboprophylaxis and Information Received on VTE*. *Percent agree/strongly agree

Discussion

The findings of our study indicate poor awareness of DVT and PE among hospitalized patients (32 and 15%, respectively). Correspondingly, they demonstrate the lack of awareness of the signs and symptoms of DVT and PE. This is consistent with the results of previous studies. A national survey conducted in the United States found that 74% of adults had a poor knowledge of DVT and its complications [14]. The lack of awareness of VTE is a common problem worldwide that is not limited to distinct patient nationalities or populations. Studies involving pregnant women, postnatal women,

and cancer patients have reached similar conclusions [15–18].

Our study also shows that more than half of respondents were unaware of the causes of DVT and that 63% do not believe that blood clots can travel to the lungs. Such findings indicate that the consequences of blood clots and the link between DVT and PE are underestimated. The lower awareness of PE compared with that of DVT may explained by the pathophysiologic nature of PE; it is a life-threatening condition considered a complication of DVT, and it is often termed the "silent killer" because of the nonspecificity of its symptoms [19]. This has also been documented in other reports [12, 13].

Most participants who correctly identified risk factors for VTE recognized immobility as a key risk factor for DVT and PE development. This result may reflect the efforts of health-care providers to encourage hospitalized patients to ambulate. However, these efforts may result in insufficient patient education on the risks associated with other health conditions, as conveyed by reports on nurses' experiences of the implementation of VTE prophylaxis [20]. A recent study on awareness of VTE during preoperative assessments reported that only 47% of patients had received verbal or written information on the condition, and that although many patients were aware of VTE, detailed information regarding its risk factors and prophylaxis was lacking [16]. This finding suggests the need to provide patients with more detailed information on VTE to ensure a better understanding of its risks and prevention.

Approximately half of patients incorrectly identified risk factors such emotional and psychologic trauma, exposure to cold air, or fever. Similarly, they were unaware of important risk factors such as cancer, which corroborates the findings of other studies in which awareness of

Table 3 Number and percentage of respondents reporting awareness of DVT or PE by respondents' characteristics

	N	Number aware	Percent	p-value[a]
All Respondents	174	65	37.4%	
Age Category (years)				0.18
18–50	77	33	42.9%	
51–70	97	32	33.0%	
Gender				0.61
Male	90	32	35.6%	
Female	84	33	39.3%	
Education Level				0.26
High school or below	134	47	35.1%	
University/Higher education	40	18	45.0%	
Personal History of VTE				0.001
Yes	25	17	68.0%	
No	149	48	32.2%	
Family History of VTE				0.046
Yes	21	12	57.1%	
No	153	53	34.6%	

[a]Based on the Chi-square test

cancer as a risk factor for VTE was poor among oncology patients [21, 22]. This information is crucial, because it helps patients to understand the rationale for thromboprophylaxis during cancer treatment; thus, cancer patients should receive more information. Our results also show that there is misperception of the signs and symptoms of DVT, as indicated by the confusion of DVT with other conditions such acute coronary syndrome (ACS). This was also noticed by interviewers when asking patients about VTE terms, and may be related to the similarity between the Arabic words for VTE and ACS. When comparing the participants in terms of the level of DVT or PE awareness, we found that demographic characteristics (age, sex, and educational level) had no impact. In contrast, awareness of DVT or PE was significantly higher among those with a personal or family history of VTE.

In this study, about 20% of respondents were unaware that they were receiving pharmacologic thromboprophylaxis, which may reflect the failure of health-care providers to provide patients with counseling in regard to their treatment during hospitalization. This may be related to respondents' poor satisfaction regarding the information they received about pharmacologic thromboprophylaxis and its adverse effects. Most respondents, however, had a positive perception of pharmacologic thromboprophylaxis, and the majority agreed that the treatment was beneficial to their health and that they were in favor of receiving it.

Better education on VTE, DVT, and PE terms, risk factors, and preventive measures is needed to encourage active involvement by patients in treatment plans, ensure their adherence particularly after hospital discharge, and promote self-diagnosis and reporting of VTE symptoms. This effort should also be extended to the general public, because we observed that level of education was unrelated to DVT awareness. Educational campaigns can be beneficial and have proven effective in increasing public awareness of VTE [17].

Our study has a number of limitations. First, its small sample size limits our ability to generalize the study results beyond our institution. The total number of participants is smaller than the calculated sample size, as some patients were not available at time of patient screening. Nevertheless, our findings were consistent with those from a number of studies, including a study utilizing a global survey administered to the general public in nine countries: Argentina, Australia, Canada, Germany, Japan, Thailand, the Netherlands, the United Kingdom, and the United States [12–16]. Secondly, closed-ended survey questions may have helped respondents to guess rather than answer with regard to their knowledge, particularly in response to questions where more than one answer was allowed (the average number of answers per question ranged from four to eight). To minimize guessing, the interviewers attempted to ask the survey questions in an open-ended manner, to allow enough time for the participants to think before providing their answer.

Conclusion

This study clearly demonstrates that awareness of VTE in general, and of DVT and PE terms—in particular, the risk factors, signs, and symptoms—among hospitalized patients is inadequate. More emphasis should be placed on the education of at-risk patients to promote adherence to treatment, self-diagnosis, recording of DVT and PE symptoms, and active involvement in safety. This study sets the stage for further research to determine the optimal approach to the education of hospitalized patients to promote safe and high-quality patient care. The findings of this study may also encourage health-care providers to deliver more education to patients and public health organizations about VTE, DVT, and PE, and their risk factors, signs and symptoms and preventive measures.

Abbreviations
ACS: Acute coronary syndrome; DVT: Deep vein thrombosis; PE: Pulmonary embolism; SC: Subcutaneously; VTE: Venous thromboembolism

Acknowledgments
We would like to show our appreciation to Alaa Elanazi, B.Sc.Pharm. and Nouf Alotaibi, B.Sc.Pharm. (postgraduate year 2 pharmacy residents at KAMC) for their valuable help with patient interviewing during data collection.

Funding
This study is not funded by any individual or institution.

Authors' contributions
Contributions: HA, LA, and NA conceived and designed the study; LA, SA, AA, AB, and NA collected and assembled the data; RB and SA analyzed and interpreted the data; and all authors wrote and provided final approval of the manuscript.

Competing interests
The authors declare that they have no competing interests.

References
1. Cohen A, Agnelli G, Anderson F, et al. Venous thromboembolism in Europe. The number of VTE events and associated morbidity and mortality. Thromb Haemost. 2007;98(4):756–64.
2. MacDougall D, Feliu A, Boccuzzi S, Lin J. Economic burden of deep-vein thrombosis, pulmonary embolism, and postthrombotic syndrome. Am J Health Syst Pharm. 2006;63:5–15.
3. Goldhaber SZ, Hennekens CH, Evans DA, Newton EC, Godleski JJ. Factors associated with correct antemortem diagnosis of major pulmonary embolism. Am J Med. 1982;73:822–6.
4. Anderson F. The prevalence of risk factors for venous thromboembolism among hospital patients. Arch Intern Med. 1992;152(8):1660.
5. Spencer F. Venous Thromboembolism in the outpatient setting. Arch Intern Med. 2007;167(14):1471–5.
6. Hill J, Treasure T. Reducing the risk of venous thromboembolism (deep vein thrombosis and pulmonary embolism) in patients admitted to hospital: summary of the NICE guideline. Heart. 2010;96(11):879–82.

7. Hodgson LJ, Emed JD. Exploring nurses' experience with the implementation of the venous thromboembolism prophylaxis protocol. Unpublished master's thesis. Montreal: McGill University; 2007.

8. Lubenow N, Hinz P, Ekkernkamp A, Greinacher A. Should patients be informed about the risk of heparin-induced thrombocytopenia before prolonged low-molecular-weight heparin thromboprophylaxis post-trauma/orthopedic surgery? Eur J Haematol. 2007;79(3):187–90.

9. Arnold DM, Kahn SR, Shrier I. Missed opportunities for prevention of venous thromboembolism: an evaluation of the use of thromboprophylaxis guidelines. Chest. 2001;120:1964–71.

10. Geerts WH, Pineo GF, Heit JA, et al. Prevention of venous thromboembolism: the seventh ACCP conference on antithrombotic and thrombolytic therapy. Chest. 2004;126(3 Suppl):338S–400S.

11. Morrison R. Venous thromboembolism: scope of the problem and the nurse's role in risk assessment and prevention. J Vasc Nurs. 2006;24:82–90.

12. Wendelboe A, McCumber M, Hylek E, Buller H, Weitz J, Raskob G. Global public awareness of venous thromboembolism. J Thromb Haemost. 2015; 13(8):1365–71.

13. Le Sage S, McGee M, Emed JD. Knowledge of venous thromboembolism (VTE) prevention among hospitalized patients. J Vasc Nurs. 2008;26(4):109–17.

14. American Public Health Association. Deep vein thrombosis: advancing awareness to protect patient lives. White paper. Washington, DC: Public Health Leadership Conference; 2003.

15. Kingman C, Economides D. Travel in pregnancy: pregnant women's experiences and knowledge of health issues. J Travel Med. 2003;10:330–3.

16. Reynolds S. Deep vein thrombosis: are postnatal women aware? Br J Midwifery. 2004;12:636–40.

17. Noble S. Acceptability of low molecular weight heparin thromboprophylaxis for inpatients receiving palliative care: qualitative study. BMJ. 2006; 332(7541):577–80.

18. Sousou TKhorana A. Cancer patients and awareness of venous thromboembolism. Cancer Investig. 2009;28(1):44–5.

19. Thrombosis, Vein. "Case management adherence guidelines version 1.0 deep vein thrombosis (DVT) Guidelines from the Case Management Society of America for improving patient adherence to DVT medication therapies." 2008.

20. Haymes A. Venous thromboembolism: patient awareness and education in the pre-operative assessment clinic. J Thromb Thrombolysis. 2015;41(3):459–63.

21. Aggarwal A, Fullam L, Brownstein A, et al. Deep vein thrombosis (DVT) and pulmonary embolism (PE): awareness and prophylaxis practices reported by patients with cancer. Cancer Investig. 2015;33(9):405–10.

22. Baglin T, Luddington R, Brown K, Baglin C. Incidence of recurrent venous thromboembolism in relation to clinical and thrombophilic risk factors: prospective cohort study. Lancet. 2003;362(9383):523–6.

23

TTP-like syndrome: novel concept and molecular pathogenesis of endotheliopathy-associated vascular microthrombotic disease

Jae C. Chang🆔

Abstract

TTP is characterized by microangiopathic hemolytic anemia and thrombocytopenia associated with brain and kidney dysfunction. It occurs due to ADAMTS13 deficiency. TTP-like syndrome occurs in critically ill patients with the similar hematologic changes and additional organ dysfunction syndromes. Vascular microthrombotic disease (VMTD) includes both TTP and TTP-like syndrome because their underlying pathology is the same disseminated intravascular microthrombosis (DIT). Microthrombi are composed of platelet-unusually large von Willebrand factor multimers (ULVWF) complexes. TTP occurs as a result of accumulation of circulating ULVWF secondary to ADAMTS13 deficiency. This protease deficiency triggers microthrombogenesis, leading to "microthrombi" formation in microcirculation. Unlike TTP, TTP-like syndrome occurs in critical illnesses due to complement activation. Terminal C5b-9 complex causes channel formation to endothelial membrane, leading to endotheliopathy, which activates two different molecular pathways (i.e., inflammatory and microthrombotic). Activation of inflammatory pathway triggers inflammation. Activation of microthrombotic pathway promotes platelet activation and excessive endothelial exocytosis of ULVWF from endothelial cells (ECs). Overexpressed and uncleaved ULVWF become anchored to ECs as long elongated strings to recruit activated platelets, and assemble "microthrombi". In TTP, circulating microthrombi typically be lodged in microvasculature of the brain and kidney, but in TTP-like syndrome, microthrombi anchored to ECs of organs such as the lungs and liver as well as the brain and kidneys, leading to multiorgan dysfunction syndrome. TTP occurs as hereditary or autoimmune disease and is the phenotype of ADAMTS13 deficiency-associated VMTD. But TTP-like syndrome is hemostatic disorder occurring in critical illnesses and is the phenotype of endotheliopathy-associated VMTD. Thus, this author's contention is TTP and TTP-like syndrome are two distinctly different disorders with dissimilar underlying pathology and pathogenesis.

Keywords: ADAMTS13, Complement, Disseminated intravascular coagulation (DIC) , Disseminated intravascular microthrombosis (DIT), Endotheliopathy, Microthrombogenesis, Thrombotic thrombocytopenic purpura (TTP), TTP-like syndrome, Unusually large von Willbrand factor multimers (ULVWF), Vascular microthrombotic disease (VMTD)

Correspondence: jaec@uci.edu
Department of Medicine, University of California Irvine School of Medicine, Irvine, CA, USA

Background

The new term vascular microthrombotic disease (VMTD) has been used [1–3], but has not been designated as a disease entity yet. Both microvascular thrombosis and vascular microthrombosis have been used interchangeably to describe the similar pathological conditions. Disseminated VMTD represents both TTP and TTP-like syndrome, but the identity of TTP-like syndrome has not been clearly defined to date.

TTP is characterized by microvascular thrombosis associated with markedly decreased ADAMTS13 activity due to mutation of ADAMTS13 gene (hereditary) or due to antibody against ADAMTS13 (acquired). Hematologic phenotype is consumptive thrombocytopenia and microangiopathic hemolytic anemia (MAHA) as a result of disseminated intravascular microthrombosis (DIT) [2, 4]. Organ involvement occurs typically in the brain and kidneys. DIT is the pathological condition caused by vascular "microthrombi", which are exclusively composed of the complexes of platelet and unusually large von Willbrand factor multimers (ULVWF) in various organs [4–6]. In 1924, Eli Moschcowitz first recognized a thrombotic blood disorder characterized by disseminated hyaline microthrombi in terminal arterioles and capillaries of organs in a young woman who died at the Beth Israel Hospital in New York City [7]. Later, Singer et al. named this disorder thrombotic thrombocytopenic purpura (TTP) [8].

Other focal, multifocal or localized microvascular thrombosis also exists without proper name designation. Appropriate medical term could be focal, multifocal or localized VMTD. These may include ischemic stroke syndrome (e.g., transient ischemic attack) [9, 10] and myocardial ischemia (e.g., angina) [10]. Also, focal endotheliopathy in HERNS disease and Susac syndrome as well as localized endotheliopathy in Kasabach-Merritt syndrome are suspected to be due to microthrombosis in smaller or larger vasculatures. These syndromes cannot be designated as TTP because their involvement in the organs is not generalized and is usually not associated with thrombocytopenia and MAHA.

More recently, TTP-like syndrome has been frequently reported. It is also characterized by vascular microthrombosis with thrombocytopenia and MAHA, but commonly atypical organ dysfunction syndromes such as acute respiratory distress syndrome (ARDS), rhabdomyolysis, acute fulminating hepatic failure, and pancreatitis have occurred. These syndromes are also characterized by DIT [1–3]. Therefore, to properly classify TTP-like syndrome in the category of VMTD, there is a need for differentiating between TTP and acquired TTP-like syndrome and identifying the pathogenesis of TTP-like syndrome since it is not associated with ADAMTS13 antibody.

TTP-like syndrome

TTP typically involves the brain and kidneys, but TTP-like syndrome prominently develops in one or more of vital organs [11–14], including the liver [15, 16], heart [17, 18], lungs [11–13, 19, 20], pancreas [21] and others with or without involvement of the brain and kidneys. Oftentimes fewer schistocytes are present on the blood film and intravascular hemolysis could have easily missed [11, 13]. Since MAHA is not overt because of fewer schistocytes, the diagnosis of TTP-like syndrome could have been masked even though thrombocytopenia was present [2]. Because of less prominent nature of schistocytes, it has been termed atypical MAHA (aMAHA) [1, 2]. The most notable observation of TTP-like syndrome is its frequent occurrence in critical illnesses such as infection, sepsis, trauma, cancer, autoimmune disease, malignant hypertension, drug and toxin, envenomation, and complications of pregnancy, surgery and transplant (Table 1).

In the early 1980s, Moake et al. made a very important discovery that ULVWF contributed to the pathogenesis of TTP [22]. Furlan et al. [23] and Tsai [24] independently published the presence of VWF-cleaving protease, and subsequently the deficient role of this protease ADAMTS13 due to anti-ADAMTS13 antibody was established.

Prior to the role of autoantibody was recognized, clinicians accepted the use of the term TTP whenever a patient presented with the dyad of thrombocytopenia and MAHA, even though obvious organ dysfunction was not present yet [12]. This dyadic feature was considered to be sufficient criteria to make the diagnosis of TTP for the purpose of initiating urgent therapeutic plasma exchange (TPE) to save lives [11–13]. The generic term TTP, encompassing both TTP and TTP-like syndrome, has served well for the patient by allowing TPE when presented with thrombocytopenia and MAHA/aMAHA even though organ dysfunction is not developed yet. TPE has been very effective and life-saving measure in both disorders when it was employed in the earliest possible time [2, 11–13, 20].

Because of common occurrence of TTP with acute renal failure/hemolytic-uremic syndrome (HUS) in clinical medicine, the combined term TTP-HUS also has been in use to include both TTP and TTP-like syndrome to date [25] even though the pathogenesis and clinical features of HUS are clearly different from TTP [3]. In retrospect, this combined term might have contributed to the masking of TTP-like syndrome and VMTD when organ dysfunction developed in other than the brain and kidneys. It also has delayed identifying the multifaceted pathogenesis of TTP-like syndromes. In addition, this terminology could have kept disseminated intravascular coagulation ("DIC") as a different disease from TTP-like

Table 1 Genesis and characteristics of VMTD in TTP and TTP-like syndrome

	Hereditary TTP (GA-VMTD) Acquired TTP (AA-VMTD)	TTP-like syndrome (EA-VMTD)
Primary causes/events	Hereditary ADAMTS13 gene mutation Acquired ADAMTS13 antibody formation ↓	Pathogen (e.g., viruses; bacteria; fungi; rickettsia; parasites) Polytrauma (e.g., chest/lung; bone; skull/brain injury) Pregnancy (e.g., preeclampsia; abruptio placenta; amniotic fluid embolism) Cancer (e.g., disseminated stomach/breast/lung cancer) Transplant (e.g., liver; kidney; bone marrow) Drug and toxin (e.g., cyclosporine; mitomycin C; Shiga toxin) ↓
Secondary event	Excessive circulating mULVWF ↓	Complement activation (C5b-9) and endothelial injury → endotheliopathy ↓
Tertiary event	Microthrombogenesis → platelet-ULVWF complexes ↓ Microthrombi lodged in arteriolar and capillary lumens ↓	Cytokine release → inflammation → SIRS Platelet activation and endothelial exocytosis of eULVWF ↓ Microthrombogenesis → platelet-ULVWF complex strings ↓
Final event	Microvascular microthrombosis ↓ DIT/VMTD ↓ TTP	Vascular microthrombosis ↓ DIT/VMTD ↓ TTP-like syndrome
Hematologic features		
Platelet	Consumptive thrombocytopenia	Consumptive thrombocytopenia
Red blood cell	MAHA	MAHA/aMAHA
Clinical syndromes		
Inflammation	Uncommon	Very common
Cytokine storm	Absent	Often present in sepsis and MODS
SIRS	Absent	Often present in sepsis and MODS
Encephalopathy	Very common	Common, especially in HUS
ARDS	Probably absent	Common
AFHF	Probably absent	Common, sometimes with hepatic coagulopathy
ARF/HUS	Very common	Common
"DIC" (see text)	Doesn't occur	Identical to TTP-like syndrome
Laboratory features		
ADAMTS13 activity	Markedly decreased (< 5% of normal)	Mild to moderately decreased (20–70% of normal)
ADAMTS13 antibody	Positive in acquired TTP	Negative
Haptoglobin	Markedly decreased	Markedly decreased
Schistocytes	++ to ++++	None to +++
Therapeutic response to		
TPE	Very good response	Excellent and fast response if treated in early stage
Platelet transfusion	Contraindicated	Contraindicated
rADAMTS13	Unknown; expected to be effective in GA-VMTD	Unknown; expected to be very effective

AFHF acute fulminant hepatic failure, *ARF/HUS* acute renal failure/hemolytic uremic syndrome, *ARDS* acute respiratory distress syndrome, *"DIC"* disseminated intravascular coagulation of McKay, *ECs*, endothelial cells, *eULVWF/mULVWF* endothelial unusually large von Willebrand factor/megakaryocytic ULVWF, *LDH* lactate dehydrogenase, *MAHA/aMAHA* microangiopathic hemolytic anemia/atypical MAHA, *rADAMTS13* recombinant ADAMTS13, *SIRS*, systemic inflammatory response syndrome, *TMA* thrombotic microangiopathy *TPE*, therapeutic plasma exchange; *TTP*, thrombotic thrombocytopenic purpura, *VMTD* vascular microthrombotic disease

syndrome [26]. Quotation marks have been placed on "DIC" to note that it is different from true DIC, which causes fibrin clots composed of fibrin meshes that is seen in acute promyelocytic leukemia (APL).

Hematologists have been puzzled when encountered acquired TTP-like syndrome with negative ADAMTS13 antibody and phenotype of thrombocytopenia and MAHA. This syndrome has occurred with atypical organ phenotypes. Such syndromes include the hemolysis, elevated liver enzymes and low platelet (HELLP) syndrome [16], acute respiratory distress syndrome (ARDS) [2, 13, 19, 20], HUS [3, 27, 28], acute myocardial infraction [17, 29, 30], acute pancreatitis [21, 31, 32], rhabdomyolysis [33, 34], encephalopathy [35, 36], viral hemorrhagic fevers [1, 37–40] and many others [2, 12–14].

TTP vs. TTP-like syndrome

TTP and TTP-like syndrome are characterized by hematologic phenotypes of VMTD presenting with consumptive thrombocytopenia and MAHA. TTP occurs in two conditions: one is gene mutation-associated VMTD (GA-VMTD) and the other is antibody-associated VMTD (AA-VMTD). GA-VMTD, known as Upshaw-Schulman syndrome, is the result of homozygous or compound heterozygous mutations of ADAMTS13 gene. However, AA-VMTD is autoimmune disease resulting from ADAMTS13 antibody.

In contrast, TTP-like syndrome develops due to endotheliopathy-associated VMTD (EA-VMTD) in critical illnesses such as sepsis and trauma [2, 16, 40–43] as illustrated in Table 1. The pathologic nature of microthrombi, which are composed of platelet and ULVWF complexes, are the same in both TTP and TTP-like syndrome [2–6]. However, the pathophysiological mechanism forming microthrombi appears to be different, and in TTP, their physical configuration in vivo is not clearly defined at this time. In TTP-like syndrome, the organ localization of microthrombi is distinctly different among different organs and within the same organ; perhaps it is due to endothelial heterogeneity and organotropism [3]. To annotate the clinical and organ dysfunction syndromes, occurring as a result of endotheliopathy in critical illnesses, a novel "two-activation theory of the endothelium" has been proposed [1, 2, 26].

Pathogenesis of TTP-like syndrome
Thrombocytopenia in critically ill patients (TCIP)

The earliest suspicion of TTP-like syndrome should come from unexplained thrombocytopenia in the critically ill patient. After exclusion of known causes of thrombocytopenia such as heparin-induced, drug or transfusion-related, consumptive coagulopathy-associated and hypersplenism-caused thrombocytopenia, and others [2], the term TCIP has been used to identify etiology-undetermined thrombocytopenia in critically ill patients. It is particularly well known in infectious diseases, including bacterial, viral, rickettsial, fungal and parasitic sepsis, are associated with TCIP [37–41, 44, 45]. It also occurs in non-infectious illnesses (e.g., severe trauma, cancer, complications of surgery, pregnancy and transplant, and immunologic and collagen vascular diseases) [2, 13, 42, 43, 46, 47].

Recently, significant correlation has been noted between the degree of thrombocytopenia, and severity and outcome of critical illnesses [48, 49]. Severer thrombocytopenia has been associated with systemic inflammatory response syndrome (SIRS) and multiorgan dysfunction syndrome (MODS) [50, 51]. These observations support TCIP is a key participant in the pathogenesis of critical illnesses, leading to VMTD. Now it is clear that TCIP is consumptive thrombocytopenia in the process of DIT in critically ill patients [1–3].

Role of complement activation on the endothelium

The activation of complement system is one of the pivotal events in innate immune defense mechanism of the host against pathogen. Its protective function for the host is to detect and eliminate invading microorganisms. Opsonization of foreign surfaces by covalently attached C3b fulfills three major functions: cell clearance by phagocytosis; amplification of complement activation by the formation of surface-bound C3 convertase; and assembly of C5 convertases [51]. Following activation of complement system through one of three pathways (classical, alternative, and lectin), cleavage of C5 induces the formation of multi-protein pore complex (C5b-9) (i.e., membrane-attack complex [MAC]), which leads to cell lysis.

However, despite its protective role for the host, when complement system becomes activated in critical illnesses [52, 53], C5b-9 also can attack innocent bystander host endothelial cells (ECs). If CD59 glycoprotein expressed on the endothelial cells [3] is downregulated due to critical illnesses, channel (pore) formation occurs in the endothelial membrane, which leads to endotheliopathy and even endothelial membrane lysis [53, 54]. Although the "imbalanced", "uncontrolled" or "dysregulated" complement activation has been implicated to be the mechanism of atypical HUS, perhaps "unprotected" endothelium due to loss of CD59 protective effect against C5b-9 could be the mechanism leading to endotheliopathy, not only in atypical HUS [53], but also in the critical illnesses.

It is interesting to note that congenital CD59 deficiency due to its gene mutation has been associated with thrombosis and hemolytic anemia [55], which also suggest the close relationship between endothelial CD-59 loss and endotheliopathy. The study of the role of CD59 in the pathogenesis of endotheliopathy is needed.

TTP-like syndrome in the critical illness

TTP-like syndrome typically occurs in critically ill patients [1, 2, 12–14, 17–21, 25–50, 56]. Inexplicably, in current clinical practice and medical literature, the most of the patients with critical illnesses presenting with VMTD with or without hemorrhagic disorder have been identified as having "DIC" with either compensated (chronic) or decompensated (acute) designation [26]. It should be emphasized that "DIC" mimics TTP-like syndrome [1] and chronic DIC is identical to TTP-like syndrome in precipitating factors (i.e., critical illnesses), pathological findings (i.e., hyaline microthrombi), and hematologic features (i.e., thrombocytopenia) [26]. Later, reinterpretation of "DIC" will be separately discussed in more detail.

"Two-activation theory of the endothelium"

Activated complement system provides a critical and multifaceted defense against infection, but it can be also activated in non-pathogen-induced critical illnesses such as polytrauma, pregnancy, surgery, transplant, autoimmune disease, and cancer [57–61]. Following the activation, complement can clear invading microorganisms by lysis or opsonization [27]. However, on the host side, the complement activation product terminal C5b-9 also could attack the host ECs and cause transmembrane channel formation on the endothelium and induce endotheliopathy. In turn, endotheliopathy triggers multiple molecular events [1–3, 55] as presented in Fig. 1.

Critical illnesses are well known to cause an injury to ECs, leading to endotheliopathy and endothelial dysfunction [62, 63]. Now, the evidence shows that complement activation plays the major role in molecular pathogenesis of inflammation and DIT [1–3, 55, 58–61, 64]. Based on endotheliopathy that promotes several biomolecular events, the "two-activation theory of

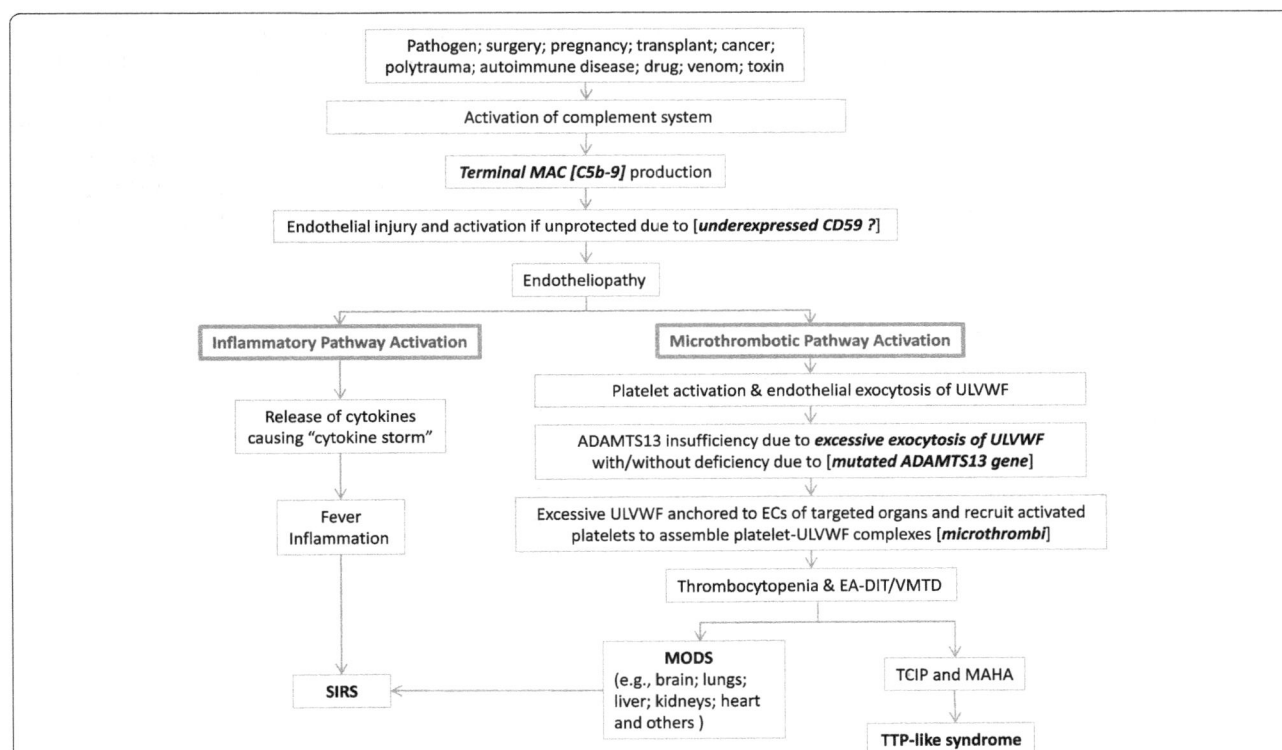

Fig. 1 Molecular pathogenesis of TTP-like syndrome Fig. 1 elaborates "two activation theory of the endothelium", which shows complement-induced endothelial molecular events, leading to endotheliopathy-associated DIT (i.e., TTP-like syndrome) and MODS. The organ phenotype syndrome in MODS includes encephalopathy, ARDS, AFHF, ARF/HUS, MI, AI, pancreatitis, rhabdomyolysis, "DIC", HELLPs, SS, and others. For example, in sepsis complement activation is the initial critical event. Complement activation can occur through one of three different pathways (i.e., classical, alternate and lectin). In addition to lysis of pathogen by terminal product C5b-9, it could induce endotheliopathy to the innocent bystander ECs of the host. C5b-9-induced endotheliopathy is suspected to occur if the endothelium is "unprotected" by CD59. Activated inflammatory pathway provokes inflammation in sepsis, but inflammation could be modest if the number of organ involvement is limited. Activated microthrombotic pathway results in endotheliopathy-associated DIT if the excess of ULVWF develops following endothelial exocytosis as a result of relative insufficiency of ADAMTS13 with/without mild to moderate ADAMTS13 deficiency, which is associated with heterozygous gene mutation or polymorphism of the gene. This theory explains all the manifestations of VMTD as illustrated in the Fig. 1. Abbreviations: AFHF, acute fulminant hepatic failure; AI, adrenal insufficiency; ARDS, acute respiratory distress syndrome; ARF, acute renal failure; "DIC", false disseminated intravascular coagulation; DIT, disseminated intravascular microthrombosis; ECs, endothelial cells; EA-DIT, endotheliopathy-associated DIT; HELLPs, hemolysis, elevated liver enzymes, and low platelet syndrome; HUS, hemolytic uremic syndrome; MI, myocardial infarction; MODS, multi-organ dysfunction syndrome; MAHA, microangiopathic hemolytic anemia; SIRS, systemic inflammatory response syndrome; SS, stroke syndrome; TCIP, thrombocytopenia in critically ill patient; TTP, thrombotic thrombocytopenic purpura; ULVWF, unusually large von Willebrand factor; VMTD, vascular microthrombotic disease

the endothelium" is proposed and illustrated in Fig. 1 [1, 2]. Endotheliopathy triggers the activation of two independent endothelial pathways (i.e., inflammatory and microthrombotic). In short, two important molecular events are: 1) release of inflammatory cytokines (e.g., interleukin [IL]-1, IL-6, tumor necrosis factor-α, and others) [63, 65, 66], and 2) activation of the platelet [67] and endothelial exocytosis of ULVWF [68, 69]. The former initiates inflammation through "activation of inflammatory pathway", and the latter mediates microthrombogenesis via "activation of microthrombotic pathway" [1–3, 26] as shown in Fig. 1.

In endotheliopathy, microthrombogenesis is a process, in which long elongated ULVWF strings are anchored to ECs after release from Weibel-Palade bodies and recruit platelets, promoting the formation of platelet-ULVWF complexes [5, 6, 70]. These microthrombi strings are the pathologic complexes formed, perhaps under the shear stress of blood flow, leading to endotheliopathy-associated DIT and hematologic features of TTP-like syndrome [2, 4].

Microthrombogenesis in VMTD
Megakaryocytic ULVWF(mULVWF) and endothelial ULVWF(eULVWF)

Two kinds of ULVWF are synthesized in two different sites (i.e., megakaryocytes and ECs) as shown in Table 2 [4, 71]. Megakaryocytic ULVWF (mULVWF) are released normally into circulation as platelet-adherent form and stored in α granules of the platelet. But endothelial ULVWF (eULVWF) are produced in ECs and stored in Weibel-Palade bodies to be available as endothelium-adherent form following release from ECs to initiate normal hemostasis in vascular injury [4, 6, 72].

Although the differences in structure and function between mULVWF and eULVWF are unknown at this time, it appears two different ULVWF multimers from different origin may have different functions [73, 74]. Microthrombogenesis of TTP occurs in microcirculation [4, 75] due to hyperactivity of circulating mULVWF in hereditary and antibody-associated ADAMTS13 deficiency. However, TTP-like syndrome is likely associated with relative insufficiency of ADAMTS13 as a result of excessive exocytosis of eULVWF in endotheliopathy [2]. In TTP, mULVWF multimers might react with platelets and assemble microthrombi in the microvasculature in situ under the shear stress, but in TTP-like syndrome eULVWF strings are anchored to ECs and get decorated with platelets to form microthrombi strings [5, 6, 70].

In severe sepsis, decreased ADAMTS13 activity is correlated with greater adhesion capacity of ULVWF and higher degree of thrombocytopenia as well as severity of critical illnesses and organ dysfunction [76]. Decreased ADAMTS13 activity in some patients with TTP-like syndrome also suggests underling partial ADAMTS13 deficiency could exist as well. In addition to endothelial exocytosis of ULVWF, partial ADAMTS13 deficiency associated with polymorphism or heterozygous mutation of the gene could contribute to the onset and degree of severity of TTP-like syndrome [77–80].

Both ULVWF lodged in capillaries and ULVWF anchored to ECs are rapidly cleaved by ADAMTS13 in vitro [4, 6, 72]. This observation is certainly consistent with the benefit of TPE for TTP due to ADAMTS13 deficiency and TTP-like syndrome with its insufficiency.

Table 2 Characteristics of two different ULVWF multimers

	mULVWF multimers	eULVWF multimers
Synthesized in	Megakaryocytes	Endothelial cells
Stored in	α granules of platelets	Weibel-Palade bodies of ECs
Primary distribution at release	In circulation	On the membrane of ECs
Availability	In microcirculation	At ECs following endothelial exocytosis
Exposure to ADAMTS13	As platelet-adherent form	As ECs-adherent form
Interaction with platelets causing	Platelet aggregation and adhesion	Platelet-ULVWF strings
Localization of platelet-ULVWF complexes	Arteriolar and capillary lumens lodged as microthrombi in situ	Endothelial membrane-anchored as microthrombi strings
Example of leading its activity	ADAMTS13 autoantibody	Sepsis-induced endotheliopathy
Endotheliopathic lesion	Microthrombotic microangiopathy	Microthrombotic angiopathy
Hematologic manifestation	Thrombocytopenia and MAHA	Thrombocytopenia and MAHA/aMAHA
Associated inflammation	None to minimal (?)	Mild to severe
Associated clinical syndrome	TTP	TTP-like syndrome

ECs endothelial cells, eULVWF/mULVWF endothelial unusually large von Willebrand factor/megakaryocytic ULVWF, MAHA/aMAHA microangiopathic hemolytic anemia/atypical MAHA, TTP thrombotic thrombocytopenic purpura

Dissimilarity between TTP and TTP-like syndrome

The dissimilar pathogenesis and different phenotypic characteristics between TTP and TTP-like syndrome are summarized in Table 1. It is hypothesized that microthrombogenesis in acquired TTP is caused by hyperactivity of mULVWF due to anti-ADAMTS13 antibody and occurs in the microvasculature *in situ*. On the other hand, microthrombogenesis in TTP-like syndrome is triggered by excessive exocytosis of eULVWF from ECs and occurs in the endothelial membrane. In both cases, deficient and or insufficient ADAMTS13 could not handle the excess of ULVWF.

This slightly different microthrombogenesis could lead to different organ localization and configuration of microthrombi, but still produce the same hematologic phenotype of VMTD. In TTP, microthrombi formed in the microvasculature become lodged within arterioles and capillaries of the brain and kidneys [4], which condition can be called "microvascular" microthrombosis. In TTP-like syndrome, it takes place on the smaller and larger vasculatures [80–83] of various organs depending upon endothelial heterogeneity that determines organ localization [83–85], which condition could be called "vascular" microthrombosis. We know more about endothelial microthrombogenesis in TTP-like syndrome, but do not know how microthrombogenesis in TTP occurs in microcirculation *in vivo* other than that it might be promoted under the condition of shear stress due to blood flow.

Without the understanding the endothelial molecular pathogenesis of TTP-like syndrome, clinicians have thought the atypical feature of different organ involvement in TTP-like syndrome is just a variant of TTP. In reality, different organ phenotypic TTP-like syndromes occur as a result of endothelial heterogeneity caused by genetic variables [3, 83–85] through endowed molecules in ECs (e.g., CD59 and Gb3 in HUS) [3, 86]. For examples, extra renal manifestations of Shiga toxin-producing *E. coli*-HUS (STEC-HUS) represent expression of endothelial heterogeneity caused by endowed molecules, localizing in the brain with encephalopathy, heart with myocardial infarction, pancreas with pancreatitis, and others [3].

Reinterpretation of "DIC"

"DIC" has been the most intriguing disease among all the human diseases because of its deadly nature and conundrums as listed follows [26]:

- No clearly defined clinical and pathological diagnostic criteria are available.
- Not a single test or set of the tests can confirm and establish the diagnosis.

- Unexplained bleeding disorders such as viral hemorrhagic fevers are often blamed to it without foundation.
- Establishing the diagnostic application has been very subjective among investigators.
- The scoring system for the diagnosis is imprecise, confusing and subjective.
- The pathogenesis (i.e., tissue factor [TF]-FVIIa activated coagulopathy) has never been proven.
- Not a single treatment has been clearly proven to be effective.
- No therapeutic benefit has occurred even after numerous clinical trials.

Only consistent clinical, pathologic and hematologic features are:

- It occurs in critical illnesses (e.g., sepsis) and APL, but with different phenotypes.
- Clinical features are VMTD (i.e., DIT).
- Pathologic features are arteriolar and capillary hyaline microthrombi.
- Hematologic features are thrombocytopenia and MAHA.

True DIC (e.g., consumption coagulopathy), which occurs in APL [87, 88], is a coagulation (hemorrhagic) disorder, developing due to activation of TF-FVIIa complex-initiated coagulation cascade. In APL, TF is strongly expressed in leukemic promyelocytic cells. TF triggers fibrinogenesis via activation of FVII. On the other hand, "DIC", which occurs in critical illnesses, has also been named as DIC based on the same TF-initiated coagulation (thrombotic) disorder [89, 90]. However, the clinical and hematologic features are very different between APL and critical illnesses. Instead, the clinical, pathological and hematological features of "DIC" are identical to endotheliopathy-associated DIT [1, 2], which is microthrombotic disorder. The differences between "DIC" (i.e., microthrombi) and true DIC (i.e., fibrin clots) are summarized in Table 3.

Pathologic coagulation (DVT) vs. microthrombogenesis (DIT)

A very important question is: "where does "DIC" belong to DVT, DIT, or true DIC of APL?" Is DIT conveniently ignored from the standpoint of hemostatic disorder?

In clinical medicine, the physiological mechanism of hemostasis and pathological mechanism of thrombosis has been considered to be the result of the same coagulation process with two different outcomes due to the different circumstance of the injury. Hemostasis is a normal protective physiological process to stop bleeding following external bodily injury, but pathologic thrombosis is the result of normal hemostatic process within

Table 3 Hematologic and Clinical Characteristics of endotheliopathy-associated DIT and true DIC

	EA-DIT/VMTD and "DIC" of McKay	True DIC
Example	TTP-like syndrome	APL
Nature of the clots	"Microthrombi strings" made of platelet-ULVWF complexes	"Fibrin clots" made of fibrin meshes
Mechanism of the genesis	Intravascular microthrombogenesis	Intravascular fibrinogenesis
Inciting causes/events	Infection; surgery; pregnancy; transplant; cancer; drug; toxin, leading to edotheliopathy	APL, leading to TF expression
Hematological manifestation	Microthrombotic disorder	Hemorrhagic disorder
Pathogenesis		
Mechanism	Activation of microthrombotic pathway	Activation of TF-initiated coagulation cascade
Site of activation	Intravascular membrane of ECs	In circulation
Thrombopathic result	Intravascular hemostasis of ULVWF path	Consumption of fibrinogen, FV and FVIII
Effect on the involved organ	Hypoxic organ dysfunction	Generalized bleeding tendency
Coagulation tests		
Fibrinogen	Normal	Decreased
PT; aPTT; TT	Normal	Prolonged
FVIII activity	Normal or markedly increased	Markedly decreased
Thrombocytopenia	Mild to moderately severe	Not consumed but decreased due to APL
Associated clinical syndrome	MODS; cytokine storm; SIRS	Hemorrhagic syndrome
Associate hematologic features		
Schistocytes	Often present	Absent
MAHA/aMAHA	Almost always present	Does not occur
Hepatic coagulopathy	Common	Does not occur
Incidence in clinical practice	Very common	Extremely rare
Management		
Platelet transfusion	Contraindicated	May be used if needed for APL
Treatment	TPE; rADAMTS13 (expected to be very effective)	Treat underlying pathology (e.g., ATRA in APL)

APL acute promyelocytic leukemia, *aPTT* activated partial thromboplastin time; *ATRA* All-trans retinoic acid, *DIC* disseminated intravascular coagulation; *DIT* disseminated intravascular microhrombosis; *FDP* fibrin degradation products, *FVIIa* activated factor VII, *FVIII* factor VIII; *MAHA/aMAHA* microangiopathic hemolytic anemia/atypical MAHA, *MODS*, multi-organ dysfunction syndrome, *PT*, prothrombin time; *rADAMTS13* recombinant ADAMTS, *SIRS* systemic inflammatory response syndrome, *TF* tissue factor, *TMA* thrombotic microangiopathy; *TPE* therapeutic plasma exchange; *TTP* thrombotic thrombocytopenic purpura, *ULVWF* unusually large von Willebrand factor multimers; *VMTD* vascular microthrombotic disease

intravascular space following intravascular injury [91]. Following TF-activated coagulation cascade, the nature of formed intravascular thrombus (e.g., deep vein thrombosis [DVT] and "DIC") has been presumed to be the same nature to the hemostatic plug (e.g., blood clots after an injury) [90, 91]. If this is the case, how can we explain that DVT is made of macrothrombus but "DIC" is made of microthrombi? Coagulation scientists have not answered this thought provoking question yet.

Intravascular microthrombosis occurring in "DIC" has been interpreted to be a pathological coagulation disorder mediated through TF-initiated FVII activation [90, 91]. This conception has been strengthened on the following grounds: 1) the term "DIC", coined by Donald McKay [91, 92], clearly implied that it is a coagulation disorder and this assumption has been accepted by clinicians and coagulation scientists without laboratory and molecular verification, and 2) unlike DIT (i.e., TTP-like

syndrome), "DIC" sometimes has occurred with severe hemorrhagic disorder associated with abnormal coagulation profile of prolonged prothrombin time, activated partial thromboplastin time, hypofibinogenemia, and increased fibrin degradation products, which is consistent with consumption of coagulation factors following TF-initiated coagulation cascade. But then, there is chronic "DIC", which is exactly the same to the feature of endotheliopathy-associated DIT.

However, this abnormal coagulation profile in acute "DIC" is non-specific even though the prevailing interpretation has blamed it to the consumption of coagulation factors in "DIC". This author differs from this assumption, which will be further discussed later, along with hepatic coagulopathy.

The concept of microthrombogenesis clearly supports that "microthrombi" in DIT are exclusively composed of platelet-ULVWF complexes [1, 2, 4–6]. In contrast, the ironclad concept of "microthrombi" in "DIC" has been "micro blood clots" made of fibrin clots with participation of platelets via TF-initiated coagulation cascade [89–91].

In fact, chronic "DIC" and endotheliopathy-associated DIT (i.e., TTP-like syndrome) are exactly the same in their underlying risk factors, pathologic and phenotypic presentation. First, clinically both disorders almost always occur in critical illnesses; second, their pathology is characterized by arteriolar and capillary hyaline microthrombi with variable fibroblastic proliferation [4, 92]; third, hematologic features are consumptive thrombocytopenia and MAHA. Thus, chronic "DIC" and endotheliopathy-associated DIT are one disease. Until now "DIC" has been incorrectly ascribed to pathological coagulation disorder initiated by TF-induced coagulation [89, 93–97]. This misconception of "DIC" has contributed to many unexplainable mysterious features of "DIC" to date. Now, it is clear that macro-thrombus of DVT and microthrombi of DIT/"DIC" occur in intravascular injury due to dissimilar hemostatic pathogenesis.

"DIC" perplexity discussed

Table 3 is self-explanatory showing the difference in hematologic and clinical characteristics between endotheliopaathy-associated DIT (i.e., TTP-like syndrome, including McKay's "DIC") and true DIC of fibrin clots occurring in APL. In contrast to "DIC"(i.e., false DIC), the predominant feature of true DIC (i.e., in APL) is always hemorrhagic disorder without microvascular thrombosis, MAHA and MODS [87, 98–101]. In regard to "DIC" mystery, a few more comments are appropriate.

First, the International Society on Thrombosis and Hemostasis (ISTH) has introduced the "DIC" scoring system to better establish the diagnosis of "DIC" [102]. It has not been used as a primary diagnostic tool, but has been applied to confirm the diagnosis using hematologic parameters only after predetermined as "DIC" with a clinical disorder known to cause "DIC". The scoring system has shown low specificity [102]. It should be emphasized that no single laboratory test or set of tests is sensitive or specific enough to allow a definitive diagnosis of "DIC" [103]. In most cases, the diagnosis is based on the combination of results of non-specific abnormal coagulation profile with a clinical condition known to be associated with "DIC" [104].

Second, coagulation scientists put their efforts to support the role of TF in "DIC", by proposing TF encryption/decryption theory [105], thiol path TF regulation theory [106], TF transfer hypothesis [107], and inflammation and coagulation interaction theory [108–111], which are all still controversial and have not proven the role of TF in "DIC". Furthermore, the negligible amount

of *in vivo* TF, even available, cannot explain the "DIC" presenting with extensive vascular microthrombosis and MODS.

Third, the abnormal coagulation profile, showing prolonged prothrombin time and activated partial thromboplastin time, hypofibrinogenemia, and increased fibrin degradation products, is non-specific, and cannot affirm the diagnosis of true DIC. Additionally, this profile oddly develops only in some patients with "DIC". Therefore, the "chronic/compensated/covert" concept [102, 112, 113], including "low grade DIC", has been introduced if the coagulation profile is normal or mildly abnormal in "DIC". This description also cannot explain inexplicably extensive microthrombosis in the absence of depleted coagulation factors.

Fourth, numerous randomized clinical trials (e.g., TF pathway inhibitor, activated protein C, anticoagulant, anti-inflammatory cytokines, and others) to modulate septic response to infection, which pathogenesis is firmly based on interaction theory between inflammation and TF-initiated coagulation, have not been successful to improve the survival in sepsis [114, 115].

It is no wonder, after extensive laboratory studies and clinical trials, why a specific diagnostic test(s) has not been established and no effective treatment discovered for "DIC" after more than half century since DIC was coined in 1950 [91, 92]. The simple answer is that the thesis of TF-initiated pathogenesis of "DIC" has been erroneous.

Acute "DIC" is due to DIT-associated hepatic coagulopathy

One remaining, very pertinent question is: "what is the correct diagnosis for acute/decompensated/overt "DIC" that is associated with abnormal coagulation profile?" The answer is clear since "DIC" is often associated with hepatic diseases [1, 15, 116–120]. In endotheliopathy-associated DIT, hepatic coagulopathy could occur as a phenotype of acute fulminant hepatic failure or acute hepatic necrosis as seen in critical illnesses [15, 90, 116–120]. The pathogenesis unknown hepato-renal syndrome [121–123] and hepatic encephalopathy [15, 121] are very much consistent with endotheliopathy-associated DIT similar to "DIC" syndrome. Thus, acute "DIC" is hepatic coagulopathy occurring in endotheliopathy-associated DIT.

Indeed, the medical literature is replete with DIT, "DIC" and/or hepatic failure, occurring in association with HELLP syndrome, HUS, acute necrotizing pancreatitis, purpura fulminans, rhabdomyolysis, acute respiratory distress syndrome, viral hemorrhagic fevers as well as hepato-renal syndrome and hepatic encephalopathy. In retrospect, when clinical phenotype of acute fulminant hepatic failure or acute hepatic necrosis presents with thrombocytopenia and coagulopathy,

Enthotheliopathy-associated DIT (i.e., TTP-like syndrome) should be suspected rather than the diagnosis of acute "DIC" [26]. Indeed, hepatic coagulopathy occurring in DIT is a life-threatening thrombo-hemorrhagic syndrome without correct diagnosis [26].

Differential diagnosis of true DIC and TTP-like syndrome

In differentiating true DIC (e.g., APL) from DIT with hepatic coagulopathy, the most reliable test is the assay of coagulation factors [1, 2, 87, 99, 124, 125] (Table 4). In true DIC, FVIII and FV are markedly decreased due to their consumption and inactivation, but, in DIT with hepatic coagulopathy (i.e., acute "DIC"), FVIII is normal or more likely markedly increased and FVII is markedly decreased. The increase of FVIII in hepatic coagulopathy is likely due to endothelial exocytosis of ULVWF, in which some of ULVWF are cleaved by ADAMTS13 to smaller VWF multimers and released into circulation to bind FVIII and protect it from degradation. A suggested guideline for laboratory tests is summarized in Table 4 to aid in the differential diagnosis among complicated thrombopathies and coagulopathies [1, 2].

Hope for the future in the treatment

VMTD presenting with both TTP and TTP-like syndrome has responded well to TPE if the treatment is initiated in the earliest possible stage [11–13, 20, 41, 42]. In medical literature, there is a plethora of case reports of successful treatment with TPE for atypical TTP and TTP-like syndrome. Once the disease progresses to the point of irreversible organ dysfunction due to tissue hypoxia, recovery is unlikely to occur in TTP-like syndrome [13]. This is particularly true in ARDS [20], encephalopathy in HUS [126], and adrenal insufficiency in sepsis (i.e., septic shock) [127].

High mortality associated with "DIC" in critically ill patients could have been related to platelet transfusions as well as masked hepatic coagulopathy and heparin treatment. The platelet transfusion is contraindicated because it aggravates on-going microthrombogenesis, and heparin treatment increases hemorrhage in hepatic coagulopathy. TPE is the treatment of choice for DIT at this time. Fresh frozen plasma or recombinant FVIIa [128] to replace the lowest FVII might have been beneficial for severe hemorrhage in hepatic coagulopathy associated with VMTD.

Table 4 Hematologic differential diagnoses among thrombopathies and coagulopathies

	TTP & TTP-like syndrome (DIT)	TTP-like syndrome (DIT) associated with HC (e.g., sepsis) equal to acute "DIC"	DIC (e.g., APL)	PF (e.g., amyloidosis)
Thrombocytopenia	Always present	Always present	Present due to APL, but not due to consumption (?)	Not present
MAHA/aMAHA	Always present	Always present	Do not occur	Not present
Fibrinogen	Normal	Decreased	Always decreased	Always decreased
Factor VIII	Normal	Normal or increased	Markedly decreased	Decreased
Factor V	Normal	Decreased	Decreased	Normal or decreased
Factor X	Normal	Decreased	Usually normal	Normal (?)
Factor VII	Normal	Markedly decreased	Normal	Normal
Factor IX	Normal	Decreased	Normal	Normal
FDP	Normal	?	Positive	Strongly positive
Prothrombin time	Normal	Prolonged	Prolonged	Prolonged
Activated partial thromboplastin time	Normal	Prolonged	Prolonged	Prolonged
Thrombin time	Normal	Prolonged	Prolonged	Prolonged
Thrombosis form	Microthrombi	Microthrombi	Friable fibrin clots (meshes)	Absent
Bleeding: Character Treatment	Petechiae; Usually no need of treatment	May cause serious bleeding; Controllable with FFP & rFVIIa	Common, serious bleeding; Abrogated with ATRA & chemotherapy	Slow & persistent bleeding; Treatable with AFA
Hypoxic organ dysfunction (MODS)	Present	Present	Not present	Not present
Platelet transfusion	Contraindicated	Contraindicated	May be used for APL	Not needed

AFA anti-fibrinolytic agent, *ATRA* all-trans retinoic acid, *"DIC"* false disseminated intravascular coagulation, *DIT* disseminated intravascular microthrombosis, *FDP* fibrin degradation products, *FFP* fresh frozen plasma; *HC* hepatic coagulopathy; *MAHA/aMAHA* microangiopathic hemolytic anemia/atypical MAHA, *PF* primary fibrinolysis, *TTP* thrombotic thrombocytopenic purpura

Theoretically, two very promising targeted therapeutic approaches for TTP-like syndrome are 1) anti-complement therapy such as eculizumab and recombinant CD59 to inhibit the first leg of the pathogenesis based on "two-activation theory of the endothelium" [3, 129–131] and 2) anti-microthrombotic therapy such as recombinant ADAMTS13 to correct or modify the second leg of the endothelial pathogenesis [3]. Indeed, eculizumab has shown promising results [129, 130]. However, anti-complement therapy should be explored with an extreme care since it could cause catastrophic harm in the septic patient by aggravating the ongoing process of sepsis and septic shock. Currently, recombinant ADAMTS13 is being investigated for the treatment of hereditary TTP. Since it has shown to cleave eULVWF [4, 6, 69], controlled clinical trials should be initiated for TTP-like syndrome as soon as possible. If it is effective, recombinant ADAMTS13 could save so many lives, especially in the critical care medicine, obstetrics, surgery, transplant and more.

Conclusion

TTP and TTP-like syndrome are two different diseases caused by dissimilar pathogenesis although their underlying pathologic feature of DIT and hematologic phenotype are similar. TTP is intravascular microthrombotic disease due to ADAMTS13 deficiency, but TTP-like syndrome is hemostatic disease associated with endotheliopathy in critical illnesses. It is essential to recognize TTP-like syndrome as a distinct disease entity, which working diagnostic criteria is summarized in Table 5. These criteria would benefit the patient through earlier unmasking of the diagnosis and life-saving TPE when presented with atypical organ phenotypic syndromes. Certainly, "two activation theory of the endothelium" has been able to clarify many unresolved issues of thrombotic microangiopathy. Among them are TTP, HUS, TTP-like syndrome, MODS, "DIC" and combined organ dysfunction syndrome with hepatic coagulopathy.

Both activation of complement through C5b-9 in critical illnesses and microthrombogenesis with participation of the platelet and ULVWF have unequivocally supported the crucial role of endotheliopathy in the pathogenesis of TTP-like syndrome. The role of endothelial protectin CD59 and C5b-9 should be evaluated to further support the endothelial molecular pathogenesis in TTP-like syndrome [131]. The future therapeutic modalities should be explored with anti-complement therapy and anti-microthrombotic therapy. This author believes anti-microthrombotic therapy is safer option.

Lastly, the designation of the term VMTD is very appropriate not only for TTP and TTP-like syndrome, but also to include hereditary focal, multifocal and localized microthrombotic diseases, and acquired microthrombotic disorders such as stroke syndromes, cardiac

Table 5 Proposed working diagnostic criteria for TTP-like syndrome

1. Thrombocytopenia and MAHA/aMAHA.
2. Underling critical illness due to such conditions as.
√ Pathogen (bacterial; viral; fungal; rickettsial; parasitic)
√ Polytrauma (chest and lung; bone; skull/brain)
√ Pregnancy (preeclampsia; abruptio placenta; amniotic fluid embolism)
√ Cancer (breast; stomach; lung)
√ Surgery (heart; bowel; uterus; bone)
√ Transplant (liver; kidney; bone marrow)
√ Disease (autoimmune vascular disease; malignant hypertension)
√ Drug (cyclosporin; mitomycin C)
√ Toxin (venom; ricin; Shiga toxin)
3. Negative antibody against ADAMTS13.
4. Mild to moderately decreased activity of ADAMTS13 (20–70% of normal).
5. One or more organ phenotype dysfunction syndromes such as.
√ Pancreatitis.
√ Myocardial infarction.
√ ARDS.
√ Acute fulminant hepatic failure.
√ Acute adrenal insufficiency.
√ Rhabdomyolysis.
√ Non-occlusive mesenteric ischemia.
√ Hepato-renal syndrome.
√ Hepatic-encephalopathy.
√ Cardio-pulmonary syndrome.
√ Tissue gangrene.
√ Peripheral digit ischemic syndrome.

+ Encephalopathy and ARF are common in both TTP and TTP-like syndrome
ARDS acute respiratory distress syndrome, *TTP* thrombotic thrombocytopenic purpura

angina, and coronary procedure-associated transient microthrombotic syndrome. The recognition of the term VMTD would further assist in the understanding of endothelial physiology and identifying of endothelial pathophysiology in many human diseases, especially in hemostasis and hemostatic disorders.

Abbreviations
ADAMTS13: A disintegrin and metalloproteinase with a thrombospondin type 1 motif, member 13; AFA: Anti-fibrinolytic agent; AFHF: Acute fulminant hepatic failure; AI: Adrenal insufficiency; APL: Acute promyelocytic leukemia; aPTT: Activated partial thromboplastin time; ARDS: Acute respiratory distress syndrome; rADAMTS13: Recombinant ADAMTS13; ARF: Acute renal failure; ATRA: All-trans retinoic acid; DIC: Disseminated intravascular coagulation; "DIC" : false disseminated intravascular coagulation; DIT: Disseminated intravascular thrombosis; ECs: Endothelial cells; FDP: Fibrin degradation products; FFP: Fresh frozen plasma; FVIIa: Activated factor VII; FVIII: Factor VIII; HC: Hepatic coagulopathy; IL: Interleukin; HELLPs: Hemolysis elevated liver enzymes and low platelet syndrome; HUS: Hemolytic uremic syndrome; LDH: Lactate dehydrogenase; MAC: Membrane attack complex; MI: Myocardial infarction; MAHA: Microangiopathic hemolytic anemia; aMAHA: Atypical MAHA; MODS: Multi-organ dysfunction syndrome;

PF: Purpura fulminans; PT: Prothrombin time; SIRS: Systemic inflammatory response syndrome; SS: Stroke syndrome; STEC: Shiga toxin producing *E. coli*; TCIP: Thrombocytopenia in critically ill patient; TF: Tissue factor; TPE: Therapeutic plasma exchange; TTP: Thrombotic thrombocytopenic purpura; vWF: von Willebrand factor; ULVWF: Unusually large von Willebrand factor multimers; eULVWF: Endothelial ULVWF; mULVWF: Megakaryocytic ULVWF; VMTD: Vascular microthrombotic disease; AA-VMTD: antibody associated VMTD; EA-VMTD: Endotheliopathy associated VMTD; GA-VMTD: Gene mutation associated VMTD

Authors' contributions

Contributed 100% by the corresponding author. The authors read and approved the final manuscript.

Authors' information

Board certified hematologist and hematopathologist, retired professor of medicine in the University of California Irvine School of Medicine, and retired professor of medicine in the Wright State University of School of Medicine.

Competing interests

The author declares that he have no competing interests.

References

1. Chang JC. A Thought on Possible Pathogenesis of Ebola Viral Hemorrhagic Disease and Potential Treatments: Could it Be Thrombotic Thrombocytopenic Purpura-like Syndrome? Ther Apher Dial. 2015;20:93-8.
2. Chang JC. Thrombocytopenia in critically ill patients due to vascular microthrombotic disease: pathogenesis based on "two activation theory of the endothelium". Vascul Dis Ther. 2017;2:1-7.
3. Chang JC. Molecular pathogenesis of STEC-HUS caused by endothelial heterogeneity and unprotected complement activation, leading to endotheliopathy and impaired ADAMTS13 activity: based on two-activation theory of the endothelium and vascular microthrombotic disease. Nephrol Renal Dis. 2017;2:1-8.
4. Tsai HM. Pathophysiology of thrombotic thrombocytopenic purpura. Int J Hematol. 2010;91:1-19.
5. Chauhan AK, Goerge T, Schneider SW, Wagner DD. Formation of platelet strings and microthrombi in the presence of ADAMTS-13 inhibitor does not require P-selectin or beta3 integrin. J Thromb Haemost. 2007;5:583-9.
6. Dong JF, Moake JL, Nolasco L, et al. ADAMTS-13 rapidly cleaves newly secreted ultralarge von Willebrand factor multimers on the endothelial surface under flowing conditions. Blood. 2002;100:4033-9.
7. Moschcowitz E. An acute febrile pleiochromic anemia with hyaline thrombosis of the terminal arterioles and capillaries: an undescribed disease. Arch Intern Med. 1925;36:89-93.
8. Singer K, Bornstein FP, Wile SA. Thrombotic thrombocytopenic purpura; hemorrhagic diathesis with generalized platelet thromboses. Blood. 1947;2:542-54.
9. Sonneveld MA, de Maat MP, Portegies ML, et al. Low ADAMTS13 activity is associated with an increased risk of ischemic stroke. Blood. 2015;126:2739-46.
10. Akyol O, Akyol S, Chen CH. Update on ADAMTS13 and VWF in cardiovascular and hematological disorders. Clin Chim Acta. 2016;463:109-18.
11. Chang JC, Newman RS. Redefining the syndromes of thrombotic microangiopathy. Ther Apher Dial. 2004;8:73-4.
12. Chang JC. The understanding of thrombotic thrombocytopenic purpura: Dyadic, triadic, pentadic, and other manifestations. J Clin Apher. 2004;19:2-4.
13. Chang JC, Kathula SK. Various clinical manifestations in patients with thrombotic microangiopathy. J Investig Med. 2002;50:201-6.
14. Sarode R. Atypical presentations of thrombotic thrombocytopenic purpura: a review. J Clin Apher. 2009;24:47-52.
15. Panackel C, Thomas R, Sebastian B, Mathai SK. Recent advances in management of acute liver failure. Indian J Crit Care Med. 2015;19:27-33.
16. Rath W, Faridi A, Dudenhausen JW. HELLP syndrome. J Perinat Med. 2000; 28:249-60.
17. Wahla AS, Ruiz J, Noureddine N, Upadhya B, Sane DC, Owen J. Myocardial infarction in thrombotic thrombocytopenic purpura: a single-center experience and literature review. Eur J Haematol. 2008;81:311-6.
18. Hawkins BM, Abu-Fadel M, Vesely SK, George JN. Clinical cardiac involvement in thrombotic thrombocytopenic purpura: a systematic review. Transfusion. 2008;48:382-92.
19. Bone RC, Henry JE, Petterson J, et al. Respiratory dysfunction in thrombotic thrombocytopenic purpura. Am J Med. 1978;65:262-70.
20. Chang JC, Aly ES. Acute respiratory distress syndrome as a major clinical manifestation of thrombotic thrombocytopenic purpura. Am J Med Sci. 2001;321:124-8.
21. Swisher KK, Doan JT, Vesely SK, et al. Pancreatitis preceding acute episodes of thrombotic thrombocytopenic purpura-hemolytic uremic syndrome: report of five patients with a systematic review of published reports. Haematologica. 2007;92:936-43.
22. Moake JL, Rudy CK, Troll JH, et al. Unusually large plasma factor VIII:von Willebrand factor multimers in chronic relapsing thrombotic thrombocytopenic purpura. N Engl J Med. 1982;307:1432-5.
23. Furlan M, Robles R, Lämmle B. Partial purification and characterization of a protease from human plasma cleaving von Willebrand factor to fragments produced by in vivo proteolysis. Blood. 1996;87:4223-34.
24. Tsai HM. Physiologic cleavage of von Willebrand factor by a plasma protease is dependent on its conformation and requires calcium ion. Blood. 1996;87:4235-4.
25. George JN. How I treat patients with thrombotic thrombocytopenic purpura-hemolytic uremic syndrome. Blood. 2000;96:1223-9.
26. Chang JC. Disseminated intravascular coagulation: is it fact or fancy? Blood Coagul Fibrinolysis. 2018;29:3030-7.
27. Ray PE, Liu XH. Pathogenesis of Shiga toxin-induced hemolytic uremic syndrome. Pediatr Nephrol. 2001;16:823-39.
28. Zhang K, Lu Y, Harley KT, Tran MH. Atypical Hemolytic Uremic Syndrome: A Brief Review. Hematol Rep. 2017;9:7053.
29. Takimoto T, Nakao M, Nakajo T, Chinen Y, Kuroda J, Taniwaki M. Acute myocardial infarction as the initial thrombotic event of thrombotic thrombocytopenic purpura. Blood Coagul Fibrinolysis. 2016;27:948-51.
30. Atreya AR, Arora S, Sivalingam SK, Giugliano GR. ST segment elevation myocardial infarction as a presenting feature of thrombotic thrombocytopenic purpura. J Cardiovasc Dis Res. 2012;3:167-9.
31. McDonald V, Laffan M, Benjamin S, Bevan D, Machin S, Scully MA. Thrombotic thrombocytopenic purpura precipitated by acute pancreatitis: a report of seven cases from a regional UK TTP registry. Br J Haematol. 2009;144:430-3.
32. Muñiz AE, Barbee RW. Thrombotic thrombocytopenic purpura (TTP) presenting as pancreatitis. J Emerg Med. 2003;24:407-11.
33. Qahtani SA. Acute renal failure and severe rhabdomyolysis in a patient with resistant thrombotic thrombocytopenic purpura. Int J Gen Med. 2011;4:687-9.
34. Ikhlaque N, Chang JC. Thrombotic Microangiopathy presenting as fulminating rhabdomyolysis with multiorgan dysfunction. Hospital Physician. 2003;39(6):51-6.
35. Burrus TM, Mandrekar J, Wijdicks EF, Rabinstein AA. Renal failure and posterior reversible encephalopathy syndrome in patients with thrombotic thrombocytopenic purpura. Arch Neurol. 2010;67:831-4.
36. Bakshi R, Shaikh ZA, Bates VE, Kinkel PR. Thrombotic thrombocytopenic purpura: brain CT and MRI findings in 12 patients. Neurology. 1999;52:1285-8.
37. Vaziri S, Navabi J, Afsharian M, et al. Crimean congo hemorrhagic fever infection simulating thrombotic thrombocytopenic purpura. Indian J Hematol Blood Transfus. 2008;24:35-8.

38. Deepanjali S, Naik RR, Mailankody S, Kalaimani S, Kadhiravan T. Dengue Virus Infection Triggering Thrombotic Thrombocytopenic Purpura in Pregnancy. Am J Trop Med Hyg. 2015;93:1028–30.

39. Ardalan MR, Tubbs RS, Chinikar S, Shoja MM. Crimean-Congo haemorrhagic fever presenting as thrombotic microangiopathy and acute renal failure. Nephrol Dial Transplant. 2006;21:2304–7.

40. Lopes da Silva R. Viral-associated thrombotic microangiopathies. Hematol Oncol Stem Cell Ther. 2011;4(2):51–9.

41. Booth KK, Terrell DR, Vesely SK, George JN. Systemic infections mimicking thrombotic thrombocytopenic purpura. Am J Hematol. 2011;86:743–51.

42. Chang JC, Shipstone A, Llenado-Lee MA. Postoperative thrombotic thrombocytopenic purpura following cardiovascular surgeries. Am J Hematol. 1996;53:11–7.

43. Naqvi TA, Baumann MA, Chang JC. Post-operative thrombotic thrombocytopenic purpura: a review. Int J Clin Pract. 2004;58:169–72.

44. Venkata C, Kashyap R, Farmer JC, Afessa B. Thrombocytopenia in adult patients with sepsis: incidence, risk factors, and its association with clinical outcome. J Intensive Care. 2013;1:9.

45. Tsirigotis P, Chondropoulos S, Frantzeskaki F, et al. Thrombocytopenia in critically ill patients with severe sepsis/septic shock: Prognostic value and association with a distinct serum cytokine profile. J Crit Care. 2016;32:9–15.

46. Kutcher ME, Redick BJ, McCreery RC, et al. Characterization of platelet dysfunction after trauma. J Trauma Acute Care Surg. 2012;73:13–9.

47. Shamseddine A, Chehal A, Usta I, Salem Z, El-Saghir N, Taher A. Thrombotic thrombocytopenic purpura and pregnancy: report of four cases and literature review. J Clin Apher. 2004;19:5–10.

48. Nguyen TC, Carcillo JA. Bench-to-bedside review: thrombocytopenia-associated multiple organ failure–a newly appreciated syndrome in the critically ill. Crit Care. 2006;10:235.

49. Stravitz RT, Ellerbe C, Durkalski V, Reuben A, Lisman T, Lee WM. Acute liver failure study group. Thromobcytopenia is associated with multi-organ system failure in patients with acute liver failure. Clin Gastroenterol Hepatol. 2016;14:613–20.

50. Nydam TL, Kashuk JL, Moore EE, et al. Refractory post-injury thrombocytopenia is associated with multiple organ failure and adverse outcomes. J Trauma 2011;70:401–406; discussion 406–7.

51. Lambris JD, Ricklin D, Geisbrecht BV. Complement evasion by human pathogens. Nat Rev Microbiol. 2008;6:132–42.

52. Markiewski MM, DeAngelis RA, Lambris JD. Complexity of complement activation in sepsis. J Cell Mol Med. 2008;12:2245–54.

53. Kerr H, Richards A. Complement-mediated injury and protection of endothelium: lessons from atypical haemolytic uraemic syndrome. Immunobiology. 2012;217:195–203.

54. Davies A, Lachmann PJ. Membrane defence against complement lysis: the structure and biological properties of CD59. Immunol Res. 1993;12:258–75.

55. Gene Cards. CD59 gene. http://www.genecards.org/cgi-bin/carddisp.pl?gene=CD59

56. Levi M, Löwenberg EC. Thrombocytopenia in critically ill patients. Semin Thromb Hemost. 2008;34:417–24.

57. Mollnes TE, Fosse E. The complement system in trauma-related and ischemic tissue damage: a brief review. Shock. 1994;2:301–10.

58. Gilbert JS, Banek CT, Katz VL, Babcock SA, Regal JF. Complement activation in pregnancy: too much of a good thing? Hypertension. 2012;60:1114–6.

59. Bruins P, te Velthuis H, Yazdanbakhsh AP, et al. Activation of the complement system during and after cardiopulmonary bypass surgery: postsurgery activation involves C-reactive protein and is associated with postoperative arrhythmia. Circulation. 1997;96:3542–8.

60. Baldwin WM, Ota H, Rodriguez ER. Complement in transplant rejection: diagnostic and mechanistic considerations. Springer Semin Immunopathol. 2003;25:181–97.

61. Afshar-Kharghan V. The role of the complement system in cancer. J Clin Invest. 2017;127:780–9.

62. Ostrowski SR, Haase N, Müller RB, et al. Association between biomarkers of endothelial injury and hypocoagulability in patients with severe sepsis: a prospective study. Crit Care. 2015;19:191.

63. Zhang C. The role of inflammatory cytokines in endothelial dysfunction. Basic Res Cardiol. 2008;103:398–406.

64. van Ierssel SH, Jorens PG, Van Craenenbroeck EM, Conraads VM. The endothelium, a protagonist in the pathophysiology of critical illness: focus on cellular markers. Biomed Res Int. 2014;2014:985813.

65. Aird WC. The role of the endothelium in severe sepsis and multiple organ dysfunction syndrome. Blood. 2003;101:3765–77.

66. Xing K, Murthy S, Liles WC, Singh JM. Clinical utility of biomarkers of endothelial activation in sepsis–a systematic review. Crit Care. 2012;16:R7.

67. van den Born BJ, Löwenberg EC, van der Hoeven NV, de Laat B, Meijers JC, Levi M, van Montfrans GA. Endothelial dysfunction, platelet activation, thrombogenesis and fibrinolysis in patients with hypertensive crisis. J Hypertens. 2011;29:922–7.

68. Bockmeyer CL, Claus RA, Budde U, et al. Inflammation-associated ADAMTS13 deficiency promotes formation of ultra-large von Willebrand factor. Haematologica. 2008;93:137–40.

69. Valentijn KM, van Driel LF, Mourik MJ, et al. Multigranular exocytosis of Weibel-Palade bodies in vascular endothelial cells. Blood. 2010;116:1807–16.

70. Bernardo A, Ball C, Nolasco L, Choi H, Moake JL, Dong JF. Platelets adhered to endothelial cell-bound ultra-large von Willebrand factor strings support leukocyte tethering and rolling under high shear stress. J Thromb Haemost. 2005;3:562–70.

71. Peyvandi F, Garagiola I, Baronciani L. Role of von Willebrand factor in the haemostasis. Blood Transfus. 2011;9(Suppl 2):s3–8.

72. Stockschlaeder M, Schneppenheim R, Budde U. Update on von Willebrand factor multimers: focus on high-molecular-weight multimers and their role in hemostasis. Blood Coagul Fibrinolysis. 2014;25:206–16.

73. Dhanesha N, Prakash P, Doddapattar P, et al. Endothelial Cell-Derived von Willebrand Factor Is the Major Determinant That Mediates von Willebrand Factor-Dependent Acute Ischemic Stroke by Promoting Postischemic Thrombo-Inflammation. Arterioscler Thromb Vasc Biol 2016. 36:1829–37.

74. Verhenne S, Denorme F, Libbrecht S, et al. Platelet-derived VWF is not essential for normal thrombosis and hemostasis but fosters ischemic stroke injury in mice. Blood. 2015;126:1715–22.

75. Crawley JT, Scully MA. Thrombotic thrombocytopenic purpura: basic pathophysiology and therapeutic strategies. Hematology Am Soc Hematol Educ Program. 2013;2013:292–9.

76. Nguyen TC, Liu A, Liu L, et al. Acquired ADAMTS-13 deficiency in pediatric patients with severe sepsis. Haematologica. 2007;92:121–4.

77. Feng S, Eyler SJ, Zhang Y, et al. Partial ADAMTS13 deficiency in atypical hemolytic uremic syndrome. Blood. 2013;122:1487–93.

78. Pourrat O, Coudroy R, Pierre F. ADAMTS13 deficiency in severe postpartum HELLP syndrome. Br J Haematol. 2013;163:409–10.

79. Gandhi C, Motto DG, Jensen M, Lentz SR, Chauhan AK. ADAMTS13 deficiency exacerbates VWF-dependent acute myocardial ischemia/reperfusion injury in mice. Blood. 2012;120:5224–30.

80. Fujioka M, Hayakawa K, Mishima K, et al. ADAMTS13 gene deletion aggravates ischemic brain damage: a possible neuroprotective role of ADAMTS13 by ameliorating postischemic hypoperfusion. Blood. 2010;115:1650–3.

81. Yu WL, Leung T, Soo Y, Lee J, Wong KS. Thrombotic thrombocytopenic purpura with concomitant small- and large-vessel thrombosis, atypical posterior reversible encephalopathy syndrome and cerebral microbleeds. Oxf Med Case Reports. 2015;2015:179–82.

82. Ibernon M, Moreso F, Carreras L, et al. Thrombotic thrombocytopenic purpura with severe large artery branch involvement. Nephrol Dial Transplant. 2005;20:467–8.

83. Obrig TG, Louise CB, Lingwood CA, Boyd B, Barley-Maloney L, Daniel TO. Endothelial heterogeneity in Shiga toxin receptors and responses. J Biol Chem. 1993;268:15484–8.

84. Nolan DJ, Ginsberg M, Israely E, et al. Molecular signatures of tissue-specific microvascular endothelial cell heterogeneity in organ maintenance and regeneration. Dev Cell. 2013;26:204–19.

85. Aird WC. Endothelial Cell Heterogeneity. Cold Spring Harb Perspect Med. 2012;2:a006429.

86. Proulx F, Seidman EG, Karpman D. Pathogenesis of Shiga toxin-associated hemolytic uremic syndrome. Pediatr Res. 2001;50:163–71.

87. Cooperberg AA. Acute promyelocytic leukemia. Can Med Assoc J. 1967;97:57–63.

88. Dunoyer-Geindre S, Rivier-Cordey AS, Tsopra O, Lecompte T, Kruithof EKO. Effect of ATRA and ATO on the expression of tissue factor in NB4 acute promyelocytic leukemia cells and regulatory function of the inflammatory cytokines TNF and IL-1β. Ann Hematol. 2017;96:905–17.

89. Levi M, van der Poll T. A short contemporary history of disseminated intravascular coagulation. Semin Thromb Hemost. 2014;40:874–80.

90. McKay DG. Progress in disseminated intravascular coagulation. Calif Med. 1969;111:186–198 contd.

91. McKay DG. Progress in disseminated intravascular coagulation part II. Calif Med. 1969;111:279–90.

92. Sueishi K, Takeuchi M. Pathology of disseminated intravascular coagulation. Nihon Rinsho. 1993;51:30–6.

93. Gando S, Levi M, Toh CH. Disseminated intravascular coagulation. Nat Rev Dis Primers. 2016;2:16037.

94. Boral BM, Williams DJ, Boral LI. Disseminated Intravascular Coagulation. Am J Clin Pathol. 2016;146:670–80.

95. Wu Y, Luo L, Niu T, et al. Evaluation of the new Chinese Disseminated Intravascular Coagulation Scoring System in critically ill patients: A multicenter prospective study. Sci Rep. 2017;7:9057.

96. Toh CH, Alhamdi Y, Abrams ST. Current Pathological and Laboratory Considerations in the Diagnosis of Disseminated Intravascular Coagulation. Ann Lab Med. 2016;36:505–12.

97. Levi M, Scully M. How I treat disseminated intravascular coagulation. Blood. 2018;131:845–54.

98. Kotiah SD. Besa EC. Acute promyelocytic leukemia clinical presentation. http://emedicine.medscape.com/article/1495306-clinical

99. Chang JC, Gross HM, Jang NS. Disseminated intravascular coagulation due to intravenous administration of hetastarch. Am J Med Sci. 1990;300:301–3.

100. He B, Hu S, Qiu G, Gu W. Clinical characteristics of acute promyelocytic leukemia manifesting as early death. Mol Clin Oncol. 2013;1:908–10.

101. Daver N, Kantarjian H, Marcucci G, et al. Clinical characteristics and outcomes in patients with acute promyelocytic leukaemia and hyperleucocytosis. Br J Haematol. 2015;168:646–53.

102. Kaneko T, Wada H. Diagnostic criteria and laboratory tests for disseminated intravascular coagulation. J Clin Exp Hematop. 2011;5:67–76.

103. Slofstra SH, Spek CA, ten Cate H. Disseminated intravascular coagulation. Hematol J. 2003;4:295–302.

104. Franchini M, Lippi G, Manzato F. Recent acquisitions in the pathophysiology, diagnosis and treatment of disseminated intravascular coagulation. Thromb J. 2006;4:4.

105. Chen VM, Hogg PJ. Encryption and decryption of tissue factor. J Thromb Haemost. 2013;11(Suppl 1):277–84.

106. Versteeg HH, Ruf W. Thiol pathways in the regulation of tissue factor prothrombotic activity. Curr Opin Hematol. 2011;18:343–8.

107. Rauch U, Bonderman D, Bohrmann B, et al. Transfer of tissue factor from leukocytes to platelets is mediated by CD15 and tissue factor. Blood. 2000;96:170–5.

108. Esmon CT. The interactions between inflammation and coagulation. Br J Haematol. 2005;131:417–30.

109. Petäjä J. Inflammation and coagulation. An overview. Thromb Res. 2011; 127(Suppl 2):S34–7.

110. Demetz G, Ott I. The Interface between Inflammation and Coagulation in Cardiovascular Disease. Int J Inflam. 2012;2012:860301.

111. Levi M, van der Poll T. Inflammation and coagulation. Crit Care Med. 2010;38(2 Suppl):S26–34.

112. Taylor FB Jr, Wada H, Kinasewitz G. Description of compensated and uncompensated disseminated intravascular coagulation (DIC) responses (non-overt and overt DIC) in baboon models of intravenous and intraperitoneal Escherichia coli sepsis and in the human model of endotoxemia: toward a better definition of DIC. Crit Care Med. 2000;28(9 Suppl):S12–9.

113. Taylor FB Jr, Kinasewitz GT. The diagnosis and management of disseminated intravascular coagulation. Curr Hematol Rep. 2002;1:34–40.

114. Fourrier F. Severe sepsis, coagulation, and fibrinolysis: dead end or one way? Crit Care Med. 2012;40:2704–8.

115. Marshall JC. Why have clinical trials in sepsis failed? Trends Mol Med. 2014; 20:195–203.

116. Kularatne SA, Imbulpitiya IV, Abeysekera RA, Waduge RN, Rajapakse RP, Weerakoon KG. Extensive haemorrhagic necrosis of liver is an unpredictable fatal complication in dengue infection: a postmortem study. BMC Infect Dis. 2014;14:141.

117. Talwani R, Gilliam BL, Howell C. Infectious diseases and the liver. Clin Liver Dis. 2011;15:111–30.

118. Samanta J, Sharma V. Dengue and its effects on liver. World J Clin Cases. 2015;3:125–31.

119. El Sayed SM, Abdelrahman AA, Ozbak HA, et al. Updates in diagnosis and management of Ebola hemorrhagic fever. J Res Med Sci. 2016;21:84.

120. Mammen EF. Coagulation abnormalities in liver disease. Hematol Oncol Clin North Am. 1992;6:1247–57.

121. Uemura M, Fujimura Y, Ko S, Matsumoto M, Nakajima Y, Fukui H. Determination of ADAMTS13 and Its Clinical Significance for ADAMTS13 Supplementation Therapy to Improve the Survival of Patients with Decompensated Liver Cirrhosis. Int J Hepatol. 2011;2011:759047.

122. van Dongen PW, Eskes TK, Gimbrère JS, Snel P. Maternal mortality due to the hepatorenal syndrome of pre-eclampsia. A case report. Eur J Obstet Gynecol Reprod Biol. 1979;9:299–306.

123. Isler CM, Rinehart BK, Terrone DA, May WL, Magann EF, Martin JN Jr. The importance of parity to major maternal morbidity in the eclamptic mother with HELLP syndrome. Hypertens Pregnancy. 2003;22:287–94.

124. Agarwal B, Wright G, Gatt A, Riddell A, Vemala V, Mallett S, Chowdary P, Davenport A, Jalan R, Burroughs A. Evaluation of coagulation abnormalities in acute liver failure. J Hepatol. 2012;57:780–6.

125. Senzolo M, Burra P, Cholongitas E, Burroughs AK. New insights into the coagulopathy of liver disease and liver transplantation. World J Gastroenterol. 2006;12:7725–36.

126. Malla K, Malla T, Hanif M. Prognostic indicators in haemolytic uraemic syndrome. Kathmandu Univ Med J (KUMJ). 2004;2:291–6.

127. Tsai MH, Peng YS, Chen YC, et al. Adrenal insufficiency in patients with cirrhosis, severe sepsis and septic shock. Hepatology. 2006;43:673–81128.

128. Franchini M, Manzato F, Salvagno GL, Lippi G. Potential role of recombinant activated factor VII for the treatment of severe bleeding associated with disseminated intravascular coagulation: a systematic review. Blood Coagul Fibrinolysis. 2007;18:589–93.

129. Román E, Mendizábal S, Jarque I, et al. Secondary thrombotic microangiopathy and eculizumab: A reasonable therapeutic option. Nefrologia. 2017;37:478–91.

130. Brocklebank V, Kavanagh D. Complement C5-inhibiting therapy for the thrombotic microangiopathies: accumulating evidence, but not a panacea. Clin Kidney J. 2017;10:600–24.

131. Nangaku M, Alpers CE, Pippin J. CD59 protects glomerular endothelial cells from immune-mediated thrombotic microangiopathy in rats. J Am Soc Nephrol. 1998;9:590–7.

24

Detecting clinically relevant rivaroxaban or dabigatran levels by routine coagulation tests or thromboelastography in a cohort of patients with atrial fibrillation

Yvonne M. C. Henskens[1], Anouk J. W. Gulpen[2,4]* iD, René van Oerle[1,2], Rick Wetzels[1], Paul Verhezen[1], Henri Spronk[2], Simon Schalla[3], Harry J. Crijns[3], Hugo ten Cate[2,4] and Arina ten Cate-Hoek[1,5]

Abstract

Background: Traditional coagulation tests are included in emergency guidelines for management of patients on direct oral anticoagulants (DOACs) who experience acute bleeding or require surgery. We determined the ability of traditional coagulation tests and fast whole blood thromboelastography (ROTEM®) to screen for anticoagulation activity of dabigatran and rivaroxaban as low as 30 ng/mL.

Methods: One hundred eighty-four citrated blood samples (75 dabigatran, 109 rivaroxaban) were collected from patients with non-valvular atrial fibrillation (NVAF), to perform screening tests from different manufacturers, (diluted, D) PT, aPTT, TT and ROTEM®. The activity of DOACs was quantitatively determined by clot detection assays: Hemoclot DTT and DiXal test (Biophen), on CS2100 (Siemens). The clotting time (CT) of INTEM and EXTEM ROTEM® (Werfen) were used as test parameters.

Results: Dabigatran, $\geq$ 30 ng/mL, was accurately detected by five coagulation tests: APTT Actin FSL (93%), PT Neoplastin (93%), APTT Cephascreen, Thromboclotin, and Thrombin (all 100%), but not by PT Innovin (49%). CT-EXTEM (91%) was sufficiently sensitive, but not CT-INTEM (52%). APTT Cephascreen and Thrombin showed good linearity ($R^2 = 0.71, R^2 = 0.72$). For the other tests linearity was moderate to poor. Rivaroxaban was accurately detected by PT Neoplastin (98%) and less so by APTT Cephascreen (85%). In addition, rivaroxaban was also accurately detected by CT-INTEM (96%). PT Neoplastin showed good linearity ($R^2 = 0.81$), all other tests had moderate to poor linearity.

Conclusion: In patients with NVAF, the ability of routine coagulation tests to detect the presence of significant levels of DOACs is test and reagent dependent. CT-INTEM and CT-EXTEM may be fast whole blood alternatives.

Keywords: Dabigatran, Rivaroxaban, Routine coagulation tests, Pt, aPTT, Tt, ROTEM®, Drug concentration (diltPT, antiXa activity)

* Correspondence: anouk.gulpen@mumc.nl
[2]Laboratory for Clinical Thrombosis and Hemostasis, Internal medicine, CARIM, Maastricht, The Netherlands
[4]Internal medicine, MUMC+, Maastricht, The Netherlands
Full list of author information is available at the end of the article

Background

For more than 60 years vitamin K antagonists (VKA) were the drugs of choice to prevent thrombosis in patients with NVAF and mechanical heart valves, as well as to treat and prevent recurrence of thrombosis in patients with venous thromboembolism (VTE).

The management of patients on anticoagulant therapy was guided by laboratory testing of prothrombin time (PT), which was internationally harmonized by the ISI factor resulting in (international normalized ratio) INR, an easily interpretable laboratory test [1]. With the introduction of direct oral anticoagulants it was emphasized that no routine laboratory testing would be needed [2–7]. However, in emergency situations the need for testing remains since residual activity of the anticoagulant treatment might introduce e.g. bleeding during surgery. Screening tests for detecting anticoagulants, which can be performed 24 h a day instead of just during working hours should therefore be available to guide treatment decisions. The concentration below 30 ng/mL is proposed as a safe-for surgical treatment threshold [8]. Thereby, this concentration is sufficient to administer antidote against DOAC if needed [9].

Activity-based drug levels in plasma can be determined but are not obtainable in all care settings [10]. Traditional routine coagulation tests are widely available and may be used for first line testing in emergency situations [11–15]. In many countries regional guidelines have been issued upon the introduction of the DOACs indicating the preferred strategies of action for both the prescription and (laboratory) management of these drugs [16–18]. These guidelines do indicate that the thrombin time (TT) is the most sensitive routine coagulation assay for detection of dabigatran and that the PT is the most sensitive routine coagulation assay for detection of rivaroxaban. Guidelines do however not (sufficiently) report on the sensitivity of the different individual TT, PT and activated partial thromboplastin Time (aPTT) tests that are commercially available. This may be due to the fact that most of these guidelines were based on laboratory data using plasma spiked with DOAC instead of samples acquired from patients using the drugs.

We therefore set out to evaluate two proposed screening algorithms [16, 18] and at the same time validate seven different routine anticoagulation tests for screening of plasma drug activity in daily practice, using plasma samples from a cohort of patients on dabigatran and rivaroxaban. In addition we evaluated ROTEM® for the same purpose in whole blood in a subsample of the study population [19].

Methods

Patients

This analysis comprises the first 76 non-valvular Atrial Fibrillation (NVAF) patients (30 on dabigatran, 46 on rivaroxaban) that were structurally followed in an observational DOAC study in the Maastricht University Medical Center (MUMC+), the Netherlands. The study is ongoing.

Study population

All patients came from a single institution, the anticoagulation clinic Maastricht, and were referred by cardiologists of the MUMC. Patients were followed in an observational cohort study, which started January 2012 and is still ongoing. The Institutional Review Board of the MUMC approved the study (December 2011, project number 114069). All patients enrolled in the follow-up signed informed consent. All consecutive patients with NVAF and a $CHADS_2$ score ≥ 2 who were initiated on a DOAC were eligible for inclusion in the study.

Study design

This laboratory study is part of a prospective observational cohort study. Patients were invited to a special structured nurse-based office visit at the anticoagulation clinic. All patients were followed for 1 year, during which 5 visits were planned (at start of DOAC therapy, 1 month after start DOAC, 3 months, 6 months and 12 months). Important parameters recorded during these visits were: thrombotic events and bleeding complications, side effects of medication, compliance to medication, intermittent illness and/or hospital admissions and renal function. Renal function was assessed at 4 points in time; additional blood for testing of a panel of laboratory tests was drawn. The panel of laboratory tests consisted of: APTT Actin FSL (Siemens), APTT Cephascreen (Stago), PT Innovin (Siemens), PT neoplastin (Stago), Diluted PT (DPT) Innovin (Siemens), TT Thromboclotin (Siemens), TT Thrombin (Stago), CT INTEM (ROTEM®), and CT EXTEM (ROTEM®, Werfen). Diluted TT Hemoclot (Biophen) was set as gold standard for the detection of dabigatran and anti Xa activity DiXal (Biophen) for the detection of rivaroxaban. For this paper clinical details are not presented because the blood samples were purely used for laboratory validation.

Blood sampling and laboratory measurements

Blood was taken by antecubital venipuncture and collected into 3,2% citrated vacutainer® tubes using a 21 gauche eclipse signal blood collection needle (BD vacutainer®), sampling was standardized and timed between 9 and 11 a.m.

Plasma was obtained after centrifugation for 10 min at 2000 g at room temperature. Plasma samples were frozen at −80 °C and thawed in a standard procedure before coagulation testing. PT and DPT Innovin, APTT Actin FSL, TT Thromboclotin and diluted TT Hemoclot

Table 1 Overview of screening tests, analysers and cut-off values used in this study

	Reagent	Analyser	Firm	Cutt-off
PT	Innovin	CS2100	Siemens	12 s
PT	Neoplastin	STA-R	Stago	15 s
aPTT	Actin FSL	CS2100	Siemens	32 s
aPTT	Cephascreen	STA-R	Stago	32 s
TT	Thromboclotin	CS2100	Siemens	25 s
TT	Thrombin	STA-R	Stago	25 s
CT	INTEM (Tem)	ROTEM	Siemens	195 s
CT	EXTEM (Tem)	ROTEM	Stago	60 s
Diluted TT	Hemoclot	CS2100	Hyphen	30 ng/mL
Anti-Xa activity	DiXaI	CS2100	Hyphen	30 ng/mL

APTT Activated partial thrombin time, *PT* Phrothrombin time, *TT* Thrombin time, *CT* Closure time, *Sec* Seconds

as well as Anti-Xa activity were performed on a CS2100 analyzer (Siemens). PT Neoplastin, APTT Cephascreen, TT Thrombin were performed on a STA-R analyzer (Stago), Whole blood was used for ROTEM® analyses. Table 1 summarizes the different methods. The cut-off for a clinical relevant detection limit was set at ≥30 ng/mL for both rivaroxaban and dabigatran as determined as anticoagulation activity by the diluted TT Hemoclot and DiXaI test (both Biophen) on CS2100 using dabigatran and rivaroxaban as calibrators.

Statistics
The statistical package of Graph Pad® (version 6) was used for statistical analysis. Correlations were analyzed by linear regression analysis and slope, intercept and R^2 were determined and presented. For the sensitivity the cut-off for detection for all routine laboratory tests was set at 30 ng/mL for both dabigatran and rivaroxaban. Sensitivity and specificity were calculated using a diagnostic test evaluation calculator (MedCalc®).

Results
In total 184 citrated blood samples (75 dabigatran samples and 109 rivaroxaban samples) were collected. Dabigatran activity in a steady state situation, determined by diluted TT Hemoclot varied considerably between patients: Mean $_{geometric}$ 104 (± 53) ng/mL. Rivaroxaban activity determined by DiXaI test showed similar variability, mean $_{geometric}$ 187 (± 139) ng/mL. Clinical relevant dabigatran activity (≥ 30 ng/mL) was detected accurately by both thrombin time assays: TT Thromboclotin (100%), and TT Thrombin (100%). In addition good sensitivity was reached for four other coagulation tests in the panel: APTT Actin FSL (93%), APTT Cephascreen (100%), PT Neoplastin (93%), but not for PT Innovin (49%). Also CT-EXTEM of ROTEM® (91%) was sufficiently sensitive, but not CT-INTEM (52%). (Table 2).

APTT Cephascreen and TT Thrombin showed good linearity (R^2 = 0.71 and R^2 = 0.72). For the other tests linearity was moderate to poor (APTT Actin FSL (R^2 = 0.59), PT Neoplastin (R^2 = 0.19), Thromboclotin (R^2 = 0.18), and PT Innovin (R^2 = 0.09). All correlations were highly significant (all <0.0001 and 0.0046 for PT Innovin; Fig. 1, Fig. 3).

Rivaroxaban activity was only accurately detected by two tests in the panel (PT Neoplastin (98%), and less so by APTT Cephascreen (85%). In addition Rivaroxaban activity was also accurately detected by CT intem of ROTEM® (96%). PT Innovin was not sufficiently sensitive (68%). PT Neoplastin showed good linearity across concentrations (R^2 = 0.81). All other tests had moderate to poor linearity; APTT Cephascreen (R^2 = 0.55), APTT Actin FSL (R^2 = 0.53), and ROTEM® CT-EXTEM (R^2 = 0.58). All correlations were significant (<0.0001). (Fig. 2, Fig. 3).

Discussion
The main findings of the present study are that in patients with NVAF, the ability of routine coagulation tests to detect the presence of significant levels of dabigatran or rivaroxaban is test and reagent dependent. Therefore,

Table 2 Sensitivity and specificity, PPV and NPV of a panel of coagulation tests for detecting > = 30 ng/mL dabigatran or rivaroxaban and correlation with the calibrated activity measurement of dabigatran or rivaroxaban

Detection ≥30 ng/mL	Dabigatran					Rivaroxaban				
	Sensitivity	Specificity	PPV	NPV	R^2	Sensitivity	Specificity	PPV	NPV	R^2
APTT Actin FSL	93	67	92	78	0.59	67	81	95	30	0.53
APTT Cephascreen	100	28	85	100	0.71	85	62	93	42	0.55
PT neoplastin	93	39	86	58	0.19	98	24	88	63	0.81
PT Innovin	49	78	90	27	0.09	68	67	92	27	0.26
TT Thrombin clotin	100	33	86	100	0.18	–	–	–	–	–
TT Thrombin	100	39	86	100	0.72	–	–	–	–	–
CT-INTEM ROTEM®	52	50	86	15	0.63	77	80	95	36	0.69
CT-EXTEM ROTEM®	91	75	86	15	0.51	96	75	96	75	0.58

PPV Positive predictive value, *NPV* Negative predictive value, *APTT* Activated partial thrombin time, *PT* Prothrombin time, *TT* Thrombin time, *CT* Closure time

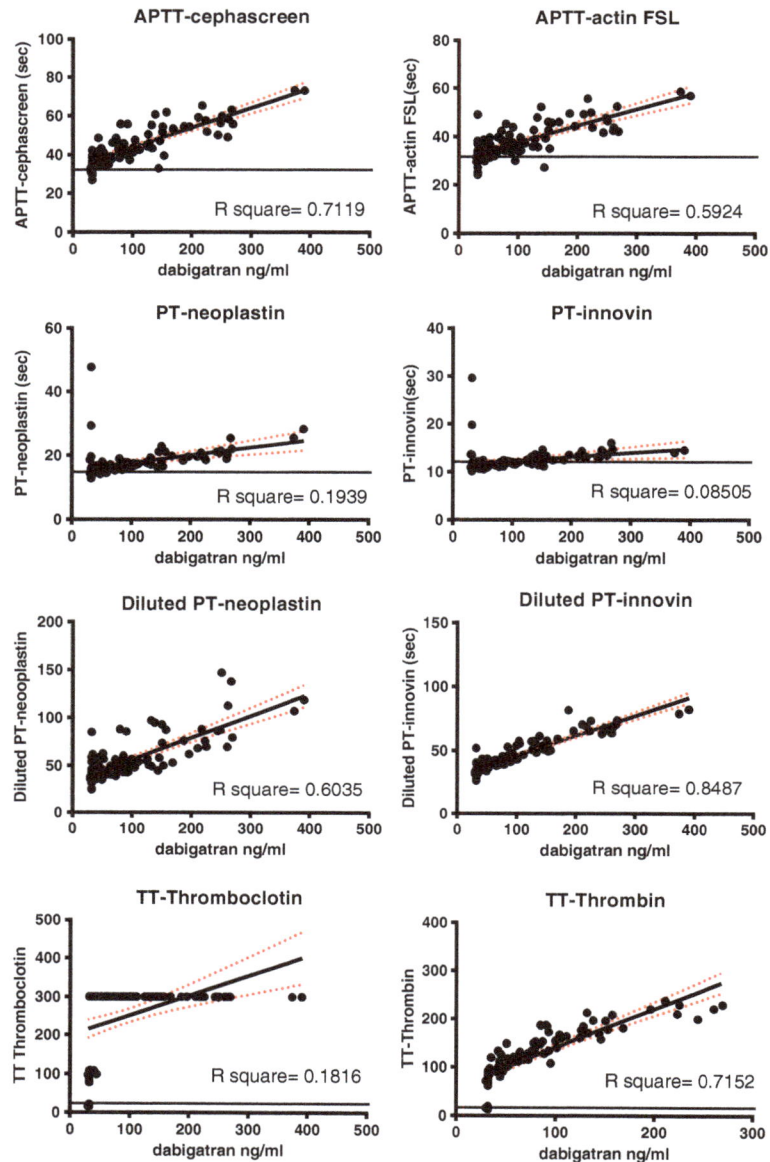

Fig. 1 Correlations for dabigatran activity determined by diluted TT Hemoclot and the panel of coagulation assays in 75 samples from patients using dabigatran. The dotted red lines represent the standard error

emergency care protocols should ensure that local test reagents are sufficiently accurate for detecting the presence of DOACs. Otherwise, the CT-INTEM and CT-EXTEM of ROTEM® may be good and fast whole blood alternatives that may be readily available on site.

In emergency situations it is crucial that routine coagulation tests are clinically validated and that the test sensitivity for the detection of minimal and clinically important levels of anticoagulation is known. In patients with serious bleeding or requiring urgent intervention with bleeding risk, a drug concentration > 30 ng/mL is proposed as clinical relevant and sufficient to administer antidote against

DOAC [9]. Emergency coagulation testing according to suggested algorithms is usually dependent on whether knowledge of the actual intake and the timing of ingestion of DOAC is available or not. If the DOAC taken by the patient is indeed known, one may choose the most appropriate test for the drug: for dabigatran the most appropriate screening test is stated to be the TT[15]. If the TT is not prolonged, the presence of dabigatran can be completely excluded. The PT is the most appropriate screening test for rivaroxaban; for most PT reagents a normal PT implies that clinical relevant concentrations of rivaroxaban can be excluded [15]. According to current

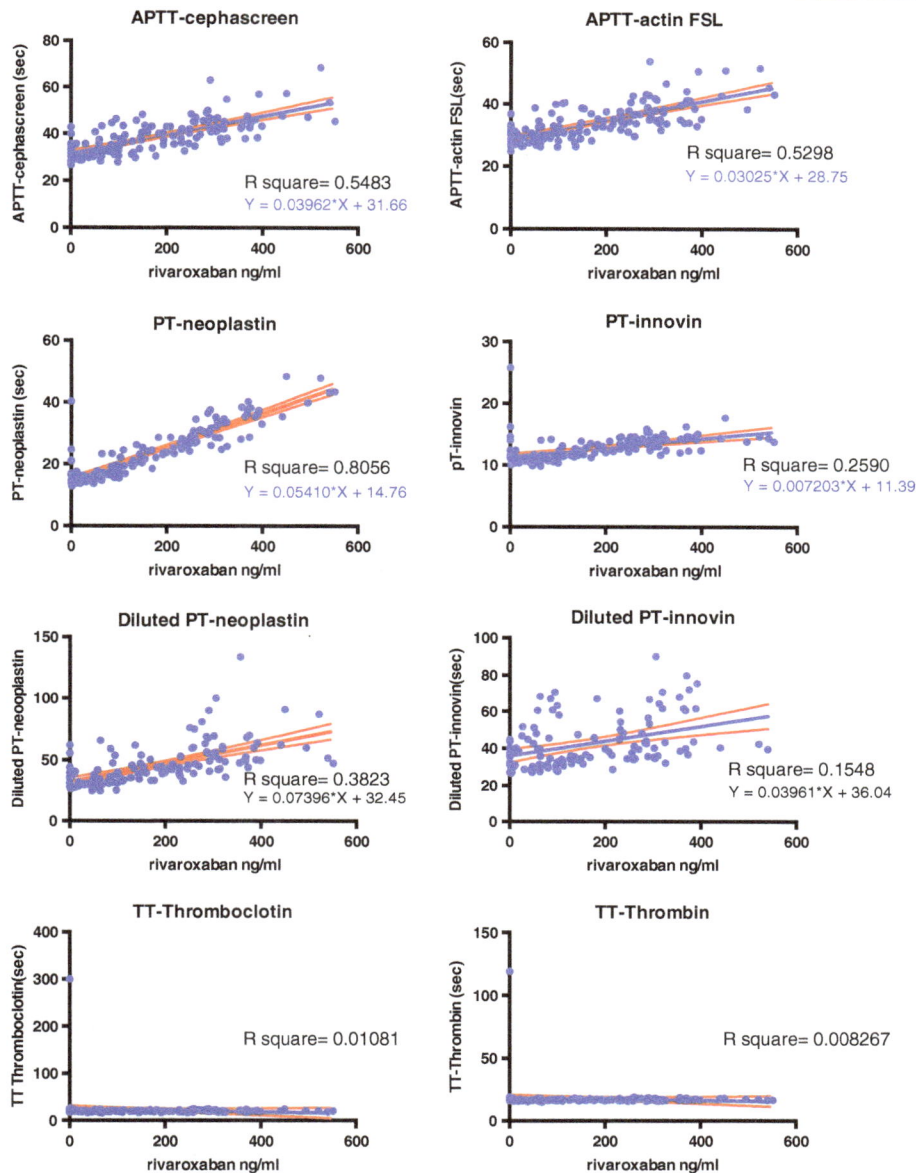

Fig. 2 Correlations for rivaroxaban activity determined by DaXa activity for the panel of coagulationassays 109 samples from patients using rivaroxaban

guidelines, a panel of conventional coagulation tests (aPTT, PT and TT) should be used in case of intake of an unknown DOAC, to thereby exclude relevant drug levels for either dabigatran or rivaroxaban. In addition, for other DOACs such as apixaban or edoxaban, calibrated drug specific anti-Xa levels still need to be measured; screening tests are not yet available [20, 21].

However, whether the suggested algorithms are actually feasible in real life situations has not been tested yet. APTT, PT and TT are both widely and rapidly available in emergency situations, but one should be careful with the interpretation of these tests [22–25]. One needs to realize that these standard coagulation tests with low

screening sensitivity might lead to a false reassurance when indicating absent drug levels. In our cohort both TT tests were able to pick up clinically relevant levels of dabigatran (≥30 ng/mL). In case of rivaroxaban however, there was a marked difference in sensitivity between the two PT tests used: PT neoplastin had a sensitivity of 97.5%, PT Innovin expressed a much lower sensitivity of only 67.7%. This may result in a underestimation of drug levels in more than 32% of patients in case PT Innovin is used for screening for active drug levels, while this is much less for PT Neoplastin (<3%). As can be appreciated from the data, most of the before mentioned tests are only useful as in- or exclusion tests (Yes, No). It

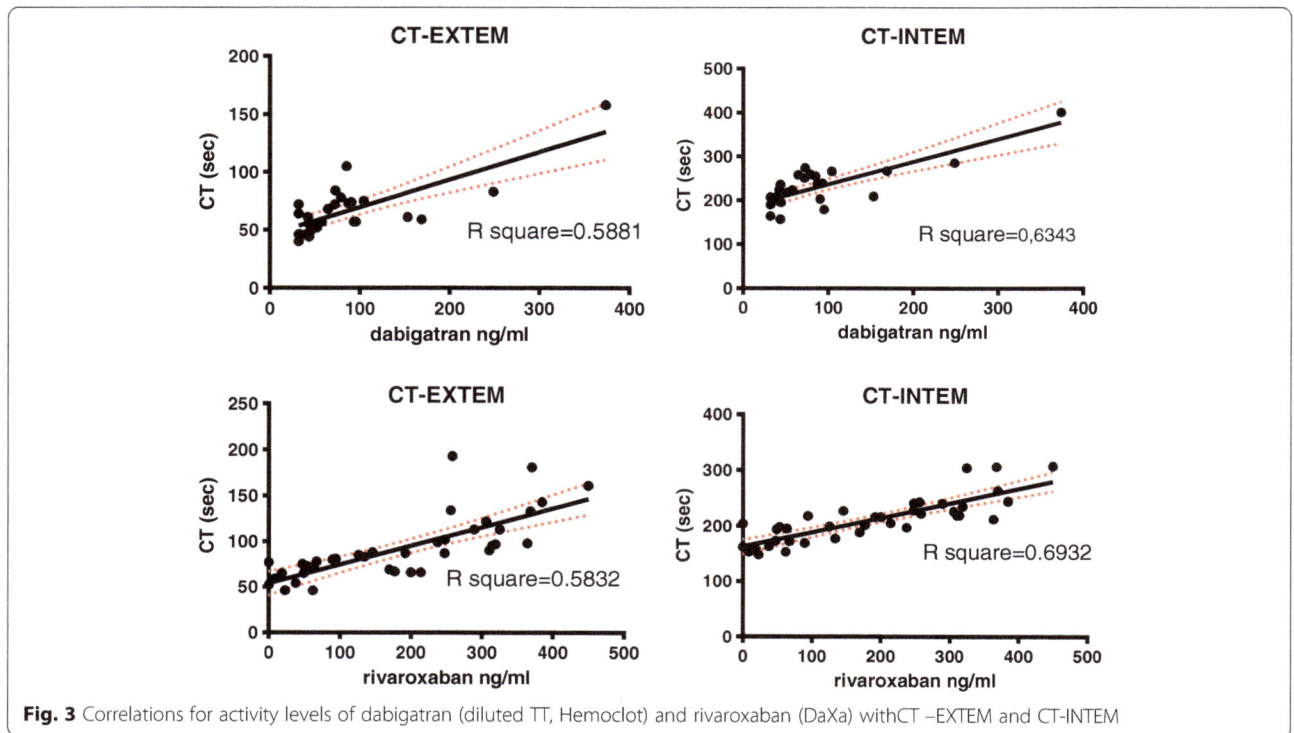

Fig. 3 Correlations for activity levels of dabigatran (diluted TT, Hemoclot) and rivaroxaban (DaXa) withCT –EXTEM and CT-INTEM

would be a great advantage if also actual drug levels could be predicted form the result of a test in an emergency situation. Therefore, the correlations between drug levels and the panel of routine coagulation tests were also assessed. For dabigatran APTT Cephascreen and Thrombin were both sensitive and accurate. For rivaroxaban only PT Neoplastin was both sensitive and level predictive. Moreover, rapid measurement of DOAC plasma concentration levels have become available and might therefore also feasible for use in emergency situations [26]. Their role in the algorithms should be evaluated in the near future. For all laboratory tests applies that handling of samples by laboratory technicians is mandatory. This is time consuming and may impact swift and adequate interventions in an emergency setting. A point of care test for which whole blood can be used would improve the decision making process.

The CT-EXTEM showed good sensitivity for both rivaroxaban and dabigatran, its linearity is however moderate. Our results differ from previous studies where ROTEM® was able to show a dose dependent increase in DOAC levels in spiked whole blood samples, but poorly performed at low DOAC levels [27]. Our study showed that the 'real life' sensitivity of ROTEM® is better in patients using DOAC and might therefore be a good candidate for emergency testing. The added advantage of ROTEM® testing is that the results are readily available (< 5 min) and there is uniform performance with worldwide standardization. ROTEM® can be used by emergency

personnel or as point of care testing in operating theaters, but also with standard situations in most hospitals laboratories. ROTEM® testing may in addition also offer the possibility of monitoring the use of antidotes.

Our study has some weaknesses: we included a relatively small number of patients and the DOACs used were limited to dabigatran and rivaroxaban, as patients in our cohort did not use apixaban or edoxaban. We furthermore did not use the accepted gold standard test, liquid chromatography with mass spectrometry (LC-MS) for quantification of DOACs [28] although the selected coagulation activity assays correlated well with LC-MS techniques.

Strengths of our study are 1) that real life samples to assess the feasibility of current guidelines on DOAC testing and 2) an extensive panel of 7 different anticoagulation tests in addition to ROTEM® testing was used.

Conclusion

We conclude that guideline proposed screening algorithms are feasible in a real life steady state NVAF population. However, the ability of routine coagulation tests to detect the presence of significant levels of dabigatran or rivaroxaban is extremely test and reagent dependent.

Emergency care protocols should ensure that local test reagents are sufficiently accurate for detecting the presence of DOACs. CT-INTEM and CT-EXTEM of ROTEM® can be considered as effective whole blood alternatives that have the advantage to be readily available on site.

Abbreviations

APTT: Activated Partial Thromboplastin Time; CT: Closure time; DOAC: Direct oral anticoagulants; INR: International Normalized Ratio; LC-MS: Liquid chromatography with mass spectrometry; MUMC +: Maastricht University Medical Center; NVAF: Non-valvular atrial fibrillation; PT: Prothrombin time; TT: Thrombin time; VKA: Vitamin K antagonists; VTE: Venous thromboembolism

Acknowledgements

None

Funding

No funding was obtained for this article.

Authors' contributions

Conceived an designed the study: YMCH, HTC, ATC, SS and HJC. Collected the data: RvO, RW, PV, HS, YMCH, ATC. Wrote the analyses plan and analyzed and interpreted the data: YMCH, ATC. Wrote and corrected the paper: YMCH, AJWG, RvO, RW, PH, HS, SS, HJC, HTC and ATC. All authors read and approved the final manuscript.

Competing interests

HTC is consultant at Stago. The other authors state that they have no conflicts of interests.

Author details

[1]Central Diagnostic Laboratory, Maastricht University Medical Centre (MUMC +), Maastricht, The Netherlands. [2]Laboratory for Clinical Thrombosis and Hemostasis, Internal medicine, CARIM, Maastricht, The Netherlands. [3]Department of Cardiology, Cardiovascular center MUMC+, Maastricht, The Netherlands. [4]Internal medicine, MUMC+, Maastricht, The Netherlands. [5]Thrombosis Expertise Centre, Vascular medicine, Cardiovascular Centre MUMC+, Maastricht, The Netherlands.

References

1. van den Besselaar AM. Standardization of the prothrombin time in oral anticoagulant control. Haemostasis. 1985;15(4):271–7.
2. van Ryn J, Stangier J, Haertter S, et al. Dabigatran etexilate–a novel, reversible, oral direct thrombin inhibitor: interpretation of coagulation assays and reversal of anticoagulant activity. Thromb Haemost. 2010;103(6): 1116–27.
3. Mueck W, Schwers S, Stampfuss J. Rivaroxaban and other novel oral anticoagulants: pharmacokinetics in healthy subjects, specific patient populations and relevance of coagulation monitoring. Thromb J. 2013;11(1):10.
4. Agency EM. Pradaxa [dabigatran etexilate], product information. http://www. ema.europa.eu/docs/en_GB/document_library/EPAR_-_Product_Information/human/000829/WC500041059.pdf. Accessed 28 september 2015.
5. Agency EM. Xarelto [rivaroxaban], product information. http://www.ema. europa.eu/docs/en_GB/document_library/EPAR_-_Product_Information/human/000944/WC500057108.pdf. Accessed 17 July 2015.
6. Agency EM. Eliquis [apixaban], product information. http://www.ema.europa. eu/docs/en_GB/document_library/EPAR_-_Product_Information/human/002148/WC500107728.pdf Accessed 29 October 2015.
7. Agency EM. Lixiana [edoxaban], product information.. http://www.ema. europa.eu/docs/en_GB/document_library/EPAR_-_Product_Information/human/002629/WC500189045.pdf. Accessed 3 July 2015.
8. Ebner M, Birschmann I, Peter A, et al. Point-of-care testing for emergency assessment of coagulation in patients treated with direct oral anticoagulants. Crit Care. 2017;21(1):32.
9. Levy JH, Ageno W, Chan NC, et al. When and how to use antidotes for the reversal of direct oral anticoagulants: guidance from the SSC of the ISTH. J Thromb Haemost. 2016;14(3):623–7.
10. Samuelson BT, Cuker A, Siegal DM, Crowther M, Garcia DA. Laboratory assessment of the anticoagulant activity of direct oral anticoagulants: a systematic review. Chest. 2017;151(1):127–38.
11. Funk DM. Coagulation assays and anticoagulant monitoring. Hematology Am Soc Hematol Educ Program. 2012;2012:460–5.
12. Letertre LR, Gudmundsdottir BR, Francis CW, et al. A single test to assay warfarin, dabigatran, rivaroxaban, apixaban, unfractionated heparin, and enoxaparin in plasma. J Thromb Haemost. 2016;14(5):1043–53.
13. Garcia D, Barrett YC, Ramacciotti E, Weitz JI. Laboratory assessment of the anticoagulant effects of the next generation of oral anticoagulants. J Thromb Haemost. 2013;11(2):245–52.
14. Lind SE, Boyle ME, Fisher S, Ishimoto J, Trujillo TC, Kiser TH. Comparison of the aPTT with alternative tests for monitoring direct thrombin inhibitors in patient samples. Am J Clin Pathol. 2014;141(5):665–74.
15. Baglin T, Keeling D, Kitchen S. British Committee for Standards in H. Effects on routine coagulation screens and assessment of anticoagulant intensity in patients taking oral dabigatran or rivaroxaban: guidance from the British Committee for Standards in Haematology. Br J Haematol. 2012;159(4):427–9.
16. Specialisten. WNvdwveOvM. Leidraad voor begeleide introductie nieuwe orale antistollingsmiddelen. 2012; https://cvgk.nl/2013/01/04/leidraad-begeleide-introductie-noacs/.
17. Salmonson T, Dogne JM, Janssen H, Garcia Burgos J, Blake P. Non-vitamin-K oral anticoagulants and laboratory testing: now and in the future: views from a workshop at the European medicines agency (EMA). Eur Heart J Cardiovasc Pharmacother. 2017;3(1):42–7.
18. Tran H, Joseph J, Young L, et al. New oral anticoagulants: a practical guide on prescription, laboratory testing and peri-procedural/bleeding management. Australasian Society of Thrombosis and Haemostasis. Intern Med J. 2014;44(6):525–36.
19. Adelmann D, Wiegele M, Wohlgemuth RK, et al. Measuring the activity of apixaban and rivaroxaban with rotational thrombelastometry. Thromb Res. 2014;134(4):918–23.
20. Skeppholm M, Al-Aieshy F, Berndtsson M, et al. Clinical evaluation of laboratory methods to monitor apixaban treatment in patients with atrial fibrillation. Thromb Res. 2015;136(1):148–53.
21. Gouin-Thibault I, Flaujac C, Delavenne X, et al. Assessment of apixaban plasma levels by laboratory tests: suitability of three anti-Xa assays. A multicentre French GEHT study. Thromb Haemost. 2014;111(2):240–8.
22. Testa S, Legnani C, Tripodi A, et al. Poor comparability of coagulation screening test with specific measurement in patients receiving direct oral anticoagulants: results from a multicenter/multiplatform study. J Thromb Haemost. 2016;14(11):2194–201.
23. Godier A, Dincq AS, Martin AC, et al. Predictors of pre-procedural concentrations of direct oral anticoagulants: a prospective multicentre study. Eur Heart J. 2017;38(31):2431–9.
24. Lessire S, Douxfils J, Pochet L, et al. Estimation of rivaroxaban plasma concentrations in the perioperative setting in patients with or without heparin bridging. Clin Appl Thromb Hemost. 2016:1076029616675968.
25. Douxfils J, Lessire S, Dincq AS, et al. Estimation of dabigatran plasma concentrations in the perioperative setting. An ex vivo study using dedicated coagulation assays. Thromb Haemost. 2015;113(4):862–9.
26. Seiffge DJ, Traenka C, Polymeris A, et al. Feasibility of rapid measurement of rivaroxaban plasma levels in patients with acute stroke. J Thromb Thrombolysis. 2017;43(1):112–6.
27. Seyve L, Richarme C, Polack B, Marlu R. Impact of four direct oral anticoagulants on rotational thromboelastometry (ROTEM). Int J Lab Hematol. 2017;
28. Gous T, Couchman L, Patel JP, Paradzai C, Arya R, Flanagan RJ. Measurement of the direct oral anticoagulants apixaban, dabigatran, edoxaban, and rivaroxaban in human plasma using turbulent flow liquid chromatography with high-resolution mass spectrometry. Ther Drug Monit. 2014;36(5):597–605.

25

Sickle cell disease, sickle trait and the risk for venous thromboembolism

Jean Jacques Noubiap[1]*, Mazou N. Temgoua[2]†, Ronni Tankeu[2]†, Joel Noutakdie Tochie[3]†, Ambroise Wonkam[4] and Jean Joël Bigna[5,6]

Abstract

Background: Globally, sickle cell disease (SCD) is one of the most common haemoglobinopathy. Considered a public health problem, it leads to vessel occlusion, blood stasis and chronic activation of the coagulation system responsible for vaso-occlussive crises and venous thromboembolism (VTE) which may be fatal. Although contemporary observational studies suggest a relationship between SCD or sickle trait (SCT) and VTE, there is lack of a summary or meta-analysis data on this possible correlation. Hence, we propose to summarize the available evidence on the association between SCD, SCT and VTE including deep vein thrombosis (DVT) and pulmonary embolism (PE).

Methods: We searched PubMed and Scopus to identify all cross-sectional, cohort and case-control studies reporting on the association between SCD or SCT and VTE, DVT or PE in adults or children from inception to April 25, 2017. For measuring association between SCD or SCT and VTE, DVT, or PE, a meta-analysis using the random-effects method was performed to pool weighted odds ratios (OR) of risk estimates.

Results: From 313 records initially identified from bibliographic databases, 10 studies were eligible and therefore included the meta-analysis. SCD patients had significantly higher risk for VTE (pooled OR 4.4, 95%CI 2.6–7.5, $p < 0.001$), DVT (OR 1.1, 95% CI 1.1–1.2, $p < 0.001$) and PE (pooled OR 3.7, 95% CI 3.6–3.8, $p < 0.001$) as compared to non SCD-adults. A higher risk of VTE (OR 33.2, 95% CI 9.7–113.4, $p < 0.001$) and DVT (OR 30.7, 95% CI 1.6–578.2, $p = 0.02$) was found in pregnant or postpartum women with SCD as compared to their counterparts without SCD. Compared to adults with SCT, the risk of VTE was higher in adults with SCD (pooled OR 3.1, 95% CI 1.8–5.3, $p < 0.001$), and specifically in SCD pregnant or postpartum women (OR 20.3, 95% CI 4.1–102, $p = 0.0003$). The risk of PE was also higher in adults with SCD (OR 3.1, 95% CCI 1.7–5.9, $p = 0.0004$) as compared to those with SCT. The risk of VTE was higher in individuals with SCT compared to controls (pooled OR 1.7, 95% CI 1.3–2.2, $p < 0.0001$), but not in pregnant or postpartum women (OR 0.9, 95% CI 0.3–2.9, $p = 0.863$). Compared to controls, SCT was associated with a higher risk of PE (pooled OR 2.1, 95% CI 1.2–3.8, $p = 0.012$) but not of DVT (pooled OR 1.2, 95% CI 0.9–1.7, $p = 0.157$).

Conclusion: Individuals with SCD, especially pregnant or postpartum women, might have a higher risk of VTE compared to the general population. SCT might also increases the risk of VTE. However, currently available data are not sufficient to allow a definite conclusion. Further larger studies are needed to provide a definitive conclusion on the association between SCD, SCT and VTE.

Keywords: Sickle cell disease, Sickle cell anemia, Sickle cell trait, Venous thromboembolism, Pulmonary embolism, Deep vein thrombosis

* Correspondence: noubiapjj@yahoo.fr
†Mazou N. Temgoua, Ronni Tankeu and Joel Noutakdie Tochie contributed equally to this work.
[1]Department of Medicine, Groote Schuur Hospital and University of Cape Town, Cape Town 7925, South Africa
Full list of author information is available at the end of the article

Background

Sickle cell disease (SCD) is one of the most common severe monogenic disorders, affecting 20–25 million people globally [1, 2]. The clinical manifestations and complications of SCD result mainly from vaso-occlusion and/or hemolysis. When deoxygenated, hemoglobin S (HbS) polymerizes to form a fibrous network responsible for red cell rigidity, hemolysis, increased blood viscosity, poor microvascular blood flow and vessel occlusion [3]. Acute and chronic vessel occlusion could cause significant complications in various organs including the brain (strokes or silent brain infarcts), the kidneys (renal infarction with papillary necrosis or medullar fibrosis), the bones (aseptic osteonecrosis, pain crises), the spleen (spleen infarcts), the retina (retinopathy), the lungs (acute chest syndrome) or the male external genitalia (priapism) [3–5]. Some studies have also suggested an increased risk of venous thromboembolism (VTE) in patients with SCD or sickle cell trait (SCT) [6–9].

VTE which includes deep vein thrombosis (DVT) and its life-threatening complication, pulmonary embolism (PE), is a major contributor to global disease burden [10]. Thrombosis and subsequently embolism results from the interaction between blood stasis, vein wall injury and hypercoagulability (Virchow's classic triad), playing on the background of genetic predispositions [11]. Vessel occlusion and blood stasis, as well as chronic activation of the coagulation system are plausible mechanisms to explain the possible increased risk of VTE in patients with SCD or SCT [12, 13].

While other thrombotic complications of SCD have been extensively studied, VTE has so far been overlooked as a major complication of SCD. Whether or not SCD and SCT are associated with VTE and the degree to which this possible association might influence our approach to the prevention of VTE in these specific populations, especially regarding anticoagulation remains unknown. Hence, we conducted this systematic review and meta-analysis to summarize existing evidence on the risk of VTE in people with SCD or SCT.

Methods

This review is reported in accordance with the Preferred Reporting Items for Systematic reviews and Meta-Analyses (PRISMA) guidelines [14].

Literature search

We performed a comprehensive and exhaustive search of Medline through PubMed and Scopus to identify all relevant articles published on VTE in individuals with SCD and SCT from inception to April 25, 2017. No language restriction was applied. We conceived and applied a search strategy for each bibliographic database based on the combination of relevant terms. Terms used for VTE included the following: "venous thromboembolism", "pulmonary embolism", and "deep venous thrombosis". For SCD, the following and their variants were used: "sickle cell disease", "sickle cell anaemia", and "sickle cell trait". We scanned the reference lists of all relevant reviews and all included studies to identify other potential eligible studies. Unpublished data were not sought for this review of observational studies because, unlike clinical trials which are now always registered, observational studies are usually not registered and unpublished data from such studies are hardly trackable.

Selection of studies for inclusion in the review

We included cross-sectional, cohort and case-control studies reporting on the association between SCD or SCT and DVT or PE in male and female adults, pregnant and post-partum women as well as children. We excluded case series and studies lacking primary data. For studies published in more than one report (duplicates), the most comprehensive reporting the largest sample size was considered. SCD was defined as having the genotypes Hb SS, Hb SC, Hb SD or Hb S-thalassemia; SCT and normal control as having the genotypes Hb AS and Hb AA, respectively. PE was defined as the presence of a thrombus in the pulmonary vessels diagnosed by either CT-pulmonary angiography, magnetic resonance imaging (MRI), ventilation-perfusion lung (V/Q) scan or autopsy. DVT was defined as thrombosis of the deep venous circulation including limb, pelvic vessels, vena cava or cerebral vein diagnosed by either Doppler echography, venography, MRI or CT-Scan.

Two investigators independently screened all identified citations from the literature search results by title and abstract to identify articles for inclusion in the review (TNM and JJN). The full-texts of all citations that potentially met the inclusion criteria were then retrieved and assessed for final inclusion. All disagreements were resolved by discussion.

Data extraction and management

Two investigators (JJB and RT) independently extracted data from each included study using the data extraction form. Information extracted included: first author's name, year of publication, period of data collection, country and corresponding WHO region, study design (cross-sectional, cohort or case-control), setting (hospital-based or community-based), sample size, mean or median age and age range, proportion of female participants, type of population (children, adults, pregnant women or postpartum women), comparators (SCD or SCT versus controls) and outcome (DVT, PE or both). Disagreements between investigators were resolved through consensus following a discussion.

Assessment of risk of bias in included studies

The methodological quality of included studies was evaluated using an adapted version of the Newcastle-Ottawa Scale (NOS) [15]. Two investigators (JJB and RT) independently assessed study quality, with disagreements resolved by discussion. A score of 0–3, 4–6, and 7–9 rated the risk of bias as high, moderate, and low.

Data synthesis and analysis

Data analyses used the *'meta'* packages of the statistical software R (version 3.5.0, The R Foundation for statistical computing, Vienna, Austria). For measuring the association between SCD or SCT and VTE, DVT, or PE, a meta-analysis using the random-effects method of Der Simonian and Laird was performed to pool weighted odds ratios (OR) of risk estimates [16]. Raw data for measuring the association were extracted from each study and ORs were recalculated. Harbord test was done to assess the presence of publication bias [17]. A *p*-value < 0.10 was considered indicative of statistically significant publication bias. Heterogeneity across included studies was assessed using the χ^2 test for heterogeneity with a 5% level of statistical significance [18], and by using the I^2 statistic for which a value of 50% was considered to imply moderate heterogeneity [19]. Inter-rater agreements between investigators for study inclusion and methodological quality assessment were assessed using Kappa Cohen's coefficient [20].

Results

The review process

Initially, 313 records were identified (79 in Scopus and 234 in PubMed). After elimination of duplicates and screening of title and abstracts, 19 records were selected and their full-texts downloaded. From the 19 full-texts scrutinized, 10 papers were found eligible and therefore included in the meta-analysis [21–30] (Additional file 1: Figure S1). The inter-rater agreement for study inclusion and data extraction between investigators was κ = 0.89 and 0.79 respectively.

Characteristics of included studies

Additional file 2: Table S1 presents the characteristics of included studies. Seven studies had low risk of bias and three had moderate risk of bias. The included studies were published from 2006 to 2017. Eight studies were conducted in general adult populations [21–27], one in pregnant women only [28] and two in both pregnant and postpartum women [29, 30]. In the seven studies carried out in the general adult populations [21–27], the proportion of female varied from 25.0 to 100%. Seven studies were from the USA [21–25, 29, 30], one from the UK [26], one from Nigeria [27], and one from Brazil [28].

Sickle cell disease versus control

Data from three studies showed that SCD patients had significantly higher risk for VTE as compared to non SCD-individuals (pooled OR 4.4, 95%CI 2.6–7.9, *p* < 0.001; Fig. 1) [23–25]. The risk of PE was also higher in individuals with SCD (pooled OR 3.7, 95% CI 3.6–3.8, p < 0.001) as demonstrated in two studies (Fig. 1) [21, 24]. One study showed a slightly increased risk of DVT associated with SCD (OR 1.1, 95% CI 1.1–1.2, *p* < 0.001; Table 1) [21].

Two studies reported higher risk of VTE (OR 33.7, 95% CI 9.7–113.4, p < 0.001) and DVT (OR 30.7, 95% CI 1.6–578.2, *p* = 0.02) in pregnant or postpartum women with SCD as compared to their counterparts without SCD (Table 1) [28, 30].

Sickle cell disease versus sickle cell trait

Compared to adults with SCT, the risk of VTE was higher in adults with SCD (pooled OR 3.1, 95% CI 1.8–5.3, *p* < 0.001) as shown in 3 studies (Fig. 2) [23–25], and in SCD pregnant or postpartum women (OR 20.3, 95% CI 4.1–102.1, *p* = 0.0003, 1 study, Table 1) [30] as compared to their counterparts with SCT. The risk of PE was also higher in adults with SCD (OR 3.1, 95% CCI 1.7–5.9, *p* = 0.0004) as found in one study (Table 1) [24]. No study reported DVT as the outcome.

Sickle cell trait versus control

Four studies showed that the risk of VTE was higher in individuals with SCT compared to controls (pooled OR 1.7, 95% CI 1.3–2.2, *p* < 0.0001, Fig. 3) [22, 23, 25, 26], but not in pregnant or postpartum women (OR 0.9, 95% CI 0.3–2.9, *p* = 0.863, Table 1 and Additional file 3: Figure S2) as reported in two studies [29, 30]. Higher risk of PE was also associated with SCT (pooled OR 2.1, 95% CI 1.2–3.8, *p* = 0.012, Fig. 3) [23, 24, 26]. However, SCT did not increase the risk of DVT (pooled OR 1.2, 95% CI 0.9–1.7, *p* = 0.157, Table 1 and Additional file 4: Figure S3) in 3 studies [23, 26, 27].

Discussion

This systematic review and meta-analysis is the first to summarize available evidence on the association between SCD or SCT and VTE, DVT and PE. We found that (1) SCD was associated with a significantly higher risk of VTE and specifically DVT and PE compared to non-SCD controls; (2) the risk of VTE and PE in adults with SCD and of VTE in SCD pregnant/postpartum women was higher than in their counterparts with SCT; (3) compared to controls, individuals with SCT had a higher risk of VTE and PE but not DVT; (4) SCT was not associated with a higher risk of VTE in women during pregnancy or postpartum.

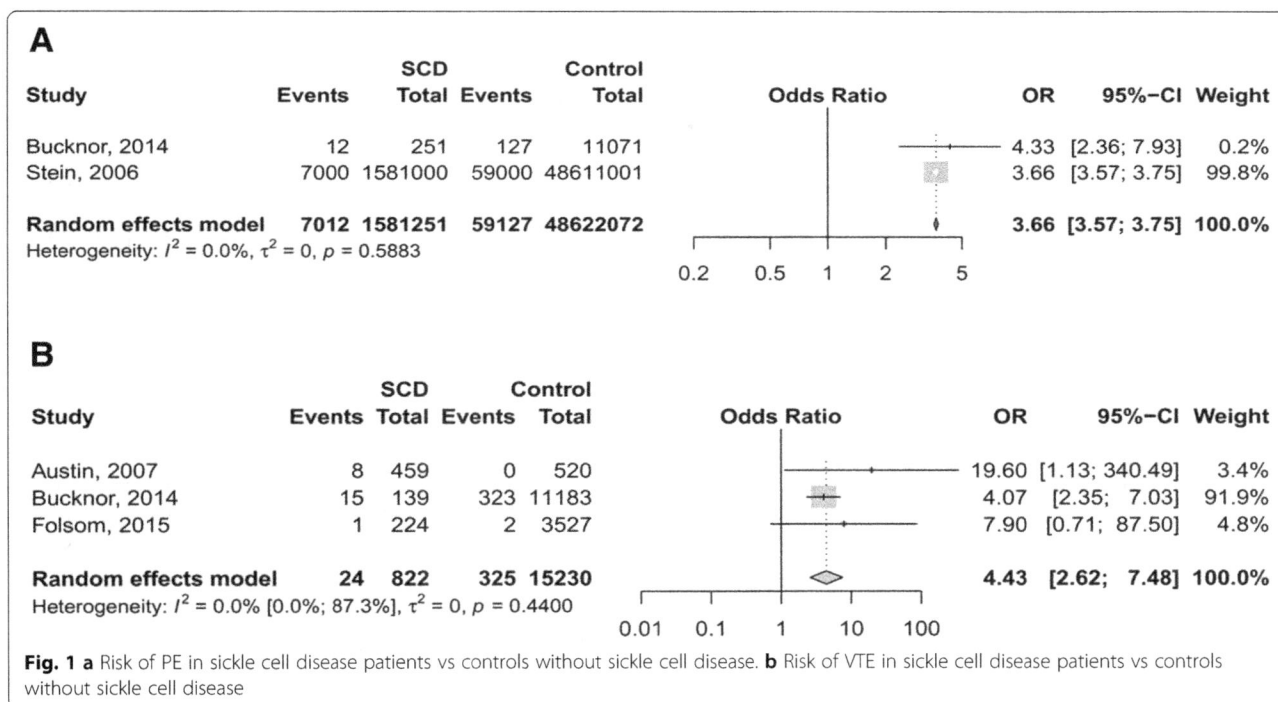

Fig. 1 a Risk of PE in sickle cell disease patients vs controls without sickle cell disease. **b** Risk of VTE in sickle cell disease patients vs controls without sickle cell disease

SCD-specific mechanisms causing hypercoagulability are believed to contribute significantly to the higher risk of VTE in the SCD population compared to the general population. Alterations of sickled red cells structure lead to haemolysis, release of prothrombotic substances such as phosphatidylserines and nitric oxide depletion [31, 32], causing platelets and coagulation cascade activation, impaired fibrinolysis, vaso-constriction, reduced blood flow and ischaemic vascular injury [32–35]. All these alterations ultimately result in hypercoagulability, endothelial dysfunction and blood stasis (Virchow's classic triad) causing thrombosis and subsequently embolism [13, 35, 36]. Furthermore, several thrombophilic abnormalities are associated with SCD. Antiphospholipid antibodies such as lupus anticoagulant, anticardiolipin and antiphosphatidylserine antibodies are highly prevalent in SCD patients,

Table 1 Summary statistics

Outcome	N studies	Population	Odds ratio (95%CI)	P value	H (95%CI)	I^2 (95%CI)	P heterogeneity	P Harbord test
SCD versus Control								
VTE	3	Adults	4.43 (2.62–7.48)	<.0001	1.0 (1.0–2.8)	0.0 (0.0–87.3)	.440	.467
DVT	1	Adults	1.12 (1.09–1.15)	<.0001	NA	NA	NA	NA
PE	2	Adults	3.66 (3.57–3.75)	<.0001	1.0	0.0	0.588	NA
VTE	1	Pregnant and PP women	33.16 (9.70–113.37)	<.0001	NA	NA	NA	NA
DVT	1	Pregnant women	30.66 (1.63–578.15)	.022	NA	NA	NA	NA
SCD versus SCT								
VTE	3	Adults	3.09 (1.79–5.33)	<.0001	1.0 (1.0–2.2)	0.0 (0.0–79.8)	.598	.524
PE	1	Adults	3.14 (1.67–5.92)	.0004	NA	NA	NA	NA
VTE	1	Pregnant and PP women	20.34 (4.05–102.05)	.0003	NA	NA	NA	NA
SCT versus Control								
VTE	4	Adults	1.71 (1.34–2.18)	<.0001	1.0 (1.0–2.5)	0.0 (0.0–83.5)	.427	.238
DVT	3	Adults	1.23 (0.92–1.65)	.157	1.0 (1.0–1.5)	0.0 (0.0–55.7)	.791	.810
PE	3	Adults	2.12 (1.18–3.80)	.012	2.3 (1.3–4.0)	80.6 (39.0–93.8)	.006	.405
VTE	2	Pregnant and PP women	0.90 (0.28–2.89)	.863	1.48	47.5	0.168	NA

CI confidence interval, *DVT* deep venous thrombosis, *VTE* venous thromboembolism, *PE* pulmonary embolism, *PP* postpartum, *SCD*, sickle cell disease, *SCT* sickle cell trait, *NA* not applicable

Study	SCD Events	SCD Total	SCT Events	SCT Total	Odds Ratio	OR	95%-CI	Weight
Austin, 2007	8	64	0	35		10.68	[0.60; 190.83]	3.6%
Bucknor, 2014	15	139	107	2641		2.86	[1.62; 5.06]	91.4%
Folsom, 2015	1	25	2	246		5.08	[0.44; 58.13]	5.0%
Random effects model	**24**	**228**		**109 2922**		**3.09**	**[1.79; 5.33]**	**100.0%**

Heterogeneity: I^2 = 0.0% [0.0%; 79.8%], τ^2 = 0, p = 0.5978

0.01   0.1   1   10   100

Fig. 2 Risk of VTE in sickle cell disease patients vs individuals with sickle cell trait

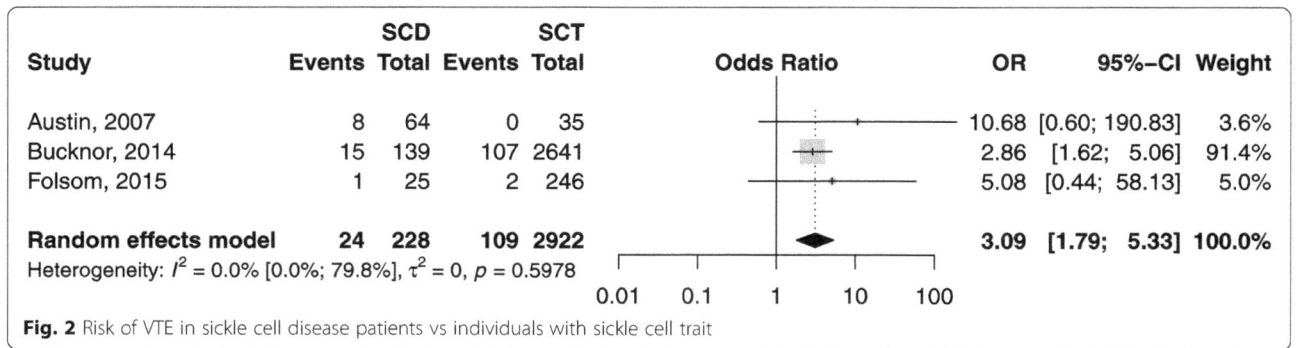

and are associated with thrombotic complications including stroke [13, 37]. The production of these auto-antibodies is thought to result from structural changes in sickled red cell membrane [37]. Genetic deficiency in Protein C and S is a known risk factor for VTE. Low circulating levels of Protein C and S found in SCD patients and which are due to chronic consumption in the context of continuous activation of coagulation cascade on the surface of sickled red blood cells, may also play a role in the thrombogenic proclivity of these patients [13, 37, 38].

Surgical splenectomy which is frequently performed in SCD patients is also potential risk factor for VTE in SCD [13]. A study which evaluated the association of surgical splenectomy with VTE in patients with sickle variant genotypes found that 27% of patients with VTE had a history of splenectomy compared to 6% without VTE, suggesting that splenic dysfunction might increase VTE risk in SCD [8]. Furthermore, few studies have revealed surgical splenectomy as a significant risk factor for VTE in the general population [39] and in hereditary haemolytic conditions such as β-thalassemia and hereditary spherocytosis [40, 41]. Few pathophysiologic mechanisms underlying the increased post-splenectomy thrombotic risk have been hypothesized, including chronic intravascular haemolysis, reduced clearance of abnormal red blood cells and hypercoagulability [36, 42, 43]. Functional asplenia secondary to splenic auto-infarction is a very common and early complication in SCD which occurs in about 90% of homozygote SS infants by age 1 and a large proportion of patients with SC

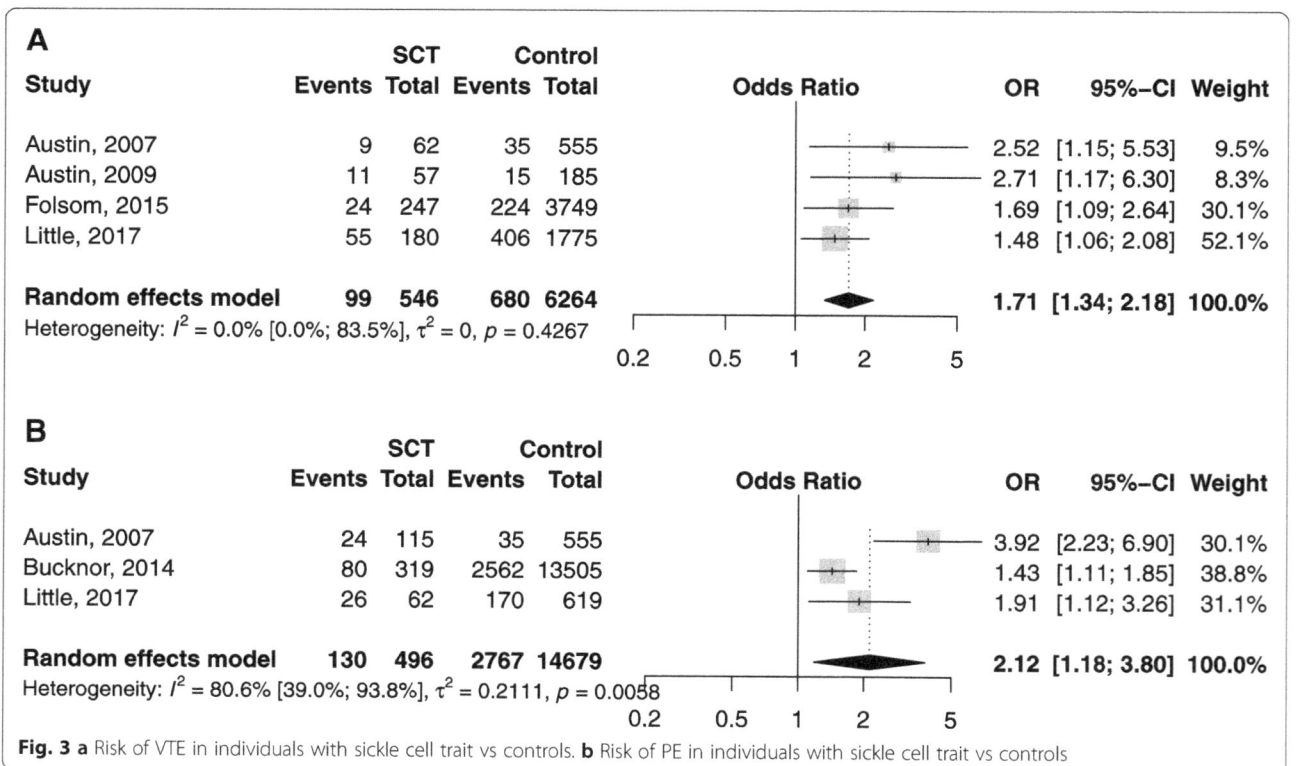

A

Study	SCT Events	SCT Total	Control Events	Control Total	Odds Ratio	OR	95%-CI	Weight
Austin, 2007	9	62	35	555		2.52	[1.15; 5.53]	9.5%
Austin, 2009	11	57	15	185		2.71	[1.17; 6.30]	8.3%
Folsom, 2015	24	247	224	3749		1.69	[1.09; 2.64]	30.1%
Little, 2017	55	180	406	1775		1.48	[1.06; 2.08]	52.1%
Random effects model	**99**	**546**	**680**	**6264**		**1.71**	**[1.34; 2.18]**	**100.0%**

Heterogeneity: I^2 = 0.0% [0.0%; 83.5%], τ^2 = 0, p = 0.4267

0.2   0.5   1   2   5

B

Study	SCT Events	SCT Total	Control Events	Control Total	Odds Ratio	OR	95%-CI	Weight
Austin, 2007	24	115	35	555		3.92	[2.23; 6.90]	30.1%
Bucknor, 2014	80	319	2562	13505		1.43	[1.11; 1.85]	38.8%
Little, 2017	26	62	170	619		1.91	[1.12; 3.26]	31.1%
Random effects model	**130**	**496**	**2767**	**14679**		**2.12**	**[1.18; 3.80]**	**100.0%**

Heterogeneity: I^2 = 80.6% [39.0%; 93.8%], τ^2 = 0.2111, p = 0.0058

0.2   0.5   1   2   5

Fig. 3 a Risk of VTE in individuals with sickle cell trait vs controls. **b** Risk of PE in individuals with sickle cell trait vs controls

genotype by mid-childhood [44]. Functional asplenia may also enhance hypercoagulability and consequentially increase the risk of VTE in SCD. However there is no available epidemiological data to support this association as it is the case for surgical splenectomy [13].

We found an increased risk of VTE in pregnant women with SCD compared to those without SCD. However, the very broad 95% CI associated to the odd ratio (~ 30) suggests a significant uncertainty of this association. Pregnancy itself is a well-recognised risk factor for VTE due to high levels of oestrogen and progesterone which are prothrombotic hormones [45, 46]. Our findings suggest that the combination of SCD and pregnancy has a multiplicative prothrombotic effect which is by far greater than the effect of each of them separately. One study showed that the prevalence of VTE was 3.5-fold greater among SCD pregnant women with a subset of complications such as vaso-occlusive crisis, acute chest syndrome and pneumonia compared to those without these complications [9]. Altogether, these data highlight the need for effective thromboprophylaxis in SCD women during pregnancy, especially those with concurrent thrombotic complications such as vaso-occlusive crisis or acute chest syndrome. Furthermore, as the majority of VTE seems to occur in the post-partum period [29], special attention should be given during this period and non-pharmacological measures such as mobilization should be encouraged early in the hospital and after discharge.

We found a higher risk of VTE and specifically PE associated with SCT in the general population. Our data suggest that not only SCD but also SCT are prothrombotic states. Interestingly, there is growing evidence underscoring a greater risk of VTE in individuals of African descent compared to Caucasians [47–50]. Considering the high prevalence of SCT in populations of African descent such as African Americans (7% to 10%) or sub-Saharan Africans (up to 30%) [51–53], it is plausible that the prothrombotic tendency of SCT may contribute to the higher incidence of VTE in individuals of African descent. However, we did not find an association between SCT and increased risk of VTE in pregnant or postpartum women. It is possible that there may be confounding factors that can drown out a possible association. Indeed, of the two studies included in this analysis, one had an age difference between the two groups compared while in the other, the compared groups differed in the distribution of the presence of diabetes at delivery. Furthermore, we observed no association between SCT and DVT, a finding in contrast with the potential link between SCT and PE. As mentioned above, it is possible that some confounding factors as well the small numbers of cases of SCT and controls hid a possible association between SCT and DVT.

Our finding of a higher risk of VTE in individuals with SCD compared to those without SCD underscore the need for a specific approach to the management of VTE in this population. Unfortunately there is no available evidence to inform anticoagulation practices in these patients. Therefore, our findings stress the need for studies to investigate anticoagulation modalities and other therapies such as hydroxyurea in the prevention and treatment of VTE in individuals with SCD including pregnant women. Before such evidence become available, it is important for clinicians to tailor their decisions regarding thromboprophylaxis and treatment to the specificities of SCD patients [13]. Hospitalized patients with SCD might benefit from thromboprophylaxis at a younger age as their risk of VTE is markedly higher than that of non-SCD individuals of the same age. While prophylactic anticoagulation is sometimes eluded in patients with low haemoglobin levels, clinicians should remember that SCD patients have lower baseline haemoglobin levels, and thus avoid an overestimation of the bleeding risk in these patients. Furthermore, the algorithms used for the diagnosis and treatment of DVT and PE should be interpreted carefully for patients with SCD. For instance, a pivotal marker like D-dimer is not reliable in these patients [13].

Our study has some limitations, mainly the limited number of studies found on the topic and included in the review. This demonstrates that VTE is still a neglected issue in the SCD population. As a consequence of the limited number of studies included and data analysed, it was not possible to assess the influence on our estimates of potential confounders such as the classic risk factors of VTE. Much more, no stratified analysis was done pertaining to the different SCD genotypes which have been shown to affect the occurrence of complications. For instance, a higher prevalence of PE was found in patients with Hb SC and Sβ + thalassemia compared to those with Hb SS [54]. Prospective studies on large cohorts of both SCD and SCT, specifically in sub-Saharan where most of patients and sickle cell carriers live are desirable. Highly elevated odds ratio found when measuring the association between DVT, VTE and exposure to SCD and SCT among pregnant women should be interpreted with caution when looking at the broad confidence interval found; the association may be lower or higher than actually presented. This large confidence interval may be explained by lack of power highlighting the need of more research in this field.

Conclusion

This review indicates that individuals with SCD, especially women during pregnancy and the postpartum period, might have a higher risk of VTE compared to the general population. SCT might also increase the risk of VTE. However, currently available data are not sufficient to allow a definite conclusion. Further larger studies are needed to provide a definitive conclusion on the association between SCD, SCT and VTE, in order to potentially inform specific approaches to the management of VTE in the SCD population.

Abbreviations
DVT: Deep vein thrombosis; PE: Pulmonary embolism; SCD: Sickle cell disease; SCT: Sickle cell trait; VTE: Venous thromboembolism

Funding
There was no funding source for this study.

Authors' contributions
JJN conceived the study. JJN did the literature search. JJN, MNT, RT and JJB selected the studies and extracted the relevant information. JJB and JJN synthesized the data. JJN, MNT, RT and JJB wrote the first draft of the paper. JJN, MNT, RT, JJB, JNT and AW critically revised successive drafts of the paper and approved its final version. JJN is the guarantor of the review.

Competing interests
The authors declare that they have no competing interests.

Author details
[1]Department of Medicine, Groote Schuur Hospital and University of Cape Town, Cape Town 7925, South Africa. [2]Department of Internal Medicine and sub-Specialties, Faculty of Medicine and Biomedical Sciences, Yaoundé, Cameroon. [3]Department of Surgery and sub-Specialties, Faculty of Medicine and Biomedical Sciences, Yaoundé, Cameroon. [4]Division of Human Genetics, Faculty of Health Sciences, University of Cape Town, Cape Town, South Africa. [5]Department of Epidemiology and Public Health, Centre Pasteur of Cameroon, Yaoundé, Cameroon. [6]Faculty of Medicine, University of Paris Sud XI, Le Kremlin Bicêtre, France.

References
1.   Modell B, Darlison M. Global epidemiology of haemoglobin disorders and derived service indicators. Bull World Health Organ. 2008;86:480–7.
2.   Aygun B, Odame I. A global perspective on sickle cell disease. Pediatr Blood Cancer. 2012;59:386–90.
3.   Bunn HF. Pathogenesis and treatment of sickle cell disease. N Engl J Med. 1997;337:762–9.
4.   Rees DC, Williams TN, Gladwin MT. Sickle-cell disease. Lancet Lond Engl. 2010;376:2018–31.
5.   Noubiap JJ, Mengnjo MK, Nicastro N, Kamtchum-Tatuene J. Neurologic complications of sickle cell disease in Africa: a systematic review and meta-analysis. Neurology. 2017;89(14):1516–24.
6.   Little I, Vinogradova Y, Orton E, Kai J, Qureshi N. Venous thromboembolism in adults screened for sickle cell trait: a population-based cohort study with nested case–control analysis. BMJ Open. 2017;7:e012665.
7.   Naik RP, Streiff MB, Haywood C Jr, Nelson JA, Lanzkron S. Venous thromboembolism in adults with sickle cell disease: a serious and under-recognized complication. Am J Med. 2013;126(5):443–9.
8.   Yu TT, Nelson J, Streiff MB, Lanzkron S, Naik RP. Risk factors for venous thromboembolism in adults with hemoglobin SC or Sß(+) thalassemia genotypes. Thromb Res. 2016;141:35–8.
9.   Seaman CD, Yabes J, Li J, Moore CG, Ragni MV. Venous thromboembolism in pregnant women with sickle cell disease: a retrospective database analysis. Thromb Res. 2014;134(6):1249–52.
10. ISTH Steering Committee for World Thrombosis. Thrombosis: a major contributor to global disease burden. J Thromb Haemost. 2014;12:1580–90.
11. Heit JA. Epidemiology of venous thromboembolism. Nat Rev Cardiol. 2015; 12:464–74.
12. Austin H, Key NS, Benson JM, Lally C, Dowling NF, Whitsett C, Hooper WC. Sickle cell trait and the risk of venous thromboembolism among blacks. Blood. 2007;110(3):908–12.
13. Naik RP, Streiff MB, Lanzkron S. Sickle cell disease and venous thromboembolism: what the anticoagulation expert needs to know. J Thromb Thrombolysis. 2013;35(3):352–8.
14. Moher D, Liberati A, Tetzlaff J, Altman DG, PRISMA group. Preferred reporting items for systematic reviews and meta-analyses: the PRISMA statement. J Clin Epidemiol. 2009;62(10):1006–12.
15. Wells GA, Shea B, O'Connell D, et al. The Newcastle-Ottawa scale (NOS) for assessing the quality of nonrandomised studies in meta-analyses. 2014. http://www.ohri.ca/programs/clinical_epidemiology/oxford.asp (accessed July 18 2016).
16. DerSimonian R, Laird N. Meta-analysis in clinical trials revisited. Contemp Clin Trials. 2015;45(Pt A):139–45.
17. Harbord RM, Egger M, Sterne JA. A modified test for small-study effects in meta-analyses of controlled trials with binary endpoints. Stat Med. 2006; 25(20):3443–57.
18. Cochran GW. The combination of estimates from different experiments. Biometrics. 1954;10(1):101–29.
19. Higgins JP, Thompson SG. Quantifying heterogeneity in a meta-analysis. Stat Med. 2002;21(11):1539–58.
20. Viera AJ, Garrett JM. Understanding interobserver agreement: the kappa statistic. Fam Med. 2005;37(5):360–3.
21. Stein PD, Beemath A, Meyers FA, Skaf E, Olson RE. Deep venous thrombosis and pulmonary embolism in hospitalized patients with sickle cell disease. Am J Med. 2006;119(10):897 e7–11.
22. Austin H, Lally C, Benson JM, Whitsett C, Hooper WC, Key NS. Hormonal contraception, sickle cell trait, and risk for venous thromboembolism among African American women, Am J Obstet Gynecol. 2009;200(6):620 e1–3.
23. Austin H, Key NS, Benson JM, Lally C, Dowling NF, Whitsett C, et al. Sickle cell trait and the risk of venous thromboembolism among blacks. Blood. 2007;110(3):908–12.
24. Bucknor MD, Goo JS, Coppolino ML. The risk of potential thromboembolic, renal and cardiac complications of sickle cell trait. Hemoglobin. 2014; 38(1):28–32.
25. Folsom AR, Tang W, Roetker NS, Kshirsagar AV, Derebail VK, Lutsey PL, Naik R, Pankow JS, Grove ML, Basu S, Key NS, Cushman M. Prospective study of sickle cell trait and venous thromboembolism incidence. J Thromb Haemost. 2015;13(1):2–9.
26. Little I, Vinogradova Y, Orton E, Kai J, Qureshi N. Venous thromboembolism in adults screened for sickle cell trait: a population-based cohort study with nested case-control analysis. BMJ Open. 2017;7(3):e012665.
27. Ahmed SG, Kagu MB, Ibrahim UA, Bukar AA. Impact of sickle cell trait on the thrombotic risk associated with non-O blood groups in northern Nigeria. Blood Transfus. 2015;13(4):639–43.
28. Costa VM, Viana MB, Aguiar RA. Pregnancy in patients with sickle cell disease: maternal and perinatal outcomes. J Matern Fetal Neonatal Med. 2015;28(6):685–9.
29. Pintova S, Cohen HW, Billett HH. Sickle cell trait: is there an increased VTE risk in pregnancy and the postpartum? PLoS One. 2013;8(5):e64141.
30. Porter B, Key NS, Jauk VC, Adam S, Biggio J, Tita A. Impact of sickle hemoglobinopathies on pregnancy-related venous thromboembolism. Am J Perinatol. 2014;31(9):805–9.
31. Chiu D, Lubin B, Roelofsen B, van Deenen LL. Sickled erythrocytes accelerate clotting in vitro: an effect of abnormal membrane lipid asymmetry. Blood. 1981;58(2):398–401.
32. Villagra J, Shiva S, Hunter LA, Machado RF, Gladwin MT, Kato GJ. Platelet activation in patients with sickle disease, hemolysis-associated pulmonary hypertension, and nitric oxide scavenging by cell-free hemoglobin. Blood. 2007;110(6):2166–72.
33. Kenny MW, George AJ, Stuart J. Platelet hyperactivity in sickle-cell disease: a consequence of hyposplenism. J Clin Pathol. 1980;33(7):622–5.
34. Westerman M, Pizzey A, Hirschman J, Cerino M, Weil-Weiner Y, Ramotar P, Eze A, Lawrie A, Purdy G, Mackie I, Porter J. Microvesicles in haemoglobinopathies offer insights into mechanisms of hypercoagulability, haemolysis and the effects of therapy. Br J Haematol. 2008;142(1):126–35.
35. Ataga KI, Orringer EP. Hypercoagulability in sickle cell disease: a curious paradox. Am J Med. 2003;115(9):721–8.
36. Ataga KI. Hypercoagulability and thrombotic complications in hemolytic anemias. Haematologica. 2009;94(11):1481–4.
37. Westerman MP, Green D, Gilman-Sachs A, Beaman K, Freels S, Boggio L, Allen S, Zuckerman L, Schlegel R, Williamson P. Antiphospholipid antibodies, proteins C and S, and coagulation changes in sickle cell disease. J Lab Clin Med. 1999;134(4):352–62.

38. Piccin A, Murphy C, Eakins E, Kinsella A, McMahon C, Smith OP, Murphy WG. Protein C and free protein S in children with sickle cell anemia. Ann Hematol. 2012;91(10):1669–71.

39. Thomsen RW, Schoonen WM, Farkas DK, Riis A, Fryzek JP, Sørensen HT. Risk of venous thromboembolism in splenectomized patients compared with the general population and appendectomized patients: a 10-year nationwide cohort study. J Thromb Haemost. 2010;8(6):1413–6.

40. Taher A, Isma'eel H, Mehio G, Bignamini D, Kattamis A, Rachmilewitz EA, Cappellini MD. Prevalence of thromboembolic events among 8,860 patients with thalassaemia major and intermedia in the Mediterranean area and Iran. Thromb Haemost. 2006;96(4):488–91.

41. Schilling RF, Gangnon RE, Traver MI. Delayed adverse vascular events after splenectomy in hereditary spherocytosis. J Thromb Haemost. 2008;6(8): 1289–95.

42. Cappellini MD, Robbiolo L, Bottasso BM, Coppola R, Fiorelli G, Mannucci AP. Venous thromboembolism and hypercoagulability in splenectomized patients with thalassaemia intermedia. Br J Haematol. 2000;111(2):467–73.

43. Cappellini MD. Coagulation in the pathophysiology of hemolytic anemias. Hematol Am Soc Hematol Educ Program. 2007:74–8.

44. Rogers ZR, Wang WC, Luo Z, Iyer RV, Shalaby-Rana E, Dertinger SD, Shulkin BL, Miller JH, Files B, Lane PA, Thompson BW, Miller ST, Ware RE, BABY HUG. Biomarkers of splenic function in infants with sickle cell anemia: baseline data from the baby hug trial. Blood. 2011;117(9):2614–7.

45. Pomp ER, Lenselink AM, Rosendaal FR, Doggen JM. Pregnancy, the postpartum period and prothrombotic defects: risk of venous thrombosis in the MEGA study. J Thromb Haemost. 2008;6:632–7.

46. James AH. Pregnancy-associated thrombosis. Hematology Am Soc Hematol Educ Program. 2009:277–85.

47. Dowling NF, Austin H, Dilley A, Whitsett C, Evatt BL, Hooper WC. The epidemiology of venous thromboembolism in Caucasians and African Americans: the GATE study. J Thromb Haemost. 2002;1:80–7.

48. White RH, Zhou H, Murin S, Harvey D. Effect of ethnicity and gender on the incidence of venous thromboembolism in a diverse population in California in 1996. Thromb Haemost. 2005;2:298–305.

49. Hooper WC. Venous thromboembolism in African-Americans: a literature-based commentary. Thrombos Res. 2010;125:12–8.

50. Danwang C, Temgoua MN, Agbor VN, Tankeu AT, Noubiap JJ. Epidemiology of venous thromboembolism in Africa: a systematic review. J Thromb Haemost. 2017;15(9):1770–81.

51. Nelson DA, Deuster PA, Carter R 3rd, Hill OT, Wolcott VL, Kurina LM. Sickle Cell Trait, Rhabdomyolysis, and Mortality among U.S. Army Soldiers. N Engl J Med. 2016;375(5):435.

52. Ojodu J, Hulihan MM, Pope SN, Grant AM, Centers for Disease Control and Prevention (CDC). Incidence of sickle cell trait--United States, 2010. MMWR Morb Mortal Wkly Rep. 2014;63(49):1155.

53. Tsaras G, Owusu-Ansah A, Boateng FO, Amoateng-Adjepong Y. Complications associated with sickle cell trait: a brief narrative review. Am J Med. 2009;122(6):507.

54. Manci EA, Culberson DE, Yang YM, Gardner TM, Powell R, Haynes J Jr, Shah AK, Mankad VN, Investigators of the cooperative study of sickle cell disease. Causes of death in sickle cell disease: an autopsy study. Br J Haematol. 2003; 123(2):359–65.

26

Prognostic assessment for patients with cancer and incidental pulmonary embolism

George Bozas[1]*[iD], Natalie Jeffery[1], Deiva Ramanujam-Venkatachala[1], Ged Avery[2], Andrew Stephens[2], Hilary Moss[1], June Palmer[1], Mandi Elliott[1] and Anthony Maraveyas[1,3]

Abstract

Background: An incidental/unsuspected diagnosis of pulmonary embolism (IPE) in cancer patients is a frequent occurrence. This single-institution analysis of uniformly managed patients investigates short and long-term outcomes and proposes a prognostic risk score, aiming to assist clinical decision-making.

Methods: Data from a prospectively recorded cohort of 234 consecutive cancer patients with IPE were analysed. Multivariate logistic regression and the Cox regression survival methods were used to identify factors with independent association with early (30-day, 3-month, 6-month) mortality and survival. Receiver operator characteristic analysis (ROC) was used to assess appropriate cut-offs for continuous variables and the fitness of prognostic scoring.

Results: 30-day, 3-month and 6-month mortality was 3.4% ($n = 8$), 15% ($n = 35$) and 31% ($n = 72$) respectively. Recurrence during anticoagulation occurred in 2.6% ($n = 6$) and major haemorrhage in 2.1% ($n = 5$) of the patients. A prognostic score incorporating performance status (0 vs 1–2 vs 3–4) and the presence of new or worsening symptoms, with and without the consideration of the presence of incurable malignancy, correlated with overall survival ($p < .001$ respectively) as well as early mortality (AUC = .821, $p = .004$ and AUC = .805, $p = 0.006$, respectively).

Conclusion: A simple prognostic score incorporating basic oncologic clinical assessment and self-reported symptomatology could reliably stratify the mortality risk of ambulant cancer patients and IPE.

Keywords: Pulmonary embolism, Cancer, Incidental finding, Unsuspected pulmonary embolism, Prognosis

Background

The widespread use of multi-slice CT in diagnosis, staging and assessment of response to treatment has resulted in an increase in the apparent incidence of what has been termed unsuspected or incidental pulmonary embolism (IPE) in cancer patients [1–3]. Notably, up to half of vascular thromboembolic events (VTE) diagnosed in Oncology centres may be incidental [1, 4]. Contrary to the assumption that these cases are asymptomatic, contemporary work shows that for a substantial majority this perception is erroneous [4, 5]. Clinicians frequently attribute relevant symptomatology to the progression of underlying cancer or to the adverse effect of cancer treatments and

often it will remain unclear indeed whether symptomatology might be attributable to the imaged PE, especially when progressive cancer is imaged concurrently. This remains a particularly unclear area as most of the data available are retrospective without nuance. Recent work seems to support the notion that cancer patients with IPE have similar outcomes to symptomatic (suspected) PE cases, their survival appearing worse compared with matched controls without PE [6–11]. Moreover, the presence of symptoms in cancer patients with IPE has been correlated with poorer outcome [12]. On the other hand it has been shown that some patients with IPE do not develop symptoms or morbidity [13].

The standard of care remains to treat all cancer patients with a PE or DVT irrespective of the manner of diagnosis [14, 15]. Outpatient care is commonly used but there is little evidence to underpin outpatient approaches, these often being empirical and based on

* Correspondence: Georgios.bozas@hey.nhs.uk
[1]Hull and East Yorkshire NHS Hospitals Trust, Queen's Centre for Oncology and Haematology, Castle Hill Hospital, Castle Road, Cottingham HU16 5JQ, UK
Full list of author information is available at the end of the article

individual clinician expertise. Care standards thus are often fragmented, poorly adhered to or vary between different specialities [16, 17]. In general it is recognised that management recommendations for IPE are extrapolated from studies on symptomatic VTE [18] and evidence from retrospective studies. Additional controversy exists for distal IPE (affecting segmental or subsegmental pulmonary artery branches); a recent meta-analysis suggests that risk of recurrence is similar to more proximal PE [9, 19].

Within this context, clinical prognostic scores may be useful in assisting clinical decision-making. Pulmonary embolism severity index (PESI) – a tool stratifying risk for all patients with PE [20] has seen wide use. Two prognostic scores have been recently suggested specifically for patients with cancer and PE: The POMPE-C tool identified patient weight, respiratory rate, O$_2$ saturation, heart rate, altered mental status, respiratory distress, unilateral limb swelling and "do not resuscitate" status as predictors of 30-day mortality. The POMPE-C score showed better prognostic accuracy than PESI for patients with active cancer [21]. The RIETE investigators [22] proposed a score utilising age > 80 years, heart rate, hypotension, low body weight, recent immobilisation, and metastatic disease, for predicting 30-day mortality. Both the above prognostic scores relate predominantly to the symptomatic PE setting.

In the present paper, we describe a prospective cohort of patients with active cancer and IPE managed uniformly under a specialised nurse-led service, with an analysis of prognostic factors for early mortality and survival. The development of a dedicated clinical prognostic score predicting early mortality and survival based on the above analysis is presented and discussed.

Methods

In our department (Queen's Centre for Oncology and Haematology, Castle Hill Hospital, Cottingham, UK, Hull and East Yorkshire Hospitals NHS Trust) all patients with cancer and IPE are managed uniformly under a nurse-led service since March 2010. The details of the development of this service have been previously published [23]. Patient-reported symptomatology at baseline was recorded through a simple dichotomous questionnaire capturing symptoms relative to this cohort of patients [12, 23]. The incorporated risk-assessment algorithm, which guides hospital admission decisions, is described in a previous publication [23] and has been based on PESI with modifications reflecting our experience regarding the outcome of these patients [24, 25]. For the calculation of the PESI score the "cancer present" variable is considered positive when cancer is measurable or evaluable and negative when not (i.e. in patients undergoing adjuvant treatment). All patients

receive Low Molecular-Weight Heparin as per institutional guidelines, following the CLOT [26] regimen for dalteparin, unless clinically contra-indicated, in which case a decision from the attending Oncologist is required. All patients on chemotherapy continue secondary prophylaxis with dalteparin; oral anticoagulants are allowed after the completion of chemotherapy at the treating physician's discretion. Duration of anticoagulation is at the physician's discretion, but a minimum of six months is recommended.

The study reported in this manuscript is the result of work that has been classified as an audit. This is a regular undertaking in UK hospitals with the primary goal of maintaining quality standards and identifying areas that need improvement if they fall below accepted standards as set by national or international guidelines. Audits can be retrospective or prospective. As per the NHS Health Research Authority guidelines our study, which can be classified within the audit / service evaluation description, does not require external Research Ethics Committee approval [27]. The NHS Trust governance body which authorises the project is doing so if the study is conducted within the regulatory framework including the Data Protection Act (1998), the Caldicott principles (1997) and the NHS Confidentiality code of practice (2003) [28]. Within this context regulatory approval is sought and obtained based on the quality of the audit and the priority of the area studied and whether it fits within the quality framework of the organization. The endorsement code for our study is No. 2013.287, issued by the Hull and East Yorkshire Hospitals NHS Trust the 29th of November 2013.

Baseline data for all patients referred and treated by the nurse-led service for the management of incidental PE were recorded in real or near real-time in an MS EXCEL®2010 (Microsoft Corp™) spreadsheet maintained in a secure virtual hard-drive with restricted access. Outcome data were collected every six months with the help of the electronic medical record system (iSOFT Patient Centre®, CSC™ and Lorenzo®, CSC™).

The database prospectively collects demographic data, weight, data regarding cancer diagnosis, current or recent cancer treatment, medical history and long-term medication, the presence of central lines, recent (30-day) surgery or hospitalisation, clinical variables included in the pulmonary embolism severity index (PESI) and the site and extent of imaged pulmonary thrombi. Patient-reported symptomatology is stratified into new, stable pre-existing and worsening pre-existing. Laboratory investigations include full blood count, biochemical profile (standard electrolyte, renal and liver function assays) and D-dimer level on diagnosis, platelet count on day 7, and records ECOG/WHO performance status (PS) (Additional file 1: Appendix A) at the time of IPE [29]. Outcomes recorded are mortality and survival, recurrence of VTE, haemorrhage and 30-day hospitalisation.

CT thorax imaging in our centre is typically obtained with a slice thickness of 1 mm. Images are reviewed in in workstations running the Phillips Extended Brilliance Workspace ® software package (currently on version V3.5.35.1011) and the Agfa PACS Impax Workstation ® software package (current version V6.5.2.657). All laboratory haematological and biochemical analyses were performed in the same laboratory and were conducted as per the standard local quality assurance protocols.

The present study analyses patients with active cancer included in the pathway between March 2010 and December 2014. The database was closed in May 31, 2015. Active cancer is defined as cancer present or current cancer treatment (i.e. adjuvant treatment) or treatment for cancer within the past six months.

Statistical considerations
All analyses were performed with SPSS ver22, IBM Corp ®.

Descriptive statistics were used to analyse patient characteristics. Survival and treatment related outcomes (VTE recurrence and haemorrhage) were calculated from the date of PE diagnosis.

Univariate correlations of continuous variables including age, WCC, Hb, PLT, D-Dimers, with 30-day, 3-month and 6-month mortality were performed with Receiver Operator Characteristics (ROC) curve analysis. ROC analysis was also used to assess cut-off points when needed. Variables which are constituents of the PESI score were not analysed as separate factors.

Survival was calculated from the date of IPE diagnosis until the date of last follow-up contact or the date of death. Only two patients were lost to follow-up and are included in the analysis. The Kaplan Meier method was utilised to explore the prognostic significance of categorical variables using the log rank test to compare factors. Multivariate analyses were performed with the logistic regression method for mortality and the Cox Proportional hazards method for survival. Case-wise exclusion was used in all analyses to handle missing data.

The Kendall tau-b test was utilised to assess correlation of risk categories with mortality event numbers at the 30-day, 3- and 6- month cut-offs.

A probability threshold of 5% was used to define statistical significance in all analyses.

Prognostic score development
The analytical process for the development of a prognostic score is illustrated in Additional file 1: Appendices B and C of the Supplementary Material. Variables with prognostic significance for early (30-day, 3-month, 6-month) mortality and overall survival were candidate for inclusion in a prognostic score predicting mortality of cancer patients with IPE. The Wald statistic from the Cox Regression analysis was used to weigh the relative prognostic significance of different variables and assign score points to each variable included in the scores. Risk score grouping was performed by assessing the Kaplan-Meier survival curve clustering for different point aggregates. ROC analysis was used to assess the fitness of different prognostic scores.

Results
234 patients are included in this analysis. Baseline characteristics and assessments of patients are shown in Table 1.

Symptoms
Symptoms recorded included: dyspnoea ($n = 121$ 51.7%), fatigue ($n = 181$, 77.4), chest pain ($n = 26$, 11.1%), lower limb oedema ($n = 78$, 33.3%), haemoptysis ($n = 8$, 3.4%). Lower limb Doppler U/S was not required as part of the work-up, nevertheless 16 patients had documented concurrent DVT. Overall 121 patients reported new or worsening pre-existing symptoms (52%).

Outcomes
Median follow-up for patients remaining alive at study closure was 36.7 months, 95%CI (27.5, 45.9).

Survival, mortality
72 patients were alive at the time of database closure; 2 patients were lost to follow-up. 30-day, 3-month and 6-month mortality was 3.4% ($n = 8$), 15% ($n = 35$) and 30.7% ($n = 72$) respectively. Median overall survival (OS) for the entire cohort was 12.6 months 95%CI (9.4, 15,8).

In ROC analysis WCC demonstrated a correlation with 30-day ($p = .005$), 3- and 6- month mortality ($p = .001$ and $p < .001$ respectively) whilst serum Creatinine demonstrated a (negative) correlation with 3- and 6-month mortality ($p < .001$ and $p = .002$), but it was not predictive of 30-day mortality ($p = .100$). Age, PLT and D-Dimer levels showed no correlation to mortality. Multivariate logistic regression analysis of clinical and laboratory factors with potential prognostic significance as selected by univariate analysis is shown in Table 2. Survival analysis indicated palliative (non-curative) setting, new and worsening symptoms (individually or combined), PS and PESI as eligible prognostic factors (Table 3).

A significant correlation of increasing WCC levels, as continuous variable, with early mortality in both univariate as well as multivariate models was observed. ROC analysis indicated a cut-off of WCC = 11.3×10^9/L as suitable for dichotomisation. Patients with WCC > 11.3×10^9/L had 30-day mortality rate of 15.4% versus 2% for patients with WCC < 11.3×10^9/L ($p = .001$). The

Table 1 Characteristics of 234 patients with cancer and IPE

	% (n)+
Age	
	[Median: 67 (Range: 27–91)]
Gender	
Male	59 (139)
Female	41 (95)
Setting	
Radical/adjuvant	20 (46)
Metastatic/incurable	80 (188)
Diagnosis	
Colorectal cancer, early	5 (12)
Colorectal cancer, metastatic	20 (46)
Oesophagogastric Cancer, early	7 (17)
Oesophagogastric Cancer, metastatic	9 (21)
Breast Cancer, Metastatic	9 (21)
Pancreaticobiliary Cancer, Advanced	9 (21)
NSCLC Metastatic/ SCLC *	12 (28)
Other	29 (68)
Treatment	
Cytotoxic chemotherapy	66 (154)
Biologic/targeted therapy **	13 (30)
Hormonal manipulation therapy***	4 (10)
Interferon	1 (2)
Risk Factors for VTE	
Recent (30d) hospitalisation	15 (36)
Recent (30d) Surgery	2 (5)
Indwelling CVC	15 (35)
PS	
0	45 (105)
1/2	43 (100)
3/4	10 (23)
MD	3 (6)
Extent of IPE	
Bilateral	39 (91)
Largest vessel: pulmonary artery (main, right, left)	20 (46)
Largest vessel: lobar branch(es)	27 (63)
Largest vessel: segmental or subsegmental	42 (99)
Largest vessel: subsegmental branches	11 (25)
Symptoms (self reported)	
Any new symptom	42 (98)
Worsening pre-existing symptoms	21 (49)
PESI group	
I/II	12 (29)
III	42 (99)
IV	37 (86)
V	8 (20)

*Extensive and limited stages, ** CD20, VEGF, EGFR, HER2 - targeted monoclonal antibodies or tyrosine kinase inhibitors., *** Tamoxifen, aromatase inhibitors, antiandrogen, GnRH
+ percentages rounded for simplicity, may not add up to 100

same cut-off appeared to correlate with overall survival (OS) ($p = .016$). Decreasing creatinine levels also showcased a relation to 3-month and 6-month mortality with a cut-off of <55 μmol/L identified as appropriate for dichotomisation in ROC analysis and in univariate survival analysis this cut-off showed a significant correlation with OS ($p = .0210$).

The distribution of PE was analysed as an ordinal categorical variable, recoded as central vs others, as subsegmental vs others with and without corrections for bilaterality. No significant effects on survival were observed.

Factors demonstrating significance in univariate survival analysis were entered in a multivariate survival model as shown in Table 3. Creatinine, WCC levels and PESI score did not retain prognostic significance.

Recurrence

In total, 20 recurrent or progressive VTE events were recorded within the follow up period [rate: 8.5%, 95%CI (5.1%, 12%)]. VTE recurrence/progression rate in the first three months was 0.9% ($n = 2$) 95%CI (0,2%, 1%), and within the first six months 2.6% ($n = 6$) 95%CI (0.9%, 4.7%). In 6 cases (2.6%) recurrent VTE occurred while on thromboprophylaxis. In one case DVT occurred in a post-operative period while on prophylactic dose of dalteparin and with an IVC filter in situ. One of the patients was on warfarin. Median time to recurrent/progressive VTE was 9.6 months 95%CI (8.5, 10.8).

Haemorrhage

13 haemorrhagic complications were recorded [5.5%, 95%CI (3%, 8.5%)] at a median of 3 months 95%CI (1.3, 4.7) from the time of IPE. Major haemorrhage as per the ISTH criteria (>2.0 g/L drop in Hb, fatal, or haemorrhage in critical area) was represented with 5 cases for an incidence of 2.1%, 95%CI (0.4%, 3.8%) and occurred at a median of 3.3 months 95%CI (1.5, 5.1). Major haemorrhage within six months occurred in 4 patients [1.7% 95%CI (.4%, 3.4%)].

Hospitalisation

23 patients in this cohort were admitted to the hospital as per protocol (9.8%). Four patients (1.7%) were inpatients at the time of IPE diagnosis. 34 patients amongst the 207 who were managed as out patients (16%) were hospitalised within 30 days of IPE. The cause for hospitalisation was recorded as "bleeding" in two (1%) and "pulmonary embolism" in two patients (1%).

Prognostic factors for haemorrhage, recurrence and 30-day hospitalisation

Multivariate logistic regression analyses were performed with clinical and laboratory factors for haemorrhage, major haemorrhage, recurrence of VTE and hospitalisation

Table 2 Logistic regression analysis

Category	30-d mortality n events: 7/219**		3-month mortality n events: 32/219**		6-month mortality n events: 64/219**	
	OR (95%CI)	p	OR (95%CI)	p	OR (95%CI)	p
Palliative setting (metastatic or incurable malignancy)	NC	.998	1.6 (.3, 1.7)	.596	1.6 (.6,4.6)	.384
PS		.239		.050		<.001
PS 0	1		1		1	
PS 1,2	1.6 (.1, 20.9)	.719	1.3 (.5, 3.7)	.932	2.7 (1.3, 5.9)	.010
PS 3,4	6.4 (.1, 87.6)	.163	4.8 (1.3, 17.9)	.019	13.7 (4, 47.2)	<.001
PESI		>.999		.096		.142
PESI Class I/II	1		1		1	
PESI III/IV	NC	.998	4.1 (.7, 22.6)	.107	0.97 (.4, 2.7)	.943
PESI V	0.7 (NC)	>.999	11.7 (1.3, 101.8)	.030	3.3 (0.7, 15.4)	.126
New/worsening symptoms	4 (.4, 40.2)	.239	1.9 (.8, 4.8)	.159	2.9 (1.4, 6)	.005
WCC (cont.) *	1.3 (1.1, 1.6)	.013	1.2 (1, 1.3)	.008	1.1 (1, 1.3)	.020
Creat (cont.) *	.98 (.9, 1)	.372	.9 (.9, .98)	<.001	.98 (.96, .99)	.014

Odds ratios are rounded to the first decimal (except when too close to 1) for simplicity. *NC* not computed. (cont.)*: continuous variable. **: number of patients with complete data in all categories

within 30 days. In these analyses PESI score class V was the only factor showing a trend for correlation with 30-day hospitalisation ($p = .0520$), HR 8.45 95%CI (.98, 72.8). Increasing creatinine levels were associated with all-grade haemorrhage ($p = .010$), HR 1.03 95%CI (1.01, 1.05), but no factor was associated with major haemorrhage. Cox regression suggested a HR of 5.40 95%CI (1.71, 17.04) for haemorrhage for Creatinine levels with a cut off of 108.5 μmol/L (>90% specificity in ROC curve analysis). No factor was associated with VTE recurrence or VTE recurrence within six months.

Prognostic score for mortality

We have previously described a feasible prognostic score for patients with cancer and IPE based on the presence of new symptoms, PS and the presence of incurable cancer, constructed on a subset of the current dataset [30]. Compared with our previous analysis, in the current cohort, PESI score class V appeared to convey an independent survival detriment compared to the reference category (PESI I/II) both in regards 3- month mortality ($p = .030$) as well as in terms of OS ($p = .026$) (Tables 2,3). On the other hand, the effect of the overall PESI variable remained non-significant on survival ($p = .081$) as well as on 30-day, 3-month and 6-month mortality ($p > .999$, $p = .096$ and $p = .142$ respectively) (Tables 2,3).

The RIETE score was also applied to this dataset. The POMPE-C score could not be considered due to missing "do not resuscitate" information. For the purposes of our analysis, hospitalisation within the past 30 days and surgery during the past 30 days were used to derive the "recent immobilisation" category of RIETE, since this was not a variable in our data recording as such.

To evaluate the feasibility of a clinical prognostic score for cancer patients with IPE deriving from our cohort we used information from logistic regression analysis on 30-day, 3-month and 6- month mortality as well as from multivariate survival analysis as shown in Tables 2 and 3. The most consistent predictors of survival in these analyses were the patient-reported symptomatology (new or worsening) and performance status at the time of IPE diagnosis. The presence of metastatic-incurable cancer had strong association with OS but not with early mortality (Tables 2 and 3). Utilising the Wald statistic for weighing significant variables and Kaplan-Meier curves for the grouping of categories, four possible scoring systems were identified; three included (a) the presence of metastatic disease, (b) the presence of new or worsening symptoms at the time of IPE diagnosis and (c) Performance status (0 vs 1,2 vs 3,4). The fourth scheme ("Hull5") excluded variable (a) since it appeared to lack association with early mortality (Additional file 1: Appendix B). All four scores were compared with ROC analysis against RIETE and PESI with all scores initially treated as continuous variables and subsequently grouped in prognostic categories (Additional file 1: Appendix C). PESI did not achieve significance in any of these analyses. The RIETE score showed an association with 3-month and 6-month mortality. The RIETE very low risk, low risk, intermediate and high risk categories retained correlation with 3- and 6-month mortality, but the HIGH/LOW grouping [22] did not. In all ROC curve analyses the Hull clinical scores appeared to outperform RIETE groups, except for 3-month mortality (Additional file 1: Appendix C).

Two of the experimental scores exhibited greater predictive consistency (Additional file 1: Appendix C); one

Table 3 Univariate (Kaplan-Meier) and multivariate (Cox Regression) analysis for overall survival.

	N*	OS (95%CI)	p	HR(95%CI)	p
Metastatic/incurable disease					
No	45		<.001	1	<.001
Yes	188	NR 10.5 (7.3, 13.7)		2.6 (1.5, 4.3)	
New Symptoms					
No	132	17 (12.7, 21.3)	.029		
Yes	98	10.1 (5.9, 14.3)			
Worsening Symptoms					
No	178	15.2 (11.9, 8.4)			
Yes	49	6.5 (5.2, 7.8)	.013		
New or Worsening symptoms					
No	111	19 (14.3, 23.8)	.004	1	.002
Yes	121	8.6 (5.3, 11.8)		1.7 (1.2, 2.4)	
WCC					
<11.3 x10^9/L	199	14 (9.9, 18.1)	.016	1	
≥11.3 x10^9/L	26	5.4 (2.4,8.3)		1.1 (.7, 1.8)	.659
Creatinine					
<55µmol/L	29	5.3 (1.5, 9.2)	.021	1	.408
>55µmol/L	195	14 (10, 17.9)		1.2 (.8, 2)	
ECOG/WHO PS			<.001		<.001
0	104	22.9 (17.9, 28.3)		1	
1,2	100	8.8 (6.5, 11)	<.001	1.9 (1.3, 2.8)	.001
3,4	23	3.3 (2.2, 4.4)	<.001	3.7 (2.2, 6.3)	<.001
PESI			<.001		.081
I,II	28	21 (6.2, 35.7)		1	
III,IV	185	13.8 (10.5, 17.1)	.222	1.5 (.8, 2.5)	.181
V	20	5.5 (4.3, 6.6)	<.001	2.3 (1.1, 4.8)	.026

Numbers are rounded to the first decimal for simplicity were possible. ROC curve analyses were used to identify candidate cut-offs for dichotomisation of continuous variable, indicating WCC 11.3 x10^9/L and Creatinine 55umol/L as useful cut-offs. 219 complete cases with 152 events available for Cox Regression

included all three clinical variables (a), (b) and (c) as above ("HULL2") and the other only (b) and (c) ("HULL5"). "HULL2" resulted in four risk groups identified by clustering of Kaplan-Meier survival curves. "HULL5" (Table 4) produced three risk clusters in Kaplan-Meier (low, intermediate, high risk, Fig. 1). Both these scores exhibited significant predictive ability for early mortality [30-day mortality: AUC = .821, 95%CI (.707, .936), p = .004 and AUC = .805, 95%CI (.675, .934), p = 0.006, respectively, as seen in Additional file 1: Appendix C]. An attempt to analyse "HULL2" grouped into three prognostic categories resulted in loss of significance in ROC analysis, therefore it was discarded in favour of "HULL5". We would like to note, though, that the initial significance of "HULL2", does demonstrate that asymptomatic/good PS patients treated for

Table 4 Derivation of the Hull5 prognostic score from a multivariate Cox regression model for OS with two selected variables exhibiting association with OS and early mortality

Variable	Categories	Wald	HR	95%(CI)	P	Points
New or worsening symptoms	Yes	10.962	1.7	(1.3, 2.4)	.001	1
	No	1	1			0
Performance status	0	1	1			0
	1/2	18.33	2.1	(1.5, 3)	< .001	2
	3/4	28.2	3.9	(2.3,6.3)	< .001	3

Grouping - Low Risk: 0, Intermediate Risk: 1–2, High Risk: 3–4

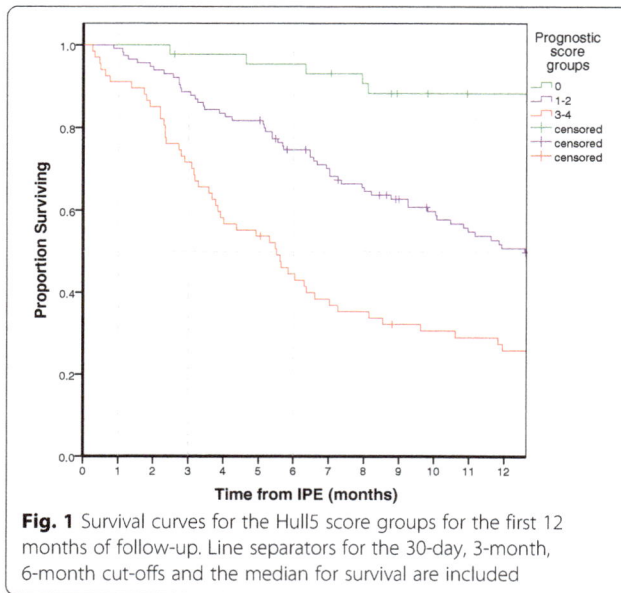

Fig. 1 Survival curves for the Hull5 score groups for the first 12 months of follow-up. Line separators for the 30-day, 3-month, 6-month cut-offs and the median for survival are included

potentially curable malignancy can be considered a particularly favourable prognostic category. Table 5 illustrates the OS and mortality rates of prognostic groups in our patient cohort as per the "HULL5" score system in comparison to the RIETE score prognostic grouping.

Discussion

The main strength of the current analysis is that it derives from a prospectively identified cohort managed uniformly under a standardised diagnostic and management protocol developed and applied in real-life conditions in a single centre. The generalisability of our observations would require validation in an external cohort.

6-month mortality in our cohort was 30.8% 95%CI (24.8, 36.8), similar, though numerically lower, to the mortality rate reported in the largest published pooled cohort of cancer patients with IPE [37% 95% CI (28%, 47%)] [19]. 30-day mortality in the cohort of 408 patients used for the derivation of the POMPE-C score was 12.5% (15% in their external validation cohort of 182 patients) and 21% in 508 patients used for the derivation of the RIETE prognostic score (24% in the external validation cohort of 261pts) [22]; both of these studies included patients with active cancer and predominantly symptomatic PE. In our cohort 30-day mortality was 3.4% 95%CI (1.3%,6,0%) possibly reflecting a difference in the outcomes of ambulatory IPE versus acute symptomatic PE patients with active cancer.

Recurrence of VTE or progressive PE within six months as well as major haemorrhage within six months were rare in our patients, comparing favourably to the report by vanderHulle et al. [19]. The reason for this difference is unclear, but it should be noted that our cohort was treated under a specific standardised protocol for treatment initiation and follow-up.

This analysis verifies the observations we previously made in a subset of this cohort suggesting that the usefulness of the standard PESI score may have reduced value in this group of patients [30]. In the current analysis, PESI class V did demonstrate statistically significant effects on mortality, as expected, since it describes patients with significant comorbidities and/or evidence of physiological

Table 5 OS, 30-day, 3-month and 6-month mortality of discussed risk scoring

Score categories	OS months (95%CI)	Mortality %(n)		
		30-d (n = 7)	3-m (n = 33)	6-m (n = 68)
Hull5 Risk Score (n = 227)				
Low (n = 45)	32(8.1,5 5.9)	0(0)	2.2(1)	4.4(2)
Intermediate (n = 115)	12.6(8.3, 16.9)	0.9(1)	11.3(13)	25.2(29)
High (n = 67)	5.5 (3.9, 7.2)	9.0(6)	28.4(19)	55.2(37)
	p < .001*	p = .004**	p < .001**	p < .001**
RIETE Risk Score (n = 205)				
Very low (n = 27)	not reached	0(0)	3.7(1)	7.4(2)
Low (n = 123)	15.9 (11.2, 20.6)	2.4(3)	9.8(12)	22.8(28)
Intermediate (n = 53)	5.4 (4.3, 6.5)	5.7(3)	32.1(17)	56.6(30)
High (n = 2)	2.7 (not calc.)	0%(0)	50(1)	50(1)
	p < .001*	p = .185**	p < .001**	p < .001**
RIETE Risk Score (n = 205)				
Low(n = 27)	not reached	0(0)	3.7(1)	7.4(2)
High (n = 178)	11.2 (7.7, 14.7)	3.4(6)	16.9(30)	33.1(59)
	p < .001*	p = .603**	p = .087**	p = .006**

*log rank (pooled)
**Kendall's tau-b exact test

compromise, nevertheless in ROC analysis PESI scoring as a continuous variable was the weakest amongst the tested risk scoring algorithms. RIETE performed better in our cohort still less consistently than the proposed clinical score. It is therefore our observation that a basic oncologic assessment of performance status at the time of IPE, combined with the self-reported presence of new or worsening symptomatology (without further elaboration) may reliably risk-stratify cancer patients with an incidental finding of pulmonary embolus.

Our analyses identify a group of patients with particularly good prognosis, namely those with an excellent prognostic status, absence of new or worsening symptoms which may be further enriched by excluding patients with metastatic disease. For this group of patients, modification of the standard management approach, for example reducing the duration of anticoagulation treatment, may be considered, still such a recommendation would require a randomised study.

Two prognostic scores have been proposed in the literature for patients with cancer and acute pulmonary embolism each utilising multiple clinical and laboratory parameters. The POMPE-C score [21] incorporates eight clinical variables and RIETE [22] six. The RIETE investigators also identified two additional laboratory variables namely $WBC > 11,000/mm^3$ and Creatinine clearance <30 ml/min. The prognostic significance of WCC was observed in our analysis regarding early mortality, nevertheless its significance was lost in multivariate OS analysis. A minor effect of serum creatinine was also observed nevertheless this effect was inverse to the RIETE observations. One interpretation of our observation could be that very low creatinine levels may correlate with cancer cachexia which itself may convey worse prognosis. We did not include WCC or Creatinine levels in the prognostic score analyses because the effects on OS were not maintained in the multivariate Cox regression model but also because their effect was relatively small as indicated with OR close to the unit and since a purely clinical prognostic score may be more readily applicable and interpretable.

Our application of RIETE in this analysis used the recorded variables of hospitalisation in the previous 30 days and surgery in the previous 30 days as surrogates for the immobilisation variable. This approximation may have introduced bias in our comparative analysis nevertheless it may also be regarded as a showcase of the inherent subjectivity of this variable. We were not able to apply POMPE-C since we did not have the information regarding Do-Not-Resuscitate orders, which in addition, is a non-standardisable variable which introduces bias. It is our view that the assessment of performance status and the self-reported presence of new or worsening symptomatology is a simple and generalizable assessment.

The presence of incurable/metastatic cancer, which may enrich the risk assessment, is also simple and objective.

Symptomatology in our analysis was a self-reported variable and did not require further elaboration to achieve prognostic significance. This observation may be considered in concert with previous publications [12]. The presence of new symptomatology and the deterioration of pre-existing symptoms exhibited a significant independent correlation with survival which may illustrate the effect of the unsuspected pulmonary embolus in patient physiology, or possibly the development of PE within the context of progressive malignancy which may cause deteriorating symptoms and also carries prothrombotic potential.

As limitations of the current work we can consider the lack of granularity of patient-reported symptom assessment as well as the lack of follow-up of symptomatology which could provide a prognostic assessment of patient-reported outcomes (PRO). We are currently piloting the utilisation of validated symptom-scale questionnaires (i.e. SF12 and PembQUOL) and plan to study patient-reported outcomes within this patient group. It should also be noted that our cohort, similarly to previously published studies, was not arithmetically powered for cancer-specific sub analyses (exploratory analyses are shown in Additional file 1: Appendix D). It is conceivable that different malignancies provide a different level of competing risk for early mortality. In addition, the relatively small number of haemorrhages, VTE recurrences and 30-day hospitalisations observed in our study population may limit the accuracy of our corresponding prognostic analysis; more accurate observations would require the analysis of these data points in larger cohorts. Moreover, since our study was based on audit data, it analysed only the baseline factors that were available as part of the standard clinical and laboratory assessments required for the safe management of the patients within our clinical pathway. Therefore, factors such as smoking history and mean platelet volume (MPV) which are known potential prognostic factors for the development of VTE or additional experimental baseline characteristics were not recorded or analysed.

Conclusion

In conclusion, our analysis suggests that a simple prognostic score based on the patient reported clinical factors -symptom assessment and contemporaneously assessed performance status - reflecting the physiological burden on a cancer patient - can be used to easily and reliably stratify the mortality outcomes of patients with IPE and cancer in the clinical setting.

Abbreviations

CLOT: Comparison of Low-molecular-weight heparin versus Oral Anticoagulant Therapy for the prevention of recurrent venous thromboembolism in patients with cancer (clinical trial acronym); CT: Computed Tomography; DVT: Deep Vein Thrombosis; ECOG: Eastern Cooperative Oncology Group; Hb: Haemoglobin; IPE: Incidental / Unsuspected Pulmonary Embolism; ISTH: International Society for Thrombosis and Haemostasis; IVC: Inferior Vena Cava; LMWH: Low Molecular Weight Heparin; OS: Overall Survival; PE: Pulmonary Embolism; PESI: Pulmonary Embolism Severity Index; PLT: Platelet count; PS: Performance Status; RIETE: Registro Informatizado de Pacientes con Enfermedad TromboEmbólica (Computerised Registry of Patients with Venous Thromboembolism); ROC: Receiver Operator Characteristics; VTE: Vascular Thromboembolic Events; WCC: White Cell Count; WHO: World Health Organisation

Acknowledgements

Julie Fountain, Quality and Safety Manager.Survival curves for the Hull5 score groups for the first 12 months of follow-up. Line separators for the 30-day, 3-month, 6-month cut-offs and the median for survival are included.

Funding

this study did not require external or internal funding.

Authors contributions

GB led the audit and designed the database, oversaw the clinical management of patients, collected data, performed the statistical analysis, and authored the manuscript. NJ critically collected data and contributed to manuscript preparation. DR-V critically collected data and contributed to the preparation of the manuscript. GA leads the diagnostic element of the service pathway and reviewed CT imaging, AS co-leads the diagnostic element of the service pathway and reviewed CT images. HM collected data and managed the database. JP carried out patient assessment and interviews and manages the service pathway. ME carried out patient assessment and interviews and collected data. AM conceived the project and leads the VTE in Cancer Steering Group in our Centre. He co-authored the manuscript and provided final approval. All authors read and approved the final manuscript.

Competing interests

All authors listed declare that they have no competing interests relevant to this manuscript.

Author details

[1]Hull and East Yorkshire NHS Hospitals Trust, Queen's Centre for Oncology and Haematology, Castle Hill Hospital, Castle Road, Cottingham HU16 5JQ, UK. [2]Hull and East Yorkshire NHS Hospitals Trust, Radiology Department, Castle Hill Hospital, Castle Road, Cottingham HU16 5JQ, UK. [3]Hull York Medical School, Academic Oncology, Castle Hill Hospital, Castle Road, Cottingham HU16 5JQ, UK.

References

1. Khorana AA, O'Connell C, Agnelli G, Liebman HA, Lee AYY, On Behalf of the Subcommittee on Hemostasis and Malignancy of the SSC of the ISTH. Incidental venous thromboembolism in oncology patients. J Thromb Haemost. 2012;10:2602–4. doi:10.1111/jth.12023.

2. Sebastian AJ, Paddon AJ. Clinically unsuspected pulmonary embolism–an important secondary finding in oncology CT. Clin Radiol. 2006;61(1):81–5. https://doi.org/10.1016/j.crad.2005.09.002.

3. Cronin CG, Lohan DG, Keane M, Roche C, Murphy JM. Prevalence and significance of asymptomatic venous thromboembolic disease found on oncologic staging CT. AJR Am J Roentgenol. 2007;189(1):162–70. https://doi.org/10.2214/AJR.07.2067.

4. van Es N, Bleker SM, Di Nisio M. Cancer-associated unsuspected pulmonary embolism. Thromb Res. 2014;133(Suppl 2):S172–8. https://doi.org/10.1016/S0049-3848(14)50028-X.

5. O'Connell CL, Boswell WD, Duddalwar V, Caton A, Mark LS, Vigen C, Liebman HA. Unsuspected pulmonary emboli in cancer patients: clinical correlates and relevance. Journal of clinical oncology : official journal of the American Society of Clinical Oncology. 2006;24(30):4928–32. https://doi.org/10.1200/JCO.2006.06.5870.

6. Dentali F, Ageno W, Becattini C, Galli L, Gianni M, Riva N, Imberti D, Squizzato A, Venco A, Agnelli G. Prevalence and clinical history of incidental, asymptomatic pulmonary embolism: a meta-analysis. Thromb Res. 2010; 125(6):518–22. https://doi.org/10.1016/j.thromres.2010.03.016.

7. den Exter PL, Hooijer J, Dekkers OM, Huisman MV. Risk of recurrent venous thromboembolism and mortality in patients with cancer incidentally diagnosed with pulmonary embolism: a comparison with symptomatic patients. Journal of clinical oncology : official journal of the American Society of Clinical Oncology. 2011;29(17):2405–9. https://doi.org/10.1200/JCO.2010.34.0984.

8. Font C, Farrus B, Vidal L, Caralt TM, Visa L, Mellado B, Tassies D, Monteagudo J, Reverter JC, Gascon P. Incidental versus symptomatic venous thrombosis in cancer: a prospective observational study of 340 consecutive patients. Annals of oncology : official journal of the European Society for Medical Oncology / ESMO. 2011;22(9):2101–6. https://doi.org/10.1093/annonc/mdq720.

9. O'Connell C, Razavi P, Ghalichi M, Boyle S, Vasan S, Mark L, Caton A, Duddalwar V, Boswell W, Grabow K, Liebman HA. Unsuspected pulmonary emboli adversely impact survival in patients with cancer undergoing routine staging multi-row detector computed tomography scanning. Journal of thrombosis and haemostasis : JTH. 2011;9(2):305–11. https://doi.org/10.1111/j.1538-7836.2010.04114.x.

10. Grigoropoulos NF, Shaw AS, Hampson FA, Baglin TP, Follows GA. Incidental pulmonary emboli in lymphoma patients are associated with aggressive disease and poor prognosis. Journal of thrombosis and haemostasis : JTH. 2010;8(12):2835–6. https://doi.org/10.1111/j.1538-7836.2010.04061.x.

11. Shteinberg M, Segal-Trabelsy M, Adir Y, Laor A, Vardi M, Bitterman H. Clinical characteristics and outcomes of patients with clinically unsuspected pulmonary embolism versus patients with clinically suspected pulmonary embolism. Respiration; international review of thoracic diseases. 2012;84(6): 492–500. https://doi.org/10.1159/000342324.

12. O'Connell CL, Razavi PA, Liebman HA. Symptoms adversely impact survival among patients with cancer and unsuspected pulmonary embolism. Journal of clinical oncology : official journal of the American Society of Clinical Oncology. 2011;29(31):4208–4209; author reply 4209-4210. https://doi.org/10.1200/JCO.2011.37.2730.

13. Bozas G, Bradley R, Avery G, Stephens A, Maraveyas A. PB3.60-3 Pre-existing pulmonary thrombi in cancer patients diagnosed with an unsuspected pulmonary embolism. Abstracts of the XXIV Congress of the International Society on Thrombosis and Haemostasis. J Thromb Haemost. 2013;11(s2): 856. doi:10.1111/jth.12284.

14. Kearon C, Akl EA, Comerota AJ, Prandoni P, Bounameaux H, Goldhaber SZ, Nelson ME, Wells PS, Gould MK, Dentali F, Crowther M, Kahn SR, American College of Chest P. Antithrombotic therapy for VTE disease: antithrombotic therapy and prevention of thrombosis, 9th ed: American College of Chest Physicians Evidence-Based Clinical Practice Guidelines. Chest. 2012;141(2 Suppl):e419S–94S. https://doi.org/10.1378/chest.11-2301.

15. Lyman GH, Khorana AA, Kuderer NM, Lee AY, Arcelus JI, Balaban EP, Clarke JM, Flowers CR, Francis CW, Gates LE, Kakkar AK, Key NS, Levine MN, Liebman HA, Tempero MA, Wong SL, Prestrud AA, Falanga A, American Society of Clinical Oncology Clinical P. Venous thromboembolism prophylaxis and treatment in patients with cancer: American Society of Clinical Oncology clinical practice guideline update. Journal of clinical oncology : official journal of the American Society of Clinical Oncology. 2013;31(17):2189–204. https://doi.org/10.1200/JCO.2013.49.1118.

16. Carrier M, Kimpton M, LEG G, Kahn SR, Kovacs MJ, Wells PS, Anderson DR, Rodger MA. The management of a sub-segmental pulmonary embolism: a cross-sectional survey of Canadian thrombosis physicians. Journal of thrombosis and haemostasis : JTH. 2011;9(7):1412–5. https://doi.org/10.1111/j.1538-7836.2011.04306.x.

17. Lim WY, Bozas G, Noble S, Hart S, Maraveyas A. Anticoagulating the subsegmental pulmonary embolism in cancer patients: a survey amongst different medical specialties. J Thromb Thrombolysis. 2015;40(1):37–41. https://doi.org/10.1007/s11239-014-1143-9.

18. Di Nisio M, Lee AYY, Carrier M, Liebman HA, Khorana AA, for the Subcommittee on Haemostasis and Malignancy. Diagnosis and treatment of incidental venous thromboembolism in cancer patients: guidance from the SSC of the ISTH. J Thromb Haemost. 2015;13:880–3. doi:10.1111/jth.12883.

19. van der Hulle T, den Exter PL, Planquette B, Meyer G, Soler S, Monreal M, Jimenez D, Portillo AK, O'Connell C, Liebman HA, Shteinberg M, Adir Y, Tiseo M, Bersanelli M, Abdel-Razeq HN, Mansour AH, Donnelly OG, Radhakrishna G, Ramasamy S, Bozas G, Maraveyas A, Shinagare AB, Hatabu H, Nishino M, Huisman MV, Klok FA. Risk of recurrent venous thromboembolism and major hemorrhage in cancer-associated incidental pulmonary embolism among treated and untreated patients: a pooled analysis of 926 patients. Journal of thrombosis and haemostasis : JTH. 2016; 14(1):105–13. https://doi.org/10.1111/jth.13172.

20. Aujesky D, Perrier A, Roy PM, Stone RA, Cornuz J, Meyer G, Obrosky DS, Fine MJ. Validation of a clinical prognostic model to identify low-risk patients with pulmonary embolism. J Intern Med. 2007;261(6):597–604. https://doi.org/10.1111/j.1365-2796.2007.01785.x.

21. Kline JA, Roy PM, Than MP, Hernandez J, Courtney DM, Jones AE, Penaloza A, Pollack CV Jr. Derivation and validation of a multivariate model to predict mortality from pulmonary embolism with cancer: the POMPE-C tool. Thromb Res. 2012;129(5):e194–9. https://doi.org/10.1016/j.thromres.2012.03.015.

22. den Exter PL, Gomez V, Jimenez D, Trujillo-Santos J, Muriel A, Huisman MV, Monreal M, Registro Informatizado de la Enfermedad TromboEmbolica I. A clinical prognostic model for the identification of low-risk patients with acute symptomatic pulmonary embolism and active cancer. Chest. 2013; 143(1):138–45. https://doi.org/10.1378/chest.12-0964.

23. Palmer J, Bozas G, Stephens A, Johnson M, Avery G, O'Toole L, Maraveyas A. Developing a complex intervention for the outpatient management of incidentally diagnosed pulmonary embolism in cancer patients. BMC Health Serv Res. 2013;13:235. https://doi.org/10.1186/1472-6963-13-235.

24. Bozas G, Palmer J, Avery G, Maraveyas A. P-TU-403. Outcome and characteristics of cancer patients with incidental pulmonary embolism managed under a specialised care pathway protocol. Abstracts of the XXIII Congress of the International Society on Thrombosis and Haemostasis. J Thromb Haemost. 2011; 9(Suppl s2):435. doi:10.1111/j.1538-7836.2011.04380_2.x.

25. Bozas G, Ramasamy S, Avery G, Maraveyas A. PO-09 Pulmonary embolism as an incidental finding in ambulatory cancer outpatients. Characteristics and outcome. Thromb Res 2010;125(Suppl 2):S168. doi:10.1016/S0049-3848(10)70059-1.

26. Lee AYY, Levine MN, Baker RI, Bowden C, Kakkar AK, Prins M, Rickles FR, Julian JA, Haley S, Kovacs MJ, Gent M. Low-molecular-weight heparin versus a Coumarin for the prevention of recurrent venous Thromboembolism in patients with cancer. N Engl J Med. 2003;349(2):146–53. https://doi.org/10.1056/NEJMoa025313.

27. HRA. Defining Research. NHS Health Rresearch Authority. 2017. http://www.hra-decisiontools.org.uk/research/docs/DefiningResearchTable_Oct2017-1.pdf. Accessed 30 Dec 2017.

28. HQIP (2016) Best practice in clinical audit. Health quality improvement partnership http://www.hqip.org.uk/resources/best-practice-in-clinical-audit-hqip-guide/. Accessed 30 Dec 2017.

29. Oken MM, Creech RH, Tormey DC, Horton J, Davis TE, McFadden ET, Carbone PP. Toxicity and response criteria of the eastern cooperative oncology group. Am J Clin Oncol. 1982;5(6):649–55.

30. Bozas G, Ramanujam-Venkatachala D, Jeffery N, Avery G, Stephens A, Algar V, Palmer J, Elliott M, Maraveyas A. Incidental pulmonary embolism in cancer: A prognostic score derived from a prospective cohort with uniform management. Abstracts from the European Cancer Congress 2015. Eur J Cancer. 2015;51(Suppl 3):S237-8. doi:10.1016/S0959-8049(16)30688-8.

27

The introduction of biosimilars of low molecular weight heparins in Europe: a critical review and reappraisal endorsed by the Italian Society for Haemostasis and Thrombosis (SISET) and the Italian Society for Angiology and Vascular Medicine (SIAPAV)

Davide Imberti[1], Marco Marietta[2], Hernan Polo Friz[3,4*] and Claudio Cimminiello[4]

Abstract

Recently, the European Medicines Agency (EMA) authorized the introduction and marketing of Thorinane® and Inhixa®, biosimilars of the Low Molecular Weight Heparin (LMWH) enoxaparin. The authorization path is considerably different from the guidelines published by the EMA in 2009, as well as from the recommendations from the International Society on Thrombosis and Haemostasis published in 2013. Indeed, both of them recommended that LMWHs biosimilars therapeutic equivalence should be demonstrated in at least one adequately designed clinical trial. Shortly after enoxaparin biosimilars approval, EMA published a revised version of its guideline, no longer requiring the execution of a clinical study in patients at risk of venous thromboembolism.

Also the assessment of safety shows some relevant flaws, as it relies only on a 20 healthy volunteers study, clearly underpowered to draw any conclusions about the safety profile of the drug.

In our opinion, the approach taken by EMA for approval of enoxaparin biosimilars raises serious concerns about their actual, clinical "similarity".

On these grounds, with the endorsement of the Italian Society for Haemostasis and Thrombosis (SISET) and the Italian Society for Angiology and Vascular Medicine (SIAPAV), we elaborated the present document aimed at reviewing and reappraising some critical points regarding the introduction of biosimilars of LMWH in Europe.

Moreover, we would strongly advise the Italian National Health Authorities not to entrust safety assessment to the post-marketing surveillance only, but to promote well designed and powered studies aimed at establish the actual efficacy and safety of LMWH biosimilars.

Keywords: Low molecular weight heparin, Biosimilar pharmaceuticals, Evidence-based practice, Therapeutic equivalency, Venous Thromboembolism

* Correspondence: hernanemilio.polofriz@asst-vimercate.it; polofriz@libero.it
[3]Internal Medicine, Medical Department, Vimercate Hospital, via Santi Cosma e Damiano 10, 20871 Vimercate, Italy
[4]Studies and Research Center of the Italian Society of Angiology and Vascular Pathology (Società Italiana di Angiologia e Patologia Vascolare, SIAPAV), via Gorizia 22, 20144 Milan, Italy
Full list of author information is available at the end of the article

Background

Low molecular weight heparins (LMWHs) are animal-derived products obtained by chemical or enzymatic depolymerization of unfractionated heparin. The efficacy and safety of LMWHs have been demonstrated in large randomized clinical trials and evidence based guidelines recommend their use for the prevention and treatment of venous and arterial thromboembolic events [1, 2].

Biological drugs are pharmaceutical products obtained by extraction from biological tissues or from biotechnological processes, constituted of larger molecules with a complex structure, thus differing from conventional small molecule medications [2]. The term "biosimilars" is used to qualify products developed to be similar to an original biological drug. Biosimilars are much more complicated to develop than a generic version of small molecule drugs and this is also true for LMWHs [3].

In the past years, patents of some LMWH have gradually expired and several copies of LMWHs have been produced and marketed in different countries. Recently, the European Commission granted a marketing authorization valid throughout the European Union for two biosimilars of LMWH enoxaparin (Thorinane and Inhixa).

The market accessibility of biosimilars is deemed to reduce costs to patients and social security systems. However, the introduction of biosimilar LMWHs have originated an intense debate since even minor differences between the biochemical and biological activities of biosimilar and originator LMWHs may have significant clinical consequences in terms of efficacy and safety [4].

Some serious concerns about the regulatory path adopted by EMA to authorize the introduction and marketing of Thorinane and Inhixa have led to the elaboration of the present document, endorsed by the Italian Society for Haemostasis and Thrombosis (SISET) and the Italian Society for Angiology and Vascular Medicine (SIAPAV), aimed at perform a review and a reappraisal of some critical points regarding the introduction of LMWH biosimilars in Europe.

Main text

Overview on guidelines, recommendations and requirements for the approval of biosimilars of LMWHs

Regulatory authorities from the United States of America (US) and Europe have taken different approaches to classify LMWH products. The Food and Drug Administration (FDA) considers LMWH semi-synthetic drugs while the European Medicines Agency (EMA) define them as biological products. Debates and controversies arising from these different positions determined the publication of several guidelines and position statements [2, 5–9]. Recommendations regarding the requirements that copies of LMWH must fulfill to be produced and marketed have been issued by the EMA [5] and the FDA [8, 9].

FDA requirements

The FDA approved the first copy of enoxaparin in 2010. Innovator LMHWs were classified as drugs under the Abbreviated New Drug Application procedure proposed for requests for marketing authorization of small molecule chemical drugs, and requiring only the demonstration of bioequivalence through pharmacokinetic studies [8]. The FDA stated that the applicant for enoxaparin demonstrated the "sameness" compared to the branded LMWH enoxaparin, by meeting five criteria: (1) physical and chemical characteristics of enoxaparin; (2) nature of the source material and the method used to cleave the polysaccharide chains into smaller fragments; (3) nature and arrangement of components that constitute enoxaparin; (4) certain laboratory measurements of anti-coagulant activity and (5) certain aspects of the drug's effect in humans [8, 9].

EMA guidelines

The EMA developed several guidelines and revisions on different aspects of the process of biosimilars LMWHs products approval.

In 2006, the EMA published the "Guideline on similar biological medicinal products containing biotechnology-derived proteins as active substance: quality issues (EMEA/CHMP/BWP/49348/2005)" [10]. Later, this document was replace by the "Guideline on similar biological medicinal products containing biotechnology-derived proteins as active substance: quality issues (revision 1). EMA/CHMP/BWP/247713/2012" [11]. Even though not specifically issued to regulate LMWHs biosimilars production, this guideline was used as reference to establish special quality aspects of biochemical LMWH characterization requirements.

In 2009, the EMA published the "Guidelines on non-clinical and clinical development of similar biological medicinal products containing low molecular weight heparin"EMEA/CHMP/BMWP/118264/2007 [5]. The document, currently in force, states as principle the need of a demonstration of the similar nature of the originator and the biosimilar in terms of safety and efficacy. Indeed, some specific criteria have to be fulfilled for a generic LMWH to be licensed, like: biochemical characterization; data on in vitro comparative bioassays (based on state of the art knowledge about clinically relevant pharmacodynamic effects of LMWH and including, at least, evaluations of anti-FXa and anti-FIIa activity); data on in vivo pharmacodynamic models comparing animal pharmacodynamic activity of the similar and the reference LMWH; data from at least one repeated dose toxicity study in a relevant species; phase I studies comparing the absorption and elimination characteristics and other pharmacodynamics tests such as Tissue Factor Pathway Inhibitor (TFPI) activity, as well as the ratio of anti-FXa and anti-FIIa activity. Moreover, the pharmacodynamic properties of biosimilars and branded LMWH must be compared in a randomized, single dose two way crossover study in healthy volunteers using subcutaneous administration, and, in case the originator product were also licensed for the intravenous or intra-arterial route, an additional comparative study should be performed via the intravenous route. In addition, the EMA guideline states that, since there is no clear correlation between pharmacodynamics parameters (anti-FXa or anti-FIIa) and clinical, a biosimilar LMWH should show equivalent efficacy and safety to a reference product approved in the EU. This therapeutic equivalence should be demonstrated in at least one adequately powered, randomized, double-blind, parallel group clinical trial. To demonstrate efficacy in the prevention of venous thromboembolism (VTE) in patients undergoing surgery with high VTE risk, the trial should be preferably conducted in major orthopedic surgery such as hip surgery and patients with hip fracture should be well represented. The study should be powered to show therapeutic equivalence on one of the two recommended endpoints and a central independent and blinded committee of experts should perform adjudication of VTE events.

Finally, the 2009 EMA guideline states that prelicensing safety data should be obtained in a number of patients sufficient to determine the adverse effect profiles of the test medicinal product, with comparative safety data from the efficacy trial being considered sufficient to provide an adequate pre-marketing safety database, and that a risk management programme plan in accordance with EU legislation and pharmacovigilance guidelines, with a particular focus on rare serious adverse events known to be associated with LMWHs such as Heparin-induced Thrombocytopenia Type II (HIT II, HITT) as well as anaphylactoid and anaphylactic reactions [5].

The EMA published a concept paper on the revision of the 2009 guideline in 2011: EMA/CHMP/BMWP/522386/2011 [12]. In the document, it was acknowledged that "the current guidance requires a comparative clinical trial demonstrating similar efficacy and safety" between the biosimilar and the reference LMWH in the prevention of VTE in patients undergoing major orthopaedic surgery, and was recommended a discussion whether a reduction in clinical data requirements could, in exceptional cases, be possible.

In 2014, the Committee for Medicinal Products for Human Use (CHMP) of the EMA issued the "Guideline on similar biological medicinal products" CHMP/437/04 Rev. 1 [13], with the purpose of describing the concept

of similar biological medicinal products and to outline the general principles to be applied. CHMP experts concluded that the biosimilar approach is more difficult to apply to biological substances arising from extraction from biological sources and/or those for which little clinical and regulatory experience has been gained, like LMWHs, when compared to products that are highly purified and can be thoroughly characterized. Furthermore, this guideline states that a biosimilar should be highly similar to the reference medicinal product in physicochemical and biological terms and that any observed differences have to be duly justified with regard to their potential impact on safety and efficacy.

International Society on thrombosis and Haemostasis (ISTH) recommendations

In 2013, the Scientific Subcommittee (SSC) on Control of Anticoagulation of the Scientific and Standardization Committee of the ISTH published an update summarizing the recommendations for the development of a biosimilar version of a branded LMWH [2]. The SSC of the ISTH recommends that the lack of significant differences between the biosimilar and originator LMWH should be demonstrated using an adequate study design, and that all results obtained in vitro, ex vivo and in clinical settings should adequately demonstrate the similarity or non-inferiority of the biosimilar LMWH relative to the originator LMWH and the confidence intervals should be defined using adequate statistical methods. Furthermore, the SSC of the ISTH clearly states that the efficacy and safety of a biosimilar LMWH should be demonstrated in comparison to the originator LMWH in clinical trials for every indication for which regulatory approval is sought. If biosimilar LMWHs claim to be as effective and safe as the originator products, a head to head comparison of the two LMWH preparations should be performed also in prospective, randomized, double blind clinical trials performed to show the non-inferiority of a biosimilar LMWH compared to the originator LMWH, in the most relevant clinical settings where LMWHs are indicated, like prophylaxis of postoperative venous thromboembolism, prophylaxis of venous thromboembolism in hospitalized patients with acute medical illness, treatment of acute deep vein thrombosis and pulmonary embolism, prevention of acute coronary events in patients with unstable or stable angina, prevention of acute coronary syndrome during and after percutaneous coronary intervention, extracorporeal circulation, and chronic haemodialysis [2].

The authorization path for the approval of biosimilars of LMWHs in Europe

In July 2016 the EMA's CHMP expressed a positive opinion for granting a marketing authorization to two biosimilars of enoxaparin sodium: Thorinane and Inhixa [14, 15]. Both European Public Assessment Reports (EPAR)s were first published on 26 October 2016. Thorinane's application was received by the EMA on 6 February 2015 and the procedure started on 25 March 2015. Inhixa's application was received on 27 May 2015 and the procedure started on 25 June 2015.

Both reports declared that the development programme of Thorinane and Inhixa had specifically considered the EU guidelines for similar biological medicinal products including the following specific guidelines for LMWH:

- CHMP Guideline on similar biological medicinal products containing biotechnology-derived proteins as active substance: quality issues (revision 1)(EMA/CHMP/BWP/247713/2012) [11]
- CHMP Guideline on Similar Biological Medicinal Products containing Biotechnology-Derived Proteins as Active Substance: Non-Clinical and Clinical Issues(EMEA/CHMP/42832/05) [16]
- Guideline on Non-Clinical and Clinical Development of Similar Biological Medicinal Products containing Low-Molecular-Weight-Heparins(EMEA/CHMP/BMWP/118264/2007) [5]
- Concept paper on the revision of the guideline on nonclinical and clinical development of similar biological medicinal products containing low molecular-weight heparins (EMA/CHMP/BMWP/522386/2011) [12]

Main conclusions reported by CHMP in the EPARs of Thorinane and Inhixa concerned non clinical aspects, clinical pharmacology, clinical efficacy and clinical safety. In general, they are the same for both products (Thorinane and Inhixa), since the rationale, authorization path and conclusions presented in both EPARs are practically identical [14, 15].

The recent approval of biosimilars of LMWHs in Europe and November 2016 revision of the EMA guidelines

Relevant concerns arise from the analysis of the authorization path that led to the recent approval of biosimilars of LMWHs by EMA, and some critical points should be clarify.

With regards to the non-clinical aspects, although some differences in the content of link region (LR) were found between Thorinane and the reference product, Thorinane EPAR authors stated that "the Applicant provided justification that the LR region is a structural feature of Enoxaparin which has no known pharmacological role that directly or indirectly affects either Heparin or Enoxaparin molecules". The same for Inhixa. No comparative or stand-alone toxicity studies were

performed to compare Thorinane and Inhixa and the reference RMP, since "toxicology studies could be not required if the quality comparability investigations of Thorinane and the RMP (addressing physicochemical parameters/analytical characterization as well as biological/biochemical parameters and similarity in biological activity) yield the expected results and did not leave open unanswered questions." The CHMP concluded that relevant assays were conducted and were not able to identify different immunogenic potential for Thorinane [14] and Inhixa [15] when compared to the reference medicinal product (RMP). Even though it was acknowledged that in vitro data with respect to immunogenicity have limitations, the most prominent safety concern associated with LMWHs, HP4 (Heparin Platelet Factor 4) complex binding was "most likely similar between the test and the RMP", and from this "it was inferred that the risk for immunogenicity is most likely also similar". This kind of inference must be better clarify, especially considering the 2008 so-called heparin crisis, where severe immune reactions were documented to be associated to the presence of oversulfated chondroitin sulfate (OSCS) as a result of a potential contamination during the extraction process of heparin from the animal source [17].

In the discussion on clinical efficacy, both Thorinane and Inhixa EPARs [14, 15] mentioned that "The EMA Guideline on non-clinical and clinical development of similar biological medicinal products containing low-molecular-weight-heparins (EMEA/CHMP/BMWP/118264/2007 + Draft Rev. 1) foresees a clinical study comparing efficacy and safety of the biosimilar candidate and the reference product unless evidence for similar efficacy and safety of the biosimilar and the reference product could be convincingly deduced from the comparison of their physicochemical characteristics, biological activity/potency, using sensitive, orthogonal and state-of-the-art analytical methods, and from comparison of their PD profiles." Instead, the 2009 "Guideline on non-clinical and clinical development of similar biological medicinal products containing low-molecular-weight-heparins", in force currently and at the time when Thorinane and Inhixa EPARs were released, clearly states that "since a clear correlation between surrogate PD parameters (anti FXa or anti FIIa) and clinical outcome has not been established"... "this therapeutic equivalence should be demonstrated in at least one adequately powered, randomized, double-blind, parallel group clinical trial", describing in detail the characteristics of that trial, like design and clinical setting. Thus, though there was no clinical efficacy studies performed to support the biosimilarity claims by Thorinane nor Inhixa, EPARs authors concluded that "it was agreed that potential efficacy study would not be sensitive enough to reveal small differences between two similar enoxaparin- containing-products showing a similar PD profile", and that "a stringent comparative quality documentation supported by a reduced (non-)clinical program was considered appropriate for showing equivalence of efficacy of LMWH".

When discussing on clinical safety issues, in both Thorinane and Inhixa EPARs, CHMP acknowledged that "the presented clinical safety data derived from a comparative PK/PD study were too scarce to conclude on a comparable safety profile of test and reference medicinal products", that "immunogenicity has not been comparatively assessed and initially" and that "the applicant did not present a strategy of in vitro and/or in vivo assays to allow for waiving of clinical safety data" [14, 15]. However, and surprisingly, the CHMP finally concluded that "the enhanced assay strategy provided by the applicant during the procedure gave reassurance that the most prominent safety concern associated with LMWHs, HP4 complex binding is most likely similar between both tested products, thus "In light of established biosimilarity on quality level, the remaining uncertainty that the safety profile of Thorinane and Clexane differs significantly was considered low enough to conclude on similarity" [17]. The same concept is expressed in the EPAR for Inhixa [11], and implies that surveillance and pharmocovigilance are the only tools to recognize potential safety issues, even though, as the case of surveillance of a biosimilar of enoxaparin in the US shows, they seems to present critical limitations [18].

A revision of the 2009 "Guidelines on non-clinical and clinical development of similar biological medicinal products containing low molecular weight heparin" was issued in November 2016 [19]. Concerning clinical efficacy, this revised guideline, expected to be coming into effect in June 2017, concludes that the evidence for similar efficacy should be derived from the similarity demonstrated in physicochemical, functional and pharmacodynamic comparisons, and that a dedicated comparative efficacy trial will be no longer considered necessary. With regards to clinical safety, the guideline states that whether "the impurity profile and the nature of excipients of the biosimilar do not create uncertainties with regard to their impact on safety/ immunogenicity, a safety/immunogenicity study may not be needed".

Thus, this guideline represent a conceptual and operative radical change respect to the previous EMA's guidelines, and does not seem their logical evolution. Moreover, we think that the timing of such a change deserves some attention.

The EMA issued the "Concept paper on the revision of the guideline on nonclinical and clinical development of similar biological medicinal products containing low-molecular-weight heparins" (EMA/CHMP/BMWP/

522386/2011) in 2011 [12], recommending a discussion about including the possibility of a modification in clinical data requirements. A draft revision was issued in 2012, but the Revision 1 of the guideline that makes effective these major modifications was adopted by CHMP on November 10th 2016, and, as mentioned, will be coming into effect on June 1st 2017.

That is, in July 2016, when EPARs authorizing the marketing of Thorinane and Inhixa were completed, the 2009 EMEA/CHMP/BMWP/118264/2007 guideline was in force, and such a guideline stated that therapeutic equivalence should be demonstrated in at least one adequately designed clinical trial.

Therefore, both enoxaparin biosimilars have been approved by using criteria quite different (and less compelling) from those required from the EMA guideline in force at that time. In our opinion, the "fast-track" approach taken by EMA for approval of enoxaparin biosimilars raises serious concerns about their actual, clinical "similarity", and can become a dangerous precedent for other drugs.

Conclusions

The authorizative path adopted by EMA for the introduction of biosimilar LMWHs in Europe raises in our opinion some relevant concerns regarding efficacy and safety of these drugs.

As far as Thorinane® and Inhixa® is concerned, the approval by the EMA was based only on in vitro preclinical assays (acknowledging that in vitro data with respect to immunogenicity have limitations) and on the outcome of a clinical PK/PD study in 20 healthy volunteers.

This approach is in keeping with the conceptual approach of FDA, which considers copies of LMWHs mostly generic drugs rather than biosimilars. However, we are unable to find any strong evidence supporting the EMA's recent position, so divergent from that advocated in the past by the same regulatory agency as well as from the recommendation of the ISTH. We think that the EMA should provide to the scientific community a more in-depth explanation of such a decision and of the rationale which led to concluding on biosimilarity for Thorinane® and Inhixa® that "in vitro preclinical assays as well as the outcome of the primary endpoints of the clinical PD study provided comprehensive information for characterisation of the biosimilar candidate to conclude similarity regarding efficacy" [14, 15].

Even stronger concerns are raised by the conclusions about safety, which are based just on a small-sized PK/PD study in healthy volunteers. Relevant to this, EMA itself acknowledges that data provided by this study are too scarce to conclude on a comparable safety profile, and entrusts the safety assessment to the post-marketing pharmacovigilance. The already cited study by Grammp et al. [18]provide interesting data to better understand how hazardous such an approach may result. These Authors compared the capabilities of claims databases and spontaneous reporting systems for monitoring the incidence of potential enoxaparin-related adverse effect (AE)s, including thrombocytopenia-related AEs, at the product-specific level, and to compare the attribution of all enoxaparin-related AEs in the FDA AE Reporting System (FAERS) database. The study found that claims data were useful for active surveillance of enoxaparin biosimilar products dispensed under pharmacy benefits but not for products administered under medical benefits. With enoxaparin, 10–35% of spontaneous reports were not attributable to a given manufacturer, and a ninefold increase in relative risk of an AE for a specific enoxaparin biosimilar could be overlooked because of the apparent underreporting to specific biosimilar manufacturers. Authors concluded that the current spontaneous reporting system will not distinguish product-specific safety signals for products distributed by multiple manufacturers, including biosimilars, and the upcoming introduction of biosimilars into the marketplace has highlighted current limitations within the data infrastructure [18]. Therefore, surveillance does not seems the final answer to LMWHs biosimilars safety concerns.

An interesting example on the scientific and regulatory debate related to biosimilars approval is represented by single-switch crossover or transition trials of biosimilar anti-TNF agents. Since no conclusive clinical trial data demonstrating the efficacy and safety of switching the therapy (originator to biosimilar) of stable patients are available, the Norwegian government decided to support a randomized, double-blind, parallel-group study, the NOR-SWITCH biosimilar study, to compare the originator infliximab with a biosimilar in patients with six immune-mediated inflammatory diseases [20].

Scientific societies such as ISTH and IUA [2, 7] have formulated recommendations about the criteria that LMWH biosimilars must fulfill to be authorized. These criteria were similar to, and even more strict than, those adopted by EMA until July to November 2016.

We think that the EMA's change of course is not supported by strong evidences, and therefore we stay on the requirements already issued by the scientific societies ISTH and IUA, thus asking for more reliable clinical data about the efficacy and safety of biosimilar LMWHs before their marketing.

Efficacy and safety assessment of biosimilars of LMWH should not be only based on post-marketing surveillance. Instead, therapeutic equivalence should be demonstrated in at least one adequately powered, randomized, double-blind, parallel group clinical trial, preferably in the prevention of VTE in patients with high VTE risk, with adjudication of VTE events by a central independent and blinded committee of experts. Prelicensing safety data should be obtained in a number of patients sufficient to determine the adverse effect profiles of the test medicinal product, with comparative safety data from the efficacy trial being considered sufficient to provide an adequate pre-marketing safety database, mainly aimed to assess endpoints such immunogenic adverse effects.

In conclusion, we agree that the development of biosimilar drugs can be an effective strategy to contain pharmaceutical expenses, thus providing more people with a wider access to treatments that are becoming more and more expensive. However, this appreciable goal should pursued by means of strict procedures, shared between stakeholders and scientific community, always placing the patient's safety in the first place.

We think that the approach taken by EMA for approval of enoxaparin biosimilars doesn't fulfill these requirements, raises serious concerns about their actual, clinical "similarity"..

On these grounds, we would strongly advise the Italian National Health Authorities not to entrust safety assessment to the post-marketing surveillance only, but to promote well designed and powered studies aimed at establish the actual efficacy and safety of LMWH biosimilars, as already performed for other molecules [20].

Abbreviations

AE's: Adverse effect; CHMP: Committee for Medicinal Products for Human Use; EMA: European Medicines Agency; EPAR's: European Public Assessment Reports; FDA: Food and Drug Administration; ISTH: International Society on Thrombosis and Haemostasis; LMWH: Low Molecular Weight Heparin; SSC: Scientific Subcommittee; VTE: Venous thromboembolism

Acknowledgements

Not applicable.

Funding

None to Declare.

Authors' contributions

DI, MM, HPF and CC certify that they have participated sufficiently in the work to take public responsibility for the content, including participation in the concept, design, analysis, writing, and revision of the manuscript. Furthermore, each author certifies that this material or similar material has not been submitted to or published in any other publication before. All authors read and approved the final manuscript.

Competing interests

Dr. Davide IMBERTI received consultancy and speaker fees from BMS- Pfizer, Boehringer Ingelheim, Sanofi, Bayer, Werfen, Medtronic, Daiichi-Sankyo, Kedrion. Dr. Marco MARIETTA has received personal fees for participation to Advisory Boards, collaborations as consultant and lectures by Novo Nordisk, Kedrion, Orphan Europe. Dr. Hernan POLO FRIZ has received personal fees for collaborations as medical writer, consultant, sponsored conferences and lectures by Bayer, Daiichi Sankyo, Pfizer, BMS, Sanofi, Boehringer Ingelheim, Health and Life, Clinical Forum, Xcape Srl, McCann Complete Medical Srl. Dr. Claudio CIMMINIELLO received consultancy and speaker fees from Pfizer, BMS, Boehringer Ingelheim, Sanofi, Bayer, MSD.

Author details

[1]Haemostasis and Thrombosis Center, Internal Medicine Department, Piacenza Hospital, Via Taverna 49, Piacenza, Italy. [2]Department of Oncology and Hematology, Section of Hematology, University of Modena and Reggio Emilia, Modena, Italy. [3]Internal Medicine, Medical Department, Vimercate Hospital, via Santi Cosma e Damiano 10, 20871 Vimercate, Italy. [4]Studies and Research Center of the Italian Society of Angiology and Vascular Pathology (Società Italiana di Angiologia e Patologia Vascolare, SIAPAV), via Gorizia 22, 20144 Milan, Italy.

References

1. Guyatt GH, Akl EA, Crowther M, Gutterman DD, Schuünemann HJ, American College of Chest Physicians Antithrombotic Therapy and Prevention of Thrombosis Panel. Executive summary: antithrombotic therapy and prevention of thrombosis, 9th ed: American College of Chest Physicians Evidence-Based Clinical Practice Guidelines. Chest. 2012;141(2 Suppl):7S–47S. doi:10.1378/chest.1412S3.

2. Harenberg J, Walenga J, Torri G, Subcommittee on Control of Anticoagulation, Scientific and Standardization Committee of the International Society on Thrombosis and Haemostasis, et al. Update of the recommendations on biosimilar low-molecular-weight heparins from the scientific Subcommittee on Control of Anticoagulation of the International Society on thrombosis and Haemostasis. J Thromb Haemost. 2013;11(7):1421–5.

3. Harenberg J, Cimminiello C, Agnelli G, et al. Biosimilars of low-molecular-weight heparin products: fostering competition or reducing 'biodiversity'? J Thromb Haemost. 2016;14(3):421–6. doi:10.1111/jth.13237. Epub 2016 Jan 30

4. Harenberg J. Differences of present recommendations and guidelines for generic low-molecular-weight heparins: is there room for harmonization. Clin Appl Thromb Hemost. 2011;17(6):E158–64. doi:10.1177/1076029610392216. Epub 2011 Mar 14

5. Guidelines on clinical and non-clinical development of medicinal products containing low-molecular-weight heparins. European Medical Agency. EMEA/CHMP/BMWP/118264/2007. http://www.ema.europa.eu/docs/en_GB/document_library/Scientific_guideline/2009/09/WC500003927.pdf. Accessed 2 Dec 2016.

6. Harenberg J, Kakkar A, Bergqvist D, on behalf of the Subcommittee on Control of Anticoagulation of the Scientific and Standardization Committee of the International Society on Thrombosis and Haemostasis, et al. Recommendations on biosimilar low-molecular-weight heparins. J Thromb Haemost. 2009;7:1222–5.

7. Kalodiki E, Fareed J, Tapson WF, et al. A consensus conference on complex biologics and low molecular weight heparin. Int Angiol. 2010;29:193–6.

8. FDA News Release, July 23, 2010. http://www.fda.gov/NewsEvents/Newsroom/PressAnnouncements/ucm220092.htm. Accessed 2 Dec 2016.

9. FDA's response to the citizen petition. http://www.fda.gov/Drugs/DrugSafety/PostmarketDrugSafetyInformationforPatientsandProviders/ucm220018.htm. Accessed 2 Dec 2016.

10. Guideline on similar biological medicinal products containing biotechnology-derived proteins as active substance: quality issues. EMEA/CHMP/BWP/49348/2005. http://www.ema.europa.eu/docs/en_GB/document_library/Scientific_guideline/2009/09/WC500003953.pdf. Accessed 2 Dec 2016.

11. Guideline on similar biological medicinal products containing biotechnology-derived proteins as active substance: quality issues (revision 1). EMEA/CHMP/BWP/247713/2012. http://www.ema.europa.eu/docs/en_GB/document_library/Scientific_guideline/2014/06/WC500167838.pdf. Accessed 2 Dec 2016.

12. Concept paper on the revision of the guideline on nonclinical and clinical development of similar biological medicinal products containing low-molecular-weight heparins. European Medical Agency. EMA/CHMP/BMWP/522386/2011 http://www.ema.europa.eu/docs/en_GB/document_library/Scientific_guideline/2011/07/WC500109588.pdf. Accessed December 2, 2016.

13. Guideline on similar biological medicinal products. European Medical Agency. CHMP/437/04 Rev 1. http://www.ema.europa.eu/docs/en_GB/document_library/Scientific_guideline/2014/10/WC500176768.pdf. Accessed 2 Dec 2016.

14. Assessment report. Thorinane. International non-proprietary name: enoxaparin sodium. Procedure No. EMEA/H/C/003795/0000. EMA/536972/2016. Committee for Medicinal Products for Human Use (CHMP). http://www.ema.europa.eu/docs/en_GB/document_library/EPAR_-_Public_assessment_report/human/003795/WC500215281.pdf. Accessed 2 Dec 2016.

15. Assessment report. Inhixa. International non-proprietary name: enoxaparin sodium. Procedure No. EMEA/H/C/004264/0000. EMA/536977/2016. Committee for Medicinal Products for Human Use (CHMP). http://www.ema.europa.eu/docs/en_GB/document_library/EPAR_-_Public_assessment_report/human/004264/WC500215211.pdf. Accessed 2 Dec 2016.

16. Guideline on similar biological medicinal products containing Biotechnology-derived proteins as active substance: Non-clinical and clinical issues. EMEA/CHMP/BMWP/42832/2005. http://www.ema.europa.eu/docs/en_GB/document_library/Scientific_guideline/2009/09/WC500003920.pdf. Accessed 2 Dec 2016.

17. Schwartz LB. Heparin comes clean. N Engl J Med. 2008;358(23):2505–9.

18. Grampp G, Bonafede M, Felix T, et al. Active and passive surveillance of enoxaparin generics: a case study relevant to biosimilars. Expert Opin Drug Saf. 2015;14(3):349–60. doi:10.1517/14740338.2015.1001364. Epub 2015 Jan 5

19. Guideline on non-clinical and clinical development of similar biological medicinal products containing low-molecular-weight-heparins. European Medical Agency. EMEA/CHMP/BMWP/118264/2007 Rev. 1. http://www.ema.europa.eu/docs/en_GB/document_library/Scientific_guideline/2016/11/WC500217126.pdf. Accessed 2 Dec 2016.

20. Faccin F, Tebbey P, Alexander E, et al. The design of clinical trials to support the switching and alternation of biosimilars. Expert Opin Biol Ther. 2016;16(12): 1445–53. Epub 2016 Sep 27

Permissions

All chapters in this book were first published in TJ, by BioMed Central; hereby published with permission under the Creative Commons Attribution License or equivalent. Every chapter published in this book has been scrutinized by our experts. Their significance has been extensively debated. The topics covered herein carry significant findings which will fuel the growth of the discipline. They may even be implemented as practical applications or may be referred to as a beginning point for another development.

The contributors of this book come from diverse backgrounds, making this book a truly international effort. This book will bring forth new frontiers with its revolutionizing research information and detailed analysis of the nascent developments around the world.

We would like to thank all the contributing authors for lending their expertise to make the book truly unique. They have played a crucial role in the development of this book. Without their invaluable contributions this book wouldn't have been possible. They have made vital efforts to compile up to date information on the varied aspects of this subject to make this book a valuable addition to the collection of many professionals and students.

This book was conceptualized with the vision of imparting up-to-date information and advanced data in this field. To ensure the same, a matchless editorial board was set up. Every individual on the board went through rigorous rounds of assessment to prove their worth. After which they invested a large part of their time researching and compiling the most relevant data for our readers.

The editorial board has been involved in producing this book since its inception. They have spent rigorous hours researching and exploring the diverse topics which have resulted in the successful publishing of this book. They have passed on their knowledge of decades through this book. To expedite this challenging task, the publisher supported the team at every step. A small team of assistant editors was also appointed to further simplify the editing procedure and attain best results for the readers.

Apart from the editorial board, the designing team has also invested a significant amount of their time in understanding the subject and creating the most relevant covers. They scrutinized every image to scout for the most suitable representation of the subject and create an appropriate cover for the book.

The publishing team has been an ardent support to the editorial, designing and production team. Their endless efforts to recruit the best for this project, has resulted in the accomplishment of this book. They are a veteran in the field of academics and their pool of knowledge is as vast as their experience in printing. Their expertise and guidance has proved useful at every step. Their uncompromising quality standards have made this book an exceptional effort. Their encouragement from time to time has been an inspiration for everyone.

The publisher and the editorial board hope that this book will prove to be a valuable piece of knowledge for researchers, students, practitioners and scholars across the globe.

List of Contributors

Erin R. Weeda and Craig I. Coleman
School of Pharmacy, University of Connecticut, 69 North Eagleville Road, Storrs, CT 06269, USA

Erin R. Weeda, Christine G. Kohn and Craig I. Coleman
University of Connecticut/Hartford Hospital Evidence-Based Practice Center, Hartford, CT, USA

Christine G. Kohn, Christopher Tanner and Daniel McGrath
University of Saint Joseph School of Pharmacy, Hartford, CT, USA

Gregory J. Fermann
Department of Emergency Medicine, University of Cincinnati, Cincinnati, OH, USA

W. Frank Peacock
Department of Emergency Medicine, Baylor College of Medicine, Houston, TX, USA. 6Janssen Scientific

Concetta Crivera and Jeff R. Schein
Affairs LLC, Raritan, NJ, USA

Joanna Cwikiel, Ingebjorg Seljeflot and Harald Arnesen
Department of Cardiology, Center for Clinical Heart Research, Oslo University Hospital Ullevaal, PB 4956 Nydalen, 0424 Oslo, Norway

Ingebjorg Seljeflot, Eivind Berge and Arnljot Flaa
Department of Cardiology, Oslo University Hospital Ullevaal, Oslo, Norway

Joanna Cwikiel, Ingebjorg Seljeflot and Harald Arnesen
Faculty of Medicine, University of Oslo, Oslo, Norway

Joanna Cwikiel and Arnljot Flaa
Section of Cardiovascular and Renal research, Oslo University Hospital Ulleval, Oslo, Norway

Kristian Wachtell
Department of Cardiology, Division of Cardiovascular and Kristian Wachtell5Pulmonary diseases, Oslo University Hospital, Oslo, Norway

Hilde Ulsaker
Modum Bad, Vikersund, Norway

Hui-Ju Tsai and Ching-Ping Tseng
Department of Medical Biotechnology and Laboratory Science, Collage of Medicine, Chang Gung University, Kweishan, Taoyuan 333, Taiwan, Republic of China Molecular Medicine Research Center, Chang Gung University, Kweishan, Taoyuan 333, Taiwan, Republic of China

Ching-Ping Tseng
Graduate Institute of Biomedical Science, Collage of Medicine, Chang Gung University, Kweishan, Taoyuan 333, Taiwan, Republic of China
Department of Laboratory Medicine, Chang Gung Memorial Hospital, Kweishan, Taoyuan 333, Taiwan, Republic of China

Lai Heng Lee
Department of Haematology, Singapore General Hospital, 20, College Road, Academia Level 3, Singapore 169856, Singapore

Hidesaku Asakura
Department of Internal Medicine (III), Kanazawa University School of Medicine, 13-1, Takaramachi, Kanazawa 920-8641, Japan

Hoyu Takahashi
Department of Internal Medicine, Niigata Prefectural Kamo Hospital, 1-9-1 Aomicho, Kamo, Niigata 959-1397, Japan

Toshimasa Uchiyama
Department of Laboratory Medicine, National Hospital Organization Takasaki General Medical Center, 36 Takamatsu-Cho, Takasaki, Gunma 370-0829, Japan

Yutaka Eguchi
Department of Critical and Intensive Care Medicine, Shiga University of Medical Science, Seta Tsukinowa-cho, Otsu, Shiga 520-2192, Japan

Kohji Okamoto
Gastroenterology and Hepatology Center, Kitakyushu City Yahata Hospital, 4-18-1, Nishihon-machi, Yahatahigashi-ku, Kitakyushu, Fukuoka 805-8534, Japan

Kazuo Kawasugi
Department of Hematology, Teikyo University School of Medicine, 2-11-1 Kaga Itabashi-Ku, Tokyo 173-8605, Japan

Seiji Madoiwa
Department of Clinical and Laboratory Medicine, Tokyo Saiseikai Central Hospital, 1-4-17, Mita, Minato-ku, Tokyo 108-0073, Japan

Hideo Wada
Department of Molecular and Laboratory Medicine, Mie University Graduate School of Medicine, Tsu, Mie 514-8507, Japan

Ren-Chieh Wu and Li-Kuang Chen
Department of Emergency Medicine, Tzu Chi Medical Center, Hualien, Taiwan

Ping-Tse Chou and Li-Kuang Chen
Department of Laboratory Diagnosis, School of Medicine, Tzu Chi University, Hualien, Taiwan

Li-Kuang Chen
Branch of Clinical Pathology, Department of Laboratory Medicine, Tzu Chi Medical Center, Hualien, Taiwan

Nina Haagenrud Schultz, Hoa Thi Tuyet Tran, Stine Bjørnsen, Per Morten Sandset and Pål Andre Holme
Research Institute of Internal Medicine, Oslo University Hospital, Box 4950 Nydalen, N-0424 Oslo, Norway

Nina Haagenrud Schultz, Per Morten Sandset and Pål Andre Holme
Department of Haematology, Oslo University Hospital, Box 4950 Nydalen, N-0424 Oslo, Norway

Nina Haagenrud Schultz and Hoa Thi Tuyet Tran
Department of Haematology, Akershus University Hospital, N-1478 Lørenskog, Norway

Nina Haagenrud Schultz, Per Morten Sandset and Pål Andre Holme
Institute of Clinical Medicine, Faculty of Medicine, University of Oslo, Box 1171 Blindern, N-0318 Oslo, Norway

Carola Elisabeth Henriksson
Department of Medical Biochemistry, Oslo University Hospital, Box 4950 Nydalen, N-0424 Oslo, Norway

Yu-Min Shen
Department of Internal Medicine, University of Texas Southwestern Medical Center, Dallas, TX 75390-8852, USA

Marco Heestermans and Bart J.M. van Vlijmen
Einthoven Laboratory for Experimental Vascular Medicine, Leiden University Medical Center, Leiden, The Netherlands
Department of Internal Medicine, Division of Thrombosis and Hemostasis, Leiden University Medical Center, Leiden, The Netherlands

Carol H. Miao
Seattle Children's Research Institute, Seattle, WA, USA
Department of Pediatrics, University of Washington, Seattle, WA, USA

Jeff R. Schein and Winnie W. Nelson
Janssen Scientific Affairs, LLC, Health Economics and Outcomes Research,
Raritan, NJ, USA

C. Michael White, Elizabeth S. Mearns and Craig I. Coleman
Department of Pharmacy Practice, University of Connecticut School of Pharmacy, 69 N. Eagleville Road, Storrs, CT 06269-3092, USA

C. Michael White, Jeffrey Kluger and Craig I. Coleman
Hartford Hospital Division of Cardiology, 80 Seymour Street, Hartford, CT 06102-5037, USA

Grigoris T. Gerotziafas, Eleftheria Lefkou, Annette K. Larsen and Ismail Elalamy
Cancer Biology and Therapeutics, Centre de Recherche Saint-Antoine, Institut National de la Santé et de la Recherche Médicale (INSERM) U938 and Université Pierre et Marie Curie (UPMC), Sorbonne Universities, Paris, France

Grigoris T. Gerotziafas, Hela Ketatni and Ismail Elalamy
Service d'Hématologie Biologique, Hôpital Tenon, Hôpitaux Universitaires Est Parisien, Assistance Publique Hôpitaux de Paris, 4, rue de la Chine, Paris Cedex 20, France

Patrick Van Dreden
Clinical Research Department, Diagnostica Stago, Gennevilliers, France

Emmanuelle Mathieu d'Argent and Marjorie Comtet
Department of Obstetrics and Gynecology, Hôpital Tenon, Hôpitaux Universitaires Est Parisien, Assistance Publique Hôpitaux de Paris, Paris, France

Siavash Piran and Sam Schulman
Department of Medicine, Division of Hematology and Thromboembolism, and Thrombosis and Atherosclerosis Research Institute, McMaster University, Hamilton, ON L8L 2X2, Canada

Man-Chiu Poon and Adrienne Lee
Department of Medicine, Cumming School of Medicine, University of Calgary, Calgary, Alberta, Canada

Man-Chiu Poon
Department of Pediatrics, Cumming School of Medicine, University of Calgary, Calgary, Alberta, Canada

Department of Oncology, Cumming School of Medicine, University of Calgary, Calgary, Alberta, Canada

Man-Chiu Poon and Adrienne Lee
Southern Alberta Rare Blood and Bleeding Disorders Comprehensive Care Program, Foothills Hospital, Alberta Health Services, Calgary, Alberta, Canada

Efthymios Arvanitidis, Sergio Bizzarro, Elena Alvarez Rodriguez, Bruno G. Loos and Elena A. Nicu
Department of Periodontology, Academic Centre for Dentistry Amsterdam (ACTA), University of Amsterdam and VU University Amsterdam, Gustav Mahlerlaan 3004, Amsterdam 1081LA, The Netherlands

Ming Chen, Shun-Ping Chang, Gwo-Chin Ma and Wen-Hsian Lin
Department of Genomic Medicine and Center for Medical Genetics, Changhua Christian Hospital, Changhua, Taiwan

Ming Chen, Shun-Ping Chang, Gwo-Chin Ma and Wen-Hsian Lin
Department of Genomic Science and Technology, Changhua Christian Hospital Healthcare System, Changhua, Taiwan

Ming Chen, Hsin-Fu Chen and Shee-Uan Chen
Department of Obstetrics and Gynecology, College of Medicine and Hospital, National Taiwan University, Taipei, Taiwan

Ming Chen
Department of Medical Genetics, National Taiwan University Hospital, Taipei, Taiwan
Department of Life Science, Tunghai University, Taichung, Taiwan
Department of Obstetrics and Gynecology, Changhua Christian Hospital, Changhua, Taiwan

Gwo-Chin Ma and Horng-Der Tsai
Institute of Biochemistry, Microbiology and Immunology, Chung Shan Medical University, Taichung, Taiwan

Gwo-Chin Ma
Department of Medical Laboratory Science and Biotechnology, Central Taiwan University of Science and Technology, Taichung, Taiwan

Feng-Po Tsai
Po-Yuan Women's Clinic and IVF Center, Changhua, Taiwan

Ming-Ching Shen
Department of Internal Medicine, and Thrombosis and Hemostasis Center, Changhua Christian Hospital, Changhua, Taiwan

Ruiqi Zhu, Yu Hu and Liang Tang
Department of Hematology, Wuhan Union Hospital of Huazhong University of Science and Technology, Wuhan 430030, China

Takahiro Kato
Departments of Pharmacy, Aichi Medical University, 1 -1 Yazakokarimata, Nagakute, Aichi 480-1195, Japan

Katsuhiko Matsuura
Laboratory of Clinical Pharmacodynamics, Aichi Gakuin University School of Pharmacy, Nagakute, Japan

Kang-Ling Wang And Chern-En Chiang
General Clinical Research Center, Taipei Veterans General Hospital, No. 201, Sec. 2, Shipai Rd., 11217 Taipei, Taiwan
School of Medicine, National Yang-Ming University, Taipei, Taiwan

Eng Soo Yap
Department of Haematology-Oncology, National University Cancer Institute, Singapore, Singapore
Department of Laboratory Medicine, National University Hospital, Singapore, Singapore

Shinya Goto
Department of Medicine, Tokai University School of Medicine, Kanagawa, Japan

Shu Zhang
Arrhythmia Center, National Center for Cardiovascular Diseases and Beijing Fuwai Hospital, Chinese Academy of Medical Sciences and Pekin Union Medical College, Beijing, China

Chung-Wah Siu
Cardiology Division, Department of Medicine, Li Ka Shing Faculty of Medicine, The University of Hong Kong, Hong Kong SAR, China

Satoshi Niijima and Kazuomi Kario
Division of Cardiovascular Medicine, Department of Medicine, Jichi Medical University School of Medicine, 3311-1 Yakushiji, Shimotsuke, Tochigi 329-0498, Japan

Tsukasa Ohmori
Department of Biochemistry, Jichi Medical University School of Medicine, 3311-1 Yakushiji, Shimotsuke, Tochigi 329-0498, Japan

Hikmat Abdel-Razeq, Hazem Abdulelah, Anas Al-Shwayat, Mohammad Makoseh, Mohammad Ibrahim, Mahmoud Abunasser, Rozan Alfar, Alaa' Abufara and Anas Bawaliz
Department of Internal Medicine, King Hussein Cancer Center, 202 Queen Rania Al-Abdulla St., Amman 11941, Jordan

Asem Mansour and Alaa Ibrahim
Radiology, King Hussein Cancer Center, Amman, Jordan

Dalia Rimawi
Scientific and Reseaerch Office, King Hussein Cancer Center, Amman, Jordan

Abeer Al-Rabaiah
Pharmacy, King Hussein Cancer Center, Amman, Jordan

Yousef Ismael
Radiation Oncology, King Hussein Cancer Center, Amman, Jordan

Hind Almodaimegh, Lama Alfehaid, Nada Alsuhebany, Rami Bustami, Shmylan Alharbi, Abdulmalik Alkatheri and Abdulkareem Albekairy
King Abdullah International Medical Research Center/ King Saud Bin Abdulaziz University for Health Sciences, College of Pharmacy, Ministry of National Guard Health Affairs, Riyadh 11426, Saudi Arabia

Hind Almodaimegh, Shmylan Alharbi, Abdulmalik Alkatheri and Abdulkareem Albekairy
Pharmaceutical Care Department, King Abdulaziz Medical City, King Abdullah International Medical Research Center/King Saud Bin Abdulaziz University for Health Sciences, Riyadh 11426, Saudi Arabia

Jae C. Chang
Department of Medicine, University of California Irvine School of Medicine, Irvine, CA, USA

Yvonne M. C. Henskens, René van Oerle, Rick Wetzels, Paul Verhezen and Arina ten Cate-Hoek
Central Diagnostic Laboratory, Maastricht University Medical Centre (MUMC +), Maastricht, The Netherlands

Anouk J. W. Gulpen, Renévan Oerle, Henri Spronk and Hugo ten Cate
Laboratory for Clinical Thrombosis and Hemostasis, Internal medicine, CARIM, Maastricht, The Netherlands

Henri Spronk, Simon Schalla and Harry J. Crijns
Department of Cardiology, Cardiovascular center MUMC+, Maastricht, The Netherlands

Anouk J. W. Gulpen and Hugo ten Cate
Internal medicine, MUMC+, Maastricht, The Netherlands

Arina ten Cate-Hoek
Thrombosis Expertise Centre, Vascular medicine, Cardiovascular Centre MUMC+, Maastricht, The Netherlands

Jean Jacques Noubiap
Department of Medicine, Groote Schuur Hospital and University of Cape Town, Cape Town 7925, South Africa

Mazou N. Temgoua and Ronni Tankeu
Department of Internal Medicine and sub-Specialties, Faculty of Medicine and Biomedical Sciences, Yaoundé, Cameroon

Joel Noutakdie Tochie
Department of Surgery and sub-Specialties, Faculty of Medicine
and Biomedical Sciences, Yaoundé, Cameroon

Ambroise Wonkam
Division of Human Genetics, Faculty of Health Sciences, University of Cape Town, Cape Town, South Africa

Jean Joël Bigna
Department of Epidemiology and Public Health, Centre Pasteur of Cameroon, Yaoundé, Cameroon
Faculty of Medicine, University of Paris Sud XI, Le Kremlin Bicêtre, France

Ged Avery and Andrew Stephens
Hull and East Yorkshire NHS Hospitals Trust, Radiology Department, Castle Hill Hospital, Castle Road, Cottingham HU16 5JQ, UK

Anthony Maraveyas
Hull York Medical School, Academic Oncology, Castle Hill Hospital, Castle Road, Cottingham HU16 5JQ, UK

Davide Imberti
Haemostasis and Thrombosis Center, Internal Medicine Department, Piacenza Hospital, Via Taverna 49, Piacenza, Italy

Marco Marietta
Department of Oncology and Hematology, Section of Hematology, University of Modena and Reggio Emilia, Modena, Italy

Hernan Polo Friz
Internal Medicine, Medical Department, Vimercate Hospital, via Santi Cosma e Damiano 10, 20871 Vimercate, Italy

Hernan Polo Friz and Claudio Cimminiello
Studies and Research Center of the Italian Society of Angiology and Vascular Pathology
(Società Italiana di Angiologia e Patologia Vascolare, SIAPAV), via Gorizia 22, 20144 Milan, Italy

Index